AI and Blockchain Applications for Privacy and Security in Smart Medical Systems

Abdul Ahad
Northwestern Polytechnical University, China

Farhan Ullah
Prince Mohammad Bin Fahd University, Saudi Arabia

IGI Global
Scientific Publishing
Publishing Tomorrow's Research Today

Vice President of Editorial Melissa Wagner
Director of Acquisitions Mikaela Felty
Director of Book Development Jocelynn Hessler
Production Manager Mike Brehm
Cover Design Phillip Shickler

Published in the United States of America by
IGI Global Scientific Publishing
701 East Chocolate Avenue
Hershey, PA, 17033, USA
Tel: 717-533-8845
Fax: 717-533-7115
Website: https://www.igi-global.com E-mail: cust@igi-global.com

Library of Congress Cataloging-in-Publication Data

LCCN: 2025000196 (CIP Data Pending)
ISBN13: 9798337305936
Isbn13Softcover: 9798337305943
EISBN13: 9798337305950

British Cataloguing in Publication Data
A Cataloguing in Publication record for this book is available from the British Library.

Table of Contents

Detailed Table of Contents

Coronary Heart Disease (CHD) continues to affect close to 145 million males and 110 million females across the globe, taking close to nine million lives each year. A new evolving framework incorporating IoT-edge computing, Explainable AI, and blockchain technology is in the process of development in order to create a secure, privacy-preserving, and interpretable automated machine learning environment to predict chronic diseases. The IoT-based system utilizes medical sensors and assistive devices for real-time monitoring of the patient. The patient information is transmitted securely using blockchain architecture so that various health practitioners have access to it with the guarantee of data integrity, confidentiality, and access control. The use of Explainable AI (XAI) enables interpretable predictions in machine learning for clinicians and fosters confidence and transparency. Physicians are able to make evidence-based decisions beyond traditional methods since XAI provides the reasons for predictions.

The Medicine Supply Chain (MSC) faces critical challenges in traceability, transparency, and counterfeit prevention. This paper proposes a Blockchain-based solution using Ethereum smart contracts (developed in Solidity, deployed via Truffle, and tested on Rinkeby and localhost networks) to enhance MSC integrity. The framework introduces consumer authentication, Universal Product Code (UPC) registration, and transaction logging to ensure end-to-end drug traceability. By embedding multilingual UPCs (e.g., Urdu, Hindi), the system improves accessibility for diverse healthcare users, who can verify medicine authenticity via QR codes or a dedicated mobile app. The study examines scalability challenges (e.g., managing 100K+ UPCs in large healthcare networks) and evaluates the shifting dynamics among stakeholders (suppliers, processors, retailers). Public Blockchain implementation demonstrates potential for decentralized, tamper-proof record-keeping, though trade-offs in efficiency and adoption barriers persist.

Blockchain technology has emerged as a transformative solution for enhancing transparency, security, and efficiency in supply chain management, particularly in the healthcare sector. This paper explores the application of blockchain for improving pharmaceutical supply chains by ensuring the traceability

This manuscript examines the transformative potential of integrating blockchain and artificial intelligence (AI) to enhance healthcare supply chain management, focusing on combating counterfeit drugs and improving product traceability. Current systems are susceptible to cyberattacks and fail to guarantee drug authenticity, posing significant risks to patient safety. Blockchain technology offers a robust solution by creating an immutable and transparent record of the entire supply chain, from manufacturing to patient delivery, enabling verification of product origin and handling at each step. Smart contracts automate these verifications, ensuring compliance and minimizing errors. Integrating AI with blockchain further amplifies these benefits. AI algorithms analyze blockchain data to identify patterns, predict disruptions, and optimize supply chain efficiency. Furthermore, blockchain provides a secure platform for medical record storage, supporting AI-driven e-health models.

Blockchain technology presents a capable solution for secure and standardized data sharing with its consensus mechanisms and smart contracts. The major objective of this study is to propose a novel blockchain architecture for secure healthcare data sharing by detecting all factors necessary for healthcare data sharing. After analyzing numerous blockchain architectures for healthcare systems, this study found three essential categories of factors called healthcare, security, and blockchain, which are vital for successful data sharing in healthcare environments. The prototypes and pseudocodes of the proposed architecture were validated by using expert opinions from 15 software experts. The study's major contribution lies in the development of this robust architecture, which not only addresses the core issues of data privacy, security, and interoperability but also lays a strong foundation for future advancements in the secure exchange of medical records using blockchain technology.

The Internet of Things (IoT) is a groundbreaking technological tool connecting devices across various industries, changing everything from how we manage our healthcare to building smart cities. However, this amalgamation brings forth significant security issues that require inventive approaches. This chapter examines the need for advanced security solutions such as Artificial Intelligence (AI) and the blockchain to mitigate the effects of vulnerabilities in IoT. It starts by analyzing the ethical implications of IoT adoption, particularly concerning privacy, consent, and equitable access. It also covers advanced security methods and demonstrates how AI-driven anomaly identification, prediction analytics, and decentralized blockchain types strengthen IoT safety. Careful case studies and real-world applications, statistical comparisons of security approaches, and analyses of the economic and social impacts of–all illustrate this point. Furthermore, the chapter outlines research gaps and future directions.

The rapid expansion of Artificial Intelligence (AI), in synergy with emerging Blockchain technologies, necessitates a departure from conventional, centralized architectures to more decentralized paradigms for privacy and security in oncology care. This chapter introduces a conceptual and theoretical framework combining AI-driven analytics, decentralized identity management, and privacy-preserving machine learning to establish robust, patient-focused smart medical systems. It examines how AI can enhance clinical decision-making, data security, and operational efficacy while addressing the limitations of traditional data handling in healthcare. Integrating foundational principles of decentralized identity—such as secure authentication, self-sovereign data ownership, and transparent access control—with AI-enabled insights, this chapter proposes a roadmap for promoting adaptable, resilient, and trust-centered oncology care.

This chapter explores the critical intersection of technology, trust, and transparency in advancing patient-centered healthcare. With digital innovations such as electronic health records, artificial intelligence, wearable devices, and blockchain, healthcare providers can now enhance patient engagement, improve care accuracy, and increase access. However, while these technologies offer unprecedented potential for personalized and proactive healthcare, they also pose challenges related to privacy, data security, and the ethical use of information. Through examining how these technologies can both build and compromise patient trust, this study identifies key strategies for enhancing transparency in healthcare delivery, fostering trust through secure and accessible digital solutions, and ensuring that healthcare remains both effective and ethically responsible. Ultimately, this paper underscores the need for a balanced approach that integrates technology with a commitment to patient autonomy, privacy, and clear communication.

Machine Learning (ML) is being adopted in the healthcare industry across diagnostics, treatment options, and analysis of patient information. The management of data increases risks to the patient's private information. This chapter explores the theoretical frameworks and consequences of privacy-enhancing ML methods, namely, differential privacy, Federated Learning (FL), and homomorphic encryption, to apply medical data for meaningful analysis while maintaining the non-disclosure of patient information. Differential privacy adds noise control to minimize identifying data corresponding to an individual. FL allows the training of models while avoiding data centralization, and homomorphic encryption will enable computations on top of encrypted data to guarantee data safety during processing. We also explain how blockchain could improve these privacy-preserving approaches; it can provide safe data sharing, models, and audit and accountability of model management.

Advances in the healthcare sector need to secure efficient and decentralized systems to handle the large number of images and test reports. Traditional cloud-based healthcare systems pose crucial challenges, such as higher maintenance costs, significant storage demand, and, most importantly, privacy concerns. This chapter introduced the comprehensive patient-centric system for decentralized storage, secure medical data sharing, integrating blockchain technology and distributed file systems. The healthcare system leverages the IPFS and Ethereum blockchain to empowering scalable privacy protection of globally available storage of medical metadata. The framework enhances the accessibility and usability of incorporating a mobile offering for the patients, hospitals, and other stakeholders to interact with the decentralized system through the blockchain-integrated mobile application.This chapter provides an innovative approach to addressing the healthcare centralized data management limitations while ensuring patient privacy and data security.

Blockchain and Artificial Intelligence (AI) together are revolutionizing healthcare by improving safety, privacy, and electronic health records' security. Adoption of private blockchain enhances accessibility and efficiency while demonstrating the industry's dedication to data protection. In addition to addressing important sector issues, this convergence offers improved illness detection, response, and overall healthcare efficacy. Additional research into cutting-edge AI features combined with blockchain promises to improve results and influence the way healthcare is delivered globally in the future while ensuring data security, privacy, and innovation. In light of the aforementioned, this chapter looks at how blockchain technology and AI can be combined to solve current issues with healthcare data security and privacy. It offers insights into best practices and strategies for utilizing blockchain and AI's revolutionary potential in healthcare by examining various recent studies and developing trends.

Preface

In an era marked by the rapid evolution of digital technologies, the healthcare sector stands at the crossroads of innovation and vulnerability. The integration of connected devices, smart systems, and digital healthcare platforms has revolutionized patient care, research, and public health initiatives. However, this transformation also presents profound challenges—particularly in safeguarding data privacy, ensuring cybersecurity, and managing sensitive medical information in compliance with stringent global regulations such as HIPAA and GDPR.

This volume delves into the transformative potential of AI and blockchain to address vulnerabilities in smart medical systems. It examines how AI can predict, detect, and respond to cyber threats with precision, while blockchain facilitates secure, decentralized, and tamper-proof data sharing. Together, these technologies offer a synergistic framework for building trust, ensuring patient consent, protecting sensitive information, and enhancing the overall integrity of healthcare systems.

Understanding that the challenges at hand are interdisciplinary, the book brings together insights from healthcare professionals, data scientists, regulatory authorities, and technology developers. It evaluates the role of AI and blockchain not only as technological solutions but also as ethical and legal instruments, ensuring that innovation in medical research, personalized care, and public health surveillance aligns with global standards of data protection and patient rights.

Our primary goal with this book is to bridge the gap between theoretical research and real-world application. Through comprehensive discussions, case studies, and practical frameworks, we aim to equip researchers, practitioners, policymakers, and innovators with the knowledge needed to implement secure, privacy-centered smart medical systems. In particular, the book offers an in-depth exploration of AI algorithms such as machine learning, neural networks, and predictive analytics for cybersecurity, alongside an examination of blockchain's potential for decentralized data governance.

Chapter 1: This chapter presents a Federated Learning (FL) framework designed to address challenges in decentralized healthcare, such as intermittent client participation and imbalanced datasets. Using distributed medical imaging datasets, the framework achieves high diagnostic accuracy while preserving data confidentiality, highlighting FL's potential to transform privacy-focused healthcare innovation.

Chapter 2: Blockchain's decentralized architecture empowers patients to control their electronic health records (EHRs), enhancing security and operational efficiency. This chapter examines blockchain's role in securing sensitive medical data, streamlining administrative processes, and combating counterfeit drugs, while also addressing regulatory hurdles.

Chapter 3: Introducing an integrated IoT, edge computing, Explainable AI (XAI), and blockchain framework, this chapter focuses on real-time CHD prediction. By leveraging medical sensors, secure data transmission, and interpretable AI predictions, the system enhances clinician trust and facilitates data integrity and confidentiality.

Chapter 4: This chapter proposes an Ethereum blockchain framework to improve medicine traceability and combat counterfeit drugs. Features like multilingual UPC registration, consumer authentication, and transaction logging enhance supply chain transparency, although scalability challenges remain.
Chapter 5: Exploring blockchain and IoT convergence, this chapter emphasizes ensuring drug authenticity, mitigating risks of counterfeit medicines, and improving supply chain efficiency. Real-time monitoring and decentralized verification strengthen patient safety and logistics operations.
Chapter 6: Through diverse case studies, this chapter demonstrates how blockchain and AI integration enhances data security, operational efficiency, and personalized care in healthcare. It also discusses regulatory, ethical, and technical barriers, anticipating future innovations like explainable AI and hybrid blockchains.
Chapter 7: Addressing the urgent need for rapid disease detection, this chapter proposes a deep learning and machine learning framework, achieving high accuracy in COVID-19 diagnosis from CT scans and X-rays. Explainable AI techniques validate the robustness and transparency of the system.
Chapter 8: This chapter discusses the integration of AI with blockchain to fortify healthcare supply chains. Smart contracts automate verification, while AI optimizes operations by analyzing blockchain data, ensuring product authenticity and efficiency throughout the supply chain.
Chapter 9: Focusing on secure and standardized healthcare data exchange, this chapter proposes a novel blockchain architecture validated by expert opinion. It identifies key healthcare, security, and blockchain factors crucial for successful implementation in healthcare data environments.
Chapter 10: Examining the vulnerabilities in IoT applications, this chapter explores how AI and blockchain integration can enhance security. Case studies, ethical considerations, and statistical analyses illustrate the potential and future directions for securing IoT-connected healthcare ecosystems.
Chapter 11: This chapter proposes a conceptual framework integrating AI analytics and decentralized identity management for oncology care. It focuses on secure authentication, self-sovereign data ownership, and privacy-preserving machine learning to promote trust-centered and resilient healthcare systems.
Chapter 12: Exploring how technology can both build and challenge patient trust, this chapter identifies strategies for fostering transparency and ethical responsibility in healthcare. It emphasizes balancing digital innovation with a commitment to patient autonomy and privacy.
Chapter 13: Differential privacy, Federated Learning, and homomorphic encryption are explored in this chapter as methods to enhance patient data privacy during AI-driven healthcare analytics. The role of blockchain in reinforcing privacy-preserving frameworks is also analyzed.
Chapter 14: Introducing a blockchain and distributed file system-based healthcare solution, this chapter presents a patient-centric framework for decentralized medical data storage and sharing, offering scalable privacy protection and improved accessibility through mobile applications.
Chapter 15: This chapter highlights the transformative potential of combining blockchain and AI to enhance healthcare data security, privacy, and operational efficiency. It provides insights into best practices, emerging trends, and strategies for future global healthcare innovation.

We also address the ethical and legal dimensions critical to the responsible integration of AI and blockchain in healthcare. Issues surrounding patient autonomy, informed consent, and data ownership are discussed, recognizing that trust in digital health technologies must be built on both technical excellence and ethical integrity.

Designed for a diverse audience—including healthcare professionals, researchers, technology developers, policymakers, educators, and industry leaders—this book aspires to serve as both a foundational resource and a forward-looking guide. It aims not only to inform but also to inspire innovation at the intersection of healthcare, technology, and privacy.

We invite readers to explore the possibilities and challenges presented in these pages, as together we chart a course toward a secure, ethical, and resilient future for smart medical systems.

Abdul Ahad
Northwestern Polytechnical University, China

Farhan Ullah
Prince Mohammad Bin Fahd University, Saudi Arabia

Chapter 1
A Federated Learning Framework for Intermittent Clients in Collaborative Smart Healthcare Systems

Ali Turab
https://orcid.org/0000-0002-5445-9728
Northwestern Polytechnical University, China

Farhan Ullah
https://orcid.org/0000-0002-1030-1275
Prince Mohammad Bin Fahd University, Saudi Arabia

Shujaat Ali Zaidi
Chiang Mai University, Thailand

ABSTRACT

The rise of cybercrime and privacy concerns in healthcare demands solutions that protect sensitive data while supporting effective machine learning (ML) models. Decentralized healthcare systems face challenges such as intermittent client participation, imbalanced datasets, and connectivity issues. This chapter presents a Federated Learning (FL) framework to address these issues by enabling privacy-preserving collaboration among healthcare institutions. Using distributed medical imaging datasets, such as chest X-rays, the framework applies data augmentation to balance class distributions and ensures consistent model updates despite client intermittency. Experiments with five to eighteen clients demonstrated its ability to achieve high accuracy and robustness across diverse scenarios. By enabling collaborative learning without sharing sensitive data, the FL framework enhances diagnostic accuracy while ensuring confidentiality. These findings underscore FL's potential to transform decentralized healthcare, enabling scalable and secure privacy-preserving innovations.

DOI: 10.4018/979-8-3373-0593-6.ch001

1. INTRODUCTION

The digital revolution and globalization have profoundly transformed the ways in which data is generated, stored, and analyzed. Across industries such as finance, manufacturing, and healthcare, data volumes are growing at an unprecedented pace, propelled by advances in digital technology, automation, and connectivity. This data deluge presents both opportunities and challenges: opportunities to extract valuable insights through sophisticated data analysis, and challenges in managing, processing, and protecting sensitive information. Mathematical techniques (Sintunavarat & Turab, 2022; Turab et al., 2024), in conjunction with machine learning (ML) and deep learning (DL), have become essential technologies for meeting these requirements, facilitating the creation of robust predictive models and inference systems adept at analyzing intricate, high-dimensional datasets (for further details, refer to Ahad et al., 2021; Ahad et al., 2025; Ullah et al., 2024).

Although their transformational capabilities, machine learning and deep learning models require extensive datasets to attain optimal performance. This data is often disseminated across several parties or groups, including healthcare institutions, financial corporations, and industrial activities. Traditionally, centralized methodologies in machine learning have been used, whereby data from several entities is consolidated onto a single server for model training. This method streamlines data consolidation but raises substantial issues with data security, privacy, and scalability (see Ali et al., 2023; Ashfaq et al., 2023).

A significant concern with centralized designs is the susceptibility of data during transmission. Confidential information, especially in sectors such as healthcare, is susceptible to interception or abuse during transmission to a central server (see Butt et al., 2023a, 2023b). Furthermore, consolidating data into a single repository heightens the danger of breaches, since attackers often target centralized systems that house substantial amounts of essential information. Regulatory frameworks, like the General Data Protection Regulation (GDPR) (Díaz & García, 2023), impose rigorous standards on data management, mandating comprehensive safeguards to protect personal and sensitive information.

One major issue is the infrastructural need for centralized machine learning. High-bandwidth, low-latency networks are crucial for the transmission of substantial datasets; nevertheless, they are often inaccessible or unreliable in distant or resource-limited environments. This issue is especially evident in developing countries or in applications related to IoT devices and edge computing, where data creation takes place in spread settings but network quality is inadequate for centralized data transmission (see Miotto et al., 2018).

To address the constraints of centralized machine learning, decentralized methodologies have garnered attention. These solutions enable data proprietors to retain authority over their datasets while collectively contributing to a collective model. Decentralized machine learning obviates the need of transmitting data to a central server, thereby diminishing network reliance and decreasing communication expenses. Nonetheless, these methodologies are not without of difficulties. Decentralized systems sometimes need an initial data transmission for model initialization, which may nevertheless present security vulnerabilities. Furthermore, the repetitive transmission of information during model training presents possible weaknesses. When data is very sensitive or disseminated across several stakeholders, such as healthcare organizations or IoT networks, these risks are exacerbated.

Figure 1. Centralized client-server architecture for traditional model training

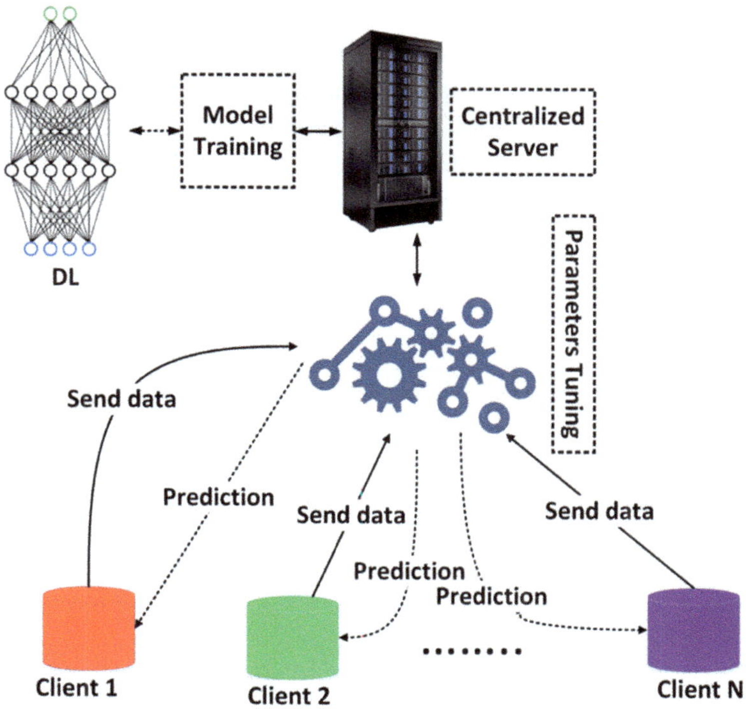

Federated Learning (FL) has evolved as an innovative paradigm to tackle the issues associated with centralized and decentralized machine learning (Rieke et al., 2020). FL enables numerous entities to cooperatively train a common model without the need of transmitting raw data to a centralized repository. Model training is conducted locally on each entity's dataset, with just the resultant model parameters or gradients sent to a central server. The server consolidates these changes to enhance the global model, which is then disseminated to the participating organizations for further local training.

FL is intentionally structured to keep sensitive data inside the local context of the data owner, hence safeguarding privacy and mitigating breach risks. This decentralized training method is especially beneficial in situations when data sharing is prohibited owing to legal, ethical, or practical limitations. For instance, consider two hospitals involved in medical research. Although both organizations possess rich datasets, privacy restrictions may inhibit the exchange of patient information. Through FL, these hospitals may collectively train a machine learning model by sharing model parameters rather than raw data, facilitating collective intelligence while preserving data security.

The use of FL in medical imaging research has considerable promise for enhancing illness detection and therapy. Medical imaging datasets, including chest X-rays, CT scans, and MRI pictures, are essential for training deep learning models capable of accurately detecting disorders. Nonetheless, these databases are often disseminated around many healthcare organizations, each possessing a distinct subset of patient information. Consolidating such datasets into a centralized repository is both impracticable and poses significant privacy issues.

FL provides an effective approach by facilitating collaborative model training across universities without necessitating data exchange. In this framework, each healthcare facility develops a local model using its dataset, and the resultant parameters are consolidated to create a global model. This method improves model accuracy by using varied datasets while ensuring adherence to privacy standards. Furthermore, FL can mitigate the issues associated with data imbalance, whereby certain illness categories may be inadequately represented in separate datasets. Data augmentation techniques may be used to equilibrate these datasets, enhancing the model's overall resilience and performance (see Brisimi et al., 2018).

This chapter concentrates on the formulation and assessment of a FL framework designed for medical imaging research. The suggested approach tackles significant issues in decentralized healthcare systems, such as privacy protection, data asymmetry, and sporadic client engagement. This chapter's principal contributions are as follows:

- A unique FL architecture is presented for collaborative medical imaging research, allowing healthcare organizations to use pooled expertise without disclosing sensitive patient information.
- The platform integrates data augmentation methods to improve dataset representation and guarantee equitable training across participating universities.
- The architecture is evaluated in scenarios with intermittent clients and unequal data distributions, mirroring real-world situations in distant healthcare environments characterized by variable patient influx.

The rest of this chapter is organized to provide a thorough overview of the proposed FL framework. Section 2 examines pertinent literature on FL and its applications within the healthcare sector. Section 3 delineates the approach, including the creation of the FL framework, data pretreatment, and augmentation strategies. Section 4 delineates the experimental results, emphasizing the framework's effectiveness across many contexts. Section 5 closes with an examination of the implications, limits, and prospective avenues for FL in medical imaging research.

2. RELATED WORK

Recent developments in machine learning have substantially improved healthcare, especially in illness identification and diagnosis using medical imaging. Numerous research have used deep learning algorithms tailored for the study of chest X-rays to effectively detect disorders (Motamed, Rogalla, & Khalvati, 2021; Hossain, Muhammad, & Guizani, 2020). Rajpurkar et al. (2017) created a Dense Convolutional Neural Network (CNN) that shown superior accuracy in identifying bacterial illnesses in chest X-rays relative to practicing doctors. XU, Wu, and Bie (2019) used a hierarchical CNN to categorize chest X-rays as healthy or pathological, therefore demonstrating the capabilities of deep learning in medical imaging.

In the framework of COVID-19, a comprehensive examination of radiological images has shown that these pictures provide essential information for early diagnosis (Shi et al., 2020). Advancements in data processing technology have enabled machine learning to assist clinicians in illness diagnosis and surgical guidance. Various methodologies have been suggested for health monitoring and illness identification, with some techniques exceeding human capabilities in medical imaging activities (Hossain & Muhammad, 2020). In addition to imaging, machine learning facilitates tailored healthcare via behavioral monitoring. For instance, first indicators of cognitive disorders may be identified via the examination of everyday activities, like alterations in gait or diminished finger dexterity, facilitating prompt intervention (Avellino, 2019; Chen et al., 2017; Ullah et al., 2022).

Notwithstanding these developments, the creation of resilient healthcare apps often necessitates access to comprehensive, annotated information. Data privacy concerns and legislative limitations, like the General Data Protection Regulation (GDPR), inhibit data exchange between people and companies (Voigt & Bussche, 2017). As a result, data is often compartmentalized, forming 'data islands' that obstruct the implementation of conventional machine learning methods dependent on centralized data consolidation. FL has arisen as a viable method for the integration of remote data while preserving privacy and security. FL facilitates collaborative model training across decentralized datasets by sharing model parameters rather than raw data. Google's FedAvg algorithm (McMahan et al., 2017) established the groundwork for FL by showcasing its capacity to train machine learning models using data from many devices without direct data transmission.

In healthcare, FL has been used across several settings, showcasing its versatility and efficacy. Elayan, Aloqaliy, and Guizani (2022) combined FL with Internet of Things (IoT) technology to provide remote patient monitoring, substantiating the efficacy of their system using ECG data analysis. Likewise, Sun et al. (2021) expanded the FL framework to augment IoT-driven intelligent automation, emphasizing its capacity to boost operational efficiency. Additionally, Rahman et al. (2020) integrated blockchain technology into FL frameworks to improve data security and dependability in industrial IoT systems. These studies highlight the adaptability of FL in tackling intricate issues within healthcare and IoT networks.

The use of FL in medical imaging has shown considerable promise in enhancing healthcare solutions. Dayan et al. (2021) used FL to detect COVID-19 infections in X-ray images using transfer learning on pre-trained models, with ResNet demonstrating the highest efficacy. Likewise, Baheti, Sikka, Arya, and Rajesh (2020) used FL to examine CT images for the identification of respiratory lung nodules, demonstrating its effectiveness in improving diagnostic accuracy. To tackle the issues posed by non-independent and identically distributed (non-IID) health data, Huang et al. (2019) used FL with clustering approaches to categorize clients into clinically relevant groups. This methodology enhanced forecasts for intensive care unit (ICU) wait times and patient mortality, underscoring FL's capacity to adjust to diverse data distributions in healthcare.

Patient similarity learning has been investigated in FL. Lee et al. (2018) devised a privacy-preserving approach to detect analogous patients across healthcare facilities without disclosing sensitive details. These studies highlight FL's capacity to surmount conventional data-sharing constraints, safeguarding privacy while promoting cooperation in healthcare. FL facilitates the creation of machine learning models without necessitating centralized data storage (McMahan et al., 2017). In FL, model training is decentralized across clients—devices or institutions—with a central server orchestrating updates. Each client locally trains the model with its data, producing updates that the central server aggregates to enhance the global model. This repeated procedure guarantees that raw data is retained locally, hence safeguarding privacy. Figure 2 illustrates that FL is very appropriate for decentralized healthcare informatics. In the FL process, clients train local models with their data and transmit the resultant changes to the server. The server consolidates these changes to formulate a global model, which is then disseminated to the clients for further local training. Encryption methods may be used to safeguard model changes, guaranteeing anonymity throughout the procedure.

Figure 2. FL framework for decentralized healthcare privacy

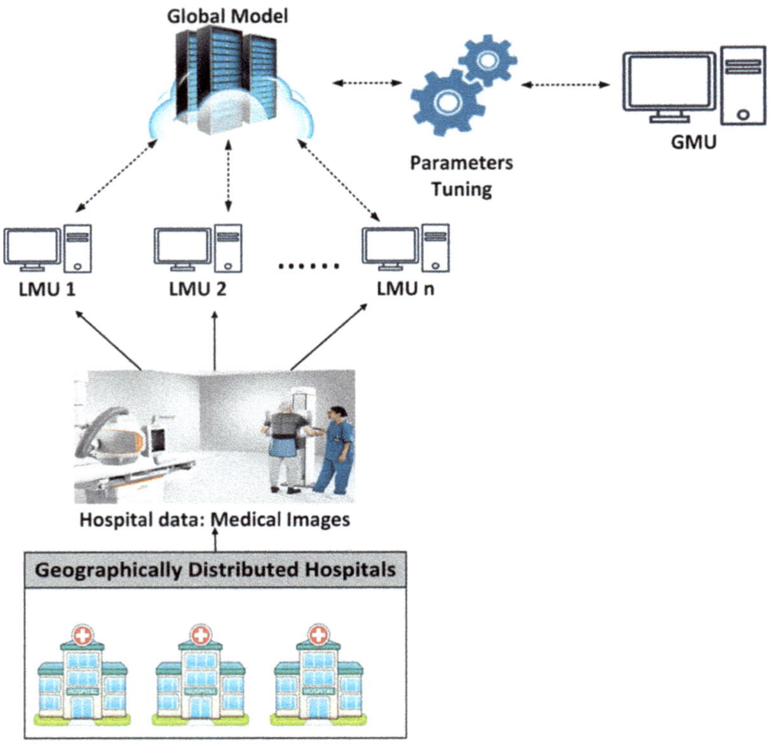

FL systems may be classified as either horizontal (homogeneous) or vertical (heterogeneous) according on data distribution. In horizontal FL, clients possess similar feature spaces but vary in data samples, as shown in picture classification tasks. In vertical FL, clients own unique feature sets while sharing common IDs, facilitating cross-silo cooperation (Yang et al., 2019). This chapter presents a FL system aimed at tackling significant issues in medical imaging, with the objective of enhancing illness detection and facilitating intelligent clinical data processing. The suggested paradigm addresses critical challenges in decentralized healthcare systems, namely with privacy, data imbalance, and sporadic client engagement. By using FL, the system guarantees the confidentiality of sensitive patient information while facilitating collaborative learning across many healthcare facilities. This decentralized method conforms to the rigorous data privacy standards in healthcare, making it a viable alternative for practical applications.

The methodology addresses the critical obstacle of imbalanced class distributions in datasets from distant hospitals and healthcare institutions. Such imbalances often yield biased models that exhibit subpar performance in underrepresented classes, hence constraining their clinical applicability. To address this, the system utilizes data augmentation approaches to enhance the representation of minority class samples. These strategies provide synthetic data points that enhance the variety and equilibrium of local datasets, facilitating improved generalization of the model across all classes. Consequently, the FL framework improves the resilience and dependability of the global model, guaranteeing its effective performance on varied and unbalanced datasets.

A further hurdle is the erratic engagement of customers in the training process, often resulting from resource limitations, restricted processing capability, or connection problems in distant regions. These disruptions may hinder the aggregation process and diminish model performance. The system includes techniques that enable the global model to adjust to sporadic client involvement. The suggested system exhibited accuracy and stability over extended testing involving five to eighteen customers and diverse data distributions, despite interruptions. The framework maintains the global model's resilience and adaptability to changing healthcare contexts by efficiently managing client inclusion and exclusion throughout training. The suggested FL architecture provides a unique method for healthcare data analysis by facilitating safe and collaborative learning without necessitating the transmission of raw data. It enables the amalgamation of scattered datasets across institutions, facilitating the creation of comprehensive and precise models that assist in illness diagnosis and treatment planning. This privacy-preserving strategy not only resolves technological and logistical issues but also fosters more cooperation among healthcare practitioners, so enhancing patient outcomes and promoting medical research. The suggested architecture provides a basis for scalable, secure, and efficient healthcare data processing. It highlights the capacity of FL to revolutionize medical imaging research and clinical decision-making by offering a viable solution to obstacles that have historically impeded the efficient use of remote data in healthcare.

3. PROPOSED METHOD

3.1. Overview of the Framework

This chapter presents a scalable FL architecture designed for decentralized smart healthcare systems. The proposed framework utilizes medical imaging data, namely chest X-ray pictures, to identify conditions like COVID-19, bacterial infections, and other viral infections. This study primarily aims to demonstrate that FL-based deep convolutional neural network (CNN) models facilitate collaborative knowledge exchange across various healthcare organizations while safeguarding patient data privacy. In contrast to traditional centralized machine learning approaches, the framework guarantees that sensitive medical data stays localized, since only model parameters are exchanged during training, thereby mitigating significant privacy and security issues. The work prioritizes the decentralized model training method above the CNN architecture, accommodating the dynamic characteristics of real-world healthcare settings. The platform is explicitly designed to address difficulties related to sporadic client engagement, a prevalent concern in distant healthcare environments owing to restricted connection or computing resources. The suggested technique improves the resilience and scalability of illness detection systems by facilitating collaborative model creation, even with varying levels of client participation. The results highlight the potential of FL to revolutionize smart healthcare systems by facilitating efficient, privacy-preserving cooperation across decentralized medical institutions, hence enhancing the use of artificial intelligence in clinical practice.

Figure 3 depicts the proposed FL architecture, which connects faraway hospitals via intermittent clients. Each hospital provides chest X-ray pictures, and categorization results may differ based on the data provided at each location. Data augmentation is used to address class imbalances prior to the local training of models. Hospitals produce local model updates (LMUs) by training models on their data and then send these changes to a central server. The server consolidates LMUs from all hospitals to generate a global model update (GMU), which is then disseminated for further training. This iterative technique guarantees precise and privacy-conserving categorization outcomes. The framework underwent thorough evaluation with different client counts and data samples to determine its robustness and classification efficacy.

Figure 3. Integration of FL framework for decentralized smart healthcare systems

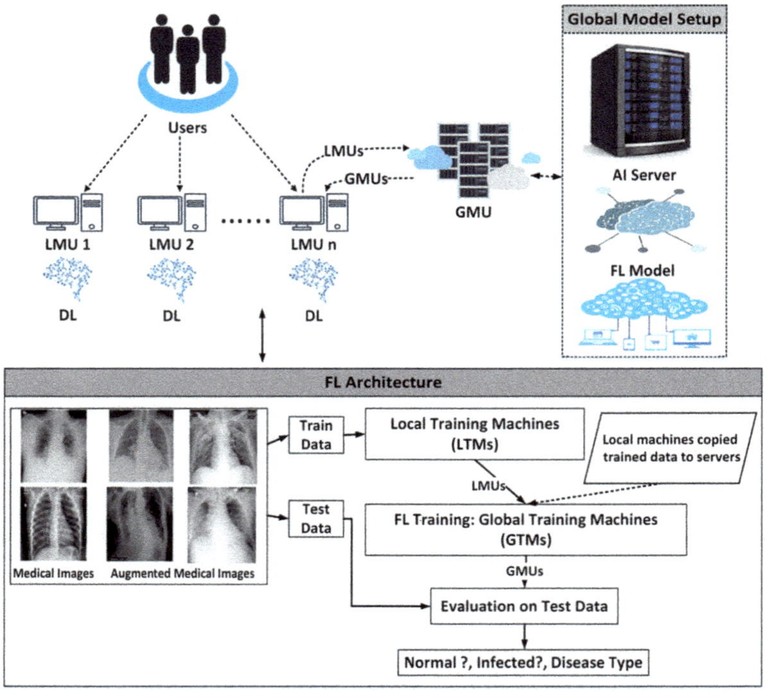

3.2. Dataset Preparation

The suggested methodology was assessed using two publicly accessible datasets from Kaggle. The first dataset, the COVID-19 Radiography Database (Chowdhury et al., 2020), was created via cooperation among researchers from Qatar University, the University of Dhaka, and several institutions in Pakistan and Malaysia. The dataset comprises 3,616 chest X-ray photos of COVID-19-positive patients, 10,192 photographs of healthy persons, 6,012 images of lung opacity due to non-COVID-related illnesses, and 1,345 images of viral pneumonia.

The second dataset, Chest X-ray pictures (Pneumonia) (Kermany et al., 2018), comprises 5,863 anterior-posterior chest X-ray pictures of pediatric patients aged 1 to 5 years. The photographs were obtained from the Guangzhou Women and Children Medical Center and are divided into three categories: 1,341 normal images, 1,345 images of viral pneumonia, and 2,530 images of bacterial pneumonia.

Figure 4 shows samples of chest X-ray scans from both datasets. In these pictures, standard X-rays reveal clean lungs devoid of obvious abnormalities, whereas bacterial pneumonia is marked by localized lobar consolidation. Conversely, viral pneumonia manifests as a widespread interstitial pattern across both lungs. These datasets provide a thorough basis for training and verifying the proposed FL architecture inside smart healthcare systems.

Figure 4. Examples of COVID-19 Radiography and Pneumonia chest X-rays

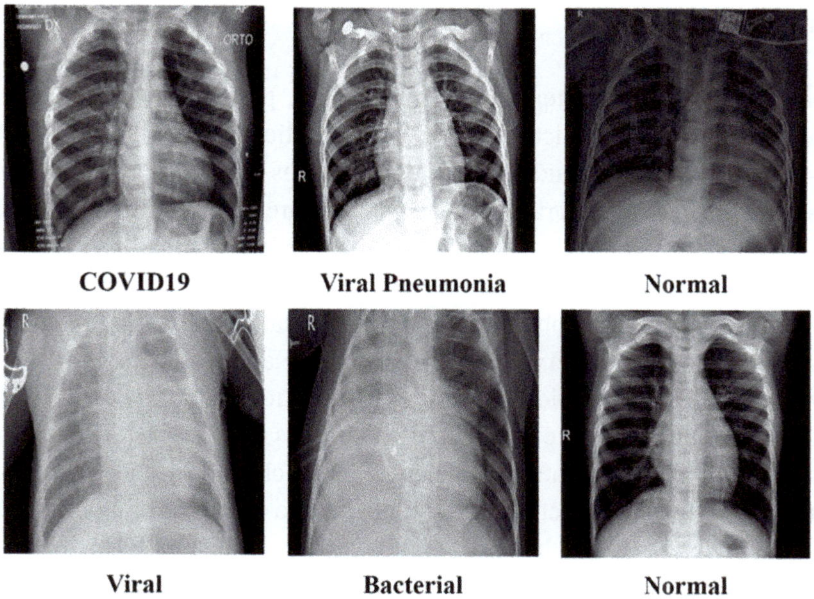

3.3. Data Augmentation

Data augmentation strategies are used to mitigate overfitting and rectify class imbalances in deep learning by enhancing sample variety (Rajotte et al., 2021). Augmentation procedures increase dataset sizes and improve model performance by adding changes in the training data. Soman and Saxena (2018) and Pant et al. (2019) proposed techniques for enhancing datasets by clustering in eigenvalue subspaces and producing samples inside these clusters. Despite recent initiatives to provide X-ray datasets, some class labels continue to be underrepresented, requiring augmentation for equitable training. The COVID-19 Radiography Database exhibits an unbalanced dataset, with the COVID-19 class including only 3,616 samples, in contrast to 10,192 normal pictures and 6,012 lung opacity images. The Pneumonia dataset demonstrates an imbalance, with bacterial pneumonia (2,530 pictures) significantly outnumbering viral pneumonia (1,345 photos) and normal cases (1,341 images). Such differences provide obstacles to categorization accuracy, especially in FL environments with sporadic client involvement.

The Synthetic Minority Oversampling Technique (SMOTE) is used to augment minority classes. In contrast to random oversampling, SMOTE creates synthetic samples using interpolation between existing minority samples and their closest neighbors. This method mitigates overfitting hazards and improves model resilience. SMOTE utilizes the k-nearest neighbor (KNN) method, which determines neighbors by Euclidean distance. For a minority class sample x_j, a new instance $\bar{x}$ is generated using Equation (1):

$$\bar{x} = x_j + |x_j + x_k| + \vartheta \quad (1)$$

Here, x_k is a randomly picked neighbor, and ϑ is a random number between 0 and 1. This approach creates realistic synthetic samples, resolving class imbalances and boosting classification accuracy.

3.4. Intermittent Clients

FL faces challenges with intermittent client engagement, particularly in collaborative healthcare. Data transmission restrictions, unpredictable network connections, and limited computer infrastructure contribute to this problem. Hospitals and healthcare institutions categorize illnesses using decentralized chest X-ray datasets in the FL framework. When new healthcare facilities join or established ones leave, frequently due to privacy or technological issues, participation is sporadic. In a FL arrangement, Clients 1, 2, and 3 have 1,244, 1,322, and 2,500 medical photos, respectively. Client 3 leaving the framework and Client 4 joining with just 28 medical photos imbalances the dataset, affecting model performance. We designed and tested two ways to preserve model performance and resilience in FL systems with intermittent client involvement. These solutions address dynamic client withdrawals and additions, which are typical in decentralized healthcare. The first technique ignores the weights of clients who leave the FL process in future global model aggregations. The aggregate includes freshly joined customers' weights. This method works well when new clients have enough data to contribute to local model training. New clients with sufficient datasets may enhance global model generalization. This method is difficult for new customers with little data, like Client 4 with 28 photos. These clients may inject bias or noise into the aggregation process, lowering model performance.

The second technique includes the latest weights from leaving customers into future aggregations. The global model receives fresh client contributions simultaneously. This strategy keeps information from leaving customers, particularly those with plenty of data, in the global model. Keeping Client 3's weights enables the global model to use its 2,500 photos to improve accuracy and stability after it leaves. This method is especially useful when leaving customers have bigger and more diversified datasets, since their absence might compromise crucial data. Both models emphasize dynamically modifying FL systems to client interaction. The approach relies on the number and quality of leaving and incoming customers' datasets and the application's needs. These methods show that FL can work in real-world healthcare settings where resource or network restrictions may limit client engagement.

Experimental findings showed that the number and quality of data stored by leaving and incoming customers considerably affects the success of FL techniques for intermittent clients. Strategy 1, which ignores leaving customers and includes only newly joined clients, worked well when the departing client had little data. In such cases, omitting the leaving client's weights avoided global model noise or bias. Strategy 2, which keeps the most current weights of outgoing customers and includes new clients, performed better when the departing clients had large datasets. Maintaining these customers' expertise guaranteed that the global model continued to benefit from their rich and varied data, improving accuracy and stability.

The system must resolve events when clients fail to send updates on time to strengthen the FL framework. We tested two adaptive case management methods. The first method is to use the latest client update until new ones arrive. This allows occasional clients to contribute to the global model without disrupting training. The second method eliminates parameters from clients that fail to update within a certain interval. Only after retraining their local models with the updated global weights can these clients rejoin the system. Thus, the framework aggregates just the most trustworthy and current weights, minimizing the influence of old or inconsistent data on the global model. These adaptive techniques show the FL framework's versatility in dynamic client engagement. Accounting for data availability and submission delays improves system performance consistently. These results emphasize the need of building FL frameworks that can withstand real-world problems, especially in healthcare settings with resource and connection restrictions.

3.5. Client-Side Model Training

Each FL client learns a local model using its dataset and computing power. After mini-batch stochastic gradient descent optimization, local CNN training follows. CNN design includes convolutional, pooling, dropout, and a fully connected softmax classification layer for all clients. This ensures training consistency and local data privacy (Frid-Adar et al., 2018). Train a local model using Algorithm 1. Initializing the local model's weights matches the server's global weights w. Training uses many local epochs and batch normalization stabilizes learning. Every client computes gradients and updates the model with its local dataset to create LMUs. Central server gets LMUs for global aggregation.

Figure 5. Algorithm

Algorithm 1: LMU: Client-side training

Input: w, w^t where w is a local weight and w^t is the global weight
Output: LMU, Where LMU is Local Model Update initialization;
Initialize $w \leftarrow w^t$;
Initially both weights are equal;
Spit $\rho_l \leftarrow P_k$, where ρ_l is the data size in batches, and P_k is set of data points on client k ;
Apply ClientUpdate($w^{(t,\rho)}$), with SGD, where SGD stands for stochastic gradient descent;
for each local epoch i from 1 to φ **do:**
while *Apply optimizer:* **do**
  for each $\rho_{(l_i)}$ in ρ_i **do:**
  Compute $G^{\rho(l_i)} \leftarrow \delta\rho(w_l, \varphi)$;
  Save $w \leftarrow w_l \leftarrow G^{\rho}_{l_i}$;
  End for
End for
Return w as a Local Model Update (LMU);
Finish

Figure 6 shows how the CNN architecture recovers features from enhanced chest X-ray images using max-pooling layers and dropout layers to reduce computational cost and overfitting. Batch normalization improves convergence and training stability.

Figure 6. Client-side training process utilizing a CNN architecture

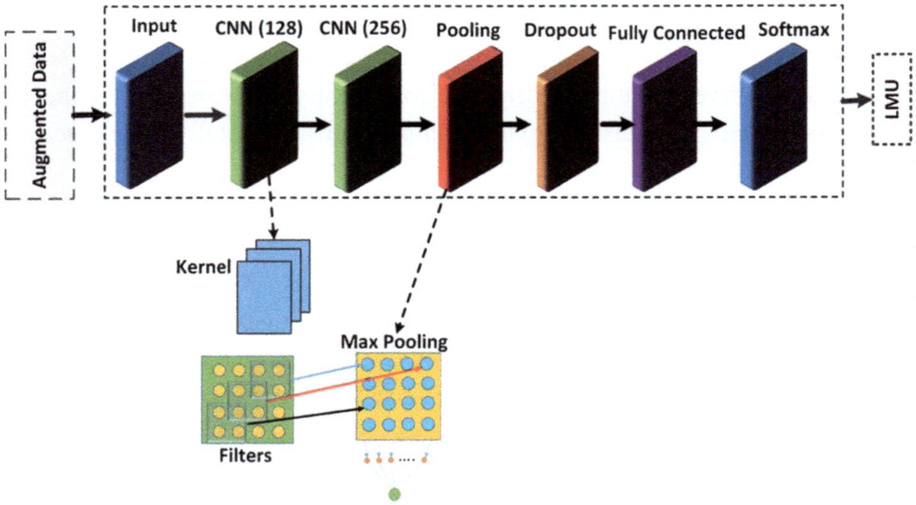

3.6. Server-Side Model Aggregation

The central server is crucial in FL by gathering Local Model Updates (LMUs) from clients, including intermittent participants, to update the global model (Rodríguez-Barroso, 2020). Federated weighted averaging ensures fairness and balanced client contributions. The percentage of data points each client has determines their contribution weight in this strategy, which compensates for local dataset sizes. Equation (2) calculates client i's weight:

$$w_i = \frac{n_1}{\sum_{i=1}^{N} n_i} \quad (2)$$

Here, w_i represents the weight of client i, n_i is the number of data points held by client i, and N is the total number of clients. The aggregated weights x_{agg} are calculated as follows

$$x_{agg} = \sum_{i=1}^{N} n_i x_i \quad (3)$$

The server uses aggregated weights to update the global model and distributes it to clients for training. The procedure is in Algorithm 2.

Figure 7. Algorithm 2

Algorithm 2: FL: Server-side aggregation

Input: w, T, where T is a $num_{feredated-rounds}$
Output: w^t as $weight_{aggregation}$
initialization;
Initialize $T \leftarrow 0, w^0$, where the number of rounds and global weight are both initially set to 0;
Compute $m \leftarrow max(C * K, 1)$, choose maximum clients from remote hospitals;
Randomly select S_t of m clients; Randomly selected clients as intermittent behavior, at each round t;
while *each client* $k \leftarrow S_t$: **do**
  Send $w^{(t-1)}$ to S_k, send last accumulated weight to selected client k;
  $w^t_{(t^k)} \leftarrow clientupdate(t^k, w^{(t-1)})$, update the current weight on client;
  End while
Compute aggregation $w^t \leftarrow \sum_{t=1}^{t^k} \frac{n_t}{n} w^t_{t^k}$, perform aggregation on global server for the selected clients;
End;
Return w^t as a $weight_{aggregation}$;
Finish

4. RESULTS AND DISCUSSION

4.1. Performance Measures

The proposed approach was evaluated using intermittent clients with varying amounts of test data to ensure its robustness and reliability. Two publicly available standard datasets, the COVID-19 Radiography Database (Dataset 1) and the Chest X-ray Pneumonia dataset (Dataset 2), as detailed in Section 3, were used for testing. These datasets were selected for their comprehensive and diverse representation of medical imaging data.

To assess the performance of the framework, four key metrics were employed: Precision, Recall, F-measure, and Accuracy. These metrics were calculated based on the counts of True Positives (TP), False Positives (FP), True Negatives (TN), and False Negatives (FN). The formulas for these performance measures are defined as follows:

$$\text{Precision} = \frac{TP}{TP + FP}$$

$$\text{Recall} = \frac{FP}{FP + TN}$$

$$\text{F} - \text{measure} = \frac{2 \times TP}{2TP + FP + FN}$$

$$\text{Kappa} = \frac{Observed_{acc} - Expected_{acc}}{1 - Expected_{acc}}$$

Here, the total number of instances is represented as

$$Total = TP + TN + FP + FN.$$

The observed accuracy is given by:

$$Observed_{acc} = \frac{TP + TN}{Total}$$

The expected accuracy accounts for the chance agreement, calculated as:

$$Expected_{acc} = \frac{(TP + TN)(TP + FP) + (FP + TN)(FN + TN)}{Total^2}.$$

4.2. Results Analysis and Comparisons

The evaluation of the proposed FL approach was conducted using server-side models trained over 50 epochs per cycle. The dynamic behavior of key performance metrics, including accuracy, loss, validation accuracy ($val_{accuracy}$), and validation loss (val_{loss}), is illustrated in Figure 6. The blue lines represent the accuracy and $val_{accuracy}$ for both training and testing datasets, while the red lines depict the loss and val_{loss} curves. These metrics provide insight into the model's learning process and its ability to generalize effectively.

In part (a) of Figure 8, the accuracy curve starts at 60%, while the loss curve begins at 75%. At the 9th epoch, a notable decline in accuracy is observed, coinciding with an increase in loss to 50%. However, both curves stabilize beyond this point, maintaining a consistent inverse relationship. The stability of these curves after the 9th epoch suggests that the model avoided overfitting, as the loss did not continue to rise with increased accuracy.

Part (b) of Figure 8 focuses on $val_{accuracy}$ and val_{loss}, both of which start at 75%. Over the initial epochs, $val_{accuracy}$ improves steadily, while val_{loss} decreases, indicating effective model training. However, minor fluctuations are observed at specific epochs. For instance, at the 5th epoch, $val_{accuracy}$ drops to 60%, accompanied by an increase in val_{loss} to 45%. Similarly, at the 23rd epoch, $val_{accuracy}$ and val_{loss} shift to 72% and 55%, respectively. These fluctuations likely reflect variations in data distribution and the model's adaptation to diverse client datasets.

Despite these minor variations, the model achieved an overall accuracy of 98% with a loss of 12%, underscoring its robust generalization capabilities. The results validate the effectiveness of the FL framework in handling decentralized and intermittent data while maintaining high performance. This demonstrates the potential of FL for applications requiring secure and collaborative learning, such as healthcare informatics.

Figure 8. Training and testing epoch curves: accuracy, loss, validation accuracy, validation loss

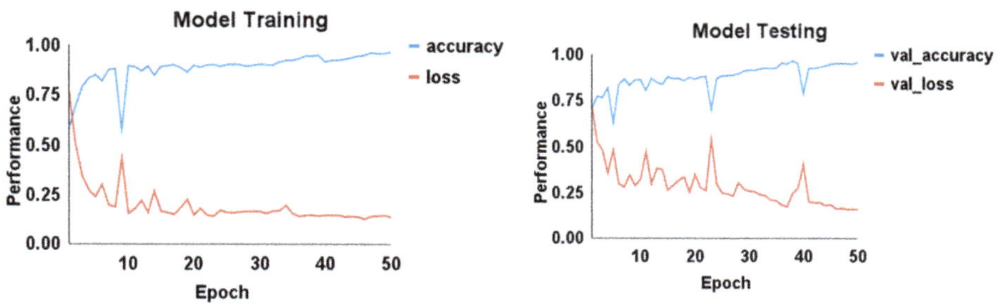

a) Model training **b)** Model testing

To evaluate the framework with intermittent clients, experiments were conducted using 200 X-ray image samples as test data for each client. As additional clients joined the FL framework, the proportion of their local data contributing to the global model decreased. This distribution of tasks mitigated data imbalance and bias issues that could arise from centralized training. Importantly, the goal was to develop models that generalized well across all clients' datasets, rather than overfitting to specific client data. After NN iterations, the global model incorporated contributions from various clients, and performance varied depending on the number of participating clients.

The effectiveness of the suggested strategy was examined for varying customer counts. Using Dataset 1, Table 1 summarizes the categorization results for five customers. Three kinds of X-ray pictures were identified: viral pneumonia, normal, and COVID. Precision, Recall, F-measure, Accuracy, and Kappa for the COVID class were 99.48%, 95.98%, 96.18%, 94%, and 96.22%, respectively. Accuracy, F-measure, and Kappa were the same across all groups. However, Precision and Recall differed somewhat between the viral pneumonia and normal pneumonia classes.

Table 2 indicates that the performance measures marginally declined when the number of customers reached seven. Kappa, Accuracy, and Overall F-measure for all courses were, for example, 95.48%, 93.25%, and 95.5%, respectively.

Table 1. Dataset 1 performance with five clients

Class	Clients	Precision	Recall	F-measure	Kappa	Accuracy (%)
COVID Normal Viral Pneumonia	5	99.48	95.98	96.18	94	96.22
		92.09	99			
		96.87	93.24			

Table 2. Dataset 1 performance with seven clients

Class	Clients	Precision	Recall	F-measure	Kappa	Accuracy (%)
COVID	7	96.98	96.50	95.48	93.25	95.5
Normal		92.12	99.50			
Viral Pneumonia		97.83	90.50			

Table 3 presents the results for ten clients. A noticeable improvement in classification accuracy was observed, with overall F-measure, Kappa, and Accuracy values reaching 95.5%, 94.77%, and 95.68%, respectively.

Table 3. Dataset 1 performance with ten clients

Class	Clients	Precision	Recall	F-measure	Kappa	Accuracy (%)
COVID	10	98.98	98.10	95.5	94.77	95.68
Normal		92.41	97.22			
Viral Pneumonia		96.25	91.38			

The efficacy of the proposed FL system was subsequently assessed with fifteen customers, and the findings are encapsulated in Table 4. The investigation revealed a considerable improvement in overall model performance with an increase in the number of participating customers. The framework attained an F-measure of 97.66%, a Kappa statistic of 96.49%, and an Accuracy of 97.94%. These metrics highlight the framework's effectiveness in sustaining superior classification performance across varied and dispersed datasets. This enhancement may be ascribed to the framework's capacity to equilibrate the contributions of local training from each client. The measures outlined in Section 3.4 were crucial in attaining this equilibrium. The approach efficiently addressed difficulties including data imbalance and sporadic client involvement, ensuring that customers with diverse data distributions and sizes contributed to the global model. The use of federated weighted averaging enabled the aggregation process to emphasize contributions in accordance with the amount and quality of each client's dataset. This mitigated the predominance of data from bigger customers and guaranteed that smaller clients with distinctive data attributes also had a significant influence on the global model.

Furthermore, the framework's capacity to alleviate data imbalances substantially enhanced the observed performance gains. The approach improved model generalization by using data augmentation methods to increase minority class samples, hence enhancing the representativeness of local datasets. The findings underscore the effectiveness of the proposed FL framework in using dispersed and heterogeneous data while maintaining fairness and stability in collaborative training, making it a feasible alternative for decentralized healthcare systems.

Table 4. Dataset 1 performance with fifteen clients

Class	Clients	Precision	Recall	F-measure	Kappa	Accuracy (%)
COVID Normal Viral Pneumonia	15	97.52 97.48 97.98	98.50 97.18 97.60	97.66	96.49	97.94

We tested the suggested FL system to categorize medical pictures correctly across different test data sets. The assessment included collaborative hospitals that trained local models with randomized test data sizes and generated Local Model Updates (LMUs) for the global model. This experimental design tested the FL framework's durability under various and dynamic test settings, mirroring real-world situations with variable test data availability and dispersion. The classification performance across different test data sizes using Dataset 1 is summarized in Table 5. Five distinct test data sizes, 200, 150, 80, 50, and 20 images, were selected to simulate varying levels of data availability. For the largest test data size of 200 image samples, the framework achieved an overall F-measure, Kappa, and Accuracy of 93.66%, 90.5%, and 93.66%, respectively. Among the classes, the COVID category demonstrated the highest classification performance, with a Precision of 96.96% and a Recall of 96.10%.

When the test data size was reduced to 150 image samples, a slight decline in classification performance was observed. The F-measure, Kappa, and Accuracy decreased marginally to 93.57%, 90.34%, and 93.55%, respectively. This minor reduction can be attributed to the decreased volume of data contributing to the training process, resulting in limited model generalization. However, an unexpected improvement in classification performance was noted when the test data size was further reduced to 80 samples. In this case, the F-measure, Kappa, and Accuracy increased to 97.89%, 96.87%, and 97.91%, respectively.

The framework achieved its best performance with 50 image samples, where the F-measure, Kappa, and Accuracy reached 97.99%, 97.2%, and 98.14%, respectively. Conversely, the lowest classification performance was recorded for the largest test data size of 200 images. These results suggest that smaller test data sizes yielded better classification outcomes. This phenomenon may be explained by the more focused impact of smaller test datasets during local model training, which reduces noise and emphasizes key features. However, it is also possible that the higher performance at smaller test sizes is influenced by the balance of data or specific dataset characteristics.

Table 5. Dataset 1 performance with test datasets

Class	Test Data	Precision	Recall	F-measure	Kappa	Accuracy (%)
COVID Normal Viral Pneumonia	200	96.96 89.72 94.68	96.10 95.42 89.78	93.66	90.5	93.66
COVID Normal Viral Pneumonia	150	97.91 88.95 94.40	94.00 96.66 90.56	93.57	90.34	93.55

continued on following page

Table 5. Continued

Class	Test Data	Precision	Recall	F-measure	Kappa	Accuracy (%)
COVID Normal Viral Pneumonia	80	100.00 96.38 97.50	96.25 100.00 97.50	97.89	96.87	97.91
COVID Normal Viral Pneumonia	50	100.00 98.00 96.97	96.00 98.00 100.00	97.99	97.20	98.14
COVID Normal Viral Pneumonia	20	100.00 94.00 100.00	100.00 100.00 93.33	97.77	96.67	97.77

To further validate the approach, Dataset 2 was used to evaluate classification performance with independent test data sizes (Table 6). Similar to Dataset 1, better results were achieved with smaller test data sizes. For example, using 20 image samples, the F-measure, Kappa, and Accuracy were 96.65%, 94.99%, and 96.66%, respectively. With 200 image samples, these metrics dropped to 79.31%, 69.25%, and 79.5%, respectively.

Table 6. Dataset 1 performance with different & independent datasets

Class	Test Data	Precision	Recall	F-measure	Kappa	Accuracy (%)
Bacterial Normal Viral	200	69.41 94.68 77.71	88.50 89.00 61.00	79.31	69.25	79.50
Bacterial Normal Viral	100	81.67 95.10 94.87	98.00 97.00 74.00	89.45	84.49	89.66
Bacterial Normal Viral	80	91.36 100.00 90.12	92.50 97.50 91.25	93.78	90.62	90.38
Bacterial Normal Viral	50	86.54 92.31 89.13	90.00 96.00 82.00	89.25	84.00	89.33
Bacterial Normal Viral	20	100.00 100.00 90.91	100.00 90.00 100.00	96.65	94.99	96.66

The classification performance for intermediate test data sizes, such as 100, 80, and 50 samples, remained consistent, achieving over 90% accuracy in most cases. These results highlight the framework's robustness in handling variations in test data sizes. However, the observed decrease in performance for larger test data sizes may be attributed to the Local Model Updates

(LMUs) being generated using test data sizes that were not part of the initial training process. This discrepancy can introduce variability in model generalization, particularly when larger datasets include more diverse and potentially unaligned samples. Despite these challenges, the proposed framework demonstrated its capacity to maintain high accuracy across varying and independent test data sizes, addressing a critical concern in FL systems where test data distributions may differ significantly from training data.

To investigate the model's classification and misclassification behavior, confusion matrices were evaluated for each class in both datasets. Figure 9 shows Dataset 1 intermittent client confusion matrices. The categorization rates for COVID, normal, and viral pneumonia with five clients were 98%, 96%, and 88%, respectively. The misclassification rates were 2%, 4%, and 12%. Despite its high classification rates, the suggested framework is more likely to misclassify viral pneumonia. Balances in class representation or slight feature changes across classes may explain this mismatch. The investigation shows the framework's ability to handle intermittent clients and different test data quantities.

Figure 9. Confusion matrices illustrating classification outcomes for intermittent clients with Dataset 1

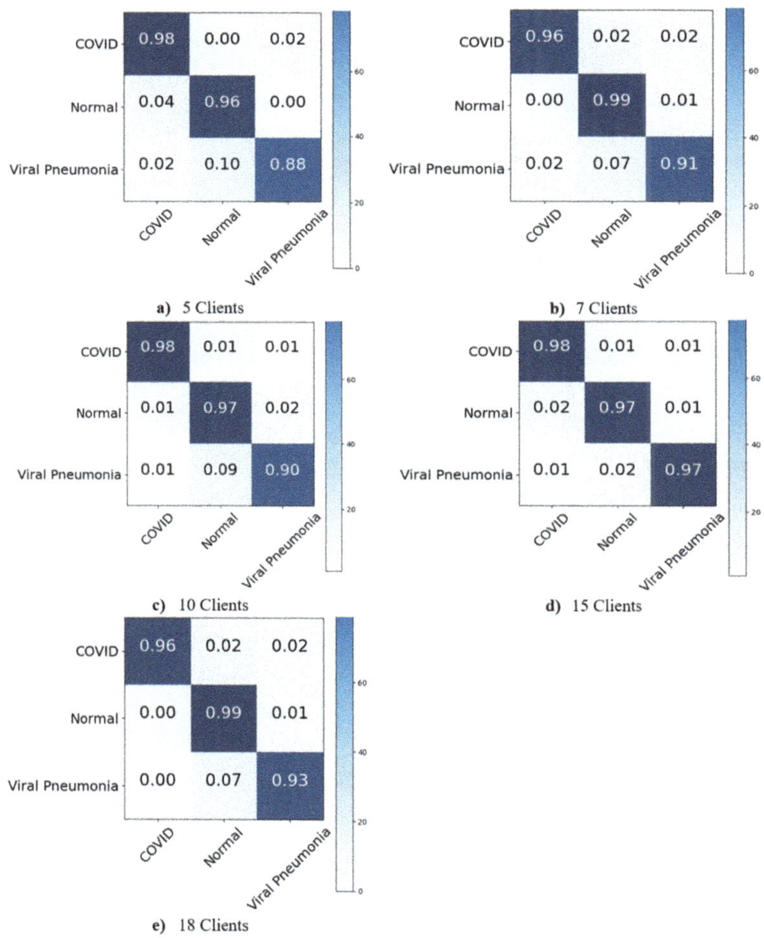

Expanding the FL architecture to seven clients marginally changed categorization and misclassification rates across the three classes. COVID, normal, and viral pneumonia classification accuracy was 96%, 99%, and 91%. The misclassification rates were 4%, 1%, and 9%. More customers may diversify the data, improving the global model's generalizability. Increasing the number of clients to 15 improved categorization rates to 98%, 97%, and 97% for COVID, normal, and viral pneumonia, respectively. Misclassification dropped to 2%, 3%, and 3%. These findings show that the FL framework can retain excellent classification accuracy despite sporadic client interaction and data distribution changes. The analysis of confusion matrices for randomized test data sizes, as shown in Figure 10 for Dataset 1, further underscores the effectiveness of the proposed framework. Using 200 image samples, classification rates for COVID, normal, and viral pneumonia classes were 96%, 96%, and 89%, respectively, with misclassification rates of 4%, 4%, and 11%. Interestingly, when the test data size was reduced to 20 samples, the classification rates improved significantly, reaching 100% for COVID and normal classes and 93% for the viral pneumonia class. Corresponding misclassification rates dropped to 0%, 0%, and 7%.

Figure 10. Variable image sample size confusion matrices using Dataset 1

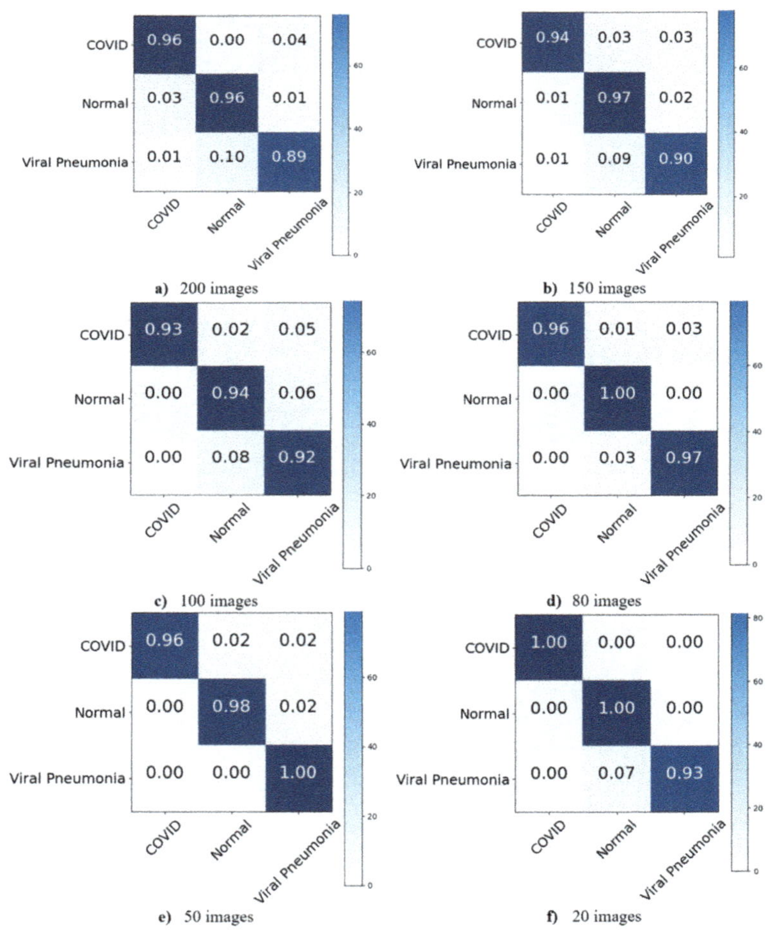

Figure 11 presents the confusion matrices for Dataset 2 with independent test sizes. For 200 image samples, classification rates for bacterial, normal, and viral classes were 89%, 89%, and 61%, with misclassification rates of 11%, 11%, and 39%. In contrast, using 20 image samples yielded the highest classification rates of 100%, 90%, and 100%, and misclassification rates of 0%, 10%, and 0%. The consistent performance across various independent test data sizes highlights the robustness of the proposed method.

Figure 11. Variable image sample size confusion matrices using Dataset 2

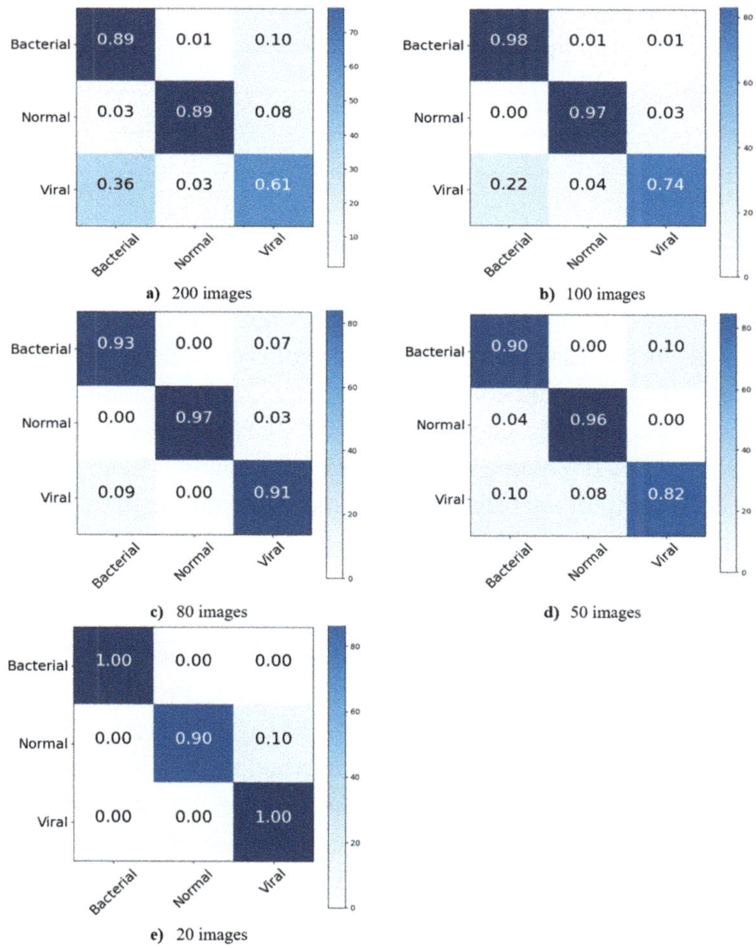

The proposed FL framework was compared with state-of-the-art methods to evaluate its effectiveness in addressing key challenges such as intermittent clients and imbalanced medical datasets. Table 7 presents a summary of these comparisons. Kumar et al. (2021) developed a blockchain-based FL framework for training global deep-learning models using CT scan images. Their method achieved a sensitivity of 98% and an accuracy of 98.68% across 182 training and 45 testing cases per hospital.

Table 7. A comparison of the suggested technique to current methods

Reference	Method	Performance (%)
Hosseini et al. (2023)	Prop-FFL	84.36
Gupta et al. (2023)	FedCare	90.32
Lu et al. (2022)	FedAP	92.02
Nair et al. (2023)	Fed-Select	94.76
Feki et al. (2021)	ResNet50 with FL	96.5
Qayyum et al. (2022)	Clustered FL	97
Elayan et al. (2022)	Deep FL	97.4
Díaz & García (2023)	2D-CNN with FL	97.52
Tian et al. (2023)	RPDFL	98
Our work	Deep CNN with FL	98.14

Díaz & García (2023) introduced a FL architecture using a 2D-CNN deep learning model, attaining a classification accuracy of 97.52% on simulated datasets with differing client quantities. Feki et al. (2021) presented an interactive FL system using VGG16 and ResNet50 to evaluate COVID-19 X-ray pictures, achieving an accuracy of 96.5%. Elayan et al. (2022) established a Deep FL system for decentralized healthcare services and automated data collection, attaining a classification accuracy of 97.4% in the diagnosis of dermatological conditions. Qayyum et al. (2022) investigated clustered FL methodologies, achieving 97% accuracy in COVID-19 diagnosis with edge computing. Lu et al. (2022) tackled domain changes in FL using FedAP, employing batch normalization measures to get a classification accuracy of 92.02%. Tian et al. (2023) introduced RPDFL, a privacy-preserving FL approach using a Ring-Allreduce algorithm, achieving 98% accuracy.

Other approaches are FedCare by Gupta et al. (2023), which used split learning to get 90.32% accuracy at the global server, and Fed-Select by Nair et al. (2023), which obtained 94.759% accuracy for Internet of Medical Things (IoMT) applications. Hosseini et al. (2023) used Prop-FLL to improve equity across healthcare institutions, achieving an accuracy of 84.36%. The suggested technique attains a classification accuracy of 98.14%, surpassing the majority of current methodologies. Its capacity to manage sporadic clients and uneven datasets underscores its applicability for use in collaborative healthcare systems. The computational complexity of the suggested algorithms was evaluated to determine their efficacy in practical applications. Table 8 delineates the complexity terms for Algorithms 1 and 2. The cost parameters include local and global model weights, batch sizes, data volume, and client count. The intricacy of Algorithm 1 is mostly determined by local calculations, while Algorithm 2 relies on global model aggregation and synchronization among clients.

Table 8. Computational complexity analysis

Cost terms	Algorithm 1 complexity	Algorithm 2 complexity
w, w^t, w_b	$\|l\|$	$\|b\| + \|m\|$
ρ_l, w^m	$\|w_\rho\| + \|\rho_i\|$	$\|c\|\|k\|$
φ, m	$\|w_{l_i}\|$	$\|s\| + \|w\|$
w, w^k	$\|l\| + \|w_\rho\| + \|\rho_i\|$	$\|S\| + \|w\|$
G, w^w	$\|\rho_{l_i}\|$	$\|k\| + \|w\|$
Total cost	$2\|l\| + 2\|\rho_i\| + 2\|w_\rho\| + 1\|w_{l_i}\|$	$1\|b\| + 3\|w\| + 2\|k\| + 2\|s\|$

In the context of the framework, here is the description of the parameters:

- w: local model weight
- w^t: global model weight
- t: training round
- b: size of a mini-batch used in training
- ρ_l: size of the data in batches
- k: specific client in the FL process
- P_k: set of data points available to client k
- m: maximum number of clients participating in training
- S: clients exhibiting intermittent behavior, meaning they may join or leave the training process dynamically
- l: weight of the local module
- C_k: subset of clients participating in training during a specific round

FL's client data heterogeneity presents statistical problems (Bottou, 2010). Using non-IID data to train a global model might cause inconsistent parameters and delayed convergence. Data distribution discrepancies between clients were measured and managed using the Earth Mover's Distance (EMD) to solve these difficulties (Zhao et al., 2018). Table 9 shows Datasets 1 and 2 EMD and classification accuracy.

Table 9. Classification accuracy versus Earth Mover's Distance (EMD) for model aggregation

EMD	0.16	0.40	0.82	1.12	1.40	1.61	1.74
Dataset 1 (Accuracy %)	97.81	96.26	95.34	94.11	93.42	91.72	90.14
Dataset 2 (Accuracy %)	94.38	92.23	89.10	86.52	81.34	77.96	71.42

As EMD increases, classification accuracy diminishes for both datasets. For instance, an EMD of 0.16 results in Dataset 1 attaining an accuracy of 97.81%, whereas an EMD of 1.74 diminishes accuracy to 90.14%. A same pattern is shown in Dataset 2, where accuracy declines from 94.38% to 71.42% with the growth of EMD. These results underscore the compromise between harmonizing non-IID data distributions and enhancing FL aggregation precision.

The experimental configuration had two non-IID scenarios: a two-class non-IID situation in which each client possessed two picture categories, and a one-class non-IID scenario where each client had a single category. Federated averaging was executed with local epochs set to 10, global epochs to 50, and batch sizes varying from 8 to 64. Learning rates were fine-tuned for each dataset and diminished exponentially throughout global model updates (GMUs).

The findings indicate that while non-IID data presents difficulties, EMD serves as a dependable indicator for addressing distribution inconsistencies. The suggested framework guarantees strong classification performance in various healthcare environments by efficiently using EMD. The comparison research verifies that the suggested FL framework achieves enhanced performance in classification accuracy while tackling significant issues such as sporadic client engagement and data heterogeneity. Its computing efficiency and capacity to handle non-IID data further emphasize its relevance for practical healthcare systems.

10. CONCLUSION

The incorporation of data-driven deep learning models into healthcare systems has emerged as a viable method for producing accurate and reliable statistical insights from medical data. Contemporary healthcare systems amass extensive data; nevertheless, the fragmented nature of this information and the related privacy issues substantially impede its comprehensive use, especially in decentralized environments. These constraints may hinder deep learning-based categorization methods from achieving their maximum efficacy, leading to subpar results.

This chapter introduces a scalable FL architecture tailored for interactive digital health services, emphasizing sporadic client interaction and unbalanced datasets. The suggested system utilizes chest X-ray pictures to tackle real-world issues, including unreliable client connections to the global server, where clients may either disengage or participate in the training process owing to technological limitations. A data augmentation method is used to equilibrate local datasets, hence improving the efficacy of local model training. To assess the framework's efficacy, experiments were performed across many situations involving five to eighteen customers and diverse test sets. Five principal performance metrics, Precision, Recall, F-measure, Kappa, and Accuracy, were used to evaluate the suggested methodology. The findings indicate that the framework attains competitive performance, achieving an overall accuracy of 98.14%, and successfully tackles the issues presented by intermittent clients and unbalanced data.

The approach guarantees data privacy by facilitating model training without necessitating the centralization of raw data. This is especially vital for protecting sensitive medical information between many organizations. Employing safe aggregation methods, including TensorFlow-based implementations, improves the privacy and security of the aggregation process during model parameter changes. Although the framework exhibits considerable advantages, certain constraints persist. In actual applications, customers may own varied data kinds or sources, resulting in difficulties in consolidating consistent and impartial model updates. This may lead to diminished accuracy or skewed forecasts, which are especially concerning for essential healthcare applications. Moreover, regular communication between clients and the central server may result in heightened overhead and delay, possibly impacting real-time applications such as emergency response systems. To mitigate these constraints and enhance the proposed FL framework, many directions for further study are recommended:

- Investigating alternate aggregation processes, such as cluster federated averaging using k-means clustering, may improve the efficiency and precision of model updates. Integrating machine learning models into the aggregation process might enhance the entire architecture.
- Analyzing possible assaults on the FL architecture, including model poisoning and data extraction, and formulating techniques to limit their effects is essential. Homomorphic encryption for safe weight transfer between clients and servers may serve as an effective option to augment data security.
- Utilizing transfer learning approaches may accelerate local training, enhancing the performance and dependability of local models. This method may potentially improve the production of Local Model Updates (LMUs) for decentralized systems.
- A significant problem in FL systems is attaining a compromise between privacy protection and model efficacy. Subsequent study need to concentrate on devising strategies that enhance this trade-off, guaranteeing that both privacy and performance criteria are satisfied in healthcare applications.
- Conducting comprehensive comparisons between centralized and distributed training methodologies inside the FL framework will provide more insights into performance and privacy trade-offs, aiding in the refinement of the framework for various healthcare applications.

REFERENCES

Ahad, A., Jiangbin, Z., Mughees, A., Puspitasari, I., & Tayyab, M. (2025). Secure Horizons: Integrating Blockchain With AI for Enhanced Smart Healthcare Systems. In *AI Techniques for Securing Medical and Business Practices* (pp. 357-390). IGI Global.

Ahad, A., Tahir, M., Sheikh, M. A. S., Mughees, A., & Ahmed, K. I. (2021, October). Optimal route selection in 5G-based smart health-care network: a reinforcement learning approach. In *2021 26th IEEE Asia-Pacific Conference on Communications (APCC)* (pp. 248-253). IEEE.

Ali, Z., Ahad, A., Madeira, F., & Shayea, I. (2023, October). Enhancing Transparency and Trustworthiness of Healthcare IoT Data with AWS: A Proposed Model. In *EAI International Conference on IoT Technologies for HealthCare* (pp. 44-56). Cham: Springer Nature Switzerland. DOI: 10.1007/978-3-031-71911-0_4

Ashfaq, F., Ahad, A., Hussain, M., & Madeira, F. (2023, October). Transforming Diabetes Care: A Review of IoT-Based Mobile Health Systems. In *EAI International Conference on IoT Technologies for HealthCare* (pp. 14-32). Cham: Springer Nature Switzerland. DOI: 10.1007/978-3-031-71911-0_2

Avellino, I., Bailly, G., Canlorbe, G., Belgihti, J., Morel, G., & Vitrani, M. A. (2019, May). Impacts of telemanipulation in robotic assisted surgery. In *Proceedings of the 2019 CHI conference on human factors in computing systems* (pp. 1-15). DOI: 10.1145/3290605.3300813

Baheti, P., Sikka, M., Arya, K. V., & Rajesh, R. (2020, February). Federated Learning on Distributed Medical Records for Detection of Lung Nodules. In *VISIGRAPP* (Vol. 4, pp. 445–451). VISAPP. DOI: 10.5220/0009144704450451

Bottou, L. (2010). Large-scale machine learning with stochastic gradient descent. In *Proceedings of-COMPSTAT'2010: 19th International Conference on Computational StatisticsParis France,August 22-27, 2010Keynote, Invited and Contributed Papers* (pp. 177-186). Physica-Verlag HD. DOI: 10.1007/978-3-7908-2604-3_16

Brisimi, T. S., Chen, R., Mela, T., Olshevsky, A., Paschalidis, I. C., & Shi, W. (2018). Federated learning of predictive models from federated electronic health records. *International Journal of Medical Informatics*, *112*, 59–67. DOI: 10.1016/j.ijmedinf.2018.01.007 PMID: 29500022

Butt, H. A., Ahad, A., Wasim, M., Madeira, F., & Chamran, M. K. (2023, October). 5G and IoT for Intelligent Healthcare: AI and Machine Learning Approaches—A Review. In *International Conference on Smart Objects and Technologies for Social Good* (pp. 107-123). Cham: Springer Nature Switzerland. DOI: 10.1007/978-3-031-52524-7_8

Butt, H. A., Ahad, A., Wasim, M., Shayea, I., Coelho, P. J., Pires, I. M., & Garcia, N. M. (2023). Federated machine learning in 5G smart healthcare: A security perspective review. *Procedia Computer Science*, *224*, 580–586. DOI: 10.1016/j.procs.2023.09.084

Chen, Y., Yang, X., Chen, B., Miao, C., & Yu, H. (2017, November). PdAssist: Objective and quantified symptom assessment of Parkinson's disease via smartphone. In *2017 IEEE International Conference on Bioinformatics and Biomedicine (BIBM)* (pp. 939-945). IEEE. DOI: 10.1109/BIBM.2017.8217783

Chowdhury, M. E., Rahman, T., Khandakar, A., Mazhar, R., Kadir, M. A., Mahbub, Z. B., Islam, K. R., Khan, M. S., Iqbal, A., Emadi, N. A., Reaz, M. B. I., & Islam, M. T. (2020). Can AI help in screening viral and COVID-19 pneumonia? *IEEE Access : Practical Innovations, Open Solutions*, *8*, 132665–132676. DOI: 10.1109/ACCESS.2020.3010287

Dayan, I., Roth, H. R., Zhong, A., Harouni, A., Gentili, A., Abidin, A. Z., Liu, A., Costa, A. B., Wood, B. J., Tsai, C.-S., Wang, C.-H., Hsu, C.-N., Lee, C. K., Ruan, P., Xu, D., Wu, D., Huang, E., Kitamura, F. C., Lacey, G., & Li, Q. (2021). Federated learning for predicting clinical outcomes in patients with COVID-19. *Nature Medicine*, *27*(10), 1735–1743. DOI: 10.1038/s41591-021-01506-3 PMID: 34526699

Díaz, J. S. P., & García, Á. L. (2023). Study of the performance and scalability of federated learning for medical imaging with intermittent clients. *Neurocomputing*, *518*, 142–154. DOI: 10.1016/j.neucom.2022.11.011

Elayan, H., Aloqaily, M., & Guizani, M. (2021). Sustainability of healthcare data analysis IoT-based systems using deep federated learning. *IEEE Internet of Things Journal*, *9*(10), 7338–7346. DOI: 10.1109/JIOT.2021.3103635

Feki, I., Ammar, S., Kessentini, Y., & Muhammad, K. (2021). Federated learning for COVID-19 screening from Chest X-ray images. *Applied Soft Computing*, *106*, 107330. DOI: 10.1016/j.asoc.2021.107330 PMID: 33776607

Frid-Adar, M., Diamant, I., Klang, E., Amitai, M., Goldberger, J., & Greenspan, H. (2018). GAN-based synthetic medical image augmentation for increased CNN performance in liver lesion classification. *Neurocomputing*, *321*, 321–331. DOI: 10.1016/j.neucom.2018.09.013

Gupta, A., Misra, S., Pathak, N., & Das, D. (2023). Fedcare: Federated learning for resource-constrained healthcare devices in iomt system. *IEEE Transactions on Computational Social Systems*, *10*(4), 1587–1596. DOI: 10.1109/TCSS.2022.3232192

Hossain, M. S., & Muhammad, G. (2020). Deep learning based pathology detection for smart connected healthcare. *IEEE Network*, *34*(6), 120–125. DOI: 10.1109/MNET.011.2000064

Hossain, M. S., Muhammad, G., & Guizani, N. (2020). Explainable AI and mass surveillance system-based healthcare framework to combat COVID-I9 like pandemics. *IEEE Network*, *34*(4), 126–132. DOI: 10.1109/MNET.011.2000458

Hosseini, S. M., Sikaroudi, M., Babaie, M., & Tizhoosh, H. R. (2023). Proportionally fair hospital collaborations in federated learning of histopathology images. *IEEE Transactions on Medical Imaging*, *42*(7), 1982–1995. DOI: 10.1109/TMI.2023.3234450 PMID: 37018335

Huang, L., Shea, A. L., Qian, H., Masurkar, A., Deng, H., & Liu, D. (2019). Patient clustering improves efficiency of federated machine learning to predict mortality and hospital stay time using distributed electronic medical records. *Journal of Biomedical Informatics*, *99*, 103291. DOI: 10.1016/j.jbi.2019.103291 PMID: 31560949

Kermany, D. (2018). Labeled optical coherence tomography (oct) and chest x-ray images for classification. *Mendeley data*.

Kumar, R., Khan, A. A., Kumar, J., Golilarz, N. A., Zhang, S., Ting, Y., & Wang, W. (2021). Blockchain-federated-learning and deep learning models for covid-19 detection using ct imaging. *IEEE Sensors Journal, 21*(14), 16301–16314. DOI: 10.1109/JSEN.2021.3076767 PMID: 35789224

Lee, J., Sun, J., Wang, F., Wang, S., Jun, C. H., & Jiang, X. (2018). Privacy-preserving patient similarity learning in a federated environment: Development and analysis. *JMIR Medical Informatics, 6*(2), e7744. DOI: 10.2196/medinform.7744 PMID: 29653917

Lu, W., Wang, J., Chen, Y., Qin, X., Xu, R., Dimitriadis, D., & Qin, T. (2022). Personalized federated learning with adaptive batchnorm for healthcare. *IEEE Transactions on Big Data*. https://doi.org//arXiv.2112.00734DOI: 10.48550

McMahan, B., Moore, E., Ramage, D., Hampson, S., & Arcas, B. A. (2017, April). Communication-efficient learning of deep networks from decentralized data. In *Artificial intelligence and statistics* (pp. 1273–1282). PMLR., DOI: 10.1109/ICDE51399.2021.00040

Miotto, R., Wang, F., Wang, S., Jiang, X., & Dudley, J. T. (2018). Deep learning for healthcare: Review, opportunities and challenges. *Briefings in Bioinformatics, 19*(6), 1236–1246. DOI: 10.1093/bib/bbx044 PMID: 28481991

Motamed, S., Rogalla, P., & Khalvati, F. (2021). RANDGAN: Randomized generative adversarial network for detection of COVID-19 in chest X-ray. *Scientific Reports, 11*(1), 8602. DOI: 10.1038/s41598-021-87994-2 PMID: 33883609

Nair, A. K., Sahoo, J., & Raj, E. D. (2023). Privacy preserving Federated Learning framework for IoMT based big data analysis using edge computing. *Computer Standards & Interfaces, 86*, 103720. DOI: 10.1016/j.csi.2023.103720

Pant, H., Sharma, M., & Soman, S. (2019). Twin neural networks for the classification of large unbalanced datasets. *Neurocomputing, 343*, 34–49. DOI: 10.1016/j.neucom.2018.07.089

Qayyum, A., Ahmad, K., Ahsan, M. A., Al-Fuqaha, A., & Qadir, J. (2022). Collaborative federated learning for healthcare: Multi-modal covid-19 diagnosis at the edge. *IEEE Open Journal of the Computer Society, 3*, 172–184. DOI: 10.1109/OJCS.2022.3206407

Rahman, M. A., Hossain, M. S., Islam, M. S., Alrajeh, N. A., & Muhammad, G. (2020). Secure and provenance enhanced internet of health things framework: A blockchain managed federated learning approach. *IEEE Access : Practical Innovations, Open Solutions, 8*, 205071–205087. DOI: 10.1109/ACCESS.2020.3037474 PMID: 34192116

Rajotte, J. F., Mukherjee, S., Robinson, C., Ortiz, A., West, C., Ferres, J. M. L., & Ng, R. T. (2021, September). Reducing bias and increasing utility by federated generative modeling of medical images using a centralized adversary. In *Proceedings of the conference on information Technology for Social Good* (pp. 79-84). DOI: 10.1145/3462203.3475875

Rieke, N., Hancox, J., Li, W., Milletari, F., Roth, H. R., Albarqouni, S., Bakas, S., Galtier, M. N., Landman, B. A., Maier-Hein, K., Ourselin, S., Sheller, M., Summers, R. M., Trask, A., Xu, D., Baust, M., & Cardoso, M. J. (2020). The future of digital health with federated learning. *NPJ Digital Medicine, 3*(1), 1–7. DOI: 10.1038/s41746-020-00323-1 PMID: 33015372

Rodríguez-Barroso, N., Stipcich, G., Jiménez-López, D., Ruiz-Millán, J. A., Martínez-Cámara, E., González-Seco, G., Luzón, M. V., Veganzones, M. A., & Herrera, F. (2020). Federated Learning and Differential Privacy: Software tools analysis, the Sherpa. ai FL framework and methodological guidelines for preserving data privacy. *Information Fusion*, *64*, 270–292. DOI: 10.1016/j.inffus.2020.07.009

Shi, H., Han, X., Jiang, N., Cao, Y., Alwalid, O., Gu, J., Fan, Y., & Zheng, C. (2020). Radiological findings from 81 patients with COVID-19 pneumonia in Wuhan, China: A descriptive study. *The Lancet. Infectious Diseases*, *20*(4), 425–434. DOI: 10.1016/S1473-3099(20)30086-4 PMID: 32105637

Sintunavarat, W., & Turab, A. (2022). Mathematical analysis of an extended SEIR model of COVID-19 using the ABC-fractional operator. *Mathematics and Computers in Simulation*, *198*, 65–84. DOI: 10.1016/j.matcom.2022.02.009 PMID: 35194306

Soman, S., & Saxena, S. (2018). EigenSample: A non-iterative technique for adding samples to small datasets. *Applied Soft Computing*, *70*, 1064–1077. DOI: 10.1016/j.asoc.2017.08.017

Sun, W., Lei, S., Wang, L., Liu, Z., & Zhang, Y. (2020). Adaptive federated learning and digital twin for industrial internet of things. *IEEE Transactions on Industrial Informatics*, *17*(8), 5605–5614. DOI: 10.1109/TII.2020.3034674

Tian, Y., Wang, S., Xiong, J., Bi, R., Zhou, Z., & Bhuiyan, M. Z. A. (2023). Robust and privacy-preserving decentralized deep federated learning training: Focusing on digital healthcare applications. *IEEE/ACM Transactions on Computational Biology and Bioinformatics*. Advance online publication. DOI: 10.1109/TCBB.2023.3243932 PMID: 37028039

Turab, A., Sintunavarat, W., Ullah, F., Zaidi, S. A., Montoyo, A., & Nescolarde-Selva, J. A. (2024). Computational modeling of animal behavior in T-mazes: Insights from machine learning. *Ecological Informatics*, *81*, 102639. DOI: 10.1016/j.ecoinf.2024.102639

Ullah, F., Moon, J., Naeem, H., & Jabbar, S. (2022). Explainable artificial intelligence approach in combating real-time surveillance of COVID19 pandemic from CT scan and X-ray images using ensemble model. *The Journal of Supercomputing*, *78*(17), 19246–19271. DOI: 10.1007/s11227-022-04631-z PMID: 35754515

Ullah, F., Turab, A., Ullah, S., Cacciagrano, D., & Zhao, Y. (2024). Enhanced network intrusion detection system for internet of things security using multimodal big data representation with transfer learning and game theory. *Sensors (Basel)*, *24*(13), 4152. DOI: 10.3390/s24134152 PMID: 39000931

Voigt, P., & Von dem Bussche, A. (2017). The eu general data protection regulation (gdpr). *A Practical Guide, 1st Ed., Cham: Springer International Publishing, 10*(3152676), 10-5555.

Xu, S., Wu, H., & Bie, R. (2018). CXNet-m1: Anomaly detection on chest X-rays with image-based deep learning. *IEEE Access : Practical Innovations, Open Solutions*, *7*, 4466–4477. DOI: 10.1109/ACCESS.2018.2885997

Yang, H. M., Duan, T., Ding, D., Bagul, A., Langlotz, C., & Shpanskaya, K. (2017). CheXNet: radiologist-level pneumonia detection on chest x-rays with deep learning. *arXiv preprint arXiv:1711.05225.*

Yang, Q., Liu, Y., Chen, T., & Tong, Y. (2019). Federated machine learning: Concept and applications. [TIST]. *ACM Transactions on Intelligent Systems and Technology*, *10*(2), 1–19. DOI: 10.1145/3298981

Zhao, Y., Li, M., Lai, L., Suda, N., Civin, D., & Chandra, V. (2018). Federated learning with non-iid data. *arXiv preprint arXiv:1806.00582*. https://doi.org//arXiv.1806.00582DOI: 10.48550

Chapter 2
Blockchain Technologies for Decentralized Medical Records

R. Gayathri
https://orcid.org/0009-0007-8937-4373
Dr. G.R. Damodaran College of Science, India

C. Bhuvaneshwari
https://orcid.org/0009-0007-7231-1448
Dr. G.R. Damodaran College of Science, India

ABSTRACT

Blockchain technology is revolutionizing healthcare through decentralization, security, and interoperability. As compared with traditional centrally stored databases, blockchain enables patients to have full control over their information through secure and efficient electronic health record (EHR) exchanges. Sensitive medical information is secured through use with cryptographic keys, minimizing cybersecurity risks through its use. Administrative processes such as consent and claims processing via smart contracts make processes efficient and less costly. In pharmacy, drugs can be validated through use with blockchain, effectively eradicating counterfeit drugs. Transparency in the supply chain is also increased, and inefficiencies resolved through its use. Regulatory barriers, however, have not yet been addressed, but a patient-first model for medical care is facilitated through increased security, efficiency, and transparency in medical information management, creating a more efficient and networked medical environment.

INTRODUCTION TO BLOCKCHAIN TECHNOLOGIES IN HEALTH CARE

Blockchain technology is an important field of study and application in many different industries since it is a revolutionary digital ledger system that provides security, decentralization, and transparency. Blockchain was first created for Bitcoin, but because of its special qualities—including privacy, security,

DOI: 10.4018/979-8-3373-0593-6.ch002

and immutability—it has spread beyond cryptocurrencies to affect industries like supply chains, healthcare, and finance (Islam et al., 2020; Bhutta et al., 2021; Jaoude & Saadé, 2019).

The decentralized structure of blockchain improves transaction security and trust by avoiding intermediaries. Its applications extend to different sectors, including the Internet of Things, energy, and government, where it offers solutions for privacy and data integrity (Cao et al., 2021; Jaoude & Saadé, 2019; Yli-Huumo et al., 2016).

Figure 1. Blockchain Technology

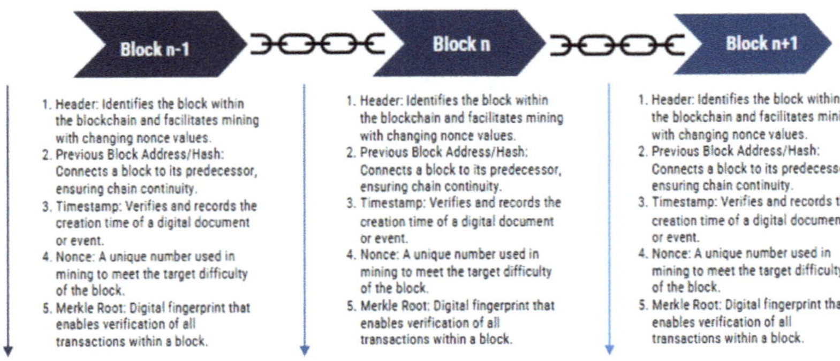

As depicted in Figure 1, Each block in a blockchain contains essential information such as a unique identifier, a timestamp, and a reference to the previous block, ensuring secure and sequential data storage.

Overview of the Blockchain technologies in health care

The increasing complexity of health systems, combined with the need for secure, transparent, and interoperable data management solutions, underlines the basic necessity to investigate advanced technologies such as blockchain. The decentralized and immutable nature of blockchain provides a revolutionary approach to overcoming the drawbacks of traditional patient record systems (Azaria et al., 2016; Zhang et al., 2018). This chapter, the authors research the possibilities of blockchain innovation for healthcare data management to fulfill the changing requirements of the health care sector.

Blockchain technology solves the challenges of today's healthcare system by using a shared digital ledger that ensures secure and efficient data management. This framework permits for the secure and instant transfer of medical information among different stakeholders while keeping the integrity and confidentiality of the data (Kuo et al., 2017). In addition, blockchain increases patient autonomy as it empowers patients to manage their health information, with a focus on transparency and patient-centered care.

This chapter explores the fundamentals of blockchain technology and its practical application in decentralized patient record systems, highlighting its associated implication on security, scalability, and regulatory frameworks. Applying a combination of theoretical perspectives with practical considerations, this analysis illustrates how blockchain technology can potentially be applied towards handling current problems with health-care data management; hence providing patients a secure and transparent methods for the administration of their patient records.

Chapter Contribution

This chapter explores how blockchain technology can be integrated into decentralized patient record management, highlighting its transformative effects on the healthcare sector. By utilizing theoretical frameworks alongside real-world examples, the chapter aims to provide the practical applications of blockchain technology. The main contributions include:

- Blockchain Fundamentals and Applications: The chapter begins with an overview of the essential features of blockchain, including transparency, immutability, and decentralization, and explores how these characteristics are utilized in managing patient data. This section positions blockchain as a key element for creating secure, interoperable, and efficient healthcare systems.
- Decentalization: The chapter highlights how decentralization allows the patient to control their data. It also gives an idea on how decentralization provides secure, transparent interoperable framework for health information exchange.
- Scalability and Hybrid Solutions: To overcome the challenges of scaling blockchain implementation, the chapter investigates hybrid solutions like off-chain storage. This part connects theoretical scalability issues with practical approaches for managing large datasets, such as medical imaging.
- Ethical and Legal Considerations: A comprehensive analysis of the ethical and legal implications of blockchain in healthcare is presented, focusing on data privacy, regulatory compliance (e.g., HIPAA, GDPR), and governance challenges. This section emphasizes the necessity of ethical frameworks to guide the adoption of blockchain technology.

Chapter Organization

The chapter is structured into 10 sections, each contributing to a comprehensive understanding of blockchain's role in decentralized patient record management:

1. Introduction

   This section highlights the urgent need for decentralized patient record systems, discussing the limitations of centralized models and the transformative potential of blockchain technology. It sets the foundation for the following discussions on blockchain's applications in healthcare.
2. Blockchain Fundamentals

   A thorough overview of blockchain technology is presented, detailing its essential features, transaction processes, and types (public, private, and consortium blockchains). This section establishes the theoretical basis for understanding its applications in healthcare.
3. Challenges in Centralized Systems

   The drawbacks of centralized patient record systems are discussed, including data barriers, security vulnerabilities, and restricted patient control. These issues make a strong case for the adoption of blockchain-based decentralized systems.
4. Decentralized Patient Records: Benefits and Use Cases

   The advantages of blockchain for enhancing data security, improving interoperability, and empowering patients are explored. Real-world examples, such as secure data sharing and real-time access, are provided to illustrate the practical benefits of blockchain.
5. Scalability and Hybrid Solutions

This section addresses the technical challenges of implementing blockchain on a large scale, focusing on hybrid models like off-chain storage for managing extensive datasets. Practical strategies for achieving scalability while maintaining security are discussed.

6. Ethical and Legal Considerations

   Ethical and legal challenges, including data privacy, consent management, and compliance with regulations such as HIPAA and GDPR, are examined. The section underscores the importance of ethical frameworks in guiding blockchain adoption in healthcare.

7. Interoperability and Real-Time Data Sharing

   This section explores how blockchain facilitates smooth data exchange among healthcare providers. It includes practical examples of blockchain-driven interoperability and discusses its effects on enhancing care coordination and improving patient outcomes.

8. Future Directions and Innovations

   This part covers emerging trends and possible advancements in blockchain technology, such as the integration of AI, cross-border interoperability, and novel healthcare applications. It offers a forward-looking view on how blockchain could influence the future of healthcare.

9. Conclusion

   The chapter wraps up with a recap of key insights and suggestions for future research and implementation. It highlights the transformative potential of blockchain in developing a secure, efficient, and patient-centered healthcare system.

2.UNDERSTANDING BLOCKCHAIN TECHNOLOGY

Blockchain technology is a distributed, digital ledger system that records transactions securely across multiple computers in a network. It is best known as the technology behind cryptocurrencies like Bitcoin, but its applications extend to various industries, including healthcare, finance, supply chain, and data security.

Decentralization, immutability, and transparency are core features of blockchain technology that collectively enhance security and trust across various applications. Decentralization eliminates the need for intermediaries, allowing peer-to-peer transactions and reducing costs while increasing efficiency (Segal et al., 2023; Alhat, 2024). Immutability ensures that once data is recorded, it cannot be altered or deleted, providing a tamper-proof record that fosters trust among participants (Monrat et al., 2019; Dong et al., 2023).

Figure 2. Features of Blockchain

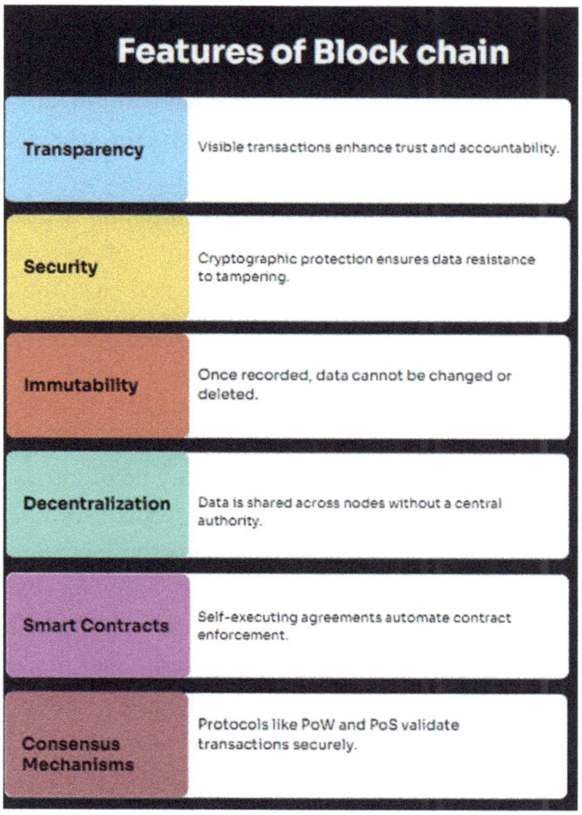

Transparency is achieved through open ledgers and real-time updates, which enhance auditability and accountability, crucial for sectors like finance and healthcare (Mukherjee et al., 2021; George et al., 2024). These attributes make blockchain a transformative tool in modern digital ecosystems (Agrawal et al., 2022; Banoth & Dave, 2022).Blockchain has the potential to become a powerful and vital tool in the healthcare arena. The special capabilities of this technology greatly determine the security, correctness, and transparency of data.

Blockchain Technology in Healthcare Management:

Blockchain technology has emerged as a promising solution for managing electronic health records (EHRs) in a decentralized, secure, and efficient manner. This distributed ledger technology offers significant advantages over traditional centralized systems by providing enhanced data security, privacy, and interoperability in healthcare (Shah et al., 2024). The use of blockchain for EHRs addresses several challenges faced by conventional systems, including data fragmentation, limited access, and poor coordination across healthcare facilities. One of the primary benefits of blockchain-based EHR systems is the ability to securely store and share patient records while maintaining anonymity and detachment. For instance, PREHEALTH, a privacy-preserving EHR management solution, utilizes distributed ledger technology and an Identity Mixer (Idemix) to effectively store patient records while ensuring privacy

(Stamatellis et al., 2020). This approach demonstrates the feasibility of implementing blockchain-based EHR systems in real-world scenarios. Blockchain technology also offers potential solutions for improving data security, privacy, and interoperability in healthcare and biomedical research.

By utilizing its decentralized, secure, and immutable nature, blockchain can prevent data breaches and cyber-attacks, which are common concerns in traditional centralized systems (Shah et al., 2024). This enhanced security is particularly crucial in the healthcare sector, where sensitive patient information must be protected from unauthorized access and interfering.

Blockchain technology also has the potential to transform public health surveillance by enhancing data security, accessibility, storage, and sharing. Its immutability proves crucial for securing healthcare data, safeguarding health records and clinical trial outcomes, and ensuring compliance with regulatory standards. This technology can lead to computerized processes for collecting and validating data, accurate information gathered from multiple sources, and reduced risk of digital crimes.

However, the implementation of blockchain in healthcare faces several challenges, including regulatory issues, technical complexity, and economic costs (Shah et al., 2024). These hurdles suggest that the adoption of blockchain technology in healthcare will likely be gradual.

Ongoing research and interdisciplinary approaches are essential for overcoming these barriers and realizing the full potential of blockchain in healthcare. Despite these challenges, blockchain technology offers numerous advantages in the healthcare sector.

It can improve data integrity, enhance collaboration, and protect intellectual property in biomedical research (Shah et al., 2024). This improved data exchange can lead to better medical diagnoses and overall healthcare outcomes. Blockchain-based EHR systems also empower patients by giving them greater control over their health records. The "Ledger of Me" concept extends Personal Health Records (PHRs) to create a new platform that combines the collection and access of medical data with digital interventions and smart contracts (Leeming et al., 2019). This approach enables patients to use their data to support their care and provides strong consent mechanisms for sharing data between different organizations and applications.

The potential applications of blockchain in healthcare extend beyond EHR management. It can be used to improve supply chain management, clinical trials, and telemedicine (Shah et al., 2024). Additionally, blockchain technology can address issues related to eligibility, enrollment, and claims processing in public health programs such as the U.S. Medicaid program.

3. CHALLENGES IN CENTRALIZED SYSTEMS

Current Challenges in Medical Record Management

The healthcare industry faces significant challenges in managing medical records effectively. Three pressing issues—fragmentation of patient records across multiple systems, security vulnerabilities in centralized systems, and inefficiencies in data sharing and interoperability—have prompted researchers to explore innovative solutions, such as blockchain technology. This section investigates into how blockchain can address these issues, with citations to support each perspective.

i. Fragmentation of Patient Records Across Multiple Systems

Fragmentation in medical record management is a widespread problem in the modern healthcare sector, where the patient's data is scattered throughout different healthcare institutions. The fragmentation of the system makes it hard to get a complete and accurate view of a patient's medical history because each provider maintains its own isolated database. Most often, these lead to data inconsistencies and redundancies. These factors contribute to critical gaps that delay patient diagnosis and hinder effective treatment of patients. An example is that a healthcare provider treating a patient in one establishment may not have information on what tests, treatments, or diagnoses were conducted at other places; hence, certain procedures are done repeatedly or perhaps early intervention was missed.

Poor interoperability among healthcare systems creates the problem, as well. In the lack of a single instance to aggregate a patient's data, providers are bound to use bits and pieces or even archaic records, which adds to the likelihood of medical mistakes. Moreover, patients lack control over their health information, posing difficulties in their ability to make their medical history available to other providers or facilities. This uncoordinated approach reduces the quality of care and increases administrative inefficiencies and costs.

This technology promises to solve the problem through a decentralized ledger system, making all patient data accessible on a unified, secure platform. Blockchain is a distributed database that records each transaction or update as a block in a chain. The blocks are immutable and timestamped, thus maintaining the integrity of the data. Unlike traditional systems that rely on centralized servers, blockchain decentralizes data storage, making it less vulnerable to breaches and system failures.

One of the main advantages of blockchain is that it empowers patients to have more control over their medical records. Through smart contracts, patients can share their data with healthcare providers on a need-to-know basis. Intermediaries are no longer needed, and data sharing and consolidation become much more streamlined. For instance, if a patient goes to see a specialist in another city, they can immediately authorize access to their medical history, thereby ensuring continuity of care without administrative delay.

Secondly, the decentralized nature of blockchain makes it more transparency and trustful for medical records management. Consensus mechanisms verify the update or transaction, ensuring that errors do not occur since no alteration is made without verification. These transparency issues help the patients and providers gain confidence since data tampering issues could be tracked back to their origin and modifications. Finally, the technique of cryptography ensures that patient information will not be disclosed since sensitive information can be encrypted securely.

Blockchain technology promises to solve the fragmentation of medical record management. By providing a secure, unified platform for patient data, blockchain enhances the accuracy and efficiency of healthcare delivery while empowering patients with greater control over their health information. As the healthcare industry continues embracing digital transformation, adopting blockchain may be a critical step toward achieving a seamless and patient-centric ecosystem.

ii. Security Vulnerabilities in Centralized Systems

Storing these medical records in centralized databases exposes them to severe security threats such as unauthorized access, data breaches, and ransomware attacks. Centralized systems make for a single point of failure, therefore making it an attractive single point that hackers want to breach.

In reality, blockchain features decentralization and cryptography, giving it a secure solution to add on and enhance security. The technology, therefore, uses encryption and shares the patient record across multiple nodes, making the malicious actor less likely to manipulate or delete records. Moreover, blockchain uses a consensus mechanism where transactions are verified and secured prior to inclusion into the ledger. This makes it highly improbable that manipulation will occur.

Xia et al. (2017) proposed a blockchain-based framework for secure medical data sharing. The study demonstrated how blockchain can ensure data integrity and confidentiality, providing an audit trail that tracks every access or modification to patient records. This approach minimizes security vulnerabilities associated with centralized systems (2).

iii. Inefficiencies in Data Sharing and Interoperability

One of the longstanding issues is interoperability y, the ability of different healthcare systems to exchange and utilize information. Most healthcare providers use incompatible data formats and protocols, which often causes delays and miscommunication. This inefficiency negatively impacts patient care and increases administrative costs.

Blockchain addresses interoperability issues by providing a standardized platform for data exchange and using smart contracts, which ensure data sharing adheres to predefined rules of permission. In addition, blockchain as an immutable system guarantees the precision and authenticity of shared data.

According to Zhang et al. (2018), a study on blockchain stressed its significance in enhancing interoperability in health ecosystems. Their study demonstrated how blockchain-based systems can ensure seamless data exchange with regulatory compliance in accordance with the Health Insurance Portability and Accountability Act (HIPAA). It concluded that blockchain would reduce redundancy and improve coordination among healthcare providers (3).

The integration of blockchain technology into medical record management holds great promise to overcome key challenges in the healthcare sector. Blockchain will revolutionize the manner in which patient data is managed and used by addressing fragmentation, enhancing security, and ensuring interoperability. Its adoption, despite its challenges, carries some issues, such as scalability and regulatory compliance, that must be grappled with for its full potential to be realized.

4. DECENTRALIZED PATIENT RECORDS: BENEFITS AND USE CASES

Centralized healthcare systems struggle with fragmented records, security risks, and inefficient data sharing, leading to delays, high costs, and limited patient control. Blockchain technology offers a decentralized solution by enhancing security, improving interoperability, and granting patients authority over their health data, ensuring seamless, secure, and transparent management of medical records.

Significance of Detailed, Correct, and Current Patient Records

Patient records are the foundation of contemporary health systems, recording in minute detail an individual's medical visits, diagnoses, treatments, laboratory findings, and medications. Effective communication among health professionals, ensures continuity of care, and lead to better patient outcomes (Adeniyi et al., 2024; Daraojimba et al., 2023). In addition, clear medical records are a critical component of clinical decision-making, allowing doctors to assess previous interventions and track chronic conditions effectively.

Aside from patient care at the individual level, the compilation of medical records is an important tool for public health studies and policy-making. Epidemiological research is dependent on the provision of good-quality and comprehensive datasets to determine trends in disease occurrence, test the effectiveness of interventions, and predict health trends (Stausberg, J., & Harkener, S., 2023). Imprecisions or patients which may result in misguided health policies or treatments.

Healthcare professionals also rely on precise records to comply with regulatory and compliance requirements. Bodies such as the Health Insurance Portability and Accountability Act (HIPAA) in the United States require patient records to be safely stored, well documented, and easily available for audits. Records are also very critical in legal and ethical situations, being used as proof in cases of malpractice or disagreement regarding treatment. Proper handling of them, therefore, is not only a clinical requirement but also a matter of law.

Difficulties of Centralized Systems

Though absolutely essential, traditional patient record management systems have several grave shortcomings. The basis of most health care organizations' operations is centralized EHR systems, which hold data in discrete, institution-specific silos. Traditionally, this system has produced a wide range of issues, including restricted access for patients, interoperability and, foremost, additional exposure to data breaches.

The key problem is the lack of interoperability of EHR systems. For example, a patient referred from primary care to a specialist may be delayed in diagnosis or treatment because their records are inaccessible without friction. Centralized systems are vulnerable to security risks as well. By definition, a centralized database is a single point of failure; should it be breached, patient information can be accessed by unauthorized parties. High-profile data breaches, including the 2015 Anthem health insurer attack, demonstrate the scope of this problem, in which personal information of close to 112 million people was compromised (Schwartz, S. 2016). These breaches not only compromise the trust of people in healthcare infrastructure but also underscore the need for improved protection from cyber threats.

Centralized systems also limit patient autonomy and access to health information about their persons. Most patients are frustrated because of delays in accessing their records, mainly because institutions delay or create unnecessary bureaucracy because of outdated administrative procedures (Shah et al., 2019). This unavailability and lack of control happen at a time when the use of precision medicine demands this kind of active participation from patients in the management of their own health.

In addition, compliance and regulatory pressures also add to the inefficiencies of central systems. To attain compliance with all privacy and data protection requirements, institutions have to shell out a lot on infrastructure and staff maintenance and may not be applied or enforced uniformly. Therefore, though digitization of medical records is possible through central systems, their limitations restrict the actual realization of an entirely patient-centered and secure model of health care.

Decentralization as a Solution

The challenges such as interoperability, security, control etc., have introduced a variety of innovative solutions in the maintenance of patient records through decentralized systems based on blockchain technology. Decentralization changes the control and ownership of medical information by providing a more secure, transparent, and interoperable framework for health information exchange.

Decentralization is the spreading of information throughout an array of nodes rather than in a centralized repository. Blockchain technology facilitates this type through a distributed ledger that retains transactions in a safe and tamper-evident manner (Zhang et al., 2018). Transactions are verified by a consensus mechanism so that only valid action is recorded, and all alterations are trackable.

One of the key advantages of decentralized patient records is improved security. By eliminating a single point of failure, blockchain lowers the risk of large-scale data breaches. Data remains secure and intact even if one node in the network is breached, providing protection against cyber-attacks (Azaria et al., 2016). Cryptographic techniques are used for maintaining the information encrypted and only viewable to authorized persons are employed as well.

Decentralization also empowers patients by providing them with ownership and control of their health information. On blockchain-based platforms, patients can control who accesses their records and for what reasons, using smart contracts to lock in and implement their preferences (Dagher et al., 2018). For instance, a patient may provide temporary access to an expert to establish a diagnosis and cancel it once the consultation is completed.

Traditional centralized systems often store large amounts of sensitive medical and personal data in a single location, exposing patient information to significant risks, especially in the event of cyberattacks or data breaches. According to a report by the U.S. Department of Health and Human Services (2020), healthcare breaches continue to increase, with millions of records being exposed each year, compromising organizational integrity and reducing patient trust. In contrast, a decentralized approach ensures there is no single point of failure by distributing data across a network of nodes. This ensures that data remains secure and intact across all nodes, even if one node is compromised.

Scalability is a problem, as blockchain networks may struggle to handle the enormous amounts of data that are generated in modern healthcare systems. To address this, hybrid models are being explored, which combine on-chain and off-chain storage, with sensitive metadata stored on the blockchain and larger files, such as imaging data, stored off-chain (Ali et al., 2023).

In addition, the implementation of decentralized systems involves a shift in approach among stakeholders in healthcare. The patients, and health care providers need to be educated on how blockchain technology functions and the advantages it can bring about in the establishment of trust and adoption. Policymakers ought to implement strict guidelines so that decentralized solutions may be easy to incorporate into existing healthcare infrastructure.

Blockchain-based decentralized patient records are the tamper-proof solution that aids in overcoming the constraints of traditional healthcare systems. Additionally, decentralization holds out the promise of increased security, empowered patients, and facilitation of interoperability for medical data management and exchange.

Benefits of Decentralized Patient Records

Enhanced Data Integrity: Blockchain's unchangeable ledger guarantees that data, once written, can't be erased or modified. This immutability enhances the integrity and reliability of medical records (Zheng et al., 2017). Every transaction or entry of data is dated and connected to the earlier one, making it a chain of records which cannot be tampered with. This aspect is extremely crucial in healthcare, where precision and dependability in patient information are essential for proper treatment.

Greater Access and Interoperability: Decentralized architecture enables simpler inter-relation data exchange between the concerned healthcare providers and, hence, enhances coordination and patient care. Interoperability is needed to enable real-time access to the patient's record (Kuo et al., 2017). Blockchain can be integrated smoothly into current EHR systems by leveraging standards like HL7 FHIR, allowing simple data exchange. The integration allows healthcare providers to access the integrated view of a patient's medical history for improved diagnosis and treatment outcomes.

Cost Efficiency: The removal of centralized data centers and the decreased dependence on third-party intermediaries decrease the operational expenses of decentralized systems (Azaria et al., 2016). The blockchain, as decentralized, lowers the cost of costly infrastructure and maintenance since data is distributed to many nodes. Additionally, the elimination of intermediaries lowers transaction costs and speeds up data exchange activities.

Patient Empowerment

The decentralized structure of blockchain also empowers patients by granting them more authority over their personal health information. In traditional healthcare systems, patients often have limited control over how their data is shared with healthcare providers. Concerns regarding data security, access, and possible misuse may arise as a result of this lack of transparency. However, people can take charge of their health information by choosing when, when, and with whom it is shared thanks to decentralization (Dagher et al., 2018).

Patients have complete control over who can access their medical records using blockchain-based technologies. Smart contracts, which are self-executing contracts having the terms of the agreement encoded directly into lines of code, can be used for this. For example, a patient may temporarily allow a specialist access for a particular diagnosis or course of therapy and then withdraw access after the session is over. This encourages a more individualized and cooperative approach to healthcare in addition to guaranteeing that individuals have complete control over their medical records (Azaria et al., 2016).

Additionally, decentralizing patient records guarantees that medical professionals have access to the most current and comprehensive medical history of a patient, enhancing clinical judgment and patient outcomes. Giving patients more control over their medical journey encourages the patients toward preventative care and raises the possibility of improved long-lasting condition management.

Fraud Prevention

The immutable and transparent ledger of blockchain technology significantly lowers the risk of fraud. The blockchain securely and permanently records every transaction, including those involving data entry, access, and modification (Zhang et al., 2018). This guarantees that any changes made to a patient's data can be tracked down, creating an audit trail that can be examined for anomalies. Blockchain makes it much more difficult to change or falsify patient data secretly by preserving an unchangeable record of diagnosis, treatments, and insurance claims.

Cost Efficiency

Finally, by decreasing administrative overhead and enhancing the effectiveness of healthcare services, decentralized patient data provide significant cost savings. In order to manage and store patient records, traditional systems may require intricate administrative procedures. Healthcare providers may find the cost of maintaining centralized EHR systems, as well as the infrastructure and personnel required to guarantee data security and compliance with laws like HIPAA, to be unaffordable (Shah et al., 2019). Because blockchain technology is decentralized, patient data may be managed more effectively and with less need on centralized IT infrastructure.

Figure 3. Decentralization of Patient Records

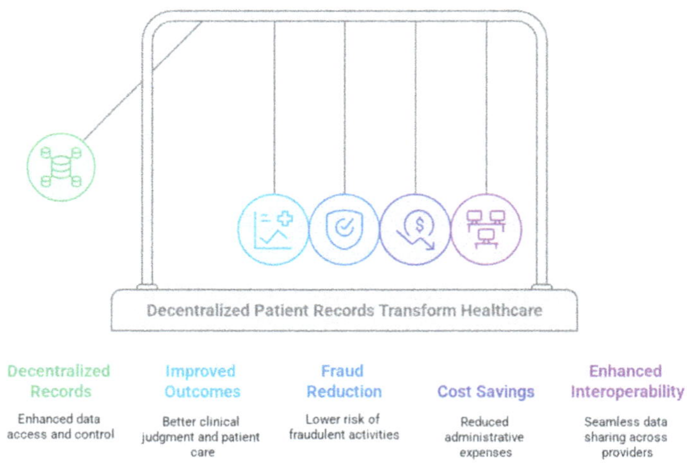

Removal of unnecessary diagnostic tests is one of the main ways that decentralized systems reduces the expenses. Repeated testing is less necessary when medical professionals have access to a patient's complete medical history, including test results, as was previously indicated. This greatly reduces healthcare expenses while also saving time for both patients and healthcare professionals. Additionally, blockchain-based systems' efficiency and transparency reduce the administrative load related to billing, insurance claims, and regulatory compliance, releasing the funds for patient treatment.

Additionally, blockchain's automation features through smart contracts can minimize the delays and administrative mistakes. For instance, blockchain improves operations and removes the need for intermediaries by automating the processing of insurance claims or the administration of patient consent. Healthcare providers may save money as a result of quicker payment cycles, less paperwork, and a need for fewer administrative staff.

The shift to decentralized patient records has enormous potential to revolutionize the way healthcare is provided. Decentralized solutions can assist in addressing some of the most important issues that traditional healthcare systems faces, such as improving interoperability, avoiding fraud, empowering patients, improving data privacy and security, and increasing cost effectiveness. These developments are made possible by blockchain technology, which offers a safe, open, and effective way to handle patient data. Decentralized patient records will be essential to build a more robust, effective, and patient-centered healthcare system as the industry continues to adopt digital revolution.

Blockchain Applications in Decentralized Patient Records

Secure, interoperable, and patient-centric data management solutions are becoming more and more necessary as healthcare institutions embrace digital technologies. Blockchain provides creative solutions to these problems because of its decentralized and impenetrable nature. Blockchain is redefining the creation, access, and sharing of patient records by disrupting conventional systems for identity management, consent tracking, interoperability, real-time data access, and storage.

Identity Management

Efficient healthcare delivery is based on safe and accurate patient identification. However, fragmented data and misidentifications result from centralized identity systems' frequent inability to reliably link people to their medical records. Decentralized identifiers (DIDs) give every patient a distinct, blockchain-secured digital identity, in contrast to conventional systems that use institution-specific identities. According to Zhang et al. (2018), this identity serves as a universal key that allows patients to maintain and access their medical records from a variety of providers.

For instance, a patient can easily access their records from many institutions utilizing a blockchain-based identity system, eliminating the need for repeated logins or requests. Decentralized identifiers ensure privacy through cryptographic encryption while also being unchangeable and verifiable. Patients can keep dissimilar information private while sharing some parts of their identification with healthcare practitioners, such as a confirmed diagnosis (Dagher et al., 2018).

Consent Tracking

Obtaining patient consent to share information is often an difficult, ad hoc, error-prone, and time-consuming process within traditional health care. Smart contracts, built on blockchain, represent a reliable technology for the automation and simplification of consent tracking. According to Azaria et al. (2016), smart contracts refer to the self-executing programs, where by predefined rules, the conditions of an agreement, such as providing or revoking consent, are enforced.

For instance, a smart contract can log a patient's permission on the blockchain when they take part in a clinical trial. This consent is unchangeable and can be automatically verified each time a researcher asks to view the patient's information. It offers an auditable record of consent transactions that has an impact on patient and provider trust because blockchain is immutable and transparent. Participants often worry about the unauthorized sharing of personal data, especially in research settings. Interoperability can be defined as the free flow of data across multiple health care systems, considered one of the critical concerns in the modern medical field. Modern EHRs are mostly isolated and do not easily connect with other systems, limiting interoperability among healthcare providers and restricting continuous patient care.

With blockchain, patient information will be stored in a standard format that is easily accessible and up-to-date without technical barriers between healthcare providers, labs, and pharmacies. For example, a blockchain interoperability solution will connect a patient's primary care physician to a specialist and a diagnostic laboratory so they can avail themselves of the most current information. It decreases redundancies, reduces errors, and improves clinical outcomes (Friedman et al., 2022).

The fact that blockchain can keep a single source of truth also improves data integrity. Most traditional interoperability efforts rely on manual data reconciliation, which may introduce errors or inconsistencies. Blockchain allows that all changes in a patient's record are recorded within an immutable ledger, thus offering a tamper-proof and reliable history of interactions (Zhang et al., 2018).

With systems like Estonia's e-Health, blockchain has the potential for developing interoperable networks across whole countries. Estonia has applied this blockchain technology for it to integrate its providers of healthcare while realizing real-time data sharing which also remains secure and private (Dagher et al., 2018). These models offer road maps towards scaling blockchain-based interoperability solutions around the world.

Blockchain technology is already transforming healthcare by offering secure and decentralized patient record management. One notable example is IBM's Hyperledger Fabric, a permissioned blockchain framework that enables healthcare organizations to securely store, share, and access patient data while ensuring privacy and compliance with regulations like HIPAA and GDPR. Unlike public blockchains, Hyperledger Fabric allows only authorized participants to access data, enhancing security and interoperability in healthcare networks.

Additionally, blockchain played a crucial role in managing COVID-19 vaccination records. Countries and healthcare providers leveraged blockchain to create tamper-proof vaccination records, preventing fraud and ensuring real-time verification of immunization status. This approach streamlined cross-border travel, public health reporting, and vaccine distribution, demonstrating blockchain's effectiveness in securing sensitive health information and improving global healthcare coordination."

5. SCALABILITY AND HYBRID SOLUTIONS

Although decentralized patient records offer enhanced security, transparency, and patient control, implementing blockchain in healthcare comes with challenges, particularly in scalability. As medical data grows exponentially, blockchain networks must handle large volumes efficiently. To address this, hybrid solutions like off-chain storage and Layer-2 scaling mechanisms optimize performance while maintaining decentralization.

Increasing volumes of data in medicine ensure that blockchain needs to have great transaction throughput handling, minimizing latencies, and cost-effectiveness..

The use of hybrid blockchain solutions-a blend of strengths in both public and private blockchain-appears to be promising for the challenge of scalability issues. The incorporation of Blockchain along with hybrid deep learning techniques offers a promising approach for scalable and secure healthcare systems (Ali et al., 2023). Using the hybrid models ensures optimization of performance with the features of decentralization and immutability in healthcare blockchains. The combination enables real-time analysis of large-scale healthcare data, facilitating timely diagnosis and treatment recommendations while ensuring data security through blockchain's decentralized framework. Likewise, the EMRI framework suggests a smart contract-based approach for privacy protection and scalable communication in electronic medical records (Mallick & Sharma, 2021).

The ZeroTrustBlock framework implements a hybrid on-chain and off-chain storage model to balance transparency with confidentiality, achieving substantial performance improvements (Thantharate & Thantharate, 2023). The ZeroTrustBlock architecture combines on-chain and off-chain storage to strike a balance between confidentiality and transparency. Key data, such as transaction metadata, are stored on-chain for transparency and immutability, while sensitive data are stored off-chain to maintain privacy and relieve blockchain congestion. The hybrid model improves performance by reducing storage costs, enhancing scalability, and tracking the transactions. With a Zero Trust approach, entry to the off-chain data is limited with cryptographic methods, ensuring security. This architecture is of value in sectors like healthcare and finance, where data privacy and adherence to regulations are critical, but it is still possible to maintain auditability and transparency on the Blockchain. Another study provides 16 solutions for addressing scalability concerns, which are categorized under storage optimization and blockchain redesign (Mazlan et al., 2020). These include blockchain modeling, read and write operations, and bi-directional networks. Hybrid technologies between blockchain and other technologies such as deep learning and smart contracts have the potential to address scalability challenges in decentralized medical record systems. In addition, enhancing blockchain design using storage optimization and redesign methods assists with enhancing scalability.

The Importance of Scalability in Blockchain-Based Medical Records

Scalability in blockchain means that a network can handle the rising number of transactions without trading off speed, cost, or security. For medical records, scalability is an important factor because patient records consist of large volumes of data including medical histories, imaging files, genetic information, and real-time monitoring data from wearable devices.

i. Guarantees Real-Time Access: In order to achieve proper diagnosis and treatment, real-time access of patient records must be granted by healthcare providers.
ii. Reduces Transaction Costs: With the congestion on the network, traditional blockchain networks, especially public ones like Ethereum, incur huge transaction fees.
iii. Interoperability between Providers: A scalable solution must allow data exchange between hospitals, clinics, insurance providers, and research institutions.

Figure 4. Scalability Solutions for Blockchain in Healthcare

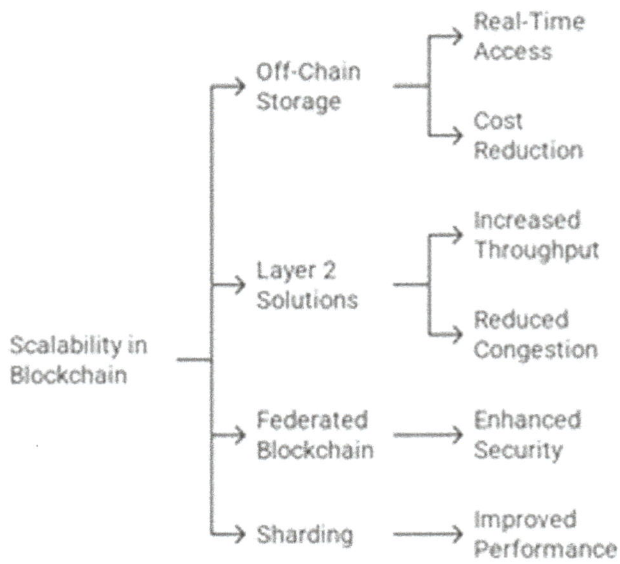

This method addresses blockchain storage limitations by keeping full medical histories in secure, decentralized storage systems off-chain.

InterPlanetary File System (IPFS) or cloud-based databases. The blockchain retains only cryptographic hashes of the medical information, maintaining integrity and security with minimal on-chain storage needs. The following are the key advantages.

i. Data Integrity: Cryptographic hashing makes sure that records do not change while enabling verification.
ii. Privacy Compliance: Sensitive patient information is never kept on a public ledger directly, which maintains HIPAA and GDPR compliance.
iii. Effective Access: Blockchain gives authentic proof of record validity without exposing private data.

This off-chain storage with on-chain validation approach is one of the most efficient blockchain scalability solutions for decentralized medical records, providing security, efficiency, and compliance.

Layer 2 Scaling Solutions

Layer 2 solutions, such as state channels and sidechains, improve blockchain scalability by processing transactions outside the main chain while maintaining its security and immutability.

State Channels

State channels enable end-to-end, private communication between participants with fewer on-chain transactions and preserving data integrity.

Side chains

Sidechains are separate blockchains that exist parallel to the parent blockchain, supporting off-chain transaction processing for hospitals. The transactions are settled at a later stage periodically on the parent blockchain.

Advantages

- **Boosts Transactional Throughput:**Supporting a greater volume of transactions per second (TPS) provides for real-time updates of medical records to avoid network clogging.
- **Reduces Congestion on the Main Blockchain Network:** Sidechains and state channels greatly reduce the computational workload on Ethereum-based or Hyperledger networks, resulting in quicker verification times.
- **Ensures Security Through Regular Settlement on the Main Chain:**Layer 2 solutions inherit security from the main blockchain by periodically committing a summary of off-chain transactions to the main network (e.g., Ethereum or Hyperledger Fabric).

Federated Blockchain Model

In a federated blockchain, different healthcare providers work together to check and approve transactions in a secure network. This method prevents unauthorized access to patient records by ensuring that only permitted entities have access, enhancing data security while ensuring decentralization.

Advantages:

- Improve scalability by lowering the number of validators on the network.
- Guarantees observance of the data privacy law.
- Offers a balance between decentralization and performance.

Sharding for Efficient Data Processing

Sharding is an approach in which the blockchain network is split into subsets of partitions (shards), and each shard is tasked with handling a subset of transactions. This increases overall network efficiency and lessens processing time.

Advantages:

- Scales workload over multiple nodes, enhancing scalability.
- Enables concurrent processing of transactions, lowering latency.
- Improve system performance without loss of security.

The medical field is challenged with effectively controlling and protecting electronic medical records because of the large volume of sensitive information and the requirement of interoperability among different healthcare organizations. Blockchain technology can change the face of healthcare by offering a secure and decentralized platform for storing medical records (Pandey & Litoriya, 2020)

One of the main benefits of blockchain technology in healthcare is the way it can guarantee the security and privacy of patient information. Centralized medical record systems are open to cyber attacks since they offer a single point of failure. (Pandey & Litoriya, 2020) On the other hand, blockchain's decentralized structure means it is more resilient against such attacks since the data is distributed across several nodes in the network. Blockchain is also immutable in nature, meaning tampering or unauthorized access can be easily identified, increasing the integrity of medical data

Scalability of blockchain technology is still a key challenge because of its extensive use in the healthcare sector. Traditional blockchain networks, like Bitcoin and Ethereum, suffer from low transaction throughput, which can limit their capacity to deal with the complete volume of medical data produced in healthcare. In response, researchers have proposed a range of hybrid solutions that merge blockchain technology with other complementary technologies, including off-chain storage and layer-2 scaling solutions.

6. INTEROPERABILITY AND REAL-TIME DATA SHARING

Healthcare interoperability is still a key challenge, making it difficult to share data among providers and affecting patient care coordination. Blockchain technology has been identified as a promising solution, providing secure, decentralized, and real-time access to health records. This chapter is a literature survey of blockchain-enabled interoperability, examining research from multiple academic sources and real-world applications. The discussion emphasizes how blockchain facilitates real-time data sharing, minimizes administrative burdens, and enhances patient outcomes.

Interoperability in healthcare involves the seamless exchange of patient information across different electronic health record (EHR) systems and institutions. The lack of standardization, security concerns, and fragmented data storage hinder the efficient transfer of medical data. Blockchain, with its immutable and transparent ledger, has been explored as a viable solution to address these challenges.

Electronic Medical Records (EMRs) have been hampered by regulatory and bureaucratic limitations, hindering interoperability and innovation. Azaria et al., 2016, proposed a decentralized system for the management of medical records using blockchain technology. The system provides a secure, unalterable record of patient medical history and facilitates transparent access across healthcare providers.

Figure 5. Interoperability and Real Time Data Sharing

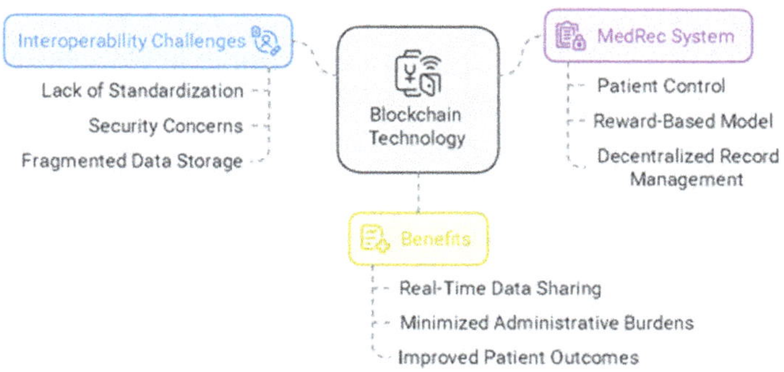

MedRec leverages blockchain's authentication, confidentiality, accountability, and data-sharing features to address EMR management issues. Its modular nature is compatible with current local storage solutions, with increased adaptability and scalability. MedRec diverges from the conventional EMR systems by putting patient control at the forefront of medical data, enhancing security and minimizing the need for intermediaries.

One of the unique features of MedRec is its reward-based model that uses Proof-of-Work consensus in which public health officials and researchers serve as blockchain participants. They verify transactions and are rewarded with untraceable medical information, encouraging data-informed research without compromising patient anonymity.

This functional prototype has shown blockchain capability in developing EMR handling through the facilitation of security, interoperability, and empowerment of patients and paving the way for ultimate field trials.

Kuo et al. (2017) investigated the use of blockchain and distributed ledger technologies in biomedical and health care fields. The chapter explains the fundamentals of blockchain, including its origins in bitcoin, key features, and alternative technologies. It emphasizes blockchain's strengths compared to conventional databases in health care, highlighting better security, interoperability, and exchange of health information. This further examines future nonfinancial applications and describes prospective issues and resolutions for the application of blockchain technology in the biomedical industry. In describing the recent implementations, this work highlights the transformative power of blockchain in enhancing data security and interoperability in medical informatics.

Chen et al. (2018) presented FHIR chain, a blockchain architecture intended to satisfy the interoperability requirements specified in the Office of the National Coordinator for Health Information Technology's (ONC) "Shared Nationwide Interoperability Roadmap."

(1) ONC requirement analysis and its implications for blockchain systems,
(2) The FHIRChain, which encapsulates the HL7 Fast Healthcare Interoperability Resources (FHIR) standard,
(3) A decentralized application using digital health identities for secure authentication in a remote cancer care case study, and

(4) Identification of key lessons learned. FHIRChain allows efficient and secure data exchange between healthcare systems, supporting collaborative decision-making while ensuring data integrity and privacy.

Radanović and Likić (2018) analyzed the possible applications of blockchain technology in medicine with an emphasis on enhancing healthcare efficiency, data protection, and patient self-determination. This article also describes how blockchain technology can facilitate electronic health records, automate administrative tasks, and secure patient data sharing. The challenges like regulatory obstacles and the necessity for scalability in blockchain applications are also discussed. By examining blockchain's strengths and limitations in medicine, this study explores its potential to drive future healthcare innovations.

Yue et al. (2016) suggested a blockchain-based system named Healthcare Data Gateways to improve privacy risk management in healthcare data management. The research targets balancing data sharing needs with stringent privacy needs, providing secure and scalable exchange of health data. Through the use of blockchain, the system seeks to reduce privacy risks while ensuring data integrity, thereby enabling efficient and secure health intelligence applications.

Engelhardt (2017) introduced the applications of blockchain technology in healthcare and how it can enhance security, data sharing, and interoperability. The article explores some of the use cases, including electronic health records, insurance claims, and clinical trials. It also highlights on the regulatory and scalability issues while emphasizing the revolutionary potential of blockchain technology in transforming healthcare processes.

McGhin et al. (2019) examined the prospective role of blockchain in healthcare, presenting major research challenges and opportunities. Security, privacy, and interoperability are critical issues that blockchain can help meet, according to the paper. It also investigates real-world use cases and possible enhancements in healthcare data handling. The research emphasizes the necessity to do more research on blockchain scalability and regulation compliance.

Meinert et al. (2019) outlined a systematic review protocol for the assessment of blockchain adoption in healthcare. The article provides methodologies to evaluate blockchain's effects on data security, interoperability, and patient control. Through systematic literature review, the study focus on the efficacy and challenges of adopting blockchain in healthcare.

Xia et al. (2017) proposed MeDShare, a blockchain-enabled framework to securely share medical data between cloud service providers. The research overcomes trust challenges in medical data exchange by using blockchain's decentralized and immutable characteristics. MeDShare provides security and integrity while facilitating effective data sharing among multiple players in the healthcare ecosystem.

Blockchain offers a innovative approach to healthcare interoperability, with the ability to securely, efficiently, and in real-time share data. Ongoing research and pilot projects will support wider adoption, ultimately improving healthcare efficiency and patient care.

7. ETHICAL AND LEGAL CONSIDERATIONS

Blockchain technology in healthcare, particularly for decentralized medical records, offers both ethical and legal opportunities and concerns. Although blockchain's decentralized structure promotes improved data security, transparency, and patient empowerment, it also brings up issues with data privacy, legal compliance, and implementation difficulties (Mayer et al., 2019; Singh et al., 2020). The preservation of patient privacy is among the most important ethical factors. Blockchain's encryption and decentralization can increase security, but there are worries about illegal access and data breaches (Wenhua et al., 2023). According to Szabo et al. (2024), the immutability of blockchain records also raises concerns over data correction and the right to be forgotten, which may be in conflict with current privacy laws like the GDPR. There are number of legal difficulties to blockchain's application in healthcare. These include jurisdictional concerns, smart contract enforceability, and adherence to current healthcare laws, such HIPAA in the US (Sahu et al., 2024; Szabo et al., 2024). In the event of mistakes or breaches, the decentralized structure of blockchain further complicates issues of accountability and fault (Odeh et al., 2022). Although blockchain technology has a lot of potential to enhance healthcare data management, its application requires careful evaluation of a wide range of ethical and legal issues.

Regulatory Issues and Privacy Law Compliance

Rolling out blockchain for health data systems entails overcoming different regulatory issues and maintaining adherence to privacy legislation:

1. HIPAA Compliance: The Health Insurance Portability and Accountability Act (HIPAA) establishes standards for safeguarding patient data. Blockchain technology must guarantee that data encryption, access controls, and audit trails are in compliance with HIPAA (HIPAA Journal, n.d.). HIPAA compliance involves technical safeguards, including encryption and access controls, as well as administrative safeguards, including policies and procedures for protecting data, in place.
2. GDPR Compliance: For healthcare providers working within the European Union, GDPR compliance is crucial. Blockchain systems need to have mechanisms to support data subject rights, including the right of access and the Right to be forgotten (off-chain storage) (European Union, 2016). GDPR compliance demands that blockchain systems adopt privacy by design principles so that data protection is embedded into the system architecture from the very beginning (European Union, 2016).

3.Regulatory Uncertainty: The dynamic character of blockchain technology and its use in healthcare may create regulatory uncertainty. Healthcare professionals are required to remain updated with respect to regulations and modify their systems accordingly (Radanović & Likić, 2018). This includes tracking changes in regulations, interacting with regulatory agencies, and contributing to industry efforts to formulate the regulatory environment. Blockchain technology has vast potential to transform the handling of medical records and health data. Decentralization of data storage and sharing, blockchain improves security, confidentiality, and data interoperability. Nevertheless, effective application depends on resolving regulatory issues as well as maintaining privacy regulations compliance.

8. FUTURE DIRECTIONS IN BLOCKCHAIN TECHNOLOGIES FOR DECENTRALIZED PATIENT DATA

Enhancing Privacy and Data Security

Because blockchain technology offers a decentralized, secured approach for handling patient data, it has the potential to significantly improve data security and privacy in the healthcare industry. One of the primary issues with healthcare data management can be resolved by utilizing blockchain technology in combination with cryptographic techniques to guarantee patient data privacy and security (Yaqoob et al., 2021; Durneva et al., 2020; Dubovitskaya et al., 2019). Future studies should concentrate on creating hybrid data storage systems that respect global rules and regulations while maintaining privacy (Dubovitskaya et al., 2019).

Improving Interoperability and Data Sharing

Blockchain can make it easier for disparate healthcare information systems to communicate with one another, allowing for smooth data exchange between platforms. By guaranteeing that medical professionals have access to complete and current patient data, this can enhance patient care (Durneva et al., 2020; Singh et al., 2023; Arbabi et al., 2023). Designing interoperable architectures and infrastructures that provide effective data interchange while preserving data security and integrity is one of the future approaches (Dubovitskaya et al., 2019).

Empowering Patients with Decentralized Identity

Blockchain-enabled self-sovereign identity gives people authority over their own medical records. This increases patient autonomy and involvement by giving patients the ability to control their data and share it with healthcare practitioners as needed (Houtan et al., 2020). Future studies should focus on developing secure identification systems that balance privacy, efficiency, and accessibility. (Houtan et al., 2020).

Resolving Issues with Scalability and Efficiency

One major problem still facing blockchain applications in the healthcare industry is scalability. Ineffective consensus algorithms and high processing power needs may prevent blockchain technology from being widely used (Durneva et al., 2020; Radanovic & Likić, 2018). Future studies should concentrate on creating consensus processes that are more effective and investigating strategies to lower the computational overhead connected to blockchain systems (Radanovic & Likić,2018)

Integrating Blockchain with Existing Healthcare Systems

There are architectural and technical difficulties when integrating blockchain technology with current healthcare systems. In order to ensure compatibility and minimize disruption, future research should focus on creating solutions that enable the smooth integration of blockchain with existing healthcare infrastructures (Arbabi et al., 2023; Mamun et al., 2022). This involves investigating how blockchain technology can be used to manage electronic health records (EHRs) and other vital medical data (Mamun et al., 2022).

Blockchain technology has the potential to completely transform healthcare data management by improving interoperability, security, and privacy. Future studies should concentrate on developing privacy-preserving systems, empowering patients with self-sovereign identities, and resolving issues with scalability and integration. Blockchain has the potential to significantly contribute to the transformation of healthcare into a more secure and patient-centered system by overcoming these obstacles.

9. CONCLUSION

Blockchain technology can transform decentralized patient data management through improved security, transparency, and patient ownership over medical records. By providing granular access control and tamper-proof, immutable records, blockchain ensures that only authorized entities can access medical data while maintaining an auditable record of transactions. This decentralized design addresses frequent problems in the flow of healthcare data by promoting trust, interoperability, and data integrity.

Nonetheless, blockchain applications in healthcare bring several disadvantages of scaling, maintaining patient privacy and their consent requirements along with proper adherence to legislation and regulatory conditions. Since blockchains are basically not mutable at some point, they raise very authentic issues as a matter of Right to be forgotten (off-chain storage). Their ability to maintain and provide transparent solution that should provide a deletion functionality. A hybrid on-chain and off-chain strategy may help to achieve a compromise between transparency and confidentiality by storing sensitive data off-chain and recording hashes or metadata on-chain for verification.

Healthcare stakeholders need to develop user-friendly consent procedures, enhance interoperability across different health systems, and ensure regulatory compliance with regulations like HIPAA and GDPR to ensure that the entire benefits of blockchain are realized. Blockchain can change healthcare by offering people more control over their health information and furthering medical research and care advancements through safe, effective, and patient-centered data management.

REFERENCES

Adeniyi, A., Arowoogun, J., Chidi, R., Okolo, C., & Babawarun, O. (2024). *The impact of electronic health records on patient care and outcomes: A comprehensive review*. World Journal of Advanced Research and Reviews.

Agrawal, K., Aggarwal, M., Tanwar, S., Sharma, G., Bokoro, P., & Sharma, R. (2022). An Extensive Blockchain Based Applications Survey: Tools, Frameworks, Opportunities, Challenges and Solutions. *IEEE Access : Practical Innovations, Open Solutions*, *10*, 116858–116906. DOI: 10.1109/ACCESS.2022.3219160

Alhat, P. (2024). *Blockchain Technology*. INTERANTIONAL JOURNAL OF SCIENTIFIC RESEARCH IN ENGINEERING AND MANAGEMENT., DOI: 10.55041/IJSREM30694

Ali, , Ali, H., Saeed, A., Ahmed Khan, A., Tin, T. T., Assam, M., Ghadi, Y. Y., & Mohamed, H. G. (2023, September). Blockchain-Powered Healthcare Systems: Enhancing Scalability and Security with Hybrid Deep Learning. *Sensors (Basel)*, *23*(18), 7740. DOI: 10.3390/s23187740 PMID: 37765797

Azaria, A., Ekblaw, A., Vieira, T., & Lippman, A. (2016, August). Medrec: Using blockchain for medical data access and permission management. In 2016 2nd international conference on open and big data (OBD) (pp. 25-30). IEEE.

Banoth, R., & Dave, M. (2022). A Survey on Decentralized Application based On Blockchain Platform. *2022 International Conference on Sustainable Computing and Data Communication Systems (ICSCDS)*, 1171-1174. DOI: 10.1109/ICSCDS53736.2022.9760861

Bhutta, M., Khwaja, A., Nadeem, A., Ahmad, H., Khan, M., Hanif, M., Song, H., Alshamari, M., & Cao, Y. (2021). A Survey on Blockchain Technology: Evolution, Architecture and Security. *IEEE Access : Practical Innovations, Open Solutions*, *9*, 61048–61073. DOI: 10.1109/ACCESS.2021.3072849

Bidve, V., Kakakde, K., Sarasu, P., Kediya, S., Tamkhade, P., & Nair, S. (2023). Patient Data Management Using Blockchain Technology. *Indonesian Journal of Electrical Engineering and Computer Science*, *32*(3), 1746–1754. DOI: 10.11591/ijeecs.v32.i3.pp1746-1754

Cao, B., Wang, Z., Zhang, L., Feng, D., Peng, M., Zhang, L., & Han, Z. (2021). Blockchain Systems, Technologies, and Applications: A Methodology Perspective. *IEEE Communications Surveys and Tutorials*, *25*(1), 353–385. DOI: 10.1109/COMST.2022.3204702

Charles, W., Van Der Waal, M., Flach, J., Bisschop, A., Van Der Waal, R., Es-Sbai, H., & McLeod, C. (2023). Blockchain-Based Dynamic Consent and its Applications for Patient-Centric Research and Health Information Sharing: Protocol for an Integrative Review. *JMIR Research Protocols*, *13*, e50339. Advance online publication. DOI: 10.2196/50339 PMID: 38315514

Dagher, G., Mohler, J., Milojkovic, M., & Marella, P. (2018). Ancile: Privacy-Preserving Framework for Access Control and Interoperability of Electronic Health Records Using Blockchain Technology. *Sustainable Cities and Society*, *39*, 283–297. DOI: 10.1016/j.scs.2018.02.014

Daraojimba, A., Enahoro, Q., Ogugua, J., Anyanwu, E., Akomolafe, O., & Odilibe, I. (2023). *The impact of electronic health records on healthcare delivery and patient outcomes: A review*. World Journal of Advanced Research and Reviews., DOI: 10.30574/wjarr.2024.21.2.0478

Dong, S., Abbas, K., Li, M., & Kamruzzaman, J. (2023). Blockchain technology and application: An overview. *PeerJ. Computer Science*, *9*, e1705. Advance online publication. DOI: 10.7717/peerj-cs.1705 PMID: 38077532

Gakire, M. (2024). *The Use of Blockchain in Securing Patient Data*. Research Output Journal of Public Health and Medicine., DOI: 10.59298/ROJPHM/2024/324750

George, E., Idemudia, C., & Ige, A. (2024). *Blockchain technology in financial services: enhancing security, transparency, and efficiency in transactions and services*. Open Access Research Journal of Multidisciplinary Studies., DOI: 10.53022/oarjms.2024.8.1.0042

Islam, I., Munim, K., Oishwee, S., Islam, A., & Islam, M. (2020). A Critical Review of Concepts, Benefits, and Pitfalls of Blockchain Technology Using Concept Map. *IEEE Access : Practical Innovations, Open Solutions*, *8*, 68333–68341. DOI: 10.1109/ACCESS.2020.2985647

Jaiman, V., & Urovi, V. (2020). A Consent Model for Blockchain-Based Health Data Sharing Platforms. *IEEE Access : Practical Innovations, Open Solutions*, *8*, 143734–143745. DOI: 10.1109/ACCESS.2020.3014565

Jaoude, J., & Saadé, R. (2019). Blockchain Applications – Usage in Different Domains. *IEEE Access : Practical Innovations, Open Solutions*, *7*, 45360–45381. DOI: 10.1109/ACCESS.2019.2902501

Kuo, T. T., Kim, H. E., & Ohno-Machado, L. (2017). Blockchain distributed ledger technologies for biomedical and health care applications. *Journal of the American Medical Informatics Association : JAMIA*, *24*(6), 1211–1220. DOI: 10.1093/jamia/ocx068 PMID: 29016974

Leeming, G., Cunningham, J., & Ainsworth, J. (2019). A Ledger of Me: Personalizing Healthcare Using Blockchain Technology. *Frontiers in Medicine*, *6*, 171. Advance online publication. DOI: 10.3389/fmed.2019.00171 PMID: 31396516

Mallick, S. R., & Sharma, S. "EMRI: A Scalable and Secure Blockchain-based IoMT Framework for Healthcare Data Transaction," 2021 *International Conference on Information and Communication Technology (OCIT)*, pp. 261-266, DOI: 10.1109/OCIT53463.2021.00060

Mayer, R., Tahir, S., & Smith, M. R. "Blockchain Technology in Healthcare: Enhancing Data Exchange and Interoperability," *Journal of Medical Systems*, vol. 43, no. 6, pp. 1-12, 2019. [Online]. Available: https://journals.sagepub.com/doi/pdf/10.1177/1460458219866350

Mazlan, A., Abas, H., Abdul Rasid, S. Z., Mohd Sam, S., Yusof, M. F., & Mohd Daud, S. (2020, January). Scalability Challenges in Healthcare Blockchain System—A Systematic Review. *IEEE Access : Practical Innovations, Open Solutions*, *8*, 23663–23673. DOI: 10.1109/ACCESS.2020.2969230

Monrat, A., Schelén, O., & Andersson, K. (2019). A Survey of Blockchain From the Perspectives of Applications, Challenges, and Opportunities. *IEEE Access : Practical Innovations, Open Solutions*, *7*, 117134–117151. DOI: 10.1109/ACCESS.2019.2936094

Mukherjee, A., Singh, R., Mishra, R., & Bag, S. (2021). Application of blockchain technology for sustainability development in agricultural supply chain: Justification framework. *Operations Management Research : Advancing Practice Through Research*, *15*(1-2), 46–61. DOI: 10.1007/s12063-021-00180-5

Omar, M., Bhuiyan, M. Z. A., Basu, A., Kiyomoto, S., & Rahman, M. S. (2019). Bhuiyan, A. Basu, S. Kiyomoto, and M. Rahman, "Privacy-Friendly Platform for Healthcare Data in Cloud Based on Blockchain Environment,". *Future Generation Computer Systems*, *95*, 511–521. DOI: 10.1016/j.future.2018.12.044

Pandey, P., & Litoriya, R. (2020). Securing and Authenticating Healthcare Records through Blockchain Technology. *Cryptologia*, *44*(4), 341–356. DOI: 10.1080/01611194.2019.1706060

Raghupathi, W., Raghupathi, V., & Saharia, A. (2023). *Analyzing Health Data Breaches: A Visual Analytics Approach*. AppliedMath., DOI: 10.3390/appliedmath3010011

Schwartz, S. (2016). Does HIPAA hit its mark. *Medical Economics*.

Segal, G., Martsiano, Y., Markinzon, A., Mayer, A., Halperin, A., & Zimlichman, E. (2023). A blockchain-based computerized network infrastructure for the transparent, immutable calculation and dissemination of quantitative, measurable parameters of academic and medical research publications. *Digital Health*, *9*, 20552076231194851. Advance online publication. DOI: 10.1177/20552076231194851 PMID: 37654719

Shah, P., Patel, C., Patel, J., Shah, A., Pandya, S., & Sojitra, B. (2024, October). Utilizing Blockchain Technology for Healthcare and Biomedical Research: A Review. *Cureus*, *16*(10). Advance online publication. DOI: 10.7759/cureus.72040 PMID: 39569280

Shahzad, W., Chen, W., Shaheen, M., Zhang, Y., & Ahmad, F. (2024). Chen, M. Shaheen, Y. Zhang, and F. Ahmad, "A Robust Algorithm for Authenticated Health Data Access via Blockchain and Cloud Computing,". *PLoS One*, *19*(9), e0307039. Advance online publication. DOI: 10.1371/journal.pone.0307039 PMID: 39312513

Stamatellis, C., Papadopoulos, P., Pitropakis, N., Katsikas, S., & Buchanan, W. (2020). A Privacy-Preserving Healthcare Framework Using Hyperledger Fabric. *Sensors (Basel)*, *20*(22), 6587. Advance online publication. DOI: 10.3390/s20226587 PMID: 33218022

Stausberg, J., & Harkener, S. (2023). High-Quality Data for Health Care and Health Research. Methods of Information in Medicine, 62, 001 - 004. DOI: 10.1055/a-2045-8287

Thantharate, P., & Thantharate, A. (2023, October). ZeroTrustBlock: Enhancing Security, Privacy, and Interoperability of Sensitive Data through ZeroTrust Permissioned Blockchain. *Big Data and Cognitive Computing*, *7*(4), 165. DOI: 10.3390/bdcc7040165

Tith, J., Lee, J.-S., Suzuki, H., Wijesundara, W. M. A. B., Taira, N., Obi, T., & Ohyama, N. (2020). Lee, H. Suzuki, W. Wijesundara, N. Taira, T. Obi, and N. Ohyama, "Patient Consent Management by a Purpose-Based Consent Model for Electronic Health Record Based on Blockchain Technology,". *Healthcare Informatics Research*, *26*(4), 265–273. DOI: 10.4258/hir.2020.26.4.265 PMID: 33190460

U.S. Department of Health and Human Services. (2020). *Breaches of Unsecured Protected Health Information* [Online]. Available. [link]

Vidhya, S., Siva Raja, P., & Sumithra, R. (2024). Blockchain-Enabled Decentralized Healthcare Data Exchange: Leveraging Novel Encryption Scheme, Smart Contracts, and Ring Signatures for Enhanced Data Security and Patient Privacy. *International Journal of Network Management*, *34*(5), e2289. Advance online publication. DOI: 10.1002/nem.2289

Vinnarasi, P. R., and K. Vadivukkarasi, "Healthcare Data Security using Blockchain Technology," *2023 International Conference on Intelligent Systems for Communication, IoT and Security (ICISCoIS)*, pp. 298-303, 2023, DOI: 10.1109/ICISCoIS56541.2023.10100572

Westphal, J., Singh, A. K., & Gupta, R. K. "Blockchain Integration in Healthcare: A Comprehensive Investigation," *Frontiers in Blockchain*, vol. 4, no. 1, pp. 1-15, 2021. [Online]. Available: https://www.frontiersin.org/journals/blockchain/articles/10.3389/fbloc.2021.732112/full

Xia, Q., Sifah, E. B., Asamoah, K. O., Gao, J., Du, X., & Guizani, M. (2017). MeDShare: Trust-Less Medical Data Sharing Among Cloud Service Providers via Blockchain. *Journal of Biomedical Informatics*, *76*, 39–52. DOI: 10.1016/j.jbi.2017.04.005

Yaqoob, K. Salah, R. Jayaraman, and Y. Al-Hammadi, "Blockchain for healthcare data management: opportunities, challenges, and future recommendations," *Neural Computing and Applications*, vol. 34, pp. 11475-11490, 2021, doi: Azaria, A., Ekblaw, A., Vieira, T., & Lippman, A. (2016). MedRec: Using Blockchain for Medical Data Access and Permission Management. *Proceedings of the 2nd International Conference on Open and Big Data (OBD 2016)*. Available at: DOI: 10.1109/OBD.2016.11

Yli-Huumo, J., Ko, D., Choi, S., Park, S., & Smolander, K. (2016). Where Is Current Research on Blockchain Technology?—A Systematic Review. *PLoS One*, *11*(10), e0163477. Advance online publication. DOI: 10.1371/journal.pone.0163477 PMID: 27695049

Zhang, P., Schmidt, D. C., White, J., & Lenz, G. (2018). Blockchain Technology Use Cases in Healthcare. *IEEE Access : Practical Innovations, Open Solutions*, *6*, 28126–28139. DOI: 10.1109/ACCESS.2018.2842265

Zhang, P., White, J., Schmidt, D. C., Lenz, G., & Rosenbloom, S. T. (2018). FHIRChain: Applying Blockchain to Securely and Scalably Share Clinical Data. *Computational and Structural Biotechnology Journal*, *16*, 267–278. DOI: 10.1016/j.csbj.2018.07.004 PMID: 30108685

Zyskind, G., & Nathan, O. (2015, May). Decentralizing privacy: Using blockchain to protect personal data. In 2015 IEEE security and privacy workshops (pp. 180-184). IEEE.

Chapter 3
Blockchain-Based Explainable AI for Secure and Privacy-Preserving Automated Machine Learning in IoT-Edge for Smart Medical Healthcare

Muqadsa Jabeen
The University of Faisalabad, Pakistan

Muhammad Ibrar
https://orcid.org/0000-0002-6813-5003
The University of Faisalabad, Pakistan

Majid Hussain
The University of Faisalabad, Pakistan

Muhammad Arshad Shehzad Hassan
https://orcid.org/0000-0003-1873-2077
The University of Faisalabad, Pakistan

ABSTRACT

Coronary Heart Disease (CHD) continues to affect close to 145 million males and 110 million females across the globe, taking close to nine million lives each year. A new evolving framework incorporating IoT-edge computing, Explainable AI, and blockchain technology is in the process of development in order to create a secure, privacy-preserving, and interpretable automated machine learning environment to predict chronic diseases. The IoT-based system utilizes medical sensors and assistive devices for real-time monitoring of the patient. The patient information is transmitted securely using blockchain architecture so that various health practitioners have access to it with the guarantee of data integrity, confidentiality, and access control. The use of Explainable AI (XAI) enables interpretable predictions in machine learning for clinicians and fosters confidence and transparency. Physicians are able to make evidence-based decisions beyond traditional methods since XAI provides the reasons for predictions.

DOI: 10.4018/979-8-3373-0593-6.ch003

1. INTRODUCTION

Integrating the latest advanced digitized technologies into health care will transform chronic care and improve patient outcomes. Among the different chronic diseases, coronary heart disease (CHD) ranks as a major burden for humanity, being one of the most common causes of death around the globe. It affects over 250 million individuals and accounts for an approximate annual death toll of nine million (Bristow, Buys et al. 2023, Lin, H., 2024). Early detection and timely management of CHD are essential to prevent severe, life-threatening complications such as heart failure. Although progress occurs in these areas, several pressing roadblocks hinder predictions and management within existing health-care systems. These include vulnerabilities related to data security, a lack of interoperability among health-care providers, and insufficient explainability associated with AI-driven decision-making systems (Deshmukh et al. 2025, Ahad et al. 2025). A novel framework proposes a solution by combining blockchain technology, XAI, and IoT-edge computing to create a secure, privacy-preserving, and interpretable Automated Machine Learning system (Ahmad, Mukhtar et al. 2021). The architecture leverages IoT-edge computing for real-time patient monitoring using medical sensors and connected devices (Abbas, Alroobaea, Krichen, Rubaiee, S, Almansour et al. 2024, Charles et al. 2024, Chattopadhyay 2024). IoT devices measure vital signs and patient activities, utilizing edge computing for local processing. This approach minimizes latency and decreases reliance on centralized cloud architecture, facilitating faster responses and quicker actions. Internet and edge computing have thus become the most favorable paradigm for adopting proactive health care delivery scenarios, such as that for coronary heart disease, when timely interventions have been proven effective.

The framework comprises a blockchain system empowered with proof of stake for validation of transactions with very little energy consumption to protect the patient data. It further employs SHA-256, a form of coding that helps transform data into a secure code for tamper detection. Hence, health records are maintained accurate and confidential.

The framework development occurs in three steps.

- **Integration of Blockchain Technology for Data Security:**
  The chapter essentially delves into how integrating blockchain technology strengthens data security within the framework of IoT-edge applications in smart medical healthcare. The decentralization of the technology not only stores sensitive medical data securely but also makes it immutable. This ensures data integrity and availability and provides a trusted platform for sharing different stakeholders in the medical community without compromising patient confidentiality.
- **Explainable AI Mechanisms:**
  Also, the introduction of XAI, which was described in the chapter, constitutes another noticeable advancement. The authors point out the transparency of AI mechanisms as being important to medical decision making where the reasons for an AI recommendation may have serious implications both for practitioners and patients. The chapter then goes on to formulate the methods that make AI models interpretable so that trust is cultivated in the users, enabling them to understand and follow AI-driven decisions in their healthcare settings.
  Automated Machine Learning (AutoML) Framework with Privacy-Preserving Nature:

The incorporation of an Automated Machine Learning framework with a strong emphasis on the protection of privacy is another significant addition. The framework integrates techniques that automatically optimize the machine learning algorithms and keep personal medical data secure. This chapter discusses certain privacy-preserving strategies like federated learning and differential privacy and demonstrates the ways in which such strategies may be effectively integrated into AutoML pipelines in order to train the model on sensitive health information without exposing the data on which it is trained. The proposed framework enhances predictive accuracy for CHD with the aid of real-time IoT data and advanced machine learning algorithms. In addition to this, it has integrated blockchain technology for data security and compliance with regulatory requirements-all major issues concerning patients and clinicians. The framework utilized XAI to provide clinicians with transparent predictions and the underlying reasons, allowing for informed, evidence-based clinical decision-making and helping to build confidence in AI solutions in the health sector.

However, the deployment is not without issues. One such issue is the reliability and quality of the IoT data because any incomplete or erroneous data will negatively affect the accuracy of the machine learning algorithms. To mitigate against such an issue, the framework is equipped with rigorous data cleansing procedures and software for detecting errors. There are also challenges regarding the computational needs of blockchain operations and XAI methods and techniques and the impact they may have on real-time functionality. Among the solutions proposed to mitigate against the challenges posed by lightweight blockchain protocols and streamlined XAI algorithms, among others, is probable resistance from the users in the form of medical practitioners who are not familiar with new technology. The deployment plan mitigates against such resistance through the offering of clinician training and technical support and the promotion of ease of use and the advantages of the system.

In total, the novel framework combines blockchain technology with IoT-edge computing and XAI in order to solve various challenges in the management of chronic diseases. It aims to ensure high-quality medical care with a focus on data protection, interpretability, and privacy in order to ensure informed decision-making. Compliance with global regulatory standards increases the dependability of the system for AI in medicine. Through real-time monitoring and secure data sharing in a clear decision-making framework, the framework aims to ensure improved health outcomes for chronic disease patients like CHD, and it is a significant step towards a technologically advanced patient-centered health system.

RELATED WORK

Historical Context of Chronic Diseases

Coronary heart disease (CHD), diabetes, and other neurological disorders are some of the most dangerous causes of morbidity and mortality worldwide. Among them, coronary heart diseases remain among the most prevalent but have the highest burdens, affecting more than 250 million across the globe and accounting for nearly nine million deaths each year. Medical science has significantly advanced in the diagnosis and treatment of chronic diseases, but neither early detection nor timely intervention is adequate. Chronic diseases now cause 70% of global deaths, which translate to 15 million premature deaths every year, leaving a huge challenge in global health. Chronic diseases like CHD lead to severe complications, such as heart failure, in the absence of proper management, thereby necessitating novel, technological innovations in care systems. Early detection mitigates the progression of CHD and other chronic illnesses; however, healthcare systems struggle due to the complexities of managing these conditions, the multitude of risk factors, and the intricate nature of disease progression. Current healthcare systems fall short amid advancements in diagnostics, treatment, and patient care to increase the provision of services. Predictive medicine must close gaps in understanding when an individual gets a disease, how it progresses, and administering early interventions. IoT, blockchain, and artificial intelligence (AI) are emerging health technology innovations for the management of chronic diseases in care units. They aim to make early intervention the norm rather than the exception. In the healthcare sector, blockchain transforms the handling of data, security, and collaboration. Blockchain's immutable and decentralized nature ensures the integrity of the health records and reduces the risk for data breaches to a significant extent. The global market for blockchain in the health sector is projected to increase to $5.6 billion in 2025, according to a BIS research report. Blockchain enables a patient-centric health environment where individuals are in control of the health data and it translates into improved care coordination, faster access to health records, and personalized care plans. Similarly, blockchain enhances the pharmaceutical supply chain with the guarantee of the genuineness and traceability of medicines and minimizes the occurrence of counterfeits. Blockchain technology introduces significant changes in the global social and economic structures and in the global health care systems worldwide. The evidence presented demonstrates the need for increased transparency, efficiency, and security and is present in all sectors.Nevertheless, challenges such as growing concerns, regulatory issues, and the need for enhanced public awareness remain significant barriers that must be addressed to fully harness the transformational power of blockchain technology. Society likely endorses the adoption and popularity of decentralized and transparent solutions in the near future, thus advancing the momentum of the blockchain revolution on the global stage to usher in an era of trust, efficiency, and inclusion. The chapter reviews the role of AI alongside blockchain in transforming healthcare services by examining how the application of blockchain promises novel solutions. The chapter also takes into consideration a full analysis of the ongoing research challenges. Both technologies empower healthcare systems to come up with reliable approaches for developing secure, effective, and personalized healthcare solutions. Blockchain represents data security and privacy, while AI is more useful with predictive analytics and decision-making-another way to enhance operational efficiency within the healthcare system.

APPLICATIONS

Role of IoT-Edge Computing in Smart Healthcare

The main aim of IoT-Edge Computing is to analyze data where it is created in the network's edge, physically closer to where it will be utilized, rather than shipping data to encompassed centralized cloud servers. Sensors, wearables, and even big machines such as MRI machines generate significant volumes of real-time data. IoT-Edge Computing turns real-time analysis into actionable transactions and decisions efficiently through the analysis of data on the device or on expert servers in the network's edge. The convergence of IoT-Edge Computing with Blockchain and XAI presents a secure, transparent, and efficient platform for the handling of healthcare data and decision-making protocols. The convergence effectively addresses significant issues in the healthcare industry on data security, privacy, interoperability, and integrity. IoT devices continuously generate data in real-time, be it from wearable devices or smart medical devices. Cryptographic technology and blockchain secure data from any form of tampering after collection. Blockchain provides a secure ledger for the registration of all the healthcare data collected at the edge with transparency, auditability, and security maintained. The healthcare data may be stored in centralized or decentralized repositories such that no entity is in control through blockchain technology. Hence, the risk of data breach is reduced and personal privacy is enhanced. IoT-Edge services process data within the local environment and reduce the risk of exposure with ongoing data transfer to a centralized server. In addition, the use of smart contracts to define the access and modification rules for data ensures data created by IoT devices is accessed or modified by qualified personnel like medical practitioners. This system facilitates easier, automated, and more transparent management of patient consent. The advantages provided by IoT-Edge Computing are tremendous. For example, reduced latency translates to faster response time as data is processed near the source. Consumption of bandwidth is less as only pertinent or summarized data is transmitted to the cloud by processing data locally, thereby conserving bandwidth. The reduction of exposure as sensitive data is processed and stored locally before transit over the network significantly improves privacy and security. Real-time analytics render the prospect of instant decisions in time-sensitive tasks such as healthcare monitoring.

IoT-Edge Computing and Blockchain in Health Care

The convergence of IoT-Edge computing and Blockchain efficiently addresses the most critical issues in healthcare regarding data security, privacy, interoperability, and data integrity. IoT devices generate real-time data in the health setting, for example, wearable sensors and advanced medical equipment. The use of cryptographic technology via blockchain secures the data from any form of tampering once collected. Blockchain works as an immutable ledger in such a setting where all the health data generated in the edge is stored securely with transparency, auditability, and protection. Health data can be stored centrally or decentralized in various locations or institutions so that no authority is in control of the data. Such a setup diminishes the possibility of a data breach and keeps the individual's privacy intact. IoT-Edge solutions process data locally and hence minimize risks due to constant data transfer to the server.

Data access control through smart contracts specifies specific rules for accessing the data generated through IoT devices. Only authorized personnel such as medical practitioners are able to view or modify the data gathered through IoT devices. The mechanism facilitates easier and automatic handling of patient consents and enhances transparency. The incorporation of XAI in IoT-Edge deployments gives clinicians insights into decision-making fundamentals in AI solutions. Such transparency is necessary in medical applications where there is a requirement for trust. IoT devices collect vital information such as heart rate and blood glucose and send it to the edge servers for real-time analysis. AI algorithms in the edge analyze the data to determine anomalies such as the risk of heart attack or diabetic events. XAI techniques such as the use of LIME or SHAP allow clinicians to view the reasoning in AI predictions through the identification of significant data points contributing to the decision and thereby establishing confidence in AI assessments. By deciphering AI decision-making patterns, XAI enables clinicians to recognize the most significant factors linked with patient medical history and real-time vitals and drive better-informed health care choices. Provides strength in evidence-based strategies with the incorporation of AI recommendations and clinical guidelines. Such strategies have the potential to bring about a revolution in health care systems with increased security and privacy, effective health management, and possible solutions for interoperability issues. The patient's data is secured through blockchain methods providing tamperproof environments and limiting information to the approved personnel. At the same time, IoT-Edge technology works to minimize risks in the transfer of data and provides local processing for privacy. Besides, XAI introduces transparency into AI-driven decision-making to enable medical practitioners to see the reasoning behind predictions and create accountability in medical practice. The coupling of real-time data processing on the edge with actionable insights through AI models secured with blockchain facilitates better decision-making and customized therapies. A wearable device for glucose monitoring, for instance, alerts the patient when levels are outside the normal and justifies insulin injection on the basis of specific context factors. Blockchain enhances interoperability among various medical systems through the provision of a secure mechanism for IoT-Edge devices to communicate with medical practitioners effectively. Utilization of blockchain's decentralized nature facilitates secure transfer of health data among institutions and interoperability in the larger health environment.

Use Case Example:

For example, in a hospital, a patient's heartbeat can be monitored by one of these smart wearables. When an abnormal incident is detected, the edge system alerts the doctor immediately. XAI then justifies the alert by indicating there was spike sudden in time, while the blockchain irreversibly records this incident. This practice promotes transparency, agility, and robust management of data. They consist of commonly used IoT devices like smart glucose meters and heart rate monitors which record real-time data, analyzed in the edge computing units. These units detect abnormalities or threats, for example, high glucose levels. An AI model at the edge processes this data and makes predictions, such as identifying potential diabetic emergencies. XAI provides justifications for these predictions, utilizing methodologies like SHAP, which might state, "The prediction results from the blood glucose level exceeding the threshold by 20%." Furthermore, blockchain technology secures data storage and validates integrity through smart contracts before any data sharing or action occurs. The inherent security of blockchain prevents hacking attempts, while IoT-edge computing ensures that sensitive data processes locally, thereby reducing exposure. This combination enhances trust: XAI enables clinicians to comprehend and trust AI-generated decisions, facilitating greater integration of AI into clinical workflows. Patients receive benefits from real-time monitoring and decision-making, significantly improving response times. The stakeholders in the healthcare ecosystem are expected to be enabled in collaboration by the secure and effortless exchange of health data via blockchain. The case study of smart healthcare monitoring presents the integration of IoT-edge computing, blockchain, and XAI in healthcare.

Table 1. Merging IoT-Edge Computing, Blockchain, and XAI in Healthcare

Technology	Role	Benefit
IoT Devices	Collect real-time data (e.g., glucose meters, heart rate monitors).	**Real-time data collection**, enabling timely detection of health abnormalities (e.g., high glucose levels).
Edge Computing	Data is processed at the edge (on local devices) to detect abnormalities (e.g., increased glucose level).	**Low-latency processing** allows real-time decision-making without sending data to centralized servers.
AI Model (AI at Edge)	Analyzes data, makes predictions (e.g., risk of diabetic emergency).	**Quick prediction** of health events (e.g., diabetic emergencies), enabling proactive response.
Explainable AI (XAI)	Provides explanations for AI predictions using techniques like SHAP.	**Transparency and trust** by explaining AI decisions, such as why a particular prediction was made (e.g., threshold breach).

continued on following page

Table 1. Continued

Technology	Role	Benefit
Blockchain	Secures and stores data, ensuring tamper-proof records. Data integrity is validated using smart contracts.	**Secure data storage and sharing,** with blockchain ensuring data authenticity and privacy.
Smart Contracts	Validate data integrity and manage access controls for data sharing.	**Automated validation and authorization,** ensuring that only authorized parties access the data.

Framework for Merging IoT-Edge Computing, Blockchain, and XAI in Healthcare:

1. Data Collection (IoT Devices)

   The actual continuous collection of patient data in real-time from IoT devices such as a smart glucose meter and heart rate monitor. These devices effectively give a continuous track of vital signs and health metrics.
2. Data Processing at the Edge (Edge Computing)

   Digital data are locally processed in edge computation units and devices, including wearables or local servers which will prompt health decisions regarding the patient. Therefore, the system can detect any deviation from glucose levels above a specified level and activate alerts immediately with the edge processing unit.
3. AI Model Analysis (AI at Edge)

   An AI model at the edge essentially processes real-time data to estimate an imminent possibility of diabetic emergencies that shall be caused due to an increase in the patient's glucose level. Such a model predicts, using the data feed, and updates the predictions based on machine learning algorithms derived from historical data for patient use.
4. Explainable Artificial Intelligence (XAI) for Transparency

   XAI techniques such as SHAP (Shapley Additive Explanations) are used to explain the system's predictions. For example, it may state that the prediction of a possible diabetic emergency should be given because the glucose level has exceeded a certain threshold by 20%. Such an explanation helps clinicians understand the AI's reasoning behind its predictions, thus building trust and enhancing transparency in its decisions.
5. Data Storage and Validation (Blockchain)

   Blockchain technology secures and stores the data generated, ensuring that the data cannot be tampered with or altered. Before sharing with authorized healthcare practitioners, the data's integrity is verified through a smart contract. This guarantees that only authenticated data is shared, preventing anyone else from accessing it.

Future Research Perspectives

The data, once authenticated, is either released to the medical personnel or is used for lots of actions like alerting a patient or doctor. Access control is ensured through smart contracts that permit access to patient data only by certain parties, namely, the doctor or the clinic.

The Future of IoT-Edge Computing

The intercommunication of devices and sensors connected to a wired or wireless network creates real-time monitoring of patients. The devices in unison acquire critical data concerning vital signs, activity levels, and environmental conditions, which are pivotal for chronic disease management. Edge computing facilitates data processing directly on the device, enhancing the relevance of the IoT in healthcare. This system processes data for its own local requirement; hence, there are no latencies, and immediate results are provided-a key consideration in the case of conditions like coronary heart disease (CHD) where every single second may matter. The union of IoT and edge computing ensures uninterrupted data collection and analysis in quasi-real-time. Health institutions can monitor the patient effectively and create relevant actions, without requiring physical visits or admission for inpatient care.

Table 2. Benefits of Merging IoT-Edge Computing, Blockchain, and XAI

Benefit	**Explanation**
Increased Security	Blockchain guarantees that the data is secure and tamper-proof, while **Edge computing** reduces the risk of sensitive data being exposed.
Improved Trust	**XAI** makes AI's decision-making transparent and understandable, which builds trust with healthcare providers.
Better Patient Care	Real-time monitoring and AI-driven predictions lead to faster interventions, improving patient outcomes.
Efficient Data Sharing	Blockchain ensures secure, seamless, and decentralized sharing of patient data among authorized stakeholders.

The health-monitoring system combines IoT-Edge computing, Blockchain, and XAI to let edge-based real-time decision-making for a timely response to possible medical emergencies.

- Provides secure, transparent, and tamper-proof data storage and sharing, which safeguards patient privacy and ensures compliance with healthcare regulations.
- Utilizes XAI to enhance clinician trust and considerate of AI-driven predictions, thereby supporting improved clinical decision-making.
- Creates a robust, secure, and trustworthy healthcare system that optimizes patient care and operational efficiency by uniting IoT-Edge computing, Blockchain, and XAI in healthcare.
- Addresses abundant challenges current healthcare faces, including data security, real-time processing, transparency, and interoperability, while effectively dealing patient data and enhancing overall experience in the health industry.

Table 3. Tabulated comparison between Blockchain-Based XAI for Secure and Privacy-Preserving Automated Machine Learning in IoT-Edge for Smart Medical Healthcare and existing applications

Aspect	Blockchain-Based XAI for Secure and Privacy-Preserving Automated Machine Learning in IoT-Edge for Smart Medical Healthcare	Existing Blockchain-Based Healthcare Solutions
Core Technology	Integration of Blockchain, XAI, and Automated Machine Learning in IoT-Edge environments for secure and privacy-preserving healthcare applications.	Primarily Blockchain and basic AI for healthcare data management and patient record sharing.
Security	Enhanced security via blockchain's decentralization, tamper-proof ledger, and privacy-preserving machine learning algorithms. Utilizes smart contracts for access control.	Security mainly through blockchain's decentralized ledger but lacks integration with privacy-preserving machine learning algorithms for data processing.
Privacy	Provides robust privacy protection by ensuring that sensitive healthcare data is processed in a privacy-preserving manner, using techniques like federated learning and differential privacy.	Privacy is addressed but generally focuses on securing the storage and sharing of patient data without incorporating advanced privacy-preserving algorithms in data processing.
Explainability	Uses XAI to provide transparent and interpretable decision-making processes, which is crucial for trust in healthcare systems.	Limited or no use of XAI for understanding model decisions, leading to opacity in automated healthcare processes.
Data Management	Blockchain allows for secure and immutable healthcare data management; AI models can allow the real time update and verification of data combined with access control via smart contracts.	Blockchain is used for securing healthcare data and ensuring transparency, but real-time data updates and automated verification may not be fully integrated.
Scalability	Highly scalable solution that can be applied to diverse healthcare applications, from patient record management to real-time IoT data processing.	Scalability is usually limited to specific areas like patient record management or supply chain tracking, but may struggle with real-time IoT data processing.
Decentralization	Fully decentralized approach, enabling control and management of healthcare data without relying on central authorities, ensuring data integrity and trust.	Blockchain ensures decentralization of patient records, but centralized aspects of the healthcare system (e.g., healthcare providers) may still control some data flows.
Use Case Examples	Real-time patient monitoring, predictive diagnostics, secure sharing of sensitive health data between providers, and IoT-enabled smart healthcare systems.	Electronic Health Records (EHR), secure sharing of patient data, drug traceability, and healthcare supply chain tracking.
Anomaly Detection & Intrusion Prevention	Utilizes automated machine learning techniques (e.g., anomaly detection models) for identifying and mitigating cybersecurity threats in IoT-enabled medical devices and systems.	Some blockchain-based healthcare applications use basic anomaly detection but lack the automated, real-time machine learning-driven security protocols integrated with IoT.
Regulatory Compliance	Blockchain and XAI ensure compliance with healthcare regulations (e.g., HIPAA, GDPR) by maintaining immutable audit trails and providing interpretable models for auditability.	Blockchain solutions help with data privacy and compliance but may lack integration with AI models that can explain decision-making processes for compliance audits.
Performance	Achieves high performance in handling large datasets and real-time processing, with a focus on secure data exchanges and AI-powered decision support.	Performance is generally good for secure record keeping but may face challenges in real-time analytics and advanced decision-making processes.

The table provides a comparative analysis of the proposed Blockchain-Based XAI designed for a secure and privacy-preserving automated machine learning system, juxtaposed with other blockchain applications in the healthcare sector. It highlights the advancements achieved by this proposed system in terms of security, privacy, explainability, and scalability. Moreover, the table illustrates applications such as real-time anomaly detection and automated machine learning tailored for IoT-edge environments, differentiating them from existing solutions. The former systems utilize blockchain for secure data management and privacy, yet they lack the advanced features offered by XAI and the integration of automated machine learning within IoT environments.

Challenges in Chronic Disease Management

New treatments for critical illnesses are still coming forth, but there are still gaps in medicine concerning early screening, patient privacy, and management of diseases. For most patients with coronary artery disease, diagnosis is done too late, at times even after the onset of some adverse events such as death. The existing health care systems are without some continuous patient care frameworks that are important for the proper treatment of chronic diseases which need timely diagnosis and treatment. Treatment regimens today are frequently fighting against data management challenges. Disorganization happens when there is a lack of ability to manage and exchange patient data with other providers and platforms and it results in incorrect diagnosis, inappropriate care, and increased risk of inappropriate care, prolonged procedures, and poor patient outcomes.

Background: Privacy, Security, and Interoperability in Health Care

The trend towards digitalization seems to reflect the increased importance of patient privacy. The rapid implementation of Electronic Health Records (EHRs) opened the doors to the debate on utmost protection of data.It raises significant concerns when nations experience breaches of health data, often resulting in the compromise of millions of patient records. The vulnerability of central systems to cyberattacks, unauthorized access, and data leaks fosters skepticism about the efficacy of digital healthcare systems. Moreover, establishing mechanisms that facilitate data sharing among healthcare providers without the burden of adhering to numerous privacy and security regulations, such as HIPAA in the United States and GDPR in Europe, becomes essential. However, the persistent incompatibility of data across healthcare systems hinders the development of unified treatment approaches for chronic diseases, particularly in cases requiring collaboration among multiple healthcare providers in a patient's treatment plan.

The Requirement of Blockchain in Healthcare

Urgent changes are required as the healthcare sector's dimensions change. Modern medicine places a strong emphasis on the value of first-rate facilities that guarantee the efficient application of cutting-edge technologies, enabling the best possible patient care and treatment results. Particular attention is given to transformative pathways in the healthcare sector in this context. Access to care and timely, accurate health information are the two main focuses of customized healthcare delivery models.

A strong and secure foundation for patient information system design is required to implement these models. In an era of wearable technology and personalized medicine, blockchain technology is well-positioned to address important privacy and data protection concerns. For both patients and healthcare professionals who require secure methods of managing sensitive health information, ensuring safety and openness in call technologies for recording, transmitting, and accessing patient information significantly reduces the chances of security breaches. Blockchain offers reliable protection against unauthorized access and tampering with patient records by decentralizing storage of data and making records immutable. Blockchain enhances healthcare resource allocation besides security, enabling patients to obtain timely and proper care. With improved Health Information Exchange (HIE), it minimizes the laborious and ineffective processes present in traditional health systems. The secure and consolidated platform for health information sharing, which this technology provides, has improved provider coordination and better treatment outcomes as its products. Enabling citizens to contribute to health studies and research is also among the prominent benefits of blockchain technology. Better and transparent public health research on the treatment procedures that are specific to heterogeneous communities is facilitated through securely stored shared data. Effective population health management in the current healthcare industry is impeded by considerable issues in data protection, data sharing, and interoperability. Blockchain emerges as the solution, providing data integrity and real-time collaboration among healthcare organizations and enabling secure, transparent, and effective data sharing. While reducing costs that are largely incurred as a result of ineffective data management, the innovative technology solves considerable challenges in the healthcare system, particularly in elevating data security and privacy and interoperability among different domains in the healthcare industry. Blockchain naturally occupies its position in different transactional domains as the healthcare industry transforms, ensuring health services remain enhanced, easily accessible, and secure.

Blockchain technologies in healthcare

Blockchain technology operates as a decentralized ledger in the health sector, keeping transactions in an immutable and transparent state. This feature is greatly needed when handling sensitive patient data. Patient data not being centralized reduces the risk of leaks and ensures patient data is safe and stored accurately. Blockchain technology saves much time, effort, and money on traditional data handling procedures in the health sector. The technology also greatly facilitates the handling of medical records through an effective system where approved parties have up-to-date and accurate access to patient data. One of the greatest concerns in the healthcare industry nowadays is confidential information leaks, which are taken advantage of by malicious individuals. Blockchain technology solves the issue by limiting access to information and keeping information confidential, avoiding misuse. Blockchain technology is a valuable component in the management of personal health information and in reducing the risks involved in data manipulation or access by unauthorized parties since it can provide transparent and traceable data and keep the patient's information private. By providing easier integration of external health and insurance information into electronic health records (EHRs) and cross-system comparison among different EHRs, blockchain technology also makes the workflow of many health procedures easier. Such a procedure fosters collaboration among healthcare practitioners, researchers, and patients through the provision of real-time and standard access to high-quality evidence-based information to all stakeholders. Blockchain technology uses a shared network to unite the therapy associates, medical practitioners, and other stakeholders in providing collaborative care, real-time information, and medical data along the patient care pathways.

Blockchain technology has the potential to revolutionize many areas in healthcare, from clinical trials, medical supply chains, and drug authenticity, to patient records. For example, by making data appropriately recorded and independently verifiable by all parties, blockchain makes clinical trials more transparent and traceable. Blockchain is being applied in the supply chain for tracking the origin of medical devices and pharmaceuticals, and ensuring they are authentic and have not been altered. Blockchain technology has several revolutionary uses in the medical field.

Figure 1. Blockchain in healthcare

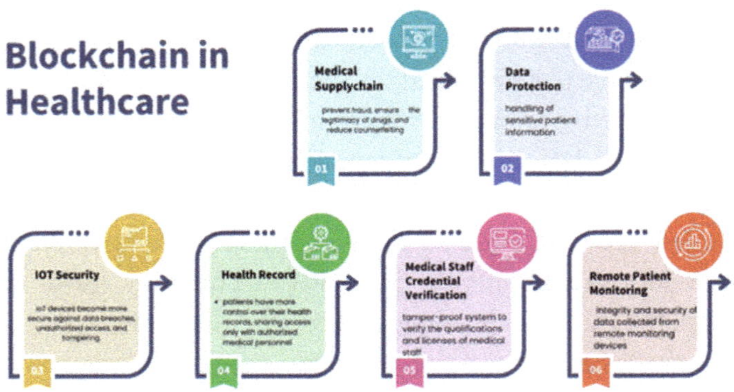

Blockchain provides a transparent, decentralized, and safe method of managing data, successfully tackling important issues in the sector like data abuse, inefficiencies, and a lack of insight. From supply chain management to clinical research and patient care, technology has the power to revolutionize many facets of healthcare practice as it develops. Blockchain technology holds great promise for the future of healthcare delivery, spurring innovation, improving patient care, and building a safer and more effective healthcare ecosystem.

Blockchain as a Solution for Healthcare

To protect patient data, the framework uses blockchain with PoS, a method that validates transactions without heavy energy use. It also applies SHA-256, a technique that converts data into a secure code to detect any tampering. This ensures health records stay accurate and private.

Figure 2. **Artificial intelligence in healthcare** *(Shinde et al., 2024)*

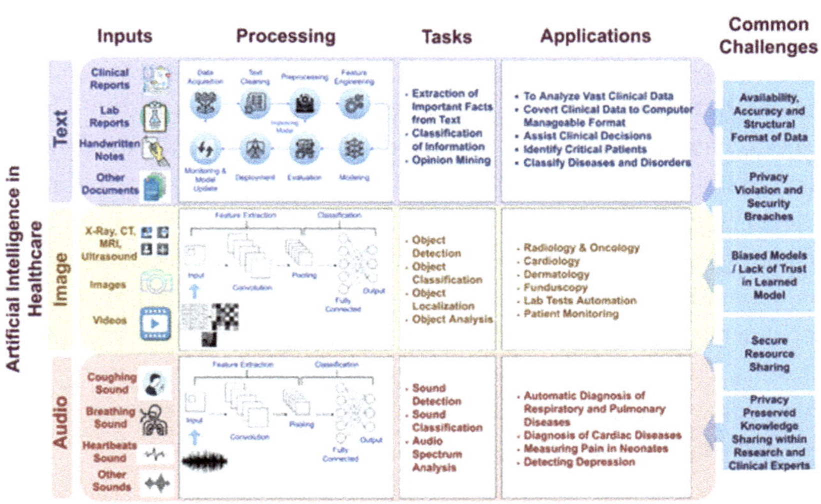

Explainable AI (XAI) for Predictive Healthcare Models

While frequently described as "black-box" systems because they lack the transparency necessary for model interpretability, traditional AI models are very accurate. The limitations of explaining AI results in ways that are meaningful to humans are especially evident in the clinical domain, where patients and physicians need to have a full understanding of predictions in order to facilitate meaningful action. XAI overcomes this limitation by rendering AI models transparent to human users and by elucidating the decision-making processes underlying such models. Healthcare practitioners will be able to better comprehend the manner in which AI algorithms develop particular predictions with the use of XAI techniques like SHAP (SHapley Additive exPlanations) and LIME (Local Interpretable Model-agnostic Explanations). It fosters confidence and enables clinicians to make educated choices in accordance with specialization and medical understanding. To interpret machine learning-based clinical decision-making models better, there is a need for XAI in risk populations' assignment to patients with chronic diseases like coronary heart disease (CHD). The use of XAI enables health practitioners to make better decisions with greater clarity, improving patient care and outcomes and increasing confidence in AI systems.

IoT-Blockchain-XAI Integrations for Smart Medical Healthcare

Blockchain technology provides significant promises in the form of secure, private, and interoperable platforms for the storage and sharing of sensitive health information among various health information systems, and XAI increases the interpretability and transparency of predictive models applicable to the diagnosis and treatment of chronic diseases. The employment of IoT devices and edge computing allows for the collection of real-time data from the patient and the processing of the data with the least possible latency for constant monitoring of the health status. This synergy resolves pressing data privacy, security, and trust concerns and greatly improves the accuracy and reliability of chronic condition diagnosis. Accordingly, transparent and actionable insights sufficient to guide evidence-based decision-making and revolutionize the treatment of chronic diseases like coronary heart disease (CHD) are delivered to health care practitioners. The remainder of the chapter describes how IoT, blockchain, and XAI separately allow the creation of secure, private, and explainable automated machine learning systems in the context of smart healthcare. The chapter establishes a new standard for secure, patient-centric care in the digital era in addition to addressing the treatment of chronic diseases.

Chapter Contribution

Data-driven technology, artificial intelligence, and machine learning are revolutionizing various disciplines, most notably the field of medicine. AI presents a revolutionized method of managing long-term diseases and other health issues. AI's use of very accurate but unexplainable black-box models is a major drawback, however. Since both clinicians and patients have to rely on the technology informing their health recommendations, the problem poses serious issues in the medical field. The main aim in this research is to integrate XAI into a secure, private, and safe automated machine learning framework. The framework is for an intelligent health solution with the use of blockchain, edge computing, and the Internet of Things. Integration with XAI addresses the necessary requirement for transparency and interpretability in AI models, specifically in the treatment of long-term diseases. The research greatly increases the confidence and trust in AI models among both patients and medical practitioners through the explanation of the functioning of the models. Unlike traditional black-box models that produce results without a comprehensible reason, explainable AI uses techniques that make AI models' processes more transparent and interpretable, providing insights into decision-making. This is particularly important in the clinical field, where AI outcomes have direct implications for patient care. To trust an AI model's clinical decisions, clinicians must be able to discern the reason why a model has made a particular diagnosis or suggested course of treatment. Furthermore, by revealing possible biases or mistakes in AI-derived decisions, XAI supports accountability and ethical compliance in medical practice. The sophistication of hospital data, which includes real-time data from wearables and electronic health records (EHR), demands AI models that are not only extremely accurate but also sufficiently interpretable for clinical practice.

Although the literature in publication demonstrates AI's superior performance in managing chronic diseases, the major problem is that such models are too opaque to be adopted in real-life healthcare practice. The present study fills the gap in explaining the manner in which XAI has improved healthcare AI systems and made them transparent, interpretable, and accurate. It makes it possible to use XAI in medical decision-making on a daily basis.

This is enabled by the IoT-edge-blockchain architecture. The IoT devices collect real-time data from the patient via wearables and sensors continuously monitoring vital signs and other health metrics to manage chronic diseases. Real-time monitoring allows for the detection of likely problems beforehand. The data is processed in the local environment through the use of edge computing instead of servers in the core, reducing latency and improving response times. Such factors are crucial in the medical field where timely interventions have a major impact on the outcome in the patient's life. Blockchain technology fosters interoperability between various health-related systems with the guarantee of the security and privacy of the collected data. It enables smooth coordination of care through the establishment of a decentralized and immutable ledger for patient data available to authorized health care providers only. Healthcare systems are enhanced in a number of ways when XAI is included in the IoT-edge-blockchain framework. First, XAI makes predictive models easier to read and comprehend. Model prediction clarity enables clinicians to trust and follow the suggestions of the AI, and it is crucial in chronic disease treatment since it demands complicated AI interpretations of big data. In order to ensure insights align with clinical expertise and include patient-specific factors, clinicians can use techniques like decision trees and attention mechanisms to discover the rationale for particular conclusions. XAI fosters patient-clinician trust, according to Thiruthuvanathan, Kumar, Swathikiran et al. (2024). Trust is necessary to break down barriers to AI use in clinical practice—often due to uncertainty about the accuracy of AI predictions. Explaining reasons for AI predictions and recommendations in terms understandable to the patient increases patient compliance with AI-based recommendations and clinician trust. Apart from the above, XAI promotes the ethical use of AI in the health sector. Since AI models themselves may be biased, be it because of biased training data or the bias embedded in the system, it is necessary to identify and counter such bias in order to ensure fairness in the output in the health sector. XAI also helps in promoting privacy and security for AI in the health sector without violating patient confidentiality and delivering valuable insights without the use of raw data. Complex techniques like blockchain not just store and transfer patient data securely but also add an additional layer of protection for the health AI systems. The combinatory approach of IoT-edge-based computing, blockchain, and XAI brings enormous benefits in the management of chronic diseases.

IoT devices enable real-time monitoring and collection of data on the patient to recognize deterioration in advance. Health practitioners are able to take preventive action against catastrophes and drive better patient outcomes through the utilization of the insights derived from XAI. Chronic conditions often require bespoke interventions and the utilization of XAI enables the use of more customized treatment plans. Clinicians are better positioned to understand the reasoning behind the predictions made by a model due to the increased transparency in AI models and the creation of better customized and effective treatment plans with improved patient outcomes. Blockchain enables easier collaboration among different caregivers in a secure manner and is significant in the handling of chronic conditions that commonly require multiple medical specialists. Through an open and intelligent health care delivery system, the integrated model promotes improved patient care and empowers the practitioners with the necessary information to make informed decisions to manage chronic diseases better. In creating a framework for the use of advanced technology, the research keeps pushing the evolutionary journey and develops patient care solutions for people with chronic diseases that are safer, clearer, and improved.

Solution

This introduction of XAI into automated machine learning systems in the healthcare field constitutes a new way of treating this subject as existing research in this arena has neglected the vital aspect of model interpretability that underlies it. Classic machine learning methods, such as Random Forests and Support Vector Machines (SVM), often form basic blocks in disease prediction due to their excellent output. Unfortunately, "black box" models do not tell how it came up with the prediction, thus making it a considerable bottleneck in healthcare scenario. Therefore, they do a wonderfull prediction but it does not tell how predicted the facts which is very critical in case of healthcare. It is extremely important for a clinician to know the grounds on which AI is taking predictions or recommendations so that the decision made is upright, evidence based, and has met clinical standards. Current models lack clarity and inhibit trust which shrinks the application of AI across the spheres of medical practice. I am closing this gap by incorporating advanced XAI methods, such as SHAP (SHapley Additive exPlanations) and LIME (Local Interpretable Model-agnostic Explanations), into machine learning models not just for having accurate but also interpretable models. SHAP and LIME helps by providing clear understandable explanations on how different factors contribute to this prediction from model. This enhances the understanding of mechanisms behind the AI system among health professionals while boosting their confidence in AI-assisted decision-making. Verification and justification of AI outputs from physicians are necessary, especially with respect to patient safety and accountability in treatment decisions. XAI help healthcare providers build that trust that should be in these predictive models for a more standard application in the clinical environment.

XAI has roles between doctors even further strengthening patient-centered care. It opens up to the patients the explanations of the AI models that empower them to understand how these decisions are reached and thus the AI models can put forth a logic-based explanation of their diagnoses or treatment recommendations. A patient who can perceive the reasoning behind an AI-supported recommendation is unlikely to trust it and to use it under the recommendation's terms. In particular, it is within the management of chronic diseases like CHD and Diabetes Mellitus that long-term patient follow-up and adherence would be likely to yield favorable outcomes. XAI helps the patients to be informed and trust the decision-making process, as this has made them more engaged in health empowerment activities.

My research also focuses on integrating XAI with federated learning and IoT-edge-blockchain architecture. Federated learning, which uses decentralization for machine learning, enables the patient data to remain on local devices instead of being transferred to a central server, and across a network, it only shares model updates-much greater privacy. But in this scenario, a big rug pulls out from under the feet of 'decentralized culture': maintaining model interpretability. My research is aimed at such integration by applying XAI techniques to ensure that federated models' predictions are transparent as well as interpretable even in highly decentralized environments. Understandably, the combination of XAI with federated learning and blockchain strengthens the privacy-security dyad of the system while at the same time going very high on interpretability-ensuring that the patient data are protected but information remains accessible to healthcare providers. The contribution that this chapter makes is that of a precedent novel integration of Explainable artificial machine learning systems into automated secure, privacy-preserving ones for healthcare. This makes important strides by critically answering the issue of the transparency of AI health solutions; predictive models develop beyond mere accuracy towards being trustworthy and clinically applicable. Therefore, this study can enhance wider adoption of artificial intelligence for real care by harmonizing AI with clinical standards. The development of XAI in these systems lays the foundation for more intelligent, safer, and patient-centered medicine for the betterment of care for people with chronic diseases. Enhancing the all-important aim of improving chronic diseases prediction, particularly for diabetes mellitus and cardiovascular diseases, involve real-time patient data from IoT devices and medical sensors being brought to explainable machine learning models. With the incorporation of XAI, (Salama, Ragab, et al. 2023) these models not only provide accurate predictions, but well-structured interpretations to ensure that they can be understood and acted upon confidently within the healthcare profession. Another concern regarding data privacy and security is addressed by deploying security measures through blockchain algorithms, which are tough against intrusions on collecting, storing, and transmitting sensitive health-related data. Because of the decentralized and tamper-proof nature of Blockchain, the patient information becomes safe and adheres with data protection regulations, like HIPAA or GDPR (Hennebelle, Ismail, Materwala, et al. 2024). Thus, it guarantees sensitive health data across different healthcare providers while shielding the patient from exposure. The primary goal is to incorporate explainability from XAI into interpreting machine learning models by healthcare professionals. With transparent reasoning for AI predictions, these models to a large degree lend themselves to clinical understanding of how decisions are made, which in turn improves trust in AI-led insights. This interpretability is the key to ensuring that AI systems are integrated within effective clinical workflow and support better patient-centered care. Multitude of medical risk factors would be identified and studied from very diverse datasets within the hospital systems by this. With further data collection from the various IoT and medical devices, this would enable the timely and accurate diagnosis of chronic illnesses. Better still, from this data, health practitioners would then have more informed backgrounds and eventually be able to also put a finger on health risks before they become risks improving actual performance of health outcomes. The system serves well evidence-based practice for healthcare professionals with high-quality diagnosis and therapy prescriptions in transparent manner about XAI models. The last one is indeed critical because it bring together AI-driven predictions with clinical knowledge to ensure that health care providers consider this system for medical decisions that are well-informed and can also be relied on for accuracy. Finally, the system be validated against real-time datasets that represent chronic diseases. Hence, the system ensured to have high accuracy and interpretability in performance and improved disease prediction and healthcare delivery and uses real data to operationalize the system into optimality by adjusting its functions to those for the healthcare practitioners. This causes better improvements for both patients and the management of chronic diseases. (Chen, Xu et al. 2021) addresses the privacy and security concerns that arise during sharing any sensitive data in the advanced healthcare systems that employs blockchain technology. (Kumar, Javeed, Aljuhani, et al. 2023) it’s possible to observe the growing trend of advanced health care systems that get built around

IoT devices such as wearables or implants that ideally allow for the tracking of a patient's health status. In Most Cases Such Systems Are More Cost-Effective and Provide More Tailored Services. The biggest disadvantage is the threat to individual privacy and data security. The main challenges are protecting massive amounts of sensitive customer health data and making it available to authorized customers because of centralization, these systems face single points of failure and a breach of all private access controls. (Ramachandran, et al. 2024). The authors and deal with this problem in the article and propose the use of blockchain, which provides a decentralized, immutable history of transactions in a distributed P2P network, rendering a one-stop shop model unnecessary. In this way the author's reliability and privacy of the data are enhanced. The author presents a 3D Data Dissemination Scheme for Smart Healthcare that relies on blockchain. It combines a certificate-based sign cryption with proxy for efficient data sharing (Shari, et al. 2024). It employs an Improved Delegated Proof-of-Stake (DPoS) for better security and decentralization as well. The applicability of the Sign-Proxy scheme guarantees the confidentiality and no tracking of health data but limits the amount of computation done. Enhanced DPoS, strengthens the voting related parts and maintains integrity of the program by discouraging and dealing with bad actors and providing measures against proof of collusion. Data reliability in that every health data sent out is the right one and has not been tampered with. Privacy through disguising the identity of individuals until such a time it is required. Accountability in the aspect of ensuring that the players in the system who engage in malicious acts are made to face the consequences. The article has security and performance review, which has proven that the scheme is tenable even with attacks targeted at it. It has proven to be effective and viable for deployment in practical situations. This chapter deepens the analysis by contrasting the proposed healthcare framework based on blockchain technology against existing applications in the area. The authors assert that their framework has been able to deal with the evident shortcomings of privacy, trust, and accountability of which most current models of healthcare built on blockchain technology are unable to eliminate. The proposed system is based on the synergies between blockchain technology and artificial intelligence (AI), which are expected to assist in dealing with these issues and improving security and efficiency in smart healthcare systems' decentralized data exchange. It is inculcated under the Internet of Healthcare Things (IoHT). It is acquiring much attention owing to its effective network of devices and systems through which patients' healthcare may be monitored and managed real-time. At the same time, (Rahman, Hossain, Showail, et al. 2021) the IoHT is easily susceptible to heavy cybersecurity threats because of its reliance on different modes of the internet and also on centralized databases. Hence, IoHT is exposed to several cyber-attacks like loss of confidential information, invasion of privacy, and alteration of data without consent. These vulnerabilities are blanket-obscured by the author by testing a novel technique that combines both blockchain technology and AI models (Upadhyay, Singh, Gupta, et al. 2024) to the maximum extent possible: enhancing anomaly detection and secure data management. The characteristics of decentralization and immutability in addition to make tamper-proof and safeguard unauthorized access to health data with the dual advantage of blockchain. AI, more particularly such machine learning models as Support Vector Machines (SVM), 1D-Convolutional Neural Networks (1D-CNN), and Long Short-Term Memory (LSTM) networks, enhance some consensus in the recognition and classification of cyber security anomalies in real-time (Gwassi, Uçan, Navarro, et al. 2024). With the integration of blockchain and AI, any suspicious activity gets identified faster, hence minimizing the chances of attacks and maintaining continuous monitoring on IoHT devices. Apart from this, the authors involve Interplanetary File System (IPFS), a decentralized storage solution, to increase data privacy. Healthcare data is kept off-chain with IPFS; thus, it reduces the likelihood of centralized data breaches, which would enable verification of any data through the blockchain. This security paradigm involves two walls that essentially render health data impossible to access during storage and transmission and hence stops unauthorized changes, thus maintaining data integrity. This technology that enables services from blockchain is a newer object and still under constant development. With blockchain, it is possible to promote the efficient and safe exchange of information and the transfer of information among health care providers, which in turn can yield greater cost-effective treatments and more sophisticated treatments for a variety of diseases. It is predicted that this potential speed healthcare advances in the next few years. Since blockchain applications are certain to expand, especially in the logistics and financial segments, they have tremendous potential in the medical sector, an industry with a material impact on the quality of life. The digitalization through blockchain is likely to revolutionize the medical sector, ensuring safer, transparent, and streamlined systems.

CONCLUSION

This chapter presents a holistic and interdisciplinary approach with the use of IoT-edge computing, XAI, and blockchain technology to address the pressing problems in managing chronic diseases like coronary heart disease (CHD). The presented system enables real-time monitoring of the patient through IoT devices with the guarantee of data protection and confidentiality and regulatory compliance through the use of blockchain-based smart contracts and cryptographic hashing. The addition of XAI enables clinicians to interpret the predictions made through machine learning and make evidence-based clinical decisions and be confident in AI-based health care solutions. The employment of federated learning enhances the patient's privacy and enables the model to be trained in a decentralized manner without the exposure of sensitive data. The scalability and modularity in the architecture ensure flexibility in diverse health care setups and provide secure and tailored medical care on a personal scale. System validation on a large scale demonstrates the success in real-life clinical applications where the accuracy in predictions, patient outcomes, and clinician confidence improved. Through the convergence of these advanced technologies, the proposed solution addresses data integrity, transparency, and interoperability challenges and elevates the standard for smart healthcare systems. This chapter thereby sets a foundational path toward patient-centered, technology-enabled, and explainable medical care, contributing meaningfully to the evolution of intelligent healthcare solutions for chronic disease prediction and management.

REFERENCES

Abbas, A., Alroobaea, R., Krichen, M., Rubaiee, S., Vimal, S., & Almansour, F. M. (2024). Blockchain-assisted secured data management framework for health information analysis based on Internet of Medical Things. *Personal and Ubiquitous Computing*, *28*(1), 59–72. DOI: 10.1007/s00779-021-01583-8

Ahad, A., Jiangbin, Z., Mughees, A., Puspitasari, I., & Tayyab, M. (2025). Secure Horizons: Integrating Blockchain With AI for Enhanced Smart Healthcare Systems. In AI Techniques for Securing Medical and Business Practices (pp. 357-390). IGI Global.

Ahmad, M., Jabeen, M., Qasim, M., & Hasnain, M. (2024). Integrating Modern Technology in Education: Enhancing Learning, Engagement, and Accessibility in the Digital Age. *International Research Journal of Management and Social Sciences*, *5*(2), 267–271.

Bala, I., Pindoo, I., Mijwil, M. M., Abotaleb, M., & Yundong, W. (2024). Ensuring security and privacy in Healthcare Systems: A Review Exploring challenges, solutions, Future trends, and the practical applications of Artificial Intelligence. *Jordan Medical Journal*, *58*(3).

Bathula, A., Gupta, S. K., Merugu, S., Saba, L., Khanna, N. N., Laird, J. R., Sanagala, S. S., Singh, R., Garg, D., Fouda, M. M., & Suri, J. S. (2024). Blockchain, artificial intelligence, and healthcare: The tripod of future—a narrative review. *Artificial Intelligence Review*, *57*(9), 238. DOI: 10.1007/s10462-024-10873-5

Bristow, A. S., Buys, K. C., & Mays, L. C. (2023). OLD CLASS: An Innovative Approach to the Chronic Disease History of Present Illness. *The Journal for Nurse Practitioners*, *19*(5), 104545. DOI: 10.1016/j.nurpra.2023.104545

Charles, S., & Natarajan, J. (2024). Identification of key gene modules and novel transcription factors in tetralogy of fallot using machine learning and network topological features. *Medinformatics*, *1*(1), 27–34. DOI: 10.47852/bonviewMEDIN32021554

Chattopadhyay, S. (2024). *Decoding medical diagnosis with machine learning classifiers*. Medinformatics. DOI: 10.47852/bonviewMEDIN42022583

Chen, Z., Xu, W., Wang, B., & Yu, H. (2021). A blockchain-based preserving and sharing system for medical data privacy. *Future Generation Computer Systems*, *124*, 338–350. DOI: 10.1016/j.future.2021.05.023

Deshmukh, V., Pathak, S., & Bhattacharya, P. (2025). Bl-Boost: A blockchain-based XG-Boost EHR scheme in Healthcare 5.0 ecosystems. *International Journal of Computing*, *17*(1), 1–15.

Dimitrov, D. V. (2019). Blockchain applications for healthcare data management. *Healthcare Informatics Research*, *25*(1), 51–56. DOI: 10.4258/hir.2019.25.1.51 PMID: 30788182

Ghadi, Y. Y., Mazhar, T., Shahzad, T., Amir khan, M., Abd-Alrazaq, A., Ahmed, A., & Hamam, H. (2024). Muhammad Amir khan, Alaa Abd-Alrazaq, Arfan Ahmed, and Habib Hamam. "The role of blockchain to secure internet of medical things.". *Scientific Reports*, *14*(1), 18422. DOI: 10.1038/s41598-024-68529-x PMID: 39117650

Gwassi, O. A. H., Uçan, O. N., & Navarro, E. A. (2024). Cyber-XAI-Block: An end-to-end cyber threat detection & fl-based risk assessment framework for iot enabled smart organization using xai and blockchain technologies. *Multimedia Tools and Applications*, •••, 1–42. DOI: 10.1007/s11042-024-20059-4

Haleem, A., Javaid, M., Singh, R. P., Suman, R., & Rab, S. (2021). Blockchain technology applications in healthcare: An overview. *International Journal of Intelligent Networks*, *2*, 130–139. DOI: 10.1016/j.ijin.2021.09.005

Hennebelle, A., Ismail, L., Materwala, H., Al Kaabi, J., Ranjan, P., & Janardhanan, R. (2024). Secure and privacy-preserving automated machine learning operations into end-to-end integrated IoT-edge-artificial intelligence-blockchain monitoring system for diabetes mellitus prediction. *Computational and Structural Biotechnology Journal*, *23*, 212–233. DOI: 10.1016/j.csbj.2023.11.038 PMID: 38169966

Hennebelle, A., Ismail, L., Materwala, H., Al Kaabi, J., Ranjan, P., & Janardhanan, R. (2024). Secure and privacy-preserving automated machine learning operations into end-to-end integrated IoT-edge-artificial intelligence-blockchain monitoring system for diabetes mellitus prediction. *Computational and Structural Biotechnology Journal*, *23*, 212–233. DOI: 10.1016/j.csbj.2023.11.038 PMID: 38169966

Jabeen, M., Hussain, M., & Rana Hassam Ahmed, H. A. A BLOCKCHAIN-BASED IPFS AUGMENTED DISTRIBUTED INFORMATION SHARING PARADIGM FOR SECURE COMMUNICATION IN NETWORKED ENVIRONMENT.

Jagatheesaperumal, S. K., Pham, Q. V., Ruby, R., Yang, Z., Xu, C., & Zhang, Z. (2022). Explainable AI over the Internet of Things (IoT): Overview, state-of-the-art and future directions. *IEEE Open Journal of the Communications Society*, *3*, 2106–2136. DOI: 10.1109/OJCOMS.2022.3215676

Jagatheesaperumal, S. K., Pham, Q. V., Ruby, R., Yang, Z., Xu, C., & Zhang, Z. (2022). Explainable AI over the Internet of Things (IoT): Overview, state-of-the-art and future directions. *IEEE Open Journal of the Communications Society*, *3*, 2106–2136. DOI: 10.1109/OJCOMS.2022.3215676

Kumar, R., Javeed, D., Aljuhani, A., Jolfaei, A., Kumar, P., & Islam, A. N. (2023). Blockchain-based authentication and explainable AI for securing consumer IoT applications. *IEEE Transactions on Consumer Electronics*.

Lin, H. (2024). Artificial intelligence with great potential in medical informatics: A brief review. *Medinformatics*, *1*(1), 2–9. DOI: 10.47852/bonviewMEDIN42022204

Liu, H., Crespo, R. G., & Martínez, O. S. (2020, July). Enhancing privacy and data security across healthcare applications using blockchain and distributed ledger concepts. []. MDPI.]. *Health Care*, *8*(3), 243. PMID: 32751325

Mahajan, P., Aujla, G. S., & Krishna, C. R. (2024, June). Explainable Edge Computing in a Distributed AI-Powered Autonomous Vehicular Networks. In *2024 IEEE International Conference on Communications Workshops (ICC Workshops)* (pp. 1195-1200). IEEE. DOI: 10.1109/ICCWorkshops59551.2024.10615824

Murthy, C. V. B., & Shri, M. L. (2024, February). Novel Architecture Integrating XAI with Blockchain and IoT Devices for Healthcare. In *2024 Second International Conference on Emerging Trends in Information Technology and Engineering (ICETITE)* (pp. 1-5). IEEE DOI: 10.1109/ic-ETITE58242.2024.10493418

Omidian, H. (2024). Synergizing blockchain and artificial intelligence to enhance healthcare. *Drug Discovery Today*, *29*(9), 104111. DOI: 10.1016/j.drudis.2024.104111 PMID: 39034026

Rahman, M. A., Hossain, M. S., Showail, A. J., Alrajeh, N. A., & Alhamid, M. F. (2021). A secure, private, and explainable IoHT framework to support sustainable health monitoring in a smart city. *Sustainable Cities and Society*, *72*, 103083. DOI: 10.1016/j.scs.2021.103083

Rane, N., Choudhary, S., & Rane, J. (2023). Explainable Artificial Intelligence (XAI) in healthcare: Interpretable Models for Clinical Decision Support. Available at *SSRN* 4637897. DOI: 10.2139/ssrn.4637897

Salama, R., & Ragab, M. (2023). Blockchain with Explainable Artificial Intelligence Driven Intrusion Detection for Clustered IoT Driven Ubiquitous Computing System. *Computer Systems Science and Engineering*, *46*(3), 2917–2932. DOI: 10.32604/csse.2023.037016

Shari, N. F. M., & Malip, A. (2024). Enhancing privacy and security in smart healthcare: A blockchain-powered decentralized data dissemination scheme. *Internet of Things : Engineering Cyber Physical Human Systems*, *27*, 101256. DOI: 10.1016/j.iot.2024.101256

Tagde, P., Tagde, S., Bhattacharya, T., Tagde, P., Chopra, H., Akter, R., Kaushik, D., & Rahman, M. H. (2021). Blockchain and artificial intelligence technology in e-Health. *Environmental Science and Pollution Research International*, *28*(38), 52810–52831. DOI: 10.1007/s11356-021-16223-0 PMID: 34476701

Thiruthuvanathan, M. M., Kumar, K. P., Nasar, N., Swathikiran, K. K., & Joseph, P. M. (2024). Security and privacy aspects in intelligence systems through blockchain and explainable AI. In *XAI Based Intelligent Systems for Society 5.0* (pp. 365–400). Elsevier. DOI: 10.1016/B978-0-323-95315-3.00011-5

Upadhyay, J., Singh, S. K., Kar, N. K., Pandey, M. K., Gupta, P., & Tiwari, P. (2024). Healthcare Data Security Using AI and Blockchain: Safeguarding Sensitive Information for a Safer Society. In *Next-Generation Cybersecurity: AI, ML, and Blockchain* (pp. 159–178). Springer Nature Singapore. DOI: 10.1007/978-981-97-1249-6_8

Williamson, S. M., & Prybutok, V. (2024). Balancing privacy and progress: A review of privacy challenges, systemic oversight, and patient perceptions in AI-driven healthcare. *Applied Sciences (Basel, Switzerland)*, *14*(2), 675. DOI: 10.3390/app14020675

Chapter 4
Blockchain-Based Medicine Supply Chain for Transparent Healthcare Tracking

Rana Muhammad Amir Latif
https://orcid.org/0000-0001-6007-6275
East China Normal University, China

Muhammad Farhan
COMSATS University Islamabad, Sahiwal, Pakistan

Jawad Ahmad
Prince Mohammad Bin Fahd University, Saudi Arabia

Leonardo Mostarda
University of Perugia, Italy

Diletta Cacciagrano
https://orcid.org/0000-0003-4491-0666
University of Camerino, Italy

ABSTRACT

The Medicine Supply Chain (MSC) faces critical challenges in traceability, transparency, and counterfeit prevention. This paper proposes a Blockchain-based solution using Ethereum smart contracts (developed in Solidity, deployed via Truffle, and tested on Rinkeby and localhost networks) to enhance MSC integrity. The framework introduces consumer authentication, Universal Product Code (UPC) registration, and transaction logging to ensure end-to-end drug traceability. By embedding multilingual UPCs (e.g., Urdu, Hindi), the system improves accessibility for diverse healthcare users, who can verify medicine authenticity via QR codes or a dedicated mobile app. The study examines scalability challenges (e.g., managing 100K+ UPCs in large healthcare networks) and evaluates the shifting dynamics among stakeholders (suppliers, processors, retailers). Public Blockchain implementation demonstrates potential for decentralized, tamper-proof record-keeping, though trade-offs in efficiency and adoption barriers persist.

DOI: 10.4018/979-8-3373-0593-6.ch004

1 INTRODUCTION

The US Centre for Disease Control (CDC) predicts that 48 million individuals will become sick with outdated drug use, 128000 people will be treated severely, and three thousand will die per year in the US alone (Sumalatha, Raghuraman, Surya, & Monisha, 2024). The successful control of the quality of medical goods will prevent epidemiological diseases, economic adulteration, and pollution (Agarwal et al., 2022; Qin, Su, Huang, Wiersma, & Liu, 2019). New Blockchain-based systems are essential to track medical goods' consistency and maximize the degree of accessibility of the tracked data to enhance security and reduce waste (Meidute-Kavaliauskiene, Yazdi, & Mehdiabadi, 2022; Moosivand, Ghatari, & Rasekh, 2019).

Blockchain in the supply chain will reduce the scarcity of quality details on actual medical device shipments, resulting in targeted business recalls (Z. Liu & Zhang, 2023). For instance, the corporation must withdraw all medical items within a specific period, where a quality management gap is found along with the MSC (Viegas, Bond, Vaz, & Bertolo, 2019). This restriction prevents the fast extraction of a defeated material at higher MSC speeds (Ahmed, Turki, Baklouti, Dammak, & Alshahrani, 2024; Havaeji, Dao, & Wong, 2023).

A more open approach to data exchange is required to shift past a 'traceability-cantered' or an 'income-centric' supply chain. There is a trade-off between providing the customer with accurate details on a particular commodity and safeguarding the organizational integrity of the MSC. The potential of Blockchain technologies to offer open, safe, and trusted data across both private and public contexts attracted interest through crypto currents (Hu, Chen, He, & Du, 2019).

Companies involved in a supply chain are less likely to exchange data even as knowledge asymmetry has been lowered and inter-organizational cooperation has been enhanced by information and communication technology (ICT) (Dhingra, Raut, Kumar, & Naik, 2024). In such a sense, blockchain is a digital certificate authority that may offer economic and organizational advantages. However, owing to its complexity and the scarcity of usage cases and implementation studies, businesses working in a supply chain appear to have no awareness of blockchain (Adarsh, Joseph, John, Lekshmi, & Asharaf, 2021; Ghadge, Bourlakis, Kamble, & Seuring, 2023). The research is focused on a decentralized coordination system where no single central authority controls the network that is not a central individual. Data is available directly in the general ledger, and a transaction applied to the blockchain after its authentication is feasible for all accepted agencies.

- The benefit of Blockchain technologies in MSC may be extended to enhance the digital data transparency attained by multiple MSC organizations.
- With the introduction of sensor-based data processing systems of Blockchain technology, the whole exposure of medical devices through various supply chain institutions will become a fact.
- The primary benefits of implementing Blockchain technology at MSC include real-time monitoring and sensing, identifying critical bottlenecks, preventing medical product adulteration, identifying low ties on occurrences, assessing the shelf life of medical products, thereby reducing waste, and providing customers with end-to-end information.
- An early version of the research on the Specific ID has been implemented. A Product package collects details concerning the commodity and the MSC that may be added to the unique integrated ID.

Beyond the alarming statistics reported by the CDC, the medical supply chain is fraught with vulnerabilities including fragmented data systems, counterfeit drugs, and inefficient recall processes. These systemic issues demand more than incremental improvement. Blockchain technology, with its capacity for immutable record-keeping, decentralized verification, and smart automation, presents a transformative opportunity to secure, streamline, and digitize the medicine supply chain. This paper explores how blockchain can be leveraged not only to meet modern compliance and safety standards but also to rebuild trust in the healthcare ecosystem.

The paper is further organized so that in the 1st section, we have a detailed introduction related to our manuscript. In the 2nd section, we discuss previous and recent work related to our manuscript with 4 subsections. In the 3rd section, we have 1 section discussing the proposed blockchain model in the Medicine Supply Chain related to our manuscript. In the 4th section, we have 5 sub-sections discussing the case study of blockchain in healthcare. In the 5th section, we have 1 section and 2 subsections discussing blockchain implementation in real-life scenarios. In the 6th section, we have discussed the conclusion. In the last 7th section, we discussed the future work on implementing Blockchain technology in the Medicine Supply Chain network.

2 LITERATURE REVIEW

Extant literature has widely stressed that confidence and knowledge exchange are advantageous to the supply chain's success, especially in a global market with an increased propensity to outsource strategic activities to gain excellent stability and resilience. It has been demonstrated that confidence is also a helpful measure of the supply chain's success and encourages cost savings, excellent stability, and robust organizational governance. Studies usually concentrate on demand and inventory details, which can be seen when evaluating confidence and knowledge exchange in the supply chain (Panda & Satapathy, 2021).

Bitcoin Nakamoto (Nakamoto, 2008) was developed as a digitally distributed digital money infrastructure leveraging Blockchain technologies in 2008. This implementation launched common Blockchain technology recognition and use. Blockchain infrastructure is focused on database technology-driven distributed ledger structures involving collaborative multi-node management, point-to-point exchange, cryptographic algorithms, and consensus-based processes. All the features of Blockchains are looked after: high security, data transparency, decentralization, and immutability, even without a trustworthy intermediary (Latif et al., 2019).

Tracking and tracking in real-time are essential for a cohesive view of global supply chains. Monitoring and tracking are mainly required in project-based organizations where many suppliers are engaged in a single project. This paper proposes a pilot system for real-time tracking and tracing of a cloud-based portal. RFID, IoT, and Blockchain systems establish a series of permanent transactions. The pilot analysis also demonstrates the drawbacks and disadvantages of such a portal method (Jamil, Ahmad, Whangbo, Muthanna, & Kim, 2022).

Blockchain technology provides a range of development areas, especially for managing the supply chain. Several transaction-based processes throughout the supply chain might eliminate intermediary operations. However, the technology's confidence advantages cannot be passed explicitly to SCM without additional requirements. Against this context, the study says active confidence protection among supply chain partners will still be necessary. The study indicates that Blockchain technology can be heavily applicable to SCM before 2035 and offers favorable feedback and exciting opportunities for policymakers in the sector (Kopyto, Lechler, Heiko, & Hartmann, 2020).

Product management significantly affects the efficiency of the supply chain. In sound product control, supply chain knowledge is often essential. Deletion of goods, rationalization, or discontinuation analysis is sometimes ignored as a significant factor. Blockchain technology can help solve smart execution and traceability, accountability, protection, consistency, and smart deployment for commodity deletion decision-making processes. Return to home internet mail. Back to the tab from which we come (Miriam, Doreen, Dahiya, & Rene Robin, 2023).

For supply chain management, these innovations' importance resides in four sectors: greater accountability and traceability, digitization and disintermediation of the supply chain, strengthened cyber protection, and smart contracts. This report discusses many problems, differences in knowledge, and the potential for more study. The configuration of a Blockchain-enabled supply chain has also been discussed from a design viewpoint (Wang, Han, & Beynon-Davies, 2019).

However, devices from the Internet of Things (IoT) are vulnerable to protection threats. Bitcoin has recently emerged as one of the most commonly recognized applications for trustworthy, safe, decentralized smart transport networks. This study aims to encourage logistics and transport by exploring the potential of IoT and IoT technologies (Humayun, Jhanjhi, Hamid, & Ahmed, 2020).

The Internet of Things (IoT) is a crucial driver of intellectual development, including intelligent houses, intelligent communities, and intelligent industries. The rapid growth of IoT-based intelligent applications requires strong protection for data safety, information integrity, and authentication control and maintenance. The study investigates the Internet by incorporating IoT technologies into blockchain for encryption solutions. The study initially centered on the platform's core Blockchain components, forms, and architecture applications. Blockchain's potential strategies for the Internet of Things remain to be decided (Ahmad et al., 2024).

IoT devices have become a fact but are prone to attacks from the defense. Bitcoin has recently been one of the most well-known technologies for safe, trusted, decentralized smart transport systems. This thesis intends to contribute to the logistics and transport sector by analyzing the potential of IoT and IoT technologies in intelligent logistics (Humayun et al., 2020).

Blockchain focuses principally on the financial industry, although some latent sectors, such as healthcare, continue to flourish. In the context of blocks, it is necessary to decentralize patient data, laboratory assessment reports, PhD expectations, and exact knowledge of health care. These blocks may be correlated with the sequence of events in clustered blocks. This method and human involvement should be replaced and substituted to streamline the healthcare sector's focus on patient reports and laboratory examination findings. The new structure is hoped to enhance the healthcare environment in the hospital environment (Latif, Hussain, Jhanjhi, Nayyar, & Rizwan, 2020).

In both fields, blockchain gathers traction. This book includes protocols, problems, protection improvements, applicability, roles, crypto-monetary technology, and production forms. It offers broad enterprise apps with accessible case studies and significant cloud, smart city, and IoT installations. The book highlights the development, state-of-the-art technology, and numerous tools and channels (Al-Marridi, Mohamed, & Erbad, 2024).

In a comprehensive literature analysis, blockchain's assessment process growth and adoption into a decentralized supply chain are crucial study recommendations in the future. The Blockchains can result in the expense, consistency, speed, stability, and gain of reduced risks. They are, therefore, resilient and have some possible effects. Many of these gains and comparative advantages from blockchain are extracted from the supply chain (Latif, Farhan, et al., 2020).

2.1 Research Gap

Despite growing interest in blockchain for supply chain management, existing research lacks practical implementations specifically tailored to the medical supply chain. Few studies explore the integration of Ethereum-based smart contracts with traceability mechanisms like Universal Product Codes (UPC). Moreover, real-world use cases demonstrating end-to-end tracking from production to consumer remain limited. This study addresses these gaps by proposing and testing a blockchain-based medicine traceability model, emphasizing transparency, authenticity, and consumer trust.

2.2 Summary

The author discussed the usage of permission blockchains to track the medicines a pharmaceutical firm uses. The author also mentioned the function that allows recording a patient's response to medication. The author's system enables only trusted actors to join the supply chain network; therefore, these users may only submit data. The author highlighted how counterfeit medications are wreaking havoc on the healthcare system and how blockchain technology might aid in establishing a medical supply chain that runs from producer to consumer. The author proposes utilizing blockchain technology with an encrypted QR code imprinted on a medication. In his article, the author attempted to describe the intricacies of a medical supply chain. The most critical entity in a medical supply chain, a pharmaceutical firm, faces many risks that may jeopardize the quality and quantity of medication. The author argued that disclosing information about medication from the manufacturer to the consumer may assist in eradicating fraud. The author has suggested a scenario-based drug tracking and authentication system, dubbed Drug Ledger, built on peer-to-peer blockchain technology. The author discussed segmenting service components into three distinct parts. He also disclosed the methods used to determine the logic of the medication supply chain.

2.3 Existing Systems in Blockchain

The current FSC management system derives from the product's web-based architecture. Food items are built on cloud architecture with a centralized mediator server to control and verify the many actions. As Figure 1 shows, the cloud-enabled Medicine Supply Chain Management System is also not particularly safe as it cannot guarantee customers end-to-end security since many intermediaries are involved.

Figure 1. Traditional Supply Chain Model illustrating the flow of goods and information from suppliers to end customers.

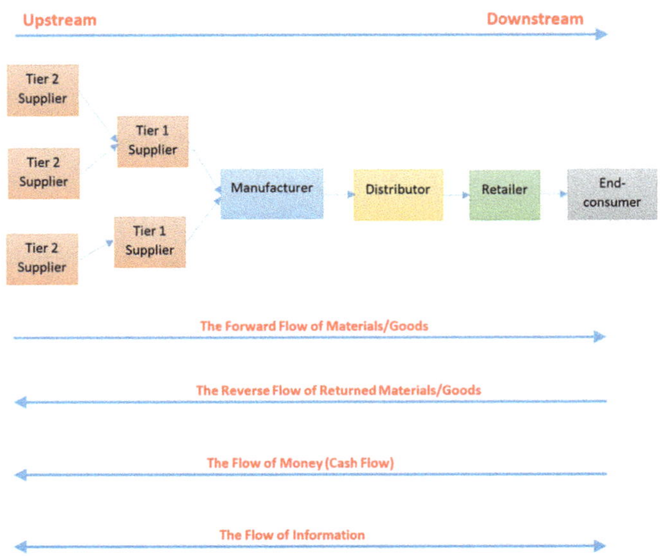

3 THE BLOCKCHAIN PLATFORM

A Blockchain platform is also a distributed publication with a digital currency structure listing all the crypto-currency transactions. Server-based solutions do not call for a central host to manage the Blockchain platform and to keep a comprehensive transaction history (Huang & Al Foysal, 2021); it is like a peer-to-peer (P2P) system. Supporting Satoshi Nakamoto's first real digital money in 2009, known as "Bitcoin," cryptography and the Blockchain platform would be the backbone technologies. On the other hand, it preserves a copy of the Blockchain Platform, therefore offering a shared archive on all nodes or entities of this system for torrent sharing of papers (Sabri, Harchi, & El Kamoun, 2022).

Every block in a Blockchain system consists of a public and a private key. Every transaction has information enough to identify the sender, time, asset information, sender, and recipient pertinent to the past ones. In a supply chain, a commodity may be a contract between a seller or buyer or a product (Adrian Gheorghe & Unal Tatar, 2021). With the public key and the pertinent material, the Secure Hash Algorithm 256 (SHA-256) generates a hexadecimal 16-digit collection known as the "hash." The generated hash blends original public key data with transaction (Shah, Verma, Sharma, Sampat, & Kulkarni, 2023) information. One element is the series of transactions. Decoding the encrypted information helps to confirm the transaction and source. Transactional data will be decoded only by sheer force. Miners are the nodes that verify these transactions; mining is the settling mechanism. Should the gadget generate an untested transaction block (Govindan, Nasr, Saeed Heidary, Nosrati-Abarghooee, & Mina, 2023), miners may verify the transaction into a cryptographical hash solution. Unlike other Blockchain systems, such Hyster edger networks, and Ethereum, Bitcoin runs on "proof of work." Consensus algorithms help explain the choice of a mining method. Three basic elements define a block on a Blockchain network: a hash, a single digital key, a timestamp, and the hash of the previous block to track account balance. The hash of this latest block is linked so that every block is jointly updated or launched by two authorized blocks, therefore defending against any block (Saha, Rathore, Parida, & Rana, 2022).

The Blockchain system marks the instant a transaction is validated. For a Blockchain network such as Bitcoin, a significant change in the recorded transaction value presents a difficulty. An attacker must get at least 51% of the total processing capacity of the database system easily available (F. Ali, Aloqaily, Alfandi, & Ozkasap, 2020). Thus, the complete Blockchain network is strengthened, and the past block is confirmed for every upgrade. As Figure 2 shows, this procedure prevents disruptive behavior and offers the necessary quality of immutability on the Blockchain Network.

Figure 2. The functioning of the Blockchain platform, demonstrating the chain of blocks and their interconnections through hashes, where each block contains its hash and the previous block's hash.

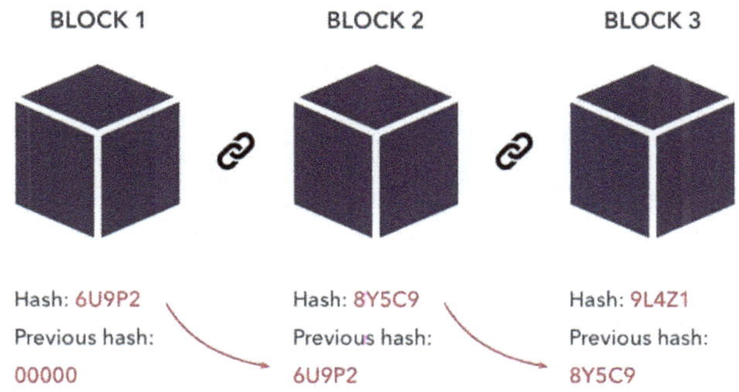

Miners are rewarded with Bitcoins according to the amount of computing power they generate. The hashing algorithm transforms the dilemma periodically by changing the minimum and maximum hash value (nonce). Miners appear to obtain too many Bitcoins, especially when electricity is measured as completely new users combine (Pablo et al., 2022) because of the value of new Blocks. The amounts of hash speed exist at PH/s (10^{15}), as shown in Figure 3. It continues to expand. Therefore, this curve is relative to Bitcoin's buying price pattern over the past nine months. A comparison between the two charts is seen in the network when more users link to this system (Quayson, Avornu, & Bediako, 2024). The problem of resolving hash is-. The standard Bitcoin Block Search time now begins at 18 zero; it also takes about 9.8 minutes to use the total network power of any mine operator on the system, as shown in Figure 4.

Figure 3. Last year graph Bitcoin Cash Hash rate historical chart (bitinfocharts, 2024)

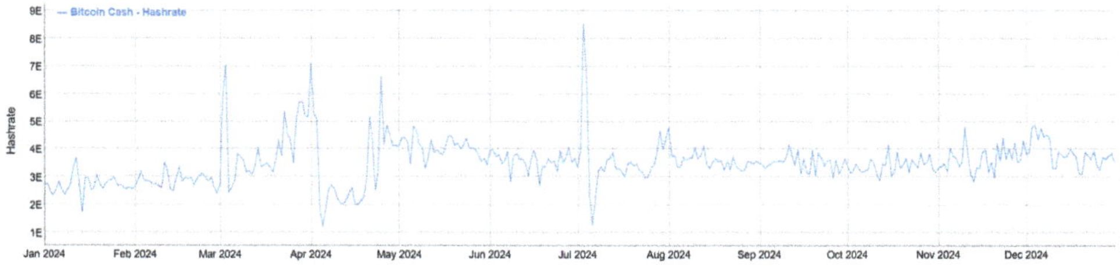

Figure 4. Bitcoin (BTC) price per day from April 6, 2022 to December 30, 2024 (statista, 2024)

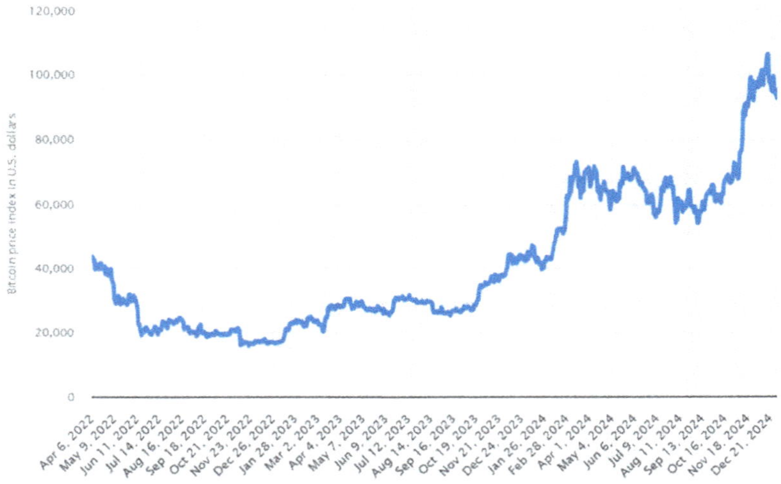

3.1 Supply Chains, Transparency, and Sustainability with Blockchain Technology

The TOE theory of the system is a theory at the organizational level that explains the adoption of decisions by three sections of the market background. The technical, operational, strategic, and environmental facets of these three components affect technological advancement and the growth of businesses. This structure was broadened to incorporate the introduction of the IT supply chain (Chattu, 2021).

Sustainability is an essential context for the climate, and we consider transparency one of disruptive technologies' most important attributes. Literature analysis indicates a spectrum of sustainable qualities has been used in previous research to discuss sustainability's natural, fiscal, operational, technical, and social facets. Because of the lack of specific exposure to different confidentiality considerations, some of these characteristics are less important for judging transformative Blockchain technologies (Senna et al., 2021). By the openness of the supply chain, Blockchains boost environmental efficiency. Furthermore, the elements of transparency are included in our attributes chart.

Transparency implies the degree to which knowledge is freely available in interaction and external observers, as well as in operational and environmental contexts. In the supply chain, flexibility applies to freely accessible knowledge inside a supply chain for end consumers and businesses (Saha, Rathore, & Gigi, 2021). In light of the new world of 'contribution fewer' correlated with Blockchains, openness will likely be a critical supply chain performance indicator.

Lack of accountability will contribute to many problems in the supply chain, particularly in matters of financial, environmental, and social responsibility. Goods are being used to produce, develop, distribute, and market across an extensive network of extractor firms, dealers and marketers, transporters, storage facilities, and other service providers (Alyami, Rahman, & Yadlapalli, 2023). Sharing more knowledge regarding sources of goods and procedures is difficult because of this importance and uncertainty.

There is little analysis of how supply chains, particularly sustainability, may quickly assess and pick precise Blockchain technologies. When supply chain operators start appreciating possibilities, changes are more likely to be made in the efficiency and durability of the supply chain. We recommend that there should be three aspects of sufficient supply chain transparency:

- The number of transparencies: including factors such as the knowledge involvement degree in the Supply Chain Participant, mode of activity, environmental and social supply chain details
- Product accountability such as commodity materials monitoring (i.e., raw material sources), commodity phase monitoring (from sources to end client), product environmental knowledge tracking (e.g., carbon recovery and emissions)
- Accountability of participants, clear criteria for participants' activities, knowledge about the circumstance and their sustainability

Firstly, organizations and supplier partners must be active in the supply chain to succeed. Provision chain openness is a significant problem, significantly above one stage of the system, as most businesses have little to no knowledge regarding second and third-tier providers themselves (Ganesan, Devi, Kumar, & Gayathri, 2022). In comparison, consumers can not accurately recognize product or service attributes, e.g., Product protection, since environmental expertise is missing in the supply chain transparency.

Secondly, accountability is associated with the monitoring and traceability of goods and the supply chain. It will involve the raw material sources, providing the background for a finished product or service. Tracking goods will give customers more trust that the items are legitimate, good quality, and ethical standards are pursued. The advantage of this openness element would improve buyer trust and raise the ability to buy a commodity substantially (Sneha, Panjwani, Lade, Randolph, & Vickery, 2021). Monitoring inventory cycles and evaluating commodity production details and network mechanisms will often allow businesses in the supply chain to realize if an inventory is incorrect, wrongly handled, or inappropriately controlled from a scheduling point of view. Tracking knowledge on product sustainability has been an essential method for encouraging green consumption. It gives customers a more in-depth view of the commodity life cycle and the product's and operation's impact.

Thirdly, there are many possible detrimental effects across all supply chain stakeholders' actions and environments, such as manufacturing problems and delays, immoral and unlawful procedures, environmental pressures, loss of resources, slave labor, and unsafe industrial conditions. In recent decades, numerous accidents have left perceived vulnerability and stability to supply chain networks (Omar et al., 2021). Several supply chain processes and situations must also be monitored, such as legal and environmental issues.

Introducing modern technologies in the supply chain networks is not straightforward because the complexities of incorporation are some of the biggest obstacles. Information and information technologies may satisfy specific criteria from a supply chain inclusion viewpoint. Blockchain would have a far-reaching effect on supply chains to meet essential standards. Blockchain would have a far-reaching effect on supply chains to meet essential standards (Chiacchio et al., 2022).

- Blockchains may boost product and process reliability and traceability to control nearly all data rates, date, place, consistency, qualification, and other related details.
- Blockchains provide smoother and cheaper transfers, meaning that the multiple parties satisfy their commitments by utilizing smart contracts, almost in a less faithful fashion.

- Thanks to this paperwork, Blockchain technology can minimize paperwork and bureaucracy.
- Blockchain will reduce future risks from errors, confusion, and exchange in grey markets.
- Blockchain may establish more significant ties between the stakeholders and the supply chain.

These attributes influence the literature's criteria and inter-agency selection variables for information technology. Inclusion: expense, time, adaptability, fairness and interoperability, processing capability, scalability, protection, efficiency, involvement, and supporting partners. We also have an outline of these technological features of inter-organizational IT evaluation.

3.2 Challenges Of the Blockchain in The Field of Medicine

Mostly, a centralized organization controls the existing medical supply chain system, which is untrustworthy. Below, we highlighted several problems connected to the current system.

- In a centralized organization or a single company, it is thought that the medical supply chain is intrinsically difficult to identify, manage, and update any magic button that will assist in eliminating inefficiencies to save costs.
- For its supply chain, it accounts for around 25% of the pharmaceutical cost. In addition, medical equipment costs up to 40%. The supply chain costs about $230 billion each year.
- It is difficult to gather reliable statistics for a centralized organization such as Fairtrade. Since a particular company controls the data, other stakeholders cannot monitor the route of medications and are, therefore, unable to optimize manufacturing and storage. Even a modest improvement may thus settle a big amount.
- In addition, depending on one entity gives it tremendous control over sensitive data. Furthermore, it creates the possibility of fraud, corruption, falsified medicines, and a single failure point.
- Finally, the customer must only rely on the third-party organization's approved logos.

4 BLOCKCHAIN IN MSC BASED ON UNIVERSAL PRODUCT CODE (UPC) MODEL

A shop is where the object is kept after development in the business. A carrier is a firm that carries the product to a particular area from a shop. In any emergency user, the user may still have the cover on the commodity in question. Importers often import medicines to market these medicines in the countries at a high cost, where only one object can be purchased in a massive volume. Wholesalers and retailers operate at a limited level every day. They are following the import into the nation of the products. Wholesalers procure the merchandise and market it at a wholesale rate to consumers. In March and some other local stores identified by a government or private corporation, this seller will scale this item at any cost. The consumer may use a shared key to search for RFID, QR codes, and any mechanical gadget. Also, the customer may get statistics on the commodity from the whole distribution region and even verify the price. Check the object details on the expiration date. Additionally, the client receives an inspection of the item before payment, a machine-generated SMS, and detailed information about the item and transaction, as shown in Figure 5.

Figure 5. Universal Product Code (UPC) based Product traceability model for blockchain

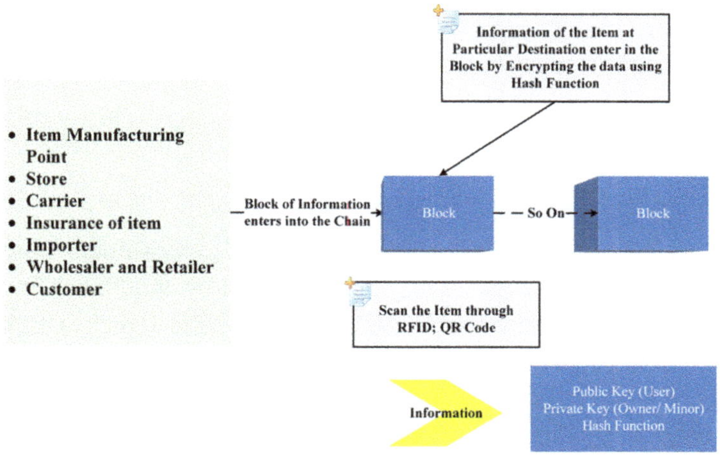

5 THE CASE STUDY OF BLOCKCHAIN IN HEALTHCARE

Today, awareness is transforming the healthcare industry. Sellers strive to strengthen their customer base and raise options for the market by relying on customized importations. The Blockchain system will help shops meet their targets economically. The blockchain from the healthcare sector will provide traders with plenty of help to progress their industry procedures to improve their enterprise and explain other methods (Jraisat, Jreissat, Upadhyay, & Kumar, 2023).

5.1 Medicine Supply Chain

Tracking shipments is an essential part of the delivery chain. Blockchain can be used to report shipping details during each tracking point, such as location, time and date, the handling of shipments, person details, fever, and product status. It allows one to determine whether the shipment has been handled accurately; it often happens on schedule in every area (Vatambeti, Krishna, Karthik, & Damera, 2024). It would also help the dealers find the facilities and goods that have been destroyed or missing on the market. Note that an official listing of this distribution sequence would enable the shops to identify the exact basis and difficulties of the products. Blockchain-related exchanges are often planned to allow vendors in the Blockchain public ledger (Yaqoob, Salah, Jayaraman, & Al-Hammadi, 2022) to buy and sell from each other and vendors (Al-Sumaidaee, Alkhudary, Zilic, & Swidan, 2023).

5.2 Customer Profiling

Blockchain may be used to gather customer-related data and to determine trend positioning. The knowledge forecasts the location and tacit product specifications to boost their trouble-free warehouse (Wan & Huang, 2023). Once again, retailers utilize Blockchain technologies to create sophisticated data management procedures, as the knowledge is invisibly backed by various analytical tools (S. Liu, Zhang,

Liu, & Shi, 2023). At delivery, the risk of illegal fiscal exchange would be minimized by blockchain. Since blockchain holds all companies, organizations can calculate costs in real time if appropriate. Price considerations, cash return, customized retail pricing deals, and other consumer cost supplies can be analyzed along with relevant supplies that a real-time base may exchange with them (Mahammad & Kumar, 2023).

5.3 Transparency

The knowledge stored in the blockchain is undoubtedly useful to consumers, stores, and manufacturers, and the stock of goods likely to be accessed may all be created by child labor. In the event of secret or unsafe pieces, the facilities and products enable retailers/Consumers to pick. This increased openness of blockchain is expected to be much more suitable for consumer behavior (Hasan et al., 2022).

5.4 Authenticity and Anti-Counterfeiting

A person may use blockchain to validate the authenticity of the object. Customers will then move through the paperwork to grant counterfeiting a massive degree of trust in the item's caliber. It can improve consumer faith (Debnath et al., 2023).

5.5 Loyalty

By retaining encoded customer data certificates, promotions, and coupons, blockchain will re-enhance the rewards policy and even get details from most shops, providing more detailed consumer documents (Centobelli, Cerchione, Del Vecchio, Oropallo, & Secundo, 2022). A Blockchain loyalty pledge will also encourage consumers to show their devotion at a specified position around the suppliers. The blockchain mentioned above processes will contribute to greater consumer loyalty, better customs purchasing, more procured companies, and more significant revenue for their merchants (Centobelli et al., 2022).

6 IMPLEMENTATION OF THE BLOCKCHAIN

The flowchart illustrates the process of managing medicine traceability through Blockchain technology. It begins with the registration of a new farm, followed by various stages like the collection of raw medicine, raw product lifecycle management, and the creation of a new medicine. The product is then packed, listed for sale, and can be sold if a buyer's offer exceeds the set price. The process continues with shipping the medicine to the new owner, who can either sell or consume the product. This flowchart emphasizes the role of blockchain in improving medicine traceability and securing transactions within the supply chain. The foundation of this paper is based on using Ethereum smart contracts, developed in solidity and tested on the 'rinkeby' test-net, as shown in Figure 6.

Figure 6. The flow chart of the implementation of the Blockchain in Medicine Supply Chain

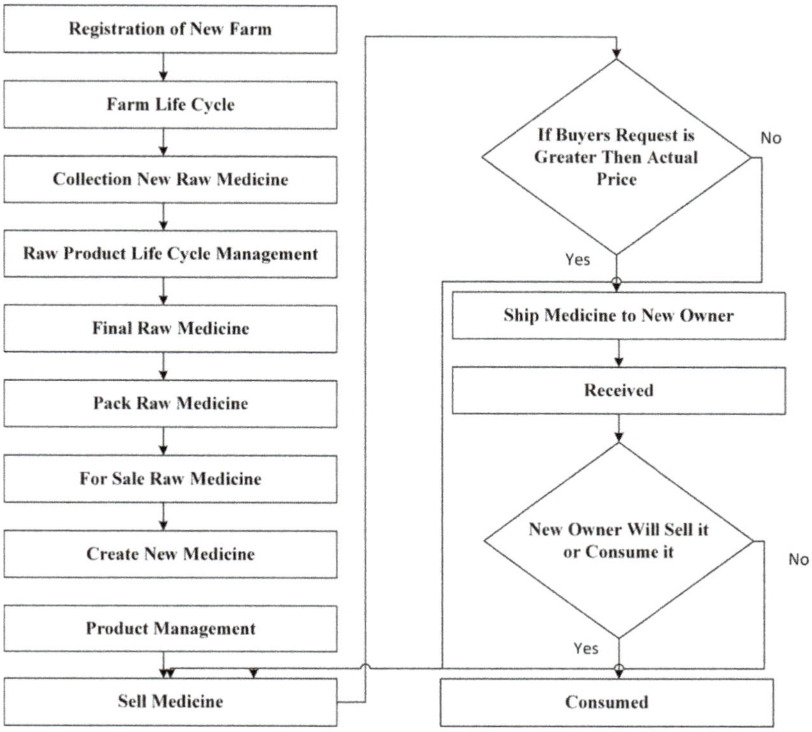

6.1 Basic Algorithm to Add One UPC in Blockchain

```
Basic algorithm to add one UPC in Blockchain
contract Consumer Role is Ownable {
using Roles for Roles Role;
event Consumer Added (address indexed account);
event Consumer Removed (address indexed account);
Roles Role private consumers;
constructor () public {
add consumer (message sender);}
modifier only consumer () {
require (is the consumer (message sender), 'Caller is not a consumer.');}
a function is Consumer (address account) public view returns (bool) {
return consumers has (account);}
function add consumer (address account) public only Owner {
add consumer (account);}
function renounce consumer () public only Owner {
remove consumer (message sender);}
function add consumer (address account) internal {
```

consumers add (account);
emit Consumer Added (account);}
function remove consumer (address account) internal {
consumers remove(account);
emit Consumer Removed (account);}}

6.2 User Login Creation in Blockchain

The user authentication process for accessing a blockchain network is depicted through eight key steps. The process begins with users entering their email and unlocking patterns on the mobile app. The mobile app generates a new Ethereum login address, which is then confirmed by the authentication server. The wallet website then prepares the transaction and sends it to the Ethereum network via MetaMask. Once the transaction is confirmed, the user is granted access to the network. These authentication measures, shown in Figure 7, ensure secure login using Ethereum-based identification. The account ID for the logged-in user is **0xca35b7d915458ef540ade6068dfe2f44e8fa733c**.

Figure 7. The login phase authentication steps for getting access to the Blockchain network

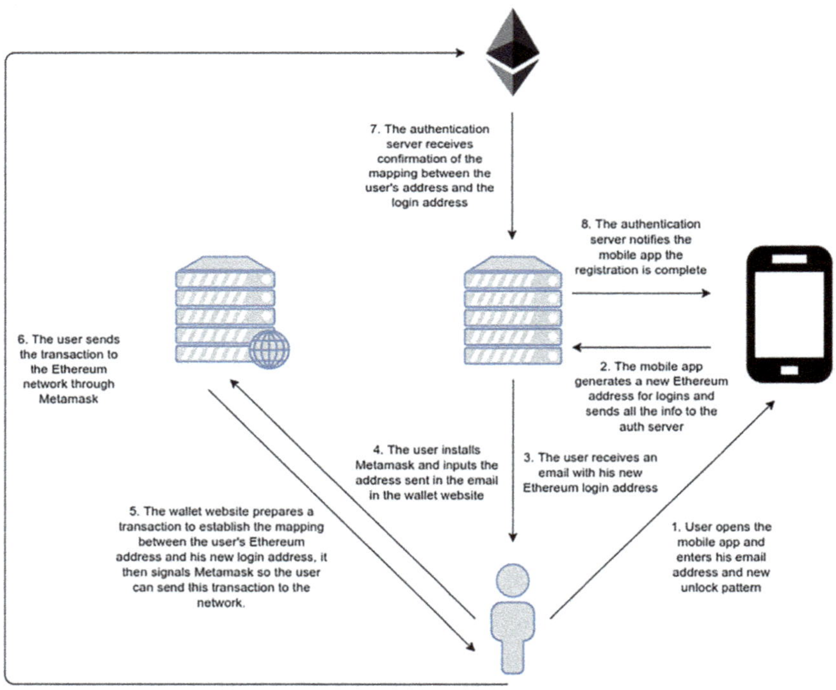

After successfully logging in, the user (the medicine owner) can register a new farm by entering essential details, such as the farm name, description, and location. The Universal Product Code (UPC) links the medicine item to the blockchain, allowing it to be tracked. Upon clicking the 'Register' button, a MetaMask popup appears, asking the user to confirm the transaction. The transaction details, including the gas fee, are shown in the popup, ensuring secure interaction with the blockchain network. This process is illustrated in Figure 8.

Figure 8. The Medicine Owner requests to register a new Farm in SC

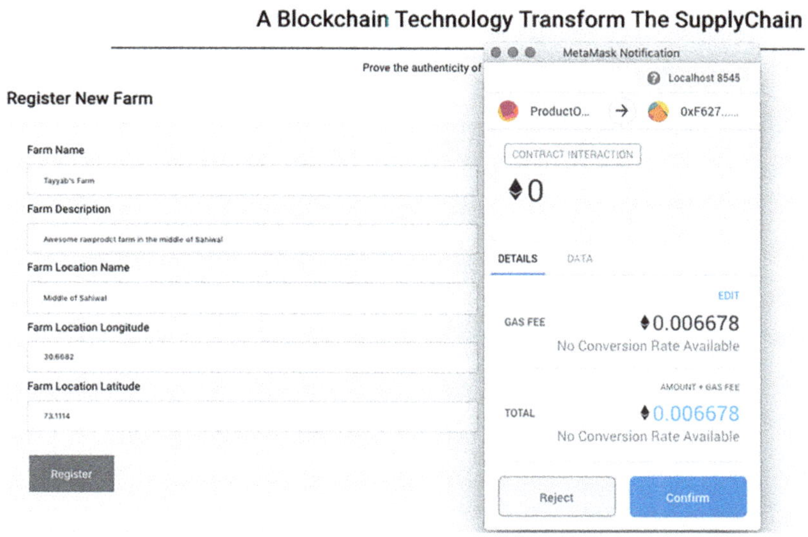

After confirming the transaction, a new farm with a unique ID is registered on the blockchain. The medicine owner can view details of all registered farms by entering the specific farm ID. The farm details include the name, location, latitude, longitude, and owner's address. Additionally, after the transaction is completed, the status, transaction hash, and gas price are shown, providing transparency regarding the transaction process. These updates are recorded in a single block on the blockchain, as illustrated in Figure 9.

Figure 9. The details of a Transaction

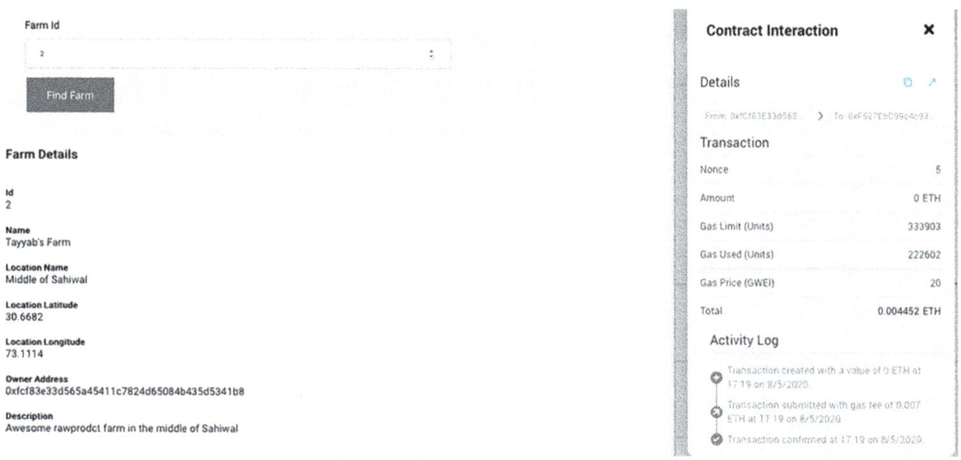

The process of managing the raw product lifecycle is demonstrated, starting with the registration of the farm and adding details about the raw product (e.g., name, vintage year, and notes). After the farm registration, the next steps, such as harvesting, packing, and listing the raw product for sale, are carried out through blockchain transactions. The transaction details on the right show MetaMask interacting with the Ethereum network for confirmation. The status of the raw product is updated as 'for sale,' as depicted in the raw product lifecycle management section, and the transaction history is recorded for transparency. These processes are further illustrated in Figure 10.

Figure 10. Harvesting, Packing, and adding for sale raw product

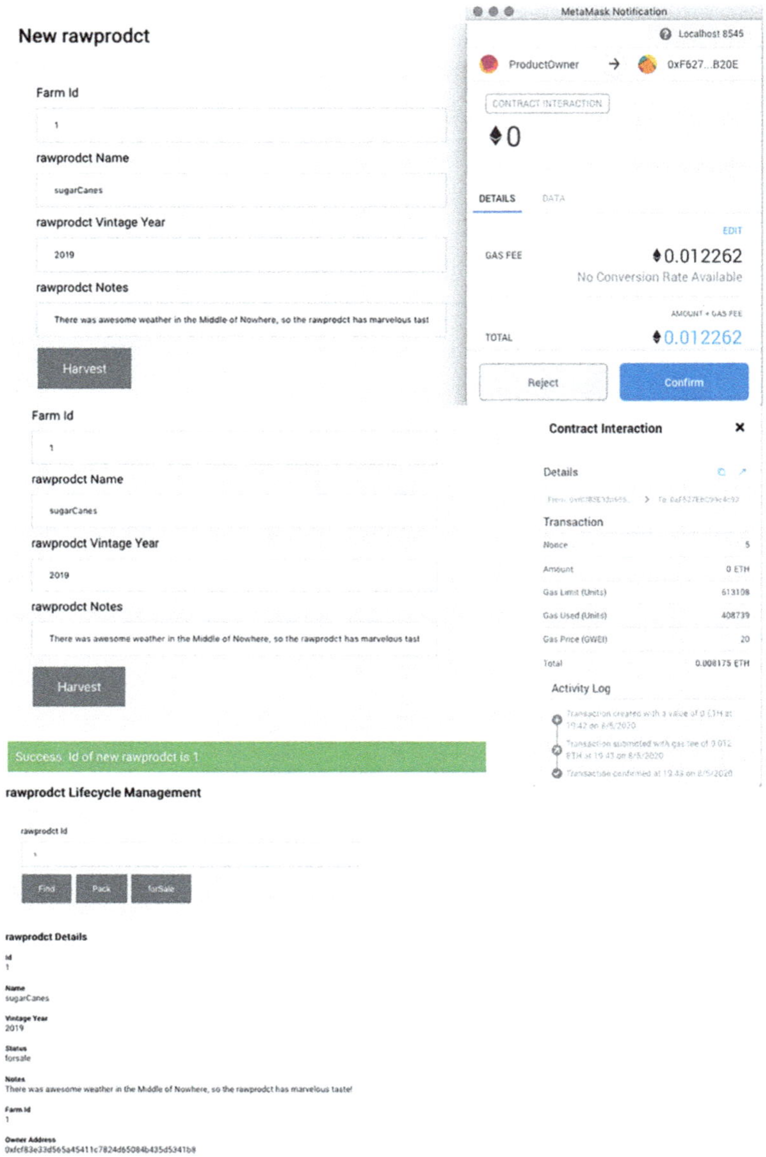

Once the raw medicine is sent to the central manufacturing unit, the product owner can create a new medicine by entering its details into the system. The owner can also find the medicine by its UPC when it is ready for further processing. Blockchain tracks this process to ensure that all product details, like ownership and transaction history, are securely recorded and accessible. The transaction details are displayed in the contract interaction section, confirming the product's creation and current status. This process is illustrated in Figure 11.

Figure 11. Creating medicines and finding them through their UPC

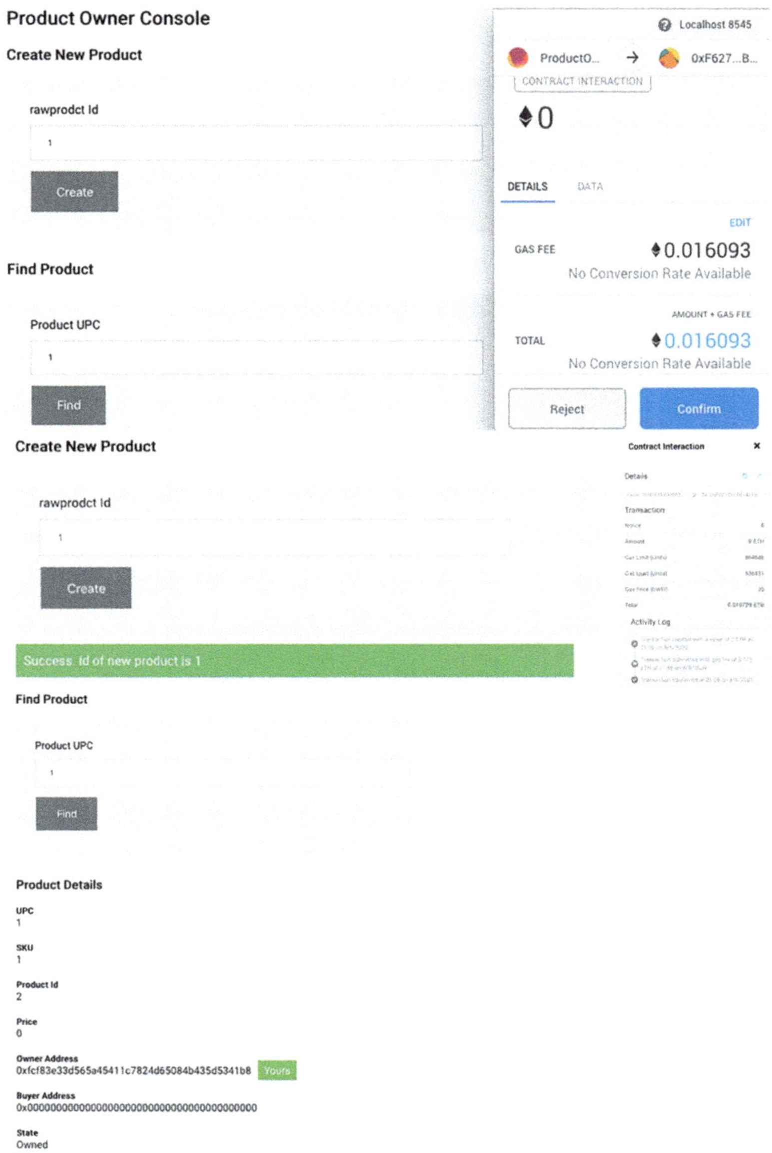

In this image, the medicine owner lists the product for sale by entering the product UPC and setting the price. The product is successfully added to the marketplace upon clicking the' Sell' button, as indicated by the message ‘ success. Products with UPC = 1 is now For sale in green. The transaction details, including the gas fee and transaction confirmation, are recorded on the blockchain, ensuring transparency. This process is depicted in Figure 12.

Figure 12. Medicine added for sale

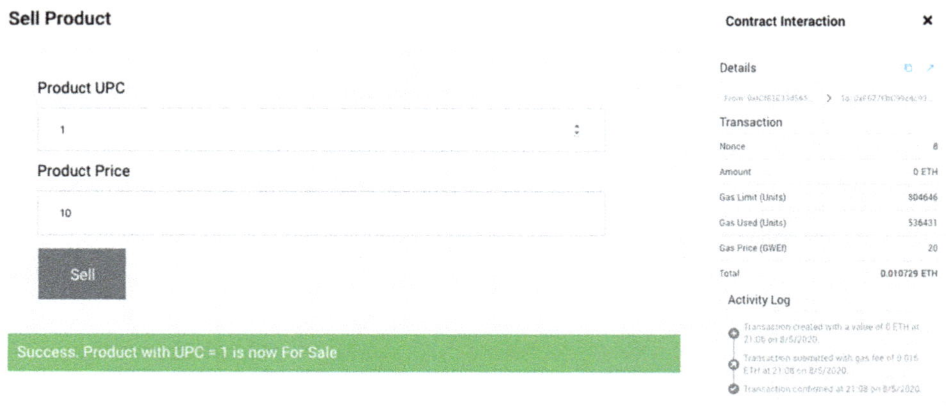

The buyer searches for available medicines for sale and enters a bid for a specific product by inputting the Product UPC and their offer. The transaction is completed if the buyer’s bid exceeds the set price. The successful transaction is confirmed with the message ‘ success. The product with UPC = 1 is now Sold’, as shown in green. The transaction details, including the amount, gas limit, gas used, and total gas fee, are recorded in the blockchain, ensuring transparency. This process is illustrated in Figure 13.

Figure 13. Medicine is sold to the buyer.

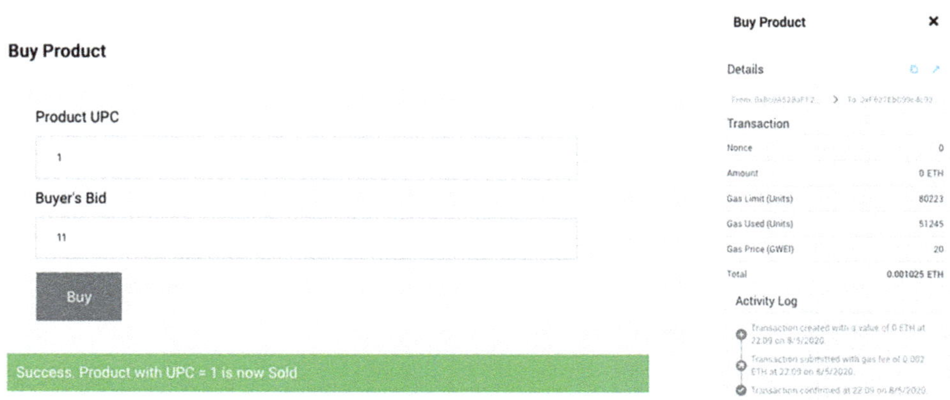
Buy Product
Product UPC
1
Buyer's Bid
11
Buy
Success. Product with UPC = 1 is now Sold
Buy Product
Details
Transaction
Nonce
0
Amount
0 ETH
Gas Limit (Units)
80223
Gas Used (Units)
51245
Gas Price (GWEI)
20
Total
0.001025 ETH
Activity Log

Figure 14 The process of managing a product is demonstrated. First, the medicine is shipped to the buyer, as indicated by the 'Ship' button. Once the buyer receives the product, the status updates to reflect that the buyer now owns the product. The buyer can then either sell or consume the product. The transactions are tracked, showcasing the entire journey of the product, from shipment to consumption or resale.

Figure 14. Shipping to buyer, receiving, and consuming of buyer

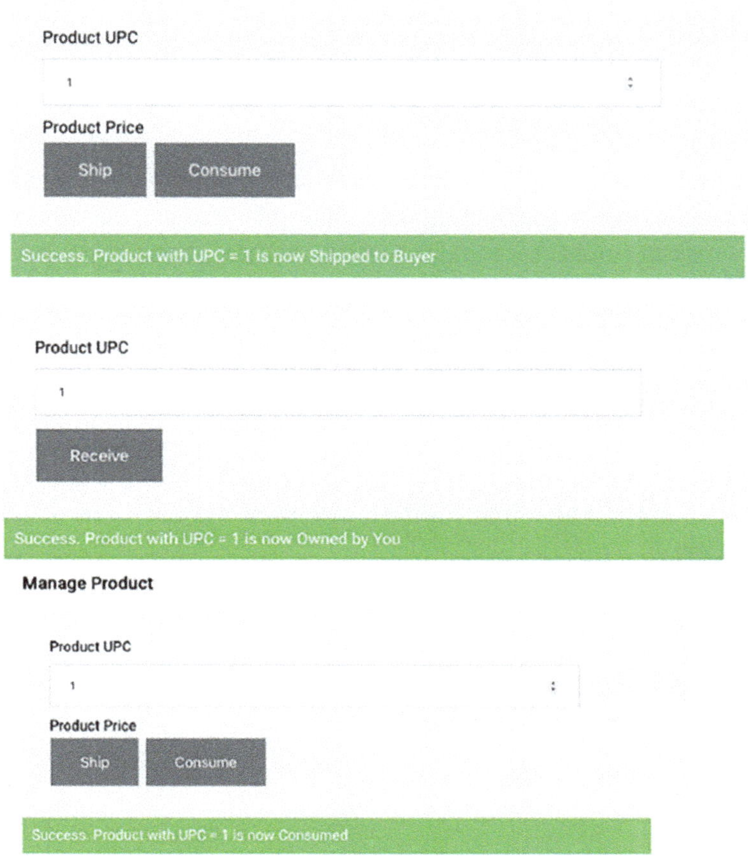

Figure 15 shows the transaction history for a supply chain process, detailing various stages of a product's lifecycle. Each entry corresponds to a specific action, such as harvesting, packing, sale, and consumption, with unique transaction hashes. This blockchain-based tracking ensures transparency and traceability throughout the supply chain.

Figure 15. Transaction History

Transaction History

- FarmRegistered - 0x456661e18077861d84034fc0b923a867aacbe25dc3a2f4b8034667506be5866a
- RawprodctHarvested - 0xc9e77e1cadd793c7212bcd890c7d99f8dc1e804fba20e3f292b31fb28ef00a37
- RawprodctPacked - 0xca344935009764433525b355582d5fcae7ae88c1ff04c3712b8c09e56f6a5f9d
- RawprodctforSaled - 0x7acc181bf514062fc6048dce42e6e07561816f9c146cf811219506920f85b01f
- ProductOwned - 0x38653fcc0d90492c967f8782059e6abc8e59a7827362fec1e0472799a9bd0b1c
- ProductForSale - 0x278d7a1de54f3af5a700964ec9a4f6b863333bc65b0e4a45f3f5a545fe05de98
- ProductSold - 0x57643f91edae99a60c25e15b3170cc7f32a219f33aad7e7a7040067745544c85
- ProductShipped - 0x7de8803efb253dfd9c80e682c506e6956680f3b9b6e71b67e07ca7e342a43f03
- ProductOwned - 0xc1cb66c9b11392406a2ad3c2d5dec0bdbbacabae5752070c488d4aa7bfbe7a19
- ProductConsumed - 0x349df56ecebce1a12b792979126f4f01fc1721ff8c1e79dac1e73f6dcb6087c4

Figure 16 displays a blockchain-detectable barcode label for a product, which includes essential information like the product name, production date, enterprise name, and website. The barcode and QR code enable easy tracking and access to product details through the blockchain system. This label ensures efficient product traceability within the supply chain.

Figure 16. Blockchain-detectable barcode label for a product

Bar Code:

(01)01234567890128supplychain-product

Product Name: Product

Product Date: 5/4/2020

Enterprise Name: XXXX

Website: XXXXXXXXX

7 CONCLUSION

In this research, we developed a Blockchain model implemented in solidity to create an Ethereum smart contract. We utilized Truffle for development and tested the smart contracts on the 'localhost' and 'rinkeby' tenets. While other testnets are available, 'rinkeby' was chosen for this study. The proposed supply chain model highlights the advantages and limitations of Blockchain technology in asset traceability compared to traditional tracking systems. Consumers can use QR codes to access detailed information about products before they are blocked in the network, fostering consumer confidence and potentially increasing customer loyalty and revenue. The balance of power between processors and retailers may shift through Blockchain implementation. Future research could explore the scalability of Blockchain systems, especially in managing a vast number of items, such as UPCs, in a large healthcare setting. This paper aims to offer valuable insights for supply chain professionals on how blockchain could disrupt existing supply chain models and address challenges to its implementation. Future work may include integrating quality control reports for each batch of medication, using embedded chips for regular location and temperature updates, and expanding the system to cover additional medical supplies.

REFERENCES

Adarsh, S., Joseph, S. G., John, F., Lekshmi, M., & Asharaf, S. (2021). A Transparent and Traceable Coverage Analysis Model for Vaccine Supply-Chain Using Blockchain Technology. *IT Professional*, *23*(4), 28–35. DOI: 10.1109/MITP.2021.3094194

Adrian Gheorghe, F. S. A. P., & Unal Tatar, O. F. K. (2021). Blockchain for a Resilient, Efficient, and Effective Supply Chain: Evidence from Cases. In: Acquisition Research Program.

Agarwal, U., Rishiwal, V., Tanwar, S., Chaudhary, R., Sharma, G., Bokoro, P. N., & Sharma, R. (2022). Blockchain technology for secure supply chain management: A comprehensive review. *IEEE Access : Practical Innovations, Open Solutions*, *10*, 85493–85517. DOI: 10.1109/ACCESS.2022.3194319

Ahmad, A. Y. B., Verma, N., Sarhan, N., Awwad, E. M., Arora, A., & Nyangaresi, V. O. (2024). An IoT and Blockchain-Based Secure and Transparent Supply Chain Management Framework in Smart Cities Using Optimal Queue Model. *IEEE Access : Practical Innovations, Open Solutions*, *12*, 51752–51771. DOI: 10.1109/ACCESS.2024.3376605

Ahmed, I., Turki, M., Baklouti, M., Dammak, B., & Alshahrani, A. (2024). Towards an Optimized Blockchain-Based Secure Medical Prescription-Management System. *Future Internet*, *16*(7), 243. DOI: 10.3390/fi16070243

Ahram, T., Sargolzaei, A., Sargolzaei, S., Daniels, J., & Amaba, B. (2017). *Blockchain technology innovations*. Paper presented at the 2017 IEEE Technology & Engineering Management Conference (TEMSCON). DOI: 10.1109/TEMSCON.2017.7998367

Al-Marridi, A. Z., Mohamed, A., & Erbad, A. (2024). Optimized blockchain-based healthcare framework empowered by mixed multi-agent reinforcement learning. *Journal of Network and Computer Applications*, *224*, 103834. DOI: 10.1016/j.jnca.2024.103834

Al-Sumaidaee, G., Alkhudary, R., Zilic, Z., & Swidan, A. (2023). Performance analysis of a private blockchain network built on Hyperledger Fabric for healthcare. *Information Processing & Management*, *60*(2), 103160. DOI: 10.1016/j.ipm.2022.103160

Ali, A., Almaiah, M. A., Hajjej, F., Pasha, M. F., Fang, O. H., Khan, R., Teo, J., & Zakarya, M. (2022). An industrial IoT-based blockchain-enabled secure searchable encryption approach for healthcare systems using neural network. *Sensors (Basel)*, *22*(2), 572. DOI: 10.3390/s22020572 PMID: 35062530

Ali, F., Aloqaily, M., Alfandi, O., & Ozkasap, O. (2020). Cyberphysical Blockchain-Enabled Peer-to-Peer Energy Trading. *arXiv*, arXiv: 2001.00746.

Alyami, A., Rahman, S., & Yadlapalli, A. (2023). The Effect of Blockchain Technology on Hospital Supply Chain Performance. Paper presented at the Proceedings of the International Conference on Industrial Engineering and Operations Management.

Centobelli, P., Cerchione, R., Del Vecchio, P., Oropallo, E., & Secundo, G. (2022). Blockchain technology for bridging trust, traceability and transparency in circular supply chain. *Information & Management*, *59*(7), 103508. DOI: 10.1016/j.im.2021.103508

Chattu, V. K. (2021). A Review of Artificial Intelligence, Big Data, and Blockchain Technology Applications in Medicine and Global Health. *Big Data and Cognitive Computing*, *5*(3), 41. DOI: 10.3390/bdcc5030041

Chiacchio, F., D'Urso, D., Oliveri, L. M., Spitaleri, A., Spampinato, C., & Giordano, D. (2022). A non-fungible token solution for the track and trace of pharmaceutical supply chain. *Applied Sciences (Basel, Switzerland)*, *12*(8), 4019. DOI: 10.3390/app12084019

Debnath, B., Shakur, M. S., Bari, A. M., Saha, J., Porna, W. A., Mishu, M. J., Islam, A. R. M. T., & Rahman, M. A. (2023). Assessing the critical success factors for implementing industry 4.0 in the pharmaceutical industry: Implications for supply chain sustainability in emerging economies. *PLoS One*, *18*(6), e0287149. DOI: 10.1371/journal.pone.0287149 PMID: 37319165

Dhingra, S., Raut, R., Kumar, M., & Naik, B. K. R. (2024). Factors impacting Indian healthcare supply chain performance and influence in the public and private sector: The mediating role of blockchain technology adoption. *Benchmarking*. Advance online publication. DOI: 10.1108/BIJ-10-2023-0687

Ganesan, R., Devi, T., Kumar, S. R., & Gayathri, N. (2022). Securing Healthcare Information Using Blockchain Technology: A Deep Insight. In *Blockchain Security in Cloud Computing* (pp. 253-263): Springer. DOI: 10.1007/978-3-030-70501-5_12

Ghadge, A., Bourlakis, M., Kamble, S., & Seuring, S. (2023). Blockchain implementation in pharmaceutical supply chains: A review and conceptual framework. *International Journal of Production Research*, *61*(19), 6633–6651. DOI: 10.1080/00207543.2022.2125595

Govindan, K., Nasr, A. K., Saeed Heidary, M., Nosrati-Abarghooee, S., & Mina, H. (2023). Prioritizing adoption barriers of platforms based on blockchain technology from balanced scorecard perspectives in healthcare industry: A structural approach. *International Journal of Production Research*, *61*(11), 3512–3526. DOI: 10.1080/00207543.2021.2013560

Hasan, K., Chowdhury, M. J. M., Biswas, K., Ahmed, K., Islam, M. S., & Usman, M. (2022). A blockchain-based secure data-sharing framework for Software Defined Wireless Body Area Networks. *Computer Networks*, *211*, 109004. DOI: 10.1016/j.comnet.2022.109004

Havaeji, H., Dao, T.-M., & Wong, T. (2023). Supervised learning by evolutionary computation tuning: An application to blockchain-based pharmaceutical supply chain cost model. *Mathematics*, *11*(9), 2021. DOI: 10.3390/math11092021

Hu, H., Chen, K., He, J., & Du, L. (2019). Whole cycle disruption analysis of petroleum supply chain (PSC) based on UASNs monitoring. *EURASIP Journal on Wireless Communications and Networking*, *2019*(1), 119. DOI: 10.1186/s13638-019-1426-0

Huang, G., & Al Foysal, A. (2021). Blockchain in Healthcare. *Technology and Investment*, *12*(3), 168–181. DOI: 10.4236/ti.2021.123010

Humayun, M., Jhanjhi, N., Hamid, B., & Ahmed, G. (2020). Emerging Smart Logistics and Transportation Using IoT and Blockchain. *IEEE Internet of Things Magazine*, *3*(2), 58–62. DOI: 10.1109/IOTM.0001.1900097

Jamil, F., Ahmad, S., Whangbo, T. K., Muthanna, A., & Kim, D.-H. (2022). Improving blockchain performance in clinical trials using intelligent optimal transaction traffic control mechanism in smart healthcare applications. *Computers & Industrial Engineering*, *170*, 108327. DOI: 10.1016/j.cie.2022.108327

Jraisat, L., Jreissat, M., Upadhyay, A., & Kumar, A. (2023). *Blockchain technology: The role of integrated reverse supply chain networks in sustainability.* Paper presented at the Supply chain forum: An international journal. DOI: 10.1080/16258312.2022.2090853

Kopyto, M., Lechler, S., Heiko, A., & Hartmann, E. (2020). Potentials of blockchain technology in supply chain management: Long-term judgments of an international expert panel. *Technological Forecasting and Social Change*, *161*, 120330. DOI: 10.1016/j.techfore.2020.120330

Latif, R. M. A., Farhan, M., Rizwan, O., Hussain, M., Jabbar, S., & Khalid, S. (2020). Retail level Blockchain transformation for product supply chain using truffle development platform. *Cluster Computing*, •••, 1–16.

Latif, R. M. A., Hussain, K., Jhanjhi, N., Nayyar, A., & Rizwan, O. (2020). A remix IDE: Smart contract-based framework for the healthcare sector by using Blockchain technology. *Multimedia Tools and Applications*, •••, 1–24.

Latif, R. M. A., Iqbal, S., Rizwan, O., Shah, S. U. A., Farhan, M., & Ijaz, F. (2019). *Blockchain transforms the retail level by using a supply chain rules and regulation.* Paper presented at the 2019 2nd International Conference on Communication, Computing and Digital systems (C-CODE).

Liu, S., Zhang, R., Liu, C., & Shi, D. (2023). P-PBFT: An improved blockchain algorithm to support large-scale pharmaceutical traceability. *Computers in Biology and Medicine*, *154*, 106590. DOI: 10.1016/j.compbiomed.2023.106590 PMID: 36736098

Liu, Z., & Zhang, X. (2023). Multimedia and multimodal sensing with edge computing for personalized healthcare supply chain system data optimization. *Personal and Ubiquitous Computing*, *27*(3), 955–972. DOI: 10.1007/s00779-022-01679-9

Mahammad, A. B., & Kumar, R. (2023). *Scalable and security framework to secure and maintain healthcare data using blockchain technology.* Paper presented at the 2023 International Conference on Computational Intelligence and Sustainable Engineering Solutions (CISES). DOI: 10.1109/CISES58720.2023.10183494

Meidute-Kavaliauskiene, I., Yazdi, A. K., & Mehdiabadi, A. (2022). Integration of blockchain technology and prioritization of deployment barriers in the blood supply chain. *Logistics (Basel)*, *6*(1), 21. DOI: 10.3390/logistics6010021

Miriam, H., Doreen, D., Dahiya, D., & Rene Robin, C. (2023). Secured Cyber Security Algorithm for Healthcare System Using Blockchain Technology. *Intelligent Automation & Soft Computing*, *35*(2).

Moosivand, A., Ghatari, A. R., & Rasekh, H. R. (2019). Supply Chain Challenges in Pharmaceutical Manufacturing Companies: Using Qualitative System Dynamics Methodology. *Iranian Journal of Pharmaceutical Research : IJPR*, *18*(2), 1103. PMID: 31531092

Nakamoto, S. (2008). Bitcoin. *A peer-to-peer electronic cash system, 21260.*

Omar, I. A., Jayaraman, R., Debe, M. S., Salah, K., Yaqoob, I., & Omar, M. (2021). Automating procurement contracts in the healthcare supply chain using blockchain smart contracts. *IEEE Access : Practical Innovations, Open Solutions*, *9*, 37397–37409. DOI: 10.1109/ACCESS.2021.3062471

Pablo, R.-G. J., Roberto, D.-P., Victor, S.-U., Isabel, G.-R., Paul, C., & Elizabeth, O.-R. (2022). Big data in the healthcare system: A synergy with artificial intelligence and blockchain technology. *Journal of Integrative Bioinformatics*, *19*(1), 20200035. DOI: 10.1515/jib-2020-0035 PMID: 34412176

Panda, S. K., & Satapathy, S. C. (2021). Drug traceability and transparency in medical supply chain using blockchain for easing the process and creating trust between stakeholders and consumers. *Personal and Ubiquitous Computing*, •••, 1–17.

Qin, X., Su, Q., Huang, S. H., Wiersma, U. J., & Liu, M. (2019). Service quality coordination contracts for online shopping service supply chain with competing service providers: Integrating fairness and individual rationality. *Operations Research*, *19*(1), 269–296. DOI: 10.1007/s12351-016-0288-z

Quayson, M., Avornu, E. K., & Bediako, A. K. (2024). Modeling the enablers of blockchain technology implementation for information management in healthcare supply chains. *Modern Supply Chain Research Applications*(ahead-of-print).

Sabri, Y., Harchi, S., & El Kamoun, N. (2022). Managing health supply chain using blockchain technology: State of art challenges and solution. *International Journal of Reconfigurable Embedded Systems*, *11*(3), 258. DOI: 10.11591/ijres.v11.i3.pp258-264

Saha, E., Rathore, P., & Gigi, A. (2021). Utilizing Blockchain Technology to Manage Functional Areas in Healthcare Systems. In *The Big Data-Driven Digital Economy: Artificial and Computational Intelligence* (pp. 125-139): Springer. DOI: 10.1007/978-3-030-73057-4_11

Saha, E., Rathore, P., Parida, R., & Rana, N. P. (2022). The interplay of emerging technologies in pharmaceutical supply chain performance: An empirical investigation for the rise of Pharma 4.0. *Technological Forecasting and Social Change*, *181*, 121768. DOI: 10.1016/j.techfore.2022.121768

Senna, P., Reis, A., Dias, A., Coelho, O., Guimarães, J., & Eliana, S. (2021). Healthcare supply chain resilience framework: Antecedents, mediators, consequents. *Production Planning and Control*, •••, 1–15.

Shah, Y., Verma, Y., Sharma, U., Sampat, A., & Kulkarni, V. (2023). *Supply chain for safe & timely distribution of medicines using blockchain & machine learning.* Paper presented at the 2023 5th International Conference on Smart Systems and Inventive Technology (ICSSIT). DOI: 10.1109/ICSSIT55814.2023.10061049

Sneha, S., Panjwani, A., Lade, B., Randolph, J., & Vickery, M. (2021). Alleviating Challenges Related to FDA-Approved Medical Wearables Using Blockchain Technology. *IT Professional*, *23*(4), 21–27. DOI: 10.1109/MITP.2021.3072535

statista. (2024). Bitcoin (BTC) price per day from April 6, 2022 to December 30, 2024 Retrieved from https://www.statista.com/statistics/326707/bitcoin-price-index/

Sumalatha, M., Raghuraman, D., Surya, S., & Monisha, V. (2024). *Secured Blockchain Technology for Medical Supply Chain (SB-MSC)*. Paper presented at the 2024 International Conference on Advances in Data Engineering and Intelligent Computing Systems (ADICS). DOI: 10.1109/ADICS58448.2024.10533582

Tseng, L., Yao, X., Otoum, S., Aloqaily, M., & Jararweh, Y. (2020). Blockchain-based database in an IoT environment: Challenges, opportunities, and analysis. *Cluster Computing*, *23*(3), 1–15. DOI: 10.1007/s10586-020-03138-7

Vatambeti, R., Krishna, E. P., Karthik, M. G., & Damera, V. K. (2024). Securing the medical data using enhanced privacy preserving based blockchain technology in Internet of Things. *Cluster Computing*, *27*(2), 1625–1637. DOI: 10.1007/s10586-023-04056-0

Viegas, C. V., Bond, A., Vaz, C. R., & Bertolo, R. J. (2019). Reverse flows within the pharmaceutical supply chain: A classificatory review from the perspective of end-of-use and end-of-life medicines. *Journal of Cleaner Production*, *238*, 117719. DOI: 10.1016/j.jclepro.2019.117719

Wan, Y., & Huang, H. (2023). Adoption and optimization of blockchain technology in the regulation of Class II vaccines. *IEEE Access : Practical Innovations, Open Solutions*, *11*, 84607–84619. DOI: 10.1109/ACCESS.2023.3301772

Wang, Y., Han, J. H., & Beynon-Davies, P. (2019). Understanding blockchain technology for future supply chains: A systematic literature review and research agenda. *Supply Chain Management*, *24*(1), 62–84. DOI: 10.1108/SCM-03-2018-0148

Yaqoob, I., Salah, K., Jayaraman, R., & Al-Hammadi, Y. (2022). Blockchain for healthcare data management: Opportunities, challenges, and future recommendations. *Neural Computing & Applications*, *34*(14), 1–16. DOI: 10.1007/s00521-020-05519-w

Chapter 5
Blockchain-Based Supply Chain Management in Healthcare

Rana Hassam Ahmed
https://orcid.org/0009-0009-7259-3283
The University of Faisalabad, Pakistan

Majid Hussain
The University of Faisalabad, Pakistan

Ashraf Khalil
College of Technological Innovation, Zayed University, UAE

ABSTRACT

Blockchain technology has emerged as a transformative solution for enhancing transparency, security, and efficiency in supply chain management, particularly in the healthcare sector. This paper explores the application of blockchain for improving pharmaceutical supply chains by ensuring the traceability of medicines from manufacturing to end-user delivery. By leveraging decentralized and immutable ledger systems, the proposed solution mitigates the risks of counterfeit drugs and enhances trust among stakeholders. Additionally, the integration of blockchain with Internet of Things (IoT) devices provides real-time monitoring of storage conditions and ensures product integrity. The system also prevents dispensing errors in pharmacies through QR code-based verification, addressing challenges posed by similar-sounding drug names. The study discusses the technical framework, implementation challenges, and the potential of blockchain to revolutionize healthcare logistics, improve patient safety, and increase operational efficiency in pharmaceutical supply chains.

1. INTRODUCTION

Supply chain management in healthcare is a critical and multifaceted process that ensures the effective delivery of medical products, devices, and services to patients while maintaining safety and reliability. It involves a series of interconnected stages, including procurement of raw materials, manufacturing of pharmaceuticals and medical devices, storage under appropriate conditions, and distribution to healthcare providers and end-users. This system ensures that essential items such as life-saving drugs, vaccines,

DOI: 10.4018/979-8-3373-0593-6.ch005

diagnostic equipment, and medical devices are delivered where they are needed, when they are needed, and in the required quantities. The ultimate goal of healthcare supply chain management is to maintain the quality and efficacy of products, ensure timely delivery to patients, and minimize wastage, particularly for perishable items like biologics and vaccines. The intricacy of this process arises from the involvement of diverse stakeholders such as manufacturers, distributors, hospitals, clinics, pharmacies, regulators, and even patients. The reliability and efficiency of this interconnected network are paramount, as any disruption or inefficiency can lead to delays, increased costs, or even life-threatening outcomes for patients. Despite its undeniable importance, traditional healthcare supply chains are plagued by numerous challenges that compromise their effectiveness. One of the most pressing issues is the lack of transparency, which hinders the ability to trace the origin, movement, and handling of products throughout their journey. This opacity fosters inefficiencies and undermines trust among stakeholders, such as manufacturers, healthcare providers, and regulators. The lack of a clear view into the supply chain also makes it vulnerable to counterfeit medicines, a widespread problem that disproportionately affects developing regions. According to global estimates, counterfeit drugs make up a significant portion of the pharmaceutical market, posing severe risks to patient health and safety. Additionally, traditional supply chains often rely on outdated manual processes and fragmented systems that fail to communicate effectively with one another. These inefficiencies lead to delays, increased operational costs, and missed opportunities for optimization. The sector also faces stringent compliance requirements that vary across jurisdictions, adding layers of complexity to operations. Moreover, sensitive items like vaccines and biologics require controlled storage and transport conditions; deviations from these conditions frequently result in significant product loss and waste. Isolated data systems further exacerbate these issues, as they limit the ability of stakeholders to collaborate and share critical information in real-time.

Blockchain technology emerges as a revolutionary solution to these long-standing challenges, offering the potential to transform healthcare supply chains. At its core, blockchain is a distributed ledger technology that records transactions securely, transparently, and immutably across a decentralized network. This means that no single entity has control over the data, and once information is recorded, it cannot be altered or deleted. Blockchain's transparency ensures that all participants in the supply chain have access to the same accurate and up-to-date information, fostering trust and collaboration. One of its most powerful features is the ability to implement smart contracts, which are self-executing agreements with predefined rules that automate processes such as payment releases, inventory updates, and regulatory compliance checks. These capabilities make blockchain particularly well-suited to addressing inefficiencies, vulnerabilities, and fragmentation in healthcare supply chains. The application of blockchain in healthcare supply chains is transformative, with benefits that directly address critical pain points. Blockchain enhances traceability by creating an immutable digital record of every product's journey, from the manufacturer to the end-user. This level of accountability ensures that stakeholders can verify the authenticity and integrity of products at every stage. Counterfeit medicines, a global menace, can be effectively combated using blockchain's ability to assign unique identifiers to products, making it nearly impossible for fake goods to infiltrate the system. Compliance with regulatory requirements is another area where blockchain excels, as it provides an auditable and tamper-proof record of transactions and activities. Furthermore, when integrated with IoT devices, blockchain enables real-time monitoring of sensitive products like vaccines, ensuring that temperature and storage conditions are maintained throughout transit. By addressing these challenges, blockchain technology has the potential to revolutionize healthcare supply chain management, creating a system that is more transparent, secure, and efficient, ultimately leading to better patient outcomes and stronger stakeholder trust.

1 KEY COMPONENTS OF BLOCKCHAIN IN SUPPLY CHAIN MANAGEMENT:

1.1 Decentralised Ledger and Transparency

A decentralized ledger is the core component of blockchain technology, offering a revolutionary approach to data management by storing information across a network of nodes instead of relying on a single centralized authority. Each node in this network maintains an identical copy of the ledger, ensuring that no single entity has control over the data. This decentralized structure eliminates the risks of data tampering, fraud, and system failure, as changes to the ledger require consensus from the network. In the healthcare supply chain, this feature is particularly valuable because it enhances trust, ensures data integrity, and provides resilience against disruptions(Aisha Nabiyeva et al., 2017). Transparency is another defining characteristic of decentralized ledgers, as every transaction recorded on the blockchain is time-stamped, immutable, and visible to all authorized participants. This creates a single source of truth, where stakeholders, such as manufacturers, distributors, regulators, and healthcare providers, can access real-time, verifiable data without intermediaries. For example, the movement of a pharmaceutical product from the manufacturer to the end user can be tracked step by step, offering full visibility into its origin, handling, and storage conditions. This level of transparency fosters trust among stakeholders and enhances collaboration across the supply chain(Sarkar, 2022b). In healthcare, the decentralized ledger is especially useful for tackling challenges like counterfeit medicines and maintaining product quality. By assigning unique identifiers to products and recording their journey on the blockchain, stakeholders can verify authenticity and ensure compliance with regulatory standards. For sensitive items like vaccines, IoT devices can monitor storage conditions such as temperature and humidity, with the data being securely recorded on the blockchain. Additionally, regulators benefit from the ability to access tamper-proof, auditable records, simplifying compliance checks and ensuring quality assurance(Cheung et al., 2011). The decentralized ledger and its transparency address critical inefficiencies in traditional healthcare supply chains. By providing a secure, trustworthy, and collaborative framework, blockchain enhances supply chain management, improves product safety, and fosters confidence among all participants.

Figure 1.

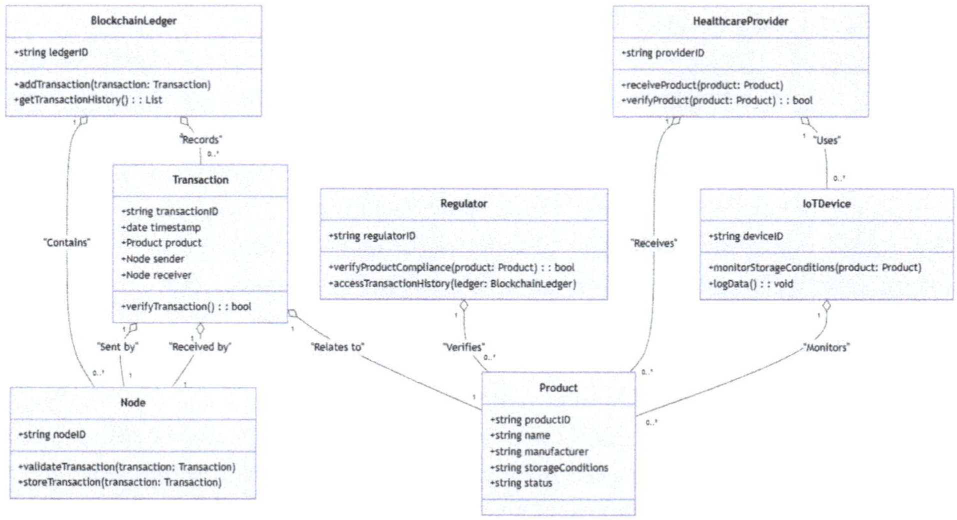

1.2 Smart Contracts for Automation

Smart contracts are self-executing agreements embedded in blockchain technology, where the terms of the contract are written directly into code. These contracts automatically execute predefined actions when specified conditions are met, without the need for intermediaries or manual intervention. In the context of healthcare supply chains, smart contracts streamline processes, enhance efficiency, and reduce errors by automating critical operations. For example, in the procurement and distribution of pharmaceuticals, a smart contract can be programmed to release payments automatically when a shipment is delivered and verified. This eliminates delays caused by manual payment processing and ensures that transactions are completed promptly and transparently(Deng et al., 2022). Similarly, in regulatory compliance, smart contracts can validate and log adherence to storage conditions for sensitive items like vaccines. If an IoT sensor records a temperature deviation, the smart contract can trigger alerts or halt further distribution, preventing compromised products from reaching patients(Pisani et al., 2021). Smart contracts also enable seamless collaboration among stakeholders. Manufacturers, distributors, and healthcare providers can operate under a unified, automated system where responsibilities and conditions are clearly defined and enforced. This reduces the risk of disputes and fosters trust among participants. Additionally, by eliminating intermediaries, smart contracts reduce operational costs and improve the overall efficiency of the supply chain(Agbo et al., 2019). The automation provided by smart contracts transforms healthcare supply chains into more reliable and secure systems. By ensuring that actions are executed precisely as intended and without delays, smart contracts enhance transparency, accountability, and efficiency, ultimately contributing to better patient care and streamlined operations(Abbas et al., 2023).

Figure 2.

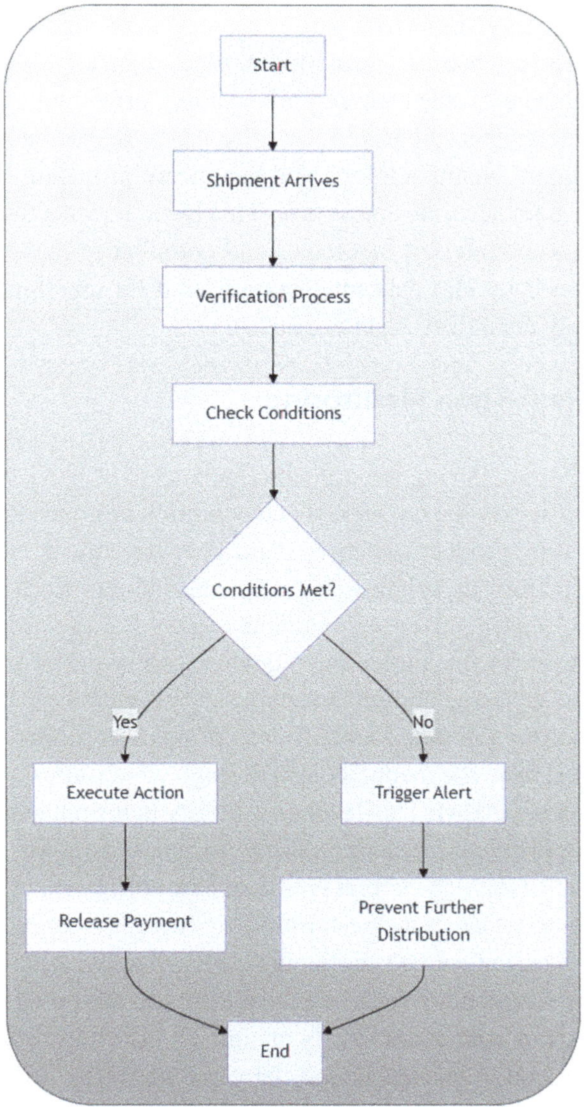

1.3 Cryptographic Security and Data Integrity

Cryptographic security and data integrity are fundamental features of blockchain technology, ensuring that the data stored and shared within the network is secure, accurate, and tamper-proof. Cryptographic techniques, such as hashing and digital signatures, play a critical role in maintaining the confidentiality and authenticity of transactions. Each block in the blockchain is linked to the previous one using a cryptographic hash, creating a secure chain of data where any attempt to alter one block would invalidate the entire chain. This immutability ensures that the information recorded on the blockchain remains reliable and resistant to unauthorized modifications. In healthcare supply chains, cryptographic security safeguards sensitive information such as product specifications, transaction records, and patient data(Jabeen et al., n.d.; Zahid et al., 2023)(Maariz et al., 2024). For instance, digital signatures verify the identities of stakeholders, ensuring that only authorized parties can access or modify specific data. This reduces the risk of fraud and unauthorized access. Furthermore, blockchain's hashing mechanisms ensure data integrity by detecting any changes to the recorded information, providing an additional layer of security(Peng et al., 2020). By leveraging cryptographic security, blockchain enhances trust and accountability among stakeholders. Regulators, manufacturers, and healthcare providers can confidently rely on the system's data, knowing it is both accurate and secure. This level of protection is particularly critical for addressing challenges such as counterfeit medicines and compliance with strict regulatory standards. Ultimately, cryptographic security and data integrity are vital for creating a transparent, secure, and trustworthy healthcare supply chain(Saxena et al., 2020).

1.4 Traceability and Real-Time Monitoring

Traceability and real-time monitoring are crucial components of blockchain technology, providing enhanced visibility and control over the movement and condition of goods throughout the supply chain. Traceability ensures that every product, whether it's a pharmaceutical, medical device, or vaccine, can be tracked at every step from its origin to the final destination. Each transaction and transfer is recorded on the blockchain, creating a secure, immutable record of the product's journey. This digital trail enables stakeholders to verify the authenticity, quality, and origin of a product, addressing issues such as counterfeit goods and ensuring compliance with safety regulations. In healthcare, traceability is especially important for ensuring the safety and efficacy of medical products. For example, a pharmaceutical product can be traced from the manufacturer, through wholesalers, to healthcare providers, and ultimately to patients(Yele et al., 2024). This level of visibility helps prevent the entry of counterfeit or expired products into the supply chain, reducing risks to patient health(Tariq et al., n.d.). Additionally, blockchain's integration with IoT devices enables real-time monitoring, allowing stakeholders to track the condition of sensitive products such as vaccines or biologics during storage and transport. Data such as temperature, humidity, and handling can be continuously recorded, with any deviation triggering alerts to prevent potential damage or spoilage. Together, traceability and real-time monitoring not only enhance the security and transparency of healthcare supply chains but also improve operational efficiency. By ensuring that products are stored, transported, and delivered according to strict standards, blockchain enables stakeholders to respond quickly to potential issues, reducing delays, waste, and costs while ensuring the safety and quality of healthcare products(Hossain et al., 2021).

2 APPLICATIONS OF BLOCKCHAIN IN HEALTHCARE SUPPLY CHAINS

2.1 Pharmaceutical Supply Chains

Blockchain technology offers significant advantages in pharmaceutical supply chains, addressing major challenges like counterfeit medicines, product traceability, and regulatory compliance. One of the key applications of blockchain in this area is **Counterfeit Medicine Detection**. Counterfeit drugs are a global issue that jeopardizes patient safety and undermines the trust in the healthcare system. Blockchain enables the creation of a transparent, tamper-proof record for each pharmaceutical product, from manufacturing to distribution. By assigning a unique identifier, such as a QR code or RFID tag, to each product, blockchain makes it nearly impossible for counterfeit drugs to enter the supply chain undetected. Every transaction or transfer of the product is recorded on the blockchain, allowing stakeholders to verify its authenticity at any point, ensuring that patients receive genuine medicines. Another important application in pharmaceutical supply chains is **Drug Traceability from Manufacturer to End User**. Blockchain ensures complete traceability of pharmaceuticals, providing a secure and auditable record of the product's journey. This traceability is critical for verifying the origin and quality of medicines, particularly in complex global supply chains. It allows healthcare providers and regulators to track drugs from the manufacturer, through distributors, and all the way to the pharmacy or healthcare provider that dispenses them. This transparency helps prevent theft, diversion, or fraud and ensures that drugs meet safety and quality standards at every step(Li et al., 2022).

Figure 3.

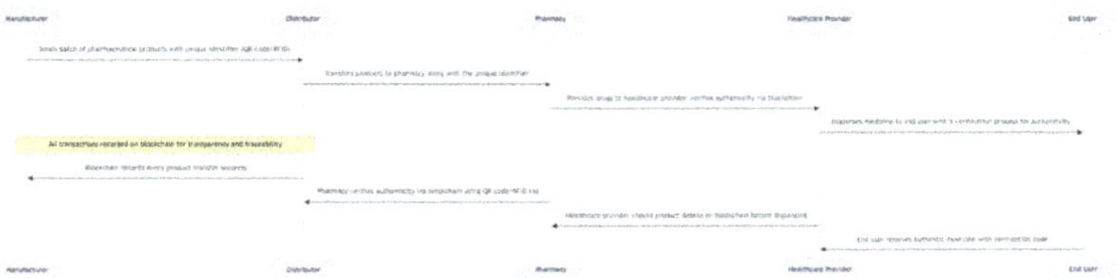

2.2 Vaccine Distribution

Vaccine distribution, especially in the case of life-saving vaccines, requires careful handling and strict adherence to temperature and storage conditions. Blockchain plays a crucial role in maintaining **Cold Chain Integrity**. Vaccines are highly sensitive to temperature fluctuations, and improper storage can render them ineffective or even harmful. Blockchain, when integrated with IoT devices that monitor temperature, can record and verify the conditions under which vaccines are stored and transported(Ahad et al., 2021). Each vaccine dose can be tracked with a unique identifier, and its temperature data is securely recorded on the blockchain. If any deviations from the required cold chain conditions occur, alerts can be triggered in real-time, preventing the use of compromised vaccines.

Real-Time Tracking and Monitoring is another essential application in vaccine distribution. With blockchain, every stage of the vaccine's journey—whether from the manufacturer to the distributor or from the distributor to the healthcare provider—can be monitored in real time. Blockchain records every transaction and transfer, and real-time data from IoT sensors provide visibility into the storage conditions of the vaccines. This ensures that stakeholders are constantly aware of the vaccine's status, helping to quickly identify and resolve issues such as delays, theft, or contamination. The integration of blockchain with real-time monitoring systems offers a comprehensive solution for the efficient and safe distribution of vaccines, particularly in critical global vaccination efforts(Lou et al., 2021; Mertz, 2018).

Figure 4.

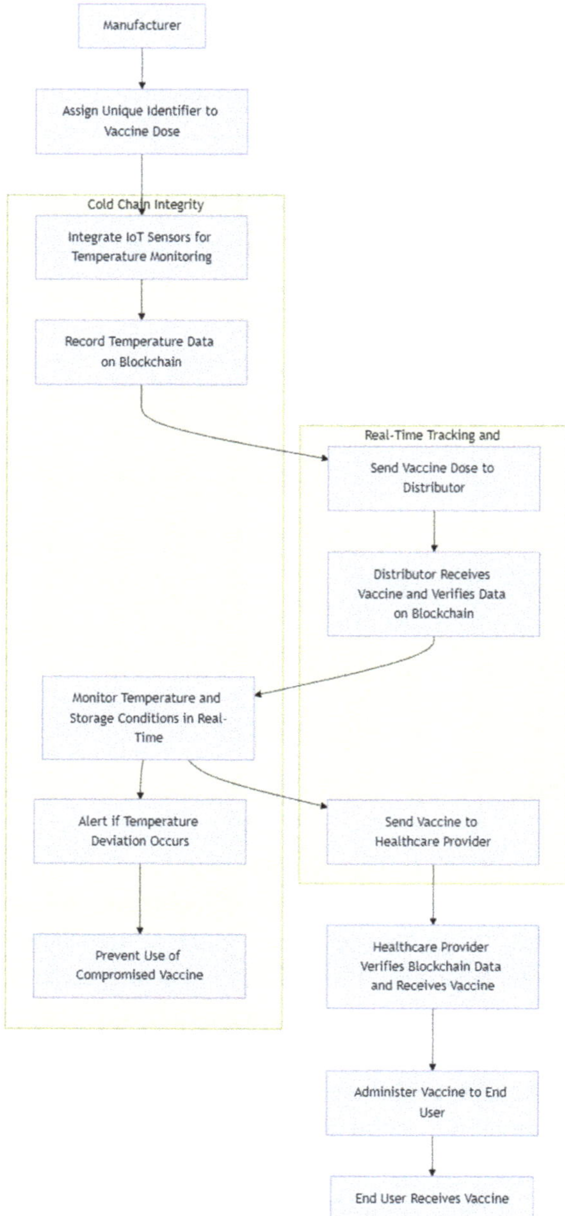

2.3 Medical Device Supply Chains

Blockchain technology has the potential to transform the management of **medical device supply chains**, offering a powerful solution to enhance **quality assurance** and enforce compliance with rigorous **regulatory standards**. Medical devices are subject to extensive testing, certification, and legal requirements to ensure their safety and efficacy before they are approved for use. Blockchain serves as an **immutable, transparent digital ledger**, meticulously recording every stage of a device's lifecycle—from manufacturing and quality control to distribution and delivery(Lou et al., 2021; Mertz, 2018). This robust system ensures that medical devices consistently meet stringent safety and quality standards, while simultaneously providing regulators with **real-time access to verified data**, offering conclusive proof of compliance at every critical juncture(Ahad et al., 2025). The importance of **quality assurance and regulatory compliance** in the medical device industry cannot be overstated, as these products directly impact patient safety and well-being. Blockchain technology empowers manufacturers and distributors to maintain a comprehensive, verifiable record of every quality control process and compliance check, establishing a reliable and transparent history for each device. In the unfortunate event of a product recall, blockchain can instantly **trace affected batches or devices**, allowing healthcare providers and end-users to respond swiftly and minimize potential risks. This rapid and precise traceability not only enhances patient safety but also reinforces trust in the system(Lou et al., 2021)(Butt et al., 2023). The immutability of blockchain records provides an added layer of security, creating a **tamper-proof audit trail** that holds all stakeholders accountable throughout the supply chain. This auditability is invaluable for demonstrating compliance during inspections, resolving disputes, and maintaining high standards of operational integrity. Additionally, blockchain fosters greater collaboration among manufacturers, distributors, and regulators by providing a unified and trustworthy source of truth. Blockchain's applications in healthcare supply chains extend beyond medical devices to include **pharmaceutical products, vaccines, and other critical healthcare items**, addressing a wide range of challenges such as **counterfeiting, traceability, cold chain management, quality assurance, and regulatory compliance**. By ensuring unparalleled levels of transparency, security, and operational efficiency, blockchain technology not only strengthens the safety and reliability of healthcare supply chains but also reduces costs, streamlines processes, and enhances accountability. This innovative technology holds the promise of **revolutionizing the healthcare sector**, ensuring that patients receive safe and effective medical devices and treatments. It fosters trust and confidence among all stakeholders—manufacturers, healthcare providers, regulators, and patients—by delivering an unshakable foundation of transparency and reliability. Blockchain is poised to become an indispensable tool in creating **resilient, efficient, and trustworthy healthcare supply chains** that safeguard patient health and uphold the highest standards of quality and compliance.

3 CASE STUDIES AND REAL-WORLD IMPLEMENTATIONS

3.1 Successful Blockchain Projects in Healthcare

Over the past few years, various successful blockchain projects have been implemented in healthcare, highlighting the potential of the technology to transform supply chains, patient care, and data management. One notable example is the **MediLedger Project**, a collaboration between pharmaceutical companies, technology providers, and regulators. The project focuses on creating a blockchain-based platform to ensure the secure and efficient flow of medicines through the supply chain. MediLedger uses blockchain to prevent counterfeit drugs from entering the system by enabling stakeholders to track and verify the authenticity of pharmaceutical products from manufacturing to distribution(Akram et al., 2024). The project also aims to streamline regulatory compliance by automating processes, such as reporting and auditing, using smart contracts(Gupta et al., n.d.). Another successful project is **PharmaLedger**, an EU-funded initiative that explores the use of blockchain to enhance pharmaceutical supply chain security and transparency. This project involves a consortium of pharmaceutical companies, regulatory bodies, and healthcare stakeholders. PharmaLedger aims to increase visibility into the supply chain, reduce fraud, and improve patient safety. By leveraging blockchain's ability to create an immutable and transparent record of drug transactions, PharmaLedger addresses concerns around counterfeit medications and provides a secure, verifiable platform for monitoring drugs' origins and movements(Balan, 2024).

3.2 Insights from Pilot Programs and Case Studies

Pilot programs and case studies in blockchain healthcare implementations provide valuable insights into the technology's effectiveness and its challenges in real-world scenarios. One such example is **The IBM Food Trust Blockchain** project, which, while not solely focused on healthcare, includes pharmaceutical traceability(Manoharan, n.d.). This pilot program demonstrated how blockchain could improve the transparency and efficiency of supply chains by enabling real-time access to data across all participants in the chain. In the context of pharmaceuticals, this technology has been adapted to track the journey of drugs from manufacturers to wholesalers, providing stakeholders with the ability to verify the product's origin and authenticity(Tiwari, 2017). Additionally, pilot programs for **vaccine distribution** have shown how blockchain can facilitate the efficient tracking of vaccines through the cold chain. One such pilot, conducted by **Chronicled**, focused on ensuring that vaccines were transported and stored at the correct temperatures to maintain their efficacy. The pilot involved using blockchain to record temperature data in real time, ensuring that any deviations from the required conditions were immediately detected. Insights from these pilots highlight blockchain's ability to address the cold chain challenges and provide immutable records that help stakeholders maintain product quality throughout the supply chain, in another pilot conducted by **Solve.Care**, blockchain technology was tested in the management of healthcare administrative processes, specifically focusing on patient care coordination and medication management(Jampani, 2024). The results of this case study showed that blockchain could improve the transparency of healthcare records, reduce fraud, and streamline the verification and validation of medical claims.

3.3 Benefits Realized in Real-World Scenarios

The real-world implementation of blockchain in healthcare has led to significant benefits across various use cases. One of the most impactful benefits is **Improved Transparency** in healthcare supply chains. Blockchain technology enables the creation of a transparent, tamper-proof record of every transaction, which enhances trust among stakeholders. Healthcare providers, regulators, and patients can easily verify the authenticity of drugs, medical devices, and vaccines, reducing the risks associated with counterfeit products and ensuring compliance with quality standards. Another benefit is **Enhanced Efficiency** in the supply chain. Blockchain reduces inefficiencies caused by manual processes, fragmented data systems, and intermediaries. Smart contracts enable automation of tasks such as payments, inventory management, and regulatory reporting, which accelerates operations and reduces human error. This streamlining of processes results in cost savings and improved operational performance for all stakeholders involved.

Improved Patient Safety is another significant benefit realized in real-world scenarios. By using blockchain for pharmaceutical traceability, real-time tracking, and quality monitoring, healthcare providers can ensure that patients receive safe, effective, and authentic products. Blockchain's role in cold chain management for vaccines and biologics is particularly vital for maintaining the efficacy and safety of these sensitive products, preventing wastage and minimizing the risk of compromised treatments(Turki et al., 2023). Finally, **Regulatory Compliance** has been streamlined through blockchain's ability to provide immutable, auditable records of every transaction and process. Regulatory bodies can access blockchain-based data in real-time, simplifying the auditing process and ensuring that healthcare organizations meet industry standards. This has proven to be particularly beneficial in highly regulated sectors such as pharmaceuticals, where maintaining compliance with safety and quality standards is crucial. Successful blockchain projects, pilot programs, and real-world implementations in healthcare have demonstrated its transformative potential. From improving transparency and efficiency to ensuring patient safety and regulatory compliance, blockchain technology has shown tangible benefits that can revolutionize healthcare supply chains and beyond. These implementations provide a blueprint for future healthcare innovations, paving the way for a more secure, efficient, and trustworthy healthcare system.

4 BLOCKCHAIN FOR SUPPLY CHAIN SUSTAINABILITY

Blockchain technology is emerging as a powerful enabler of sustainability within supply chains, particularly in the healthcare sector. By fostering transparency, enhancing traceability, and improving resource management, blockchain helps organizations adopt environmentally friendly practices while reducing operational inefficiencies. This section delves into the various ways blockchain supports sustainability goals.

4.1 Environmental Impact of Blockchain in Supply Chain Management

While traditional blockchain systems like those based on proof-of-work (PoW) have drawn criticism for their energy-intensive operations, advancements in blockchain technology are addressing these concerns. Modern consensus mechanisms such as proof-of-stake (PoS) and energy-efficient blockchain solutions consume significantly less energy, making them more suitable for sustainable applications. Additionally, by digitizing supply chain records and reducing dependency on paper-based documentation, blockchain contributes to reducing waste(R. H. Ahmed et al., 2023). Furthermore, its ability to optimize logistics and transportation minimizes fuel usage and greenhouse gas emissions, demonstrating its potential to mitigate environmental impact(Shambhu Sarkar, 2022).

4.2 Promoting Sustainability Through Transparent and Ethical Sourcing

Blockchain technology ensures that all stakeholders in the supply chain have access to an immutable record of sourcing practices. This transparency guarantees that raw materials used in healthcare products, such as medical devices or pharmaceuticals, are ethically and sustainably sourced. For example, blockchain can verify compliance with environmental and labor standards by tracking materials from their point of origin to the final product. Such visibility not only fosters trust among consumers and regulators but also encourages organizations to uphold ethical sourcing practices and align with global sustainability standards.

4.3 Blockchain's Role in Reducing Waste and Improving Resource Efficiency

Efficient inventory management is a key benefit of blockchain in reducing waste. With real-time visibility into stock levels and expiration dates, healthcare organizations can avoid overproduction and minimize the disposal of expired products. Smart contracts further enhance efficiency by automating processes, ensuring resources are allocated and utilized only as needed. Moreover, blockchain supports recycling efforts by providing detailed records of product components, enabling the recovery and reuse of materials, and promoting the adoption of circular economy principles.

4.4 Green Blockchain Solutions for the Healthcare Industry

Green blockchain initiatives are paving the way for a more sustainable future. By integrating renewable energy sources into blockchain networks, healthcare organizations can significantly lower the environmental footprint of their operations. Blockchain systems also enable tracking and managing energy consumption within the supply chain, ensuring adherence to sustainability targets. Additionally, the implementation of blockchain-based carbon credit systems incentivizes eco-friendly practices across manufacturing and distribution processes. These innovations position blockchain as a cornerstone of green transformation in the healthcare industry(Pham et al., 2019). Blockchain's capabilities not only improve operational transparency and efficiency but also empower healthcare organizations to address environmental challenges. By embracing sustainable practices and adopting green technologies, blockchain contributes to building resilient and eco-friendly supply chains in the healthcare sector.

5 BLOCKCHAIN-BASED DIGITAL IDENTITY IN HEALTHCARE SUPPLY CHAINS

Blockchain technology offers a transformative approach to managing digital identities within healthcare supply chains, providing secure, transparent, and immutable systems that enhance authentication and traceability. By integrating digital identities for healthcare products, patients, and medical records, blockchain addresses critical challenges related to counterfeit prevention, operational efficiency, and patient safety.

5.1 Creating Digital Identities for Healthcare Products

Each healthcare product, whether a pharmaceutical, vaccine, or medical device, can be assigned a unique digital identity on the blockchain. This digital identity serves as a secure and tamper-proof record that tracks the product from manufacturing to the end user. It includes detailed information such as the product's origin, batch number, expiration date, and compliance with regulatory standards. By enabling real-time access to this information, blockchain prevents counterfeiting, ensures quality assurance, and fosters trust among stakeholders.

5.2 Enhancing Patient and Product Authentication Using Blockchain

Blockchain-based digital identities play a pivotal role in authenticating both patients and products within healthcare systems. Patients can be assigned unique digital identities that securely store their medical history, prescriptions, and treatment records. Simultaneously, healthcare products can be authenticated at each stage of the supply chain to ensure they are genuine and safe for use. For example, pharmacists and healthcare providers can use blockchain to verify the authenticity of medicines and medical devices before they are dispensed, thereby preventing errors and ensuring patient safety(IEEE Computer Society et al., n.d.).

5.3 Digital Identity's Role in Medical Device Supply Chains

In medical device supply chains, digital identities facilitate comprehensive tracking and monitoring throughout the device's lifecycle. Each device's digital identity can document its manufacturing process, quality control checks, regulatory approvals, and maintenance history. This ensures compliance with stringent safety and quality standards, reduces the risk of defective devices reaching patients, and simplifies the process of recalls when necessary. Furthermore, blockchain enables seamless interoperability between manufacturers, distributors, and healthcare providers, enhancing overall supply chain efficiency.

5.4 Blockchain-Enabled Digital Health Records

Digital health records powered by blockchain provide patients with secure and decentralized control over their medical data. By linking these records to a patient's unique digital identity, blockchain ensures that only authorized parties can access sensitive health information. This approach reduces the risk of data breaches and unauthorized access while improving the accuracy and continuity of care(Zahid et al., 2023). Blockchain also facilitates secure sharing of health records between different healthcare providers and institutions, streamlining diagnoses, treatments, and research efforts. Blockchain-based digital identities revolutionize healthcare supply chains by enhancing traceability, ensuring product and patient authentication, and enabling secure and interoperable health data management. This innovative approach not only improves operational efficiency but also strengthens patient trust and safety across the entire healthcare ecosystem.

6 BENEFITS OF BLOCKCHAIN-BASED SUPPLY CHAIN MANAGEMENT

6.1 Enhanced Transparency and Traceability

One of the most significant benefits of blockchain-based supply chain management in healthcare is **Enhanced Transparency and Traceability**. Blockchain provides a decentralized, immutable ledger where every transaction is securely recorded and time-stamped. This allows stakeholders—manufacturers, distributors, healthcare providers, regulators, and patients—to access real-time data on the movement of products through the supply chain. Each step in the journey of a product, from the manufacturer to the end user, is transparently recorded on the blockchain, offering full visibility into its origin, handling, and storage conditions. For pharmaceuticals, this means that drugs can be traced from production through distribution and ultimately to the patient, ensuring authenticity and compliance with safety regulations. The ability to track products in real-time significantly reduces the risk of fraud, theft, and errors, providing a higher level of accountability across the supply chain(Sarkar, 2022a).

6.2 Improved Patient Safety

Blockchain technology improves **Patient Safety** by ensuring that healthcare products, including medicines, vaccines, and medical devices, are authentic, safe, and properly handled throughout their journey. With blockchain, each product is assigned a unique identifier that is recorded on the blockchain, making it nearly impossible for counterfeit or substandard products to enter the supply chain undetected. This is especially important in the pharmaceutical industry, where counterfeit drugs pose a significant risk to patient health. Additionally, blockchain's integration with IoT devices allows for real-time monitoring of temperature-sensitive products, such as vaccines, ensuring they are stored and transported under optimal conditions. If any deviation occurs, blockchain's immutable records provide immediate alerts, preventing compromised products from reaching patients. By offering full traceability and verification at every step, blockchain ensures that patients receive safe, high-quality products, reducing the chances of medication errors and improving overall care outcomes.

6.3 Cost Reduction and Efficiency

The adoption of blockchain in healthcare supply chains results in **Cost Reduction and Efficiency** by streamlining processes and eliminating inefficiencies. Traditional supply chains often rely on paper-based systems, manual processes, and multiple intermediaries, which can introduce delays, errors, and additional costs. Blockchain automates many of these processes through smart contracts, which execute predefined actions automatically when specific conditions are met. This eliminates the need for intermediaries and manual checks, reducing operational costs and the potential for human error. Furthermore, blockchain provides a single, secure platform for all stakeholders to access and share information, reducing the risk of duplicated efforts and information silos. The ability to track products in real time also helps minimize inventory losses and optimize stock management, leading to more efficient resource allocation. By improving operational efficiency and reducing administrative burdens, blockchain contributes to significant cost savings and enhances the overall effectiveness of the healthcare supply chain.

6.4 Strengthened Trust Among Stakeholders

Strengthened Trust Among Stakeholders is another critical benefit of blockchain-based supply chain management. The transparency and immutability of blockchain create a secure and reliable environment for all parties involved. Since all transactions and product movements are recorded in a tamper-proof manner, stakeholders can trust the data they are accessing, knowing it cannot be altered or manipulated. This transparency fosters collaboration and reduces the chances of disputes or misunderstandings between parties, such as manufacturers, distributors, and healthcare providers. Moreover, patients and regulators can have greater confidence in the safety and authenticity of healthcare products, knowing that every transaction is securely documented. By ensuring that every step in the supply chain is verifiable and auditable, blockchain establishes a foundation of trust that strengthens relationships and promotes greater cooperation among all parties. This increased trust can also lead to improved regulatory compliance and a more resilient, accountable healthcare system overall.

7 BLOCKCHAIN AND HEALTHCARE SUPPLY CHAIN METRICS

Blockchain technology introduces a data-driven approach to evaluating and improving the performance of healthcare supply chains. By leveraging its transparency, traceability, and real-time data capabilities, organizations can define and measure key metrics that ensure efficiency, effectiveness, and sustainability. This section explores the role of blockchain in healthcare supply chain metrics, emphasizing its transformative potential in performance monitoring and reporting(A. Ahmed et al., 2021).

7.1 Key Performance Indicators (KPIs) for Blockchain Supply Chain Management

Blockchain enables the identification and tracking of specific KPIs that reflect the efficiency and reliability of supply chains. Common KPIs include product traceability rates, delivery accuracy, compliance with regulatory standards, and inventory turnover ratios. Blockchain's immutable ledger ensures that these metrics are consistently updated and accessible, allowing organizations to monitor supply chain performance in real-time. Additionally, KPIs related to sustainability, such as carbon footprint reduction and waste management, can also be tracked to align with environmental goals.

7.2 Measuring the Effectiveness of Blockchain in Healthcare

The effectiveness of blockchain in healthcare supply chains can be assessed through its impact on critical areas such as fraud prevention, counterfeit detection, and operational efficiency. Metrics like reduction in counterfeit products, faster recall processes, and improved product authentication times provide tangible evidence of blockchain's value. Furthermore, blockchain's ability to enhance compliance reporting and reduce administrative burdens significantly contributes to its effectiveness in ensuring the safety and integrity of healthcare products.

7.3 Analytics and Reporting Using Blockchain Data

Blockchain's real-time data capabilities enable advanced analytics and reporting, offering actionable insights into supply chain operations. Stakeholders can use these insights to identify bottlenecks, predict demand, and optimize resource allocation. The secure and transparent nature of blockchain ensures that data used for analytics is reliable and tamper-proof. Automated reporting tools powered by blockchain simplify compliance audits and performance reviews, allowing organizations to make informed decisions with confidence.

7.4 Long-Term Performance Tracking and Blockchain Adoption Success

Blockchain facilitates long-term performance tracking by maintaining an immutable record of historical data, enabling organizations to analyze trends and assess the success of blockchain adoption over time. Metrics such as return on investment (ROI), cost savings, and improvements in stakeholder satisfaction provide a clear picture of blockchain's long-term impact. By tracking adoption rates and integration milestones, organizations can refine their strategies for scaling blockchain implementations and achieving sustainable improvements. Blockchain enhances healthcare supply chain metrics by enabling precise, transparent, and actionable performance monitoring. Through robust KPI tracking, effectiveness measurement, advanced analytics, and long-term performance evaluation, blockchain empowers healthcare organizations to optimize their supply chain operations, ensuring greater safety, efficiency, and accountability(Alam et al., 2021).

8 BLOCKCHAIN FOR INVENTORY AND STOCK MANAGEMENT IN HEALTHCARE

Effective inventory and stock management are critical for ensuring the availability of essential healthcare products while minimizing waste and inefficiencies. Blockchain technology offers transformative solutions by providing real-time visibility, automated processes, and secure data management. This section explores the various applications of blockchain in revolutionizing inventory and stock management within the healthcare industry.

8.1 Blockchain for Real-Time Inventory Tracking

Blockchain enables real-time tracking of inventory levels across the entire supply chain, from manufacturers to healthcare providers. Each product is assigned a unique digital identifier on the blockchain, allowing stakeholders to monitor its movement, location, and status in real time. This transparency ensures that healthcare facilities are always informed about stock availability, reducing delays and improving the reliability of supply chains. The decentralized nature of blockchain also facilitates seamless collaboration among multiple stakeholders, ensuring accurate inventory data across the network.

8.2 Managing Expiration Dates and Product Lifecycles Using Blockchain

Blockchain provides a robust solution for managing the expiration dates and lifecycles of healthcare products. By recording detailed information such as manufacturing dates, shelf lives, and storage conditions, blockchain ensures that stakeholders can easily identify products nearing their expiration. Automated alerts and smart contracts can trigger actions such as prioritizing the distribution of near-expiry products, reducing waste and ensuring that expired items are removed from circulation promptly. This capability is particularly valuable in managing sensitive products like vaccines and perishable medical supplies.

8.3 Inventory Optimization and Blockchain-Based Smart Contracts

Blockchain-powered smart contracts automate key aspects of inventory management, such as replenishment and order processing. When stock levels fall below a predefined threshold, smart contracts can automatically initiate orders with suppliers, ensuring timely restocking without manual intervention. This reduces the risk of human error and streamlines procurement processes. Additionally, blockchain's real-time data capabilities allow for demand forecasting and inventory optimization, ensuring that healthcare facilities maintain adequate supplies without overstocking(Mangala et al., 2024).

8.4 Reducing Overstock and Shortages with Blockchain

Blockchain technology minimizes both overstock and shortages by providing accurate and up-to-date inventory data. Overstocking leads to unnecessary costs and waste, while shortages can compromise patient care and safety. By enabling transparent communication and collaboration among supply chain stakeholders, blockchain ensures that inventory levels are balanced according to demand. Predictive analytics powered by blockchain data further enhances inventory planning, allowing healthcare organizations to anticipate needs and adjust stock levels proactively(Khedr, 2024). Blockchain transforms inventory and stock management in healthcare by offering real-time tracking, efficient lifecycle management, and automated processes. By reducing waste, preventing shortages, and optimizing inventory levels, blockchain enhances the reliability and efficiency of healthcare supply chains, ultimately improving patient outcomes and operational performance.

9 CHALLENGES AND BARRIERS TO ADOPTION

9.1 Technical Challenges Scalability and Integration

One of the primary technical challenges to adopting blockchain in healthcare supply chains is **Scalability and Integration**. Blockchain networks, particularly public blockchains, can face limitations in terms of processing large volumes of transactions quickly. The need for consensus across decentralized nodes can slow down transaction processing speeds, which may be problematic for a high-demand healthcare supply chain that requires real-time or near-real-time data. As blockchain grows, the size of the ledger increases, and the time required to process new transactions may increase as well. To ensure blockchain can handle large-scale data and provide fast transaction processing, significant advancements in blockchain infrastructure are necessary, such as developing more scalable consensus mechanisms or implementing layer-2 solutions(Alam et al., 2021). Moreover, **Integration** with existing healthcare systems presents a major challenge. Healthcare organizations often rely on legacy systems, such as Electronic Health Records (EHR), inventory management systems, and billing systems, which may not be compatible with blockchain technology. Integrating blockchain with these existing systems involves significant technical expertise, system upgrades, and data migration efforts. Interoperability between blockchain platforms and healthcare systems is essential for seamless communication and data exchange, but achieving this integration can be complex and resource-intensive.

9.2 Regulatory and Compliance Issues

The **Regulatory and Compliance Issues** surrounding blockchain adoption in healthcare are a major concern. Healthcare is a highly regulated industry with strict compliance requirements for data protection, patient privacy, and product safety. Blockchain technology, being decentralized and transparent, presents challenges in meeting these regulatory standards, especially those related to data privacy laws such as HIPAA in the U.S. or GDPR in Europe. The immutable nature of blockchain also creates challenges when it comes to data deletion or modification, which may conflict with the right to be forgotten or other privacy-related regulations. Furthermore, as blockchain adoption is still in its early stages, there is a lack of clear and consistent regulatory frameworks to govern its use in healthcare. Regulators need to develop guidelines that ensure blockchain solutions align with existing healthcare laws and standards. The uncertainty surrounding how regulators will handle blockchain technology can discourage organizations from adopting it, especially if they fear legal complications or non-compliance with industry regulations.

9.3 Resistance to Change in Traditional Systems

Resistance to Change in Traditional Systems is a common barrier to the adoption of blockchain technology in healthcare. Many healthcare organizations, such as hospitals, pharmaceutical companies, and distributors, have deeply entrenched legacy systems and practices that are familiar to their staff and have been in place for years. Shifting to a blockchain-based system requires significant changes in organizational workflows, employee training, and the overhaul of existing processes. This transition can be met with resistance, particularly from stakeholders who are hesitant to adopt new technologies due to concerns about the disruption it may cause to their established operations(M. Ahmed et al., 2022). Moreover, blockchain implementation requires collaboration between multiple parties across the healthcare ecosystem, each with different priorities, technologies, and systems. Getting all stakeholders to agree on a shared vision for blockchain adoption and to invest the necessary time and resources can be a major hurdle. This resistance to change can slow down or even prevent the widespread adoption of blockchain in healthcare, especially in an industry that is often slow to embrace new technologies.

9.4 High Initial Costs of Implementation

The **High Initial Costs of Implementation** are another significant barrier to adopting blockchain in healthcare supply chains. Setting up a blockchain system, particularly one that involves multiple stakeholders, can be costly. The infrastructure required to deploy and maintain a blockchain network, including hardware, software, and personnel, can represent a substantial financial investment. Additionally, healthcare organizations need to train their staff and update existing systems to integrate with blockchain technology, which further adds to the cost. While blockchain has the potential to reduce costs over the long term by improving efficiency, transparency, and reducing fraud, the upfront investment can be a major deterrent, particularly for smaller organizations or those with limited budgets. Many healthcare providers and manufacturers may be reluctant to commit to the high initial costs without guaranteed returns on investment. Furthermore, the lack of a proven track record in healthcare-specific blockchain solutions adds an element of risk to the investment, making decision-makers cautious about allocating significant resources to this technology.

10 FUTURE PROSPECTS AND INNOVATIONS

10.1 Integration with IoT and AI for Smarter Supply Chains

The future of blockchain in healthcare supply chains looks particularly promising when combined with **Internet of Things (IoT)** and **Artificial Intelligence (AI)**. These technologies, when integrated with blockchain, can create **smarter supply chains** that are not only more transparent but also more automated and intelligent. IoT devices play a pivotal role in the future of healthcare supply chains by enabling real-time data collection and monitoring. For example, sensors embedded in packaging or storage facilities can continuously track temperature, humidity, and location for sensitive products like vaccines or biologics(Ali et al., 2023). This data can be securely recorded on the blockchain, ensuring the integrity of the product's journey and preventing tampering or fraud. IoT-enabled devices can also trigger automated actions, such as alerts if products deviate from optimal storage conditions, improving the overall management of the supply chain(Jum'a et al., 2024).

When combined with **AI**, the potential of blockchain is significantly enhanced. AI can process the vast amounts of data generated by IoT devices to make predictions and optimize supply chain operations. For instance, AI can analyze blockchain records to detect patterns in product movements and identify inefficiencies, ultimately recommending solutions for better resource allocation, demand forecasting, and inventory management. AI-powered smart contracts can also automate complex workflows, such as product recalls or compliance checks, reducing human error and operational delays. Together, these technologies create a more efficient, responsive, and resilient healthcare supply chain capable of adapting to real-time changes.

10.2 Potential for Global Standardization

Global Standardization is another key area of future growth for blockchain in healthcare supply chains. Currently, supply chain processes across different countries and regions are often fragmented, with varying standards for data security, product traceability, and regulatory compliance. This lack of standardization complicates the flow of goods across borders and increases the risks of fraud, inefficiency, and regulatory non-compliance. Blockchain technology holds the potential to address these challenges by providing a universally accessible, transparent, and secure platform for sharing data across borders. A global standard for blockchain-enabled supply chains could help harmonize practices and regulations across countries, making it easier for stakeholders to collaborate, verify product authenticity, and comply with local laws. Blockchain's immutable ledger ensures that all parties in the supply chain have access to the same version of the truth, which is crucial for regulatory bodies and international organizations that require consistent and verifiable data. Efforts to create a **global blockchain framework** for healthcare supply chains are already underway, with multiple industry groups, governments, and international organizations exploring how to make blockchain a standard for tracking and securing medical products. If successful, this could lead to more streamlined, efficient, and secure global healthcare supply chains, improving access to essential medicines and products across the world, especially in regions with limited infrastructure(Ramasamy et al., 2024).

11 EMERGING TRENDS AND TECHNOLOGIES IN BLOCKCHAIN

As blockchain continues to evolve, several emerging trends and technologies are poised to further enhance its capabilities in healthcare supply chains.

- **Layer-2 Solutions:** One of the biggest challenges with blockchain is scalability. Current public blockchains may not be able to handle the volume of transactions required for large-scale supply chains. To address this, **Layer-2 solutions** are being developed to allow faster transactions off the main blockchain, which are later confirmed on the main chain. These solutions enable greater scalability without sacrificing the security and transparency provided by the underlying blockchain.
- **Interoperability and Cross-Chain Communication:** Blockchain networks are typically siloed, which can limit their effectiveness when data needs to be shared between different blockchain systems. New developments in **interoperability** aim to create seamless communication between different blockchain platforms, enabling a more integrated and cohesive healthcare supply chain. This would allow stakeholders using different blockchain technologies to access and verify data from other networks, further enhancing transparency and trust.
- **Blockchain for Digital Identity and Authentication:** Another emerging trend is the use of blockchain for **digital identity management** and **authentication** in healthcare. By securely storing and managing the identities of patients, healthcare providers, and other stakeholders on the blockchain, organizations can ensure that only authorized entities can access sensitive data or handle critical products. This could improve both privacy and security while also enhancing the trustworthiness of the supply chain.
- **Zero-Knowledge Proofs (ZKPs): Zero-Knowledge Proofs** are a cryptographic method that allows one party to prove to another that a statement is true without revealing any additional information. ZKPs have the potential to improve blockchain's privacy features by allowing stakeholders to verify transactions or the authenticity of products without exposing sensitive information, such as medical history or business contracts. This can enhance privacy protections while maintaining the transparency and security of the blockchain.
- **Decentralized Autonomous Organizations (DAOs): DAOs** represent a trend toward fully decentralized decision-making systems, which could extend to the governance of blockchain networks. In a DAO, stakeholders in a healthcare supply chain could participate in governance decisions through voting mechanisms, which could lead to more democratic, transparent, and efficient decision-making processes(*scholar (1)*, n.d.).

12 SUMMARY OF BLOCKCHAIN'S ROLE IN HEALTHCARE SUPPLY CHAINS

Blockchain technology has the potential to transform healthcare supply chains by providing enhanced transparency, traceability, and security. It addresses several critical issues faced by traditional healthcare supply chains, including counterfeiting, inefficiencies, lack of real-time visibility, and fragmented data systems. By leveraging the immutable and decentralized nature of blockchain, stakeholders can securely track and verify the movement of medical products from manufacturers to end users. This ensures the authenticity of pharmaceuticals, vaccines, and medical devices, reducing the risk of counterfeit products entering the supply chain. Additionally, blockchain improves operational efficiency by streamlining processes through automation via smart contracts and reducing the need for intermediaries. Blockchain's ability to integrate with other emerging technologies such as the Internet of Things (IoT) and Artificial Intelligence (AI) further enhances the supply chain's ability to track products in real time, monitor sensitive items (such as vaccines) for compliance with storage conditions, and automate complex workflows. As a result, blockchain offers a comprehensive solution for improving both the security and efficiency of healthcare supply chains, ensuring better patient safety, reducing costs, and building trust among stakeholders.

12.1 Key Takeaways and Recommendations

- **Transparency and Trust:** Blockchain provides unmatched transparency by creating an immutable ledger that tracks every transaction in the supply chain. This fosters trust between stakeholders, including manufacturers, distributors, healthcare providers, and regulators, by ensuring that data cannot be altered or tampered with.
- **Counterfeit Prevention:** Blockchain's ability to verify product authenticity and trace the movement of goods is crucial in preventing counterfeit drugs, which is a major issue in global healthcare. This feature enhances patient safety by ensuring that only verified and safe products reach the end-user.
- **Improved Efficiency and Cost Reduction:** By automating key processes through smart contracts and eliminating the need for intermediaries, blockchain reduces operational costs and inefficiencies. Moreover, it enhances inventory management and reduces losses due to mismanagement or fraud.
- **Real-time Monitoring and Compliance:** Integration with IoT allows for continuous monitoring of sensitive products, such as vaccines, ensuring they are stored and transported under optimal conditions. Blockchain ensures that all changes in the product's status are securely recorded, enabling full compliance with regulatory standards.
- **Challenges to Overcome:** Despite its potential, blockchain adoption faces challenges such as scalability, integration with existing systems, regulatory hurdles, and high initial implementation costs. Overcoming these barriers requires collaboration between stakeholders, technical advancements, and the development of clear regulatory frameworks.

Recommendations for healthcare organizations include investing in pilot programs to assess blockchain's feasibility, collaborating with regulatory bodies to establish clear guidelines, and focusing on the integration of blockchain with other technologies like IoT and AI to maximize its potential. Additionally, healthcare organizations should develop training programs to address the resistance to change and encourage adoption across the sector.

12.2 The Future of Blockchain in Healthcare

The future of blockchain in healthcare supply chains holds tremendous potential for innovation and improvement. As the technology matures, blockchain is likely to become a cornerstone of modern healthcare systems, facilitating a global ecosystem of trust, security, and efficiency. One of the most promising aspects is the potential for **global standardization**, which could harmonize regulatory practices and facilitate smoother cross-border transactions, enabling more efficient international supply chains. Future advancements in blockchain will likely focus on **scalability** and **interoperability**, enabling blockchain systems to handle larger datasets and integrate more seamlessly with existing healthcare infrastructure. Innovations such as **zero-knowledge proofs** and **smart contracts** could further enhance blockchain's privacy, security, and automation features, making it a more powerful tool for supply chain management. With the increasing integration of **AI** and **IoT** with blockchain, supply chains will become even smarter, able to predict demand, optimize inventory management, and automatically trigger actions based on real-time data. These advancements will help create a more responsive, resilient, and automated healthcare ecosystem, ensuring that critical supplies and products are delivered efficiently and securely.

REFERENCES

Abbas, H., Hussain, M., Zahid, S., & Ahmed, R. H. (2023). Enhancing Food Security: A Blockchain-Enabled Traceability Framework to Mitigate Stockpiling of Food Commodities. *2023 International Conference on IT and Industrial Technologies (ICIT)*, 1–7. DOI: 10.1109/ICIT59216.2023.10335828

Agbo, C. C., Mahmoud, Q. H., & Eklund, J. M. (2019). Blockchain technology in healthcare: A systematic review. In Healthcare (Switzerland) (Vol. 7, Issue 2). MDPI. DOI: 10.3390/healthcare7020056

Ahad, A., Jiangbin, Z., Mughees, A., Puspitasari, I., & Tayyab, M. (2025). Secure Horizons: Integrating Blockchain With AI for Enhanced Smart Healthcare Systems. In AI Techniques for Securing Medical and Business Practices (pp. 357–390). IGI Global.

Ahad, A., Tahir, M., Sheikh, M. A. S., Mughees, A., & Ahmed, K. I. (2021). Optimal route selection in 5G-based smart health-care network: a reinforcement learning approach. *2021 26th IEEE Asia-Pacific Conference on Communications (APCC)*, 248–253.

Ahmed, A., Aamir, A., Raza, T., & Khan, M. H. D. (2021). Blockchain Based RFID Prototype For Medicine Traceability along the Healthcare Supply Chain. *2021 7th International Conference on Aerospace Science and Engineering, ICASE 2021*. DOI: 10.1109/ICASE54940.2021.9904249

Ahmed, M., Reno, S., Ferdous, M., & Shama, R. M. (2022). Detection of Counterfeit Medicine Using a Private and Permissioned Blockchain. *2022 2nd Asian Conference on Innovation in Technology, ASIANCON 2022*. DOI: 10.1109/ASIANCON55314.2022.9909424

Ahmed, R. H., Hussain, M., & Zahid, S. (2023). Transforming Blood Donation Processes with Blockchain and IoT Integration: A augmented Approach to Secure and Efficient Healthcare Practices. *2023 International Conference on IT and Industrial Technologies (ICIT)*, 1–8. DOI: 10.1109/ICIT59216.2023.10335787

Akram, W., Joshi, R., Haider, T., Sharma, P., Jain, V., Garud, N., & Narwaria, N. S. (2024). Blockchain technology: A potential tool for the management of pharma supply chain. *Research in Social & Administrative Pharmacy*, *20*(6), 156–164. DOI: 10.1016/j.sapharm.2024.02.014 PMID: 38423927

Alam, N., Hasan Tanvir, M. R., Shanto, S. A., Israt, F., Rahman, A., & Momotaj, S. (2021). Blockchain based counterfeit medicine authentication system. *ISCAIE 2021 - IEEE 11th Symposium on Computer Applications and Industrial Electronics*, 214–217. DOI: 10.1109/ISCAIE51753.2021.9431789

Ali, Z., Ahad, A., Madeira, F., & Shayea, I. (2023). Enhancing Transparency and Trustworthiness of Healthcare IoT Data with AWS: A Proposed Model. *EAI International Conference on IoT Technologies for HealthCare*, 44–56.

Balan, A. (2024). Revolutionizing Medical Data Management with Secure Self-Sovereign Applications for Patient Empowerment. *2024 E-Health and Bioengineering Conference (EHB)*, 1–4.

Butt, H. A., Ahad, A., Wasim, M., Shayea, I., Coelho, P. J., Pires, I. M., & Garcia, N. M. (2023). Federated machine learning in 5G smart healthcare: A security perspective review. *Procedia Computer Science*, *224*, 580–586. DOI: 10.1016/j.procs.2023.09.084

Cheung, H. H., & Choi, S. H. (2011). Implementation issues in RFID-based anti-counterfeiting systems. *Computers in Industry*, *62*(7), 708–718. DOI: 10.1016/j.compind.2011.04.001

Deng, X., & Ouyang, Y. (2022). Cross-Border Supply Chain System Constructed by Complex Computer Blockchain for International Cooperation. *Computational Intelligence and Neuroscience*, *2022*, 1–10. Advance online publication. DOI: 10.1155/2022/6221211 PMID: 35449736

Gupta, S., Bali, A., & Singh, A. (n.d.). *Fake Product Detection System Using Blockchain Fake Product Detection Using Blockchain View project Fake Product Detection System Using Blockchain*. Retrieved from https://www.researchgate.net/publication/366064456

Hossain, M. J., Wadud, M. A. H., & Alamin, M. (2021). HDM-Chain: A Secure Blockchain-based Healthcare Data Management framework to ensure Privacy and Security in the Health Unit. *2021 5th International Conference on Electrical Engineering and Information and Communication Technology, ICEEICT 2021*. DOI: 10.1109/ICEEICT53905.2021.9667820

IEEE. Computer Society, & Green University of Bangladesh. (n.d.). *2021 3rd International Conference on Sustainable Technologies for Industry 4.0 (STI) 18-19 December, Dhaka*.

Jabeen, M., Hussain, M., & Rana Hassam Ahmed, H. A. (n.d.). *A BLOCKCHAIN-BASED IPFS AUGMENTED DISTRIBUTED INFORMATION SHARING PARADIGM FOR SECURE COMMUNICATION IN NETWORKED ENVIRONMENT*.

Jampani, R. (2024). *Blockchain Technology in Global Healthcare: A Paradigm Shift*.

Jum'a, L., Ikram, M., & Jabbour, C. J. C. (2024). Towards circular economy: A IoT enabled framework for circular supply chain integration. *Computers & Industrial Engineering*, *192*, 110194. DOI: 10.1016/j.cie.2024.110194

Khedr, A. M., & S, S. R. (2024). Enhancing supply chain management with deep learning and machine learning techniques: A review. *Journal of Open Innovation*, *10*(4), 100379. DOI: 10.1016/j.joitmc.2024.100379

Li, D., Gong, Y., Zhang, X., & Huang, M. (2022). An Exploratory Study on the Design and Management Model of Traditional Chinese Medicine Quality Safety Traceability System Based on Blockchain Technology. *Security and Communication Networks*, *2022*, 1–24. Advance online publication. DOI: 10.1155/2022/7011145

Lou, M., Dong, X., Cao, Z., & Shen, J. (2021). SESCF: A Secure and Efficient Supply Chain Framework via Blockchain-Based Smart Contracts. *Security and Communication Networks*, *2021*, 1–18. Advance online publication. DOI: 10.1155/2021/8884478

Maariz, A., Wiputra, M. A., & Armanto, M. R. D. (2024). Blockchain technology: Revolutionizing data integrity and security in digital environments. [ITEE]. *International Transactions on Education Technology*, *2*(2), 92–98. DOI: 10.33050/itee.v2i2.435

Mangala, N., Naveen, D. R., Reddy, B. E., Buyya, R., Venugopal, K. R., Iyengar, S. S., & Patnaik, L. M. (2024). Secure pharmaceutical supply chain using blockchain in iot cloud systems. *Internet of Things : Engineering Cyber Physical Human Systems*, *26*, 101215. DOI: 10.1016/j.iot.2024.101215

Manoharan, A. (n.d.). *BLOCKCHAIN TECHNOLOGY: REINVENTING TRUST AND SECURITY IN THE DIGITAL WORLD*.

Mertz, L. (2018). (Block) Chain Reaction: A Blockchain Revolution Sweeps into Health Care, Offering the Possibility for a Much-Needed Data Solution. *IEEE Pulse*, *9*(3), 4–7. DOI: 10.1109/MPUL.2018.2814879 PMID: 29757744

Nabiyeva, A., & Wu, D. Z. (2017). Serialization of prescription drugs in the USA: a centralized view (Doctoral dissertation, Massachusetts Institute of Technology).

Peng, S., Hu, X., Zhang, J., Xie, X., Long, C., Tian, Z., & Jiang, H. (2020). An Efficient Double-Layer Blockchain Method for Vaccine Production Supervision. *IEEE Transactions on Nanobioscience*, *19*(3), 579–587. DOI: 10.1109/TNB.2020.2999637 PMID: 32603300

Pham, H. L., Tran, T. H., & Nakashima, Y. (2019, December 1). Practical Anti-Counterfeit Medicine Management System Based on Blockchain Technology. *TIMES-ICON 2019 - 2019 4th Technology Innovation Management and Engineering Science International Conference*. DOI: 10.1109/TIMES-iCON47539.2019.9024674

Pisani, E., Hasnida, A., Rahmi, M., Kok, M. O., Harsono, S., & Anggriani, Y. (2021). Substandard and falsified medicines: Proposed methods for case finding and sentinel surveillance. In JMIR Public Health and Surveillance (Vol. 7, Issue 8). JMIR Publications Inc. DOI: 10.2196/29309

Ramasamy, L. K., & Khan, F. (2024). *Blockchain for Global Education*. Springer. DOI: 10.1007/978-3-031-52123-2

Sarkar, S. (2022). Supply chain security act 2023: Interoperable data exchange for drug traceability. *Int. J. Sci. Res. Comput. Sci. Eng. Inf. Technol*, *8*(3), 471–477.

Sarkar, S. (2022a). Digital Traceability of pharmaceutical drugs in supply chain. *International Journal of Advance Research in Computer Science and Management Studies*, *10*(2). www.ijarcsms.com

Sarkar, S. (2022b). *International Journal of Advance Research in Computer Science and Management Studies Online Drug trade-a threat to pharmaceutical industry*. Retrieved from www.ijarcsms.com

Saxena, N., Thomas, I., Gope, P., Burnap, P., & Kumar, N. (2020). Pharmacrypt: Blockchain for critical pharmaceutical industry to counterfeit drugs. *Computer*, *53*(7), 29–44. DOI: 10.1109/MC.2020.2989238

Tariq, M. H., Hussain, M., Zahid, S., & Ahmed, R. H. (n.d.). *DECENTRALIZED APPLICATION FOR AUTO-INSURANCE INDUSTRY: AN INTERPLANETARY FILE SYSTEM AND BLOCKCHAIN-BASED PARADIGM FOR OPTIMAL DATA AND CLAIM MANAGEMENT*.

Tiwari, S. (2017). An introduction to QR code technology. *Proceedings - 2016 15th International Conference on Information Technology, ICIT 2016*, 39–44. doi: DOI: 10.1109/ICIT.2016.38

Turki, M., Cheikhrouhou, S., Dammak, B., Baklouti, M., Mars, R., & Dhahbi, A. (2023). NFT-IoT Pharma Chain: IoT Drug traceability system based on Blockchain and Non Fungible Tokens (NFTs). *Journal of King Saud University. Computer and Information Sciences*, *35*(2), 527–543. Advance online publication. DOI: 10.1016/j.jksuci.2022.12.016

Yele, S., & Litoriya, R. (2024). Blockchain-based secure dining: Enhancing safety, transparency, and traceability in food consumption environment. *Blockchain: Research and Applications*, 100187.

Zahid, S., Hussain, M., Ahmed, R. H., Shahid, M. R., & Abbas, H. (2023). Blockchain-based Health Insurance Model Using IPFS: A Solution for Improved Optimization, Trustability, and User Control. *2023 International Conference on IT and Industrial Technologies (ICIT)*, 1–7. DOI: 10.1109/ICIT59216.2023.10335701

Chapter 6
Case Studies of Blockchain and AI Integration in Medical Systems

Bhanu Dwivedi
https://orcid.org/0000-0002-7306-4414
Manav Rachna International Institute of Research and Studies, India

Nandini Newar
https://orcid.org/0009-0009-5658-9495
Manav Rachna International Institute of Research and Studies, India

Amiti Mahajan
https://orcid.org/0009-0009-9490-2817
Manav Rachna International Institute of Research and Studies, India

Abha Susan Jimmy
https://orcid.org/0009-0008-4534-8015
Manav Rachna International Institute of Research and Studies, India

ABSTRACT

This chapter explores how the integration of blockchain and artificial intelligence (AI) can revolutionize healthcare systems by addressing pressing challenges such as data security, operational inefficiencies, and the demand for personalized care. By presenting diverse case studies, the chapter highlights practical applications like secure patient data management, transparent supply chain monitoring, and ethical clinical trial practices. Blockchain offers decentralized, tamper-proof data storage, while AI enhances predictive analytics, decision-making, and operational insights, creating a synergistic framework. Moreover, the chapter discusses the technical, ethical, and regulatory barriers to adoption and anticipates future advancements, such as explainable AI (XAI) and hybrid blockchain networks, that promise to elevate healthcare innovation. The findings serve as a resource for healthcare professionals, technologists, policymakers, and researchers aiming to harness these technologies for improved patient outcomes and system efficiency.

DOI: 10.4018/979-8-3373-0593-6.ch006

1. INTRODUCTION

1.1. Overview of Blockchain and AI in Healthcare

The integration of Blockchain and Artificial Intelligence (AI) is revolutionizing healthcare by redefining how patient data is managed, analyzed, and utilized. Unlike conventional databases, blockchain operates on a decentralized network, eliminating single points of failure and ensuring continuous data availability. Once recorded, information on the blockchain remains immutable, preserving the authenticity and integrity of sensitive medical records. Advanced cryptographic methods safeguard data, minimizing unauthorized access and significantly reducing the risk of security breaches. By enhancing privacy, integrity, and traceability, blockchain presents a robust solution to critical security challenges, particularly in managing electronic health records (EHRs). Its decentralized structure plays a crucial role in mitigating data breaches and unauthorized access, addressing the pressing need for patient confidentiality in modern healthcare.

Artificial Intelligence (AI) is transforming healthcare by enabling data-driven decision-making, predictive analytics, and process automation. It can analyze vast amounts of medical data to identify patterns and generate valuable insights that support diagnostics, personalized treatment strategies, and operational improvements. By enhancing decision-making and automating routine tasks, AI increases the accuracy and efficiency of healthcare services. Key applications include real-time monitoring of chronic conditions, predictive models for patient outcomes, and advanced medical imaging analysis. The integration of AI's data-driven capabilities with blockchain's secure and transparent storage system has the potential to revolutionize healthcare, offering enhanced data accessibility, improved clinical decision-making, and strengthened patient privacy.

The integration of blockchain and AI creates a powerful synergy that enhances the security and efficiency of managing vast volumes of medical data. Together, they address critical challenges such as ensuring the accuracy of AI-driven diagnoses, enabling secure and interoperable data exchange across healthcare institutions, and improving the scalability of healthcare systems. This convergence has the potential to transform multiple facets of healthcare, including patient record management, clinical trials, supply chain monitoring, and real-time clinical decision-making.

1.2. Significance of the Topic

The healthcare sector is under increasing pressure to enhance data security, optimize operational efficiency, and improve patient care, particularly as medical data continues to grow at an unprecedented rate. Globally, healthcare systems face challenges such as fragmented patient records, concerns over data privacy, interoperability issues, and difficulties in scaling services to meet rising demands. Additionally, patient data is often isolated within different institutions, creating barriers to seamless information exchange and slowing down critical decision-making processes.

The need for secure, efficient, and scalable solutions to manage and analyze healthcare data has become more critical than ever. The healthcare sector produces massive volumes of data, including electronic health records (EHRs), medical imaging, and genomic information. However, this data is often dispersed across multiple systems, creating challenges in accessibility, sharing, and analysis.

Data security and privacy have become major concerns in the healthcare industry. With cyberattacks on the rise, healthcare organizations are increasingly being targeted, putting confidential patient information at risk. A recent report revealed that over 1,000 data breaches occurred within a single year, compromising millions of patient records.

In an era where cyberattacks on healthcare organizations are becoming more frequent, blockchain's ability to enhance data security and privacy is invaluable. By leveraging blockchain technology, healthcare providers can establish a secure and transparent system for managing patient records, safeguarding sensitive information from unauthorized access.

Moreover, blockchain's smart contract capabilities can streamline processes such as supply chain management and insurance claims, minimizing administrative burdens and enhancing operational efficiency. For example, healthcare organizations can implement blockchain-based smart contracts to monitor the movement of medical supplies, ensuring timely and accurate deliveries to the intended destinations.

At the same time, AI's ability to process and analyze vast amounts of data can ease the workload on healthcare providers, enabling quicker and more accurate diagnoses and treatment decisions. By examining extensive medical datasets including electronic health records (EHRs), medical imaging, and genomic information AI algorithms can detect patterns and trends that might go unnoticed by human clinicians.

The combination of blockchain and AI has the potential to optimize healthcare operations, lower costs, and enhance patient outcomes, ultimately elevating the overall quality of care. By harnessing the strengths of both technologies, healthcare organizations can establish a secure, transparent, and efficient system that places patient well-being at the forefront.

In summary, the importance of this topic cannot be underestimated. The healthcare sector continues to grapple with critical issues related to data security, operational efficiency, and patient care. Integrating blockchain and AI presents a promising solution to these challenges, allowing healthcare organizations to build a secure, transparent, and efficient system that prioritizes patient well-being and improved outcomes.

1.3. Chapter Contribution

This chapter serves a multifaceted purpose, aiming to explore the transformative impact of integrating blockchain and artificial intelligence (AI) in healthcare. Its primary objectives include:

1. **Explore real-world applications:** This chapter aims to provide an in-depth analysis of how blockchain and AI are being utilized to tackle key challenges in healthcare. Through practical case studies, it examines their role in securing decentralized storage of electronic health records, preventing counterfeit drugs through supply chain tracking, predicting disease risks, reducing hospital readmissions, and accelerating drug development by analyzing molecular structures.
2. **Highlight key areas of application:** This chapter examines the integration of blockchain and AI in critical areas such as patient data management, supply chain transparency, clinical trial integrity, and predictive analytics. Blockchain ensures secure, decentralized storage of patient records, preventing unauthorized modifications, while AI enables rapid retrieval and advanced analysis to enhance treatment decisions. Additionally, AI processes vast healthcare datasets to generate predictive insights, while blockchain upholds data authenticity and transparency throughout the process.
3. **Identify challenges and opportunities:** By acknowledging the technical, ethical, and regulatory challenges associated with the integration of blockchain and AI in healthcare, this chapter aims to stimulate discussion and encourage innovation. Challenges are scalability, interoperability, and

high computational loads. Ethical issues include data privacy, AI bias, and transparency, whereas regulatory challenges are compliance, legal responsibility, and data sovereignty. These are addressed through strong frameworks, ethical AI, and responsive regulations.
4. **Inform and educate stakeholders:** This chapter seeks to serve as a valuable resource for healthcare professionals, technologists, researchers, and policymakers, providing practical knowledge and insights on leveraging blockchain and AI to address the most pressing challenges facing the healthcare industry. Stakeholders benefit from blockchain and AI through secure data sharing, fraud detection, automated processes, and personalized care. Healthcare providers employ AI for diagnostics, while patients have control over their data. Pharma companies guarantee open supply chains, insurers make claims easier, and regulators improve compliance. These technologies improve efficiency, security, and transparency in healthcare.
5. **Anticipate future innovations:** By exploring the current state of blockchain and AI in healthcare, this chapter aims to anticipate future innovations and advancements that could further transform healthcare delivery.

Ultimately, this chapter aims to expand the growing body of knowledge at the intersection of blockchain, AI, and healthcare. It seeks to inspire further research, innovation, and collaboration in this dynamic and rapidly evolving field.

2. FUNDAMENTALS OF BLOCKCHAIN AND AI IN MEDICAL SYSTEMS

2.1. Blockchain Essentials for Healthcare

Blockchain technology offers a secure, tamper-proof ledger that upholds data integrity and transparency without relying on intermediaries. In the healthcare sector, it can be utilized to manage electronic health records (EHRs) by decentralizing storage and allowing direct yet confidential access to patient information. Blockchain holds potential for resolving persistent problems such as fragmented patient data, lack of interoperability, security vulnerabilities, and inefficient administrative procedures. The key features of blockchain in healthcare include:

- **Decentralization**: Data is not stored in a single location but across multiple nodes, making it resistant to single points of failure and ensuring data integrity without a central authority. This makes it harder for cybercriminals to access sensitive information. For instance, patient medical records may be distributed among several network nodes in a healthcare blockchain system (Thatikonda et al., 2024). Patient records are protected because the integrity of the data on other nodes is not compromised in the event that one node is attacked or compromised.
- **Immutability**: Once data is recorded on a blockchain, it cannot be altered or deleted without leaving a detectable, permanent record of the alteration ensuring the accuracy and integrity of medical records and patient data. In clinical trials, for instance, it is possible to prevent results from being changed or reported selectively since all data must be documented in a manner that is resistant to tampering. Because blockchain technology has a visible audit trail, any attempts to alter data will be evident.

- **Transparency:** Blockchain's transparent nature allows all participants in a network to access and verify data, creating trust among stakeholders. It offers a transparent and open record of who has accessed patient data, when, and why. To ensure complete transparency, patients themselves have the ability to grant or withdraw access to their records, and every access event is recorded on the blockchain. In addition to giving individuals more control over their health information, this can assist prevent illegal use of their data.
- **Smart Contracts:** These self-executing agreements operate based on predefined rules and conditions, automating processes such as patient consent for data access and billing in healthcare services. In insurance claims, smart contracts can streamline the entire process from claim submission to reimbursement by automatically verifying service details (such as medical codes and service dates), confirming insurance coverage, and initiating payments once all conditions are met.

These blockchain capabilities can optimize healthcare operations, minimize fraud, empower patients with greater control over their medical records, and ensure compliance with regulations such as HIPAA.

2.2. AI Foundations in Healthcare

Artificial Intelligence (AI) is revolutionizing the healthcare industry by enhancing patient care, streamlining administrative processes, and enabling more personalized treatment options. AI encompasses various methodologies, including machine learning, natural language processing, and predictive analytics, all of which contribute to optimizing healthcare operations and improving overall outcomes.

The key components of AI in healthcare include:

- **Machine Learning**: Machine learning is a type of AI that allows systems to learn from data and improve over time. This approach allows healthcare professionals to process vast amounts of data, recognize patterns, and forecast patient outcomes. Machine learning aids in suggesting tailored treatment plans, detecting high-risk individuals, and estimating the probability of disease progression.
- **Deep Learning**: Deep learning is a sophisticated subset of machine learning that utilizes multi-layered neural networks to recognize and replicate complex patterns within large datasets. It is especially effective in handling unstructured data, such as text, audio, and medical images. For example, radiologists often use convolutional neural networks (CNNs) in deep learning to examine medical images and detect conditions like cancer or fractures.
- **Natural Language Processing:** NLP is a branch of artificial intelligence focused on enabling machines to understand, analyze, and generate human language effectively. NLP can be used to extract relevant information from unstructured clinical notes, EHRs, and research papers, making it easier for clinicians to access important data. NLP models are capable of automatically identifying important problems like drug interactions or unusual test findings and extracting relevant data from patient notes to assist clinicians in making well-informed decisions.
- **Predictive Analytics:** In the healthcare industry, predictive analytics uses advanced statistical models, machine learning, and artificial intelligence algorithms to evaluate past data and forecast future results. Predictive analytics is frequently used to forecast the onset of chronic diseases like diabetes, heart disease, and high blood pressure (Tagde et al., 2021). AI models are able to detect

high-risk individuals and suggest preventive steps by evaluating patient data, including lifestyle, genetic factors, and lab outcomes. It is also possible to identify patients who are at a higher risk for developing cancer by using predictive analytics. For instance, AI models that evaluate family history and genomic data to determine the risk of breast cancer allow for early detection and more personalized screening schedules.

- **Robotic Process Automation:** Robotic Process Automation (RPA) is the use of AI- powered software robots to automate repetitive, rule-based operations including data entry, scheduling, and claims processing. RPA is employed in the healthcare industry to automate administrative activities, lowering errors and freeing up staff for higher-value work. Healthcare organizations, for instance, utilize RPA to automatically process insurance claims, confirm a patient's insurance eligibility, or respond to billing inquiries.

Figure 1. AI and Blockchain Integration Framework.

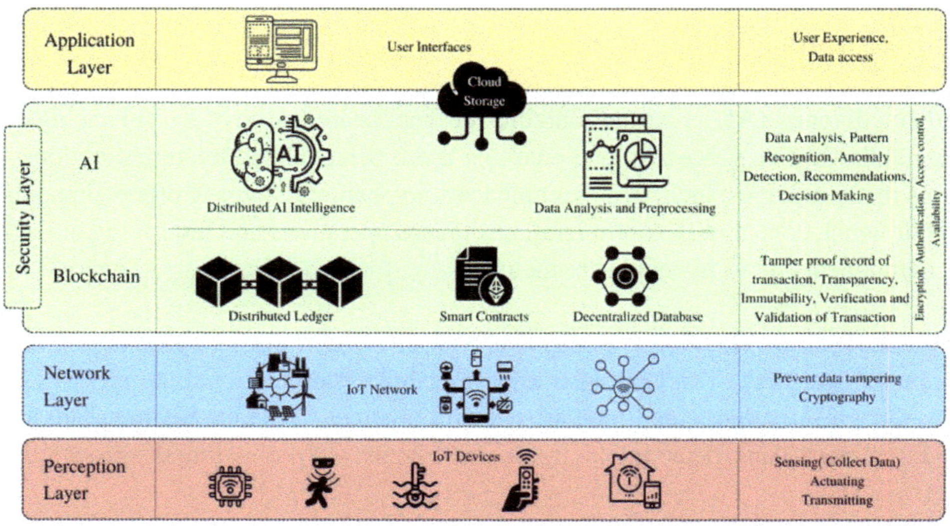

- **Reinforcement Learning:** It is a type of Machine Learning where an AI agent learns to make decisions by performing actions and receiving feedback from the environment. Reinforcement Learning is used in areas like robotic surgery or optimizing hospital operations. In the medical field, for instance, RL can optimize therapies by suggesting the most effective medication depending on patient feedback and responses.

Artificial Intelligence in healthcare has the potential to completely transform the sector, benefiting patients, providers, and the healthcare system overall by improving decision- making, streamlining healthcare processes, and increasing patient outcomes (Sai et al., 2022). Together, AI and machine learning techniques empower healthcare providers with the tools to offer more personalized, efficient, and data-driven care.

2.3. Blockchain and AI Synergy

Blockchain and AI integration in healthcare has the potential to completely transform the sector by combining the advantages of both technologies to solve difficult problems, strengthen security, enhance decision-making, and streamline processes. Integration of blockchain and artificial intelligence in healthcare creates a synergistic system in which blockchain provides decentralized, transparent, secure and tamper-proof data storage, while AI uses that data to generate advanced analytics, automation, predictive capabilities and actionable insights. The blockchain-AI synergy can lead to:

• **Data Integrity and Real-Time Decision-Making**: Some Challenges faced in Traditional Healthcare Data Management are patient records are split between hospitals, labs, and insurers, various healthcare systems use incompatible formats and centralized databases are susceptible to hacking and data breaches. Blockchain ensures that the health data (Electronic Health Records, diagnostic results, medical imaging, treatment plans) remains accurate, consistent, and tamper-proof. It also records all instances of data access, modification, and sharing (such as test results or medication prescription information) in an immutable manner, enabling patients and healthcare professionals to monitor data history in real time. Data reliability is further increased by decentralization in blockchain, which guarantees that AI systems can access data from a network of reliable nodes. By utilizing Distributed Ledger Technology (DLT), patient records are encrypted and stored across multiple nodes, ensuring data integrity and preventing unauthorized alterations. Smart contracts automate data access based on patient consent, allowing seamless and secure data exchange between hospitals, insurers, and researchers. Additionally, blockchain APIs support interoperability by integrating Electronic Health Records using standards like FHIR (Fast Healthcare Interoperability Resources. With the help of blockchain technology, people can take charge of their own data and grant or deny access to specific medical professionals, researchers, or AI systems. Patients can manage their consent through smart contracts or health data wallets, guaranteeing that AI systems only process the data they are permitted to access.

On the other hand, Artificial Intelligence models are able to automatically identify errors, discrepancies, or missing values in patient data, guaranteeing that only reliable, authentic data is sent to the blockchain for further use by AI systems. AI can obtain comprehensive records of data sources, modifications, and timestamps by utilizing blockchain's data provenance function. This guarantees that the algorithms are operating with current and legitimate data and AI algorithms process real-time vitals, medical images, and lab reports. For decision-making, deep learning models such as Convolutional Neural Networks (CNNs) and are used to identify cancerous nodules in CT scans and Recurrent Neural Networks (RNNs) are used to detect diseases by analysing patient data trends. Patients can manage access to their own data ensuring that AI operates ethically and within privacy regulations (like HIPAA or GDPR).

• **Enhanced Patient Privacy**: Blockchain keeps cryptographic proofs of the data i.e., hashes rather than the actual data on a central server. This improves privacy and lowers the chance of breaches by limiting access to the actual data to authorized persons or systems. "Blockchain decentralizes data storage, distributing encrypted medical records across multiple nodes in a peer-to-peer network. Using cryptographic hashing (SHA- 256), patient data remains immutable ensuring that no unauthorized party can alter medical records."

Using smart contracts or personal health data wallets, patients can grant access to specific medical professionals or researchers while maintaining complete control over their data. Blockchain ensures that any changes to patient records are easily traceable and auditable by providing an immutable proof of data access and updates. Blockchain technology can track when a medical professional accesses a patient's records, giving the patient insight into who has seen their information and when. This guarantees the validity and traceability of the data. Sensitive patient information is encrypted using both public and private keys to guarantee that only the designated receiver can read it. Access can be restricted using blockchain's permissioned models, which offer varying degrees of control for different healthcare stakeholders. On the blockchain, a patient's confidential health information might be encrypted so that only the doctor with the right private key could see all of the information. Smart contracts (deployed on Ethereum, or Hyperledger) regulate access to patient data. These self- executing contracts define who can access what data, under what conditions, ensuring compliance with HIPAA (USA), GDPR (Europe), or other regulations. For example, a smart contract can grant temporary access to a researcher for AI model training, ensuring data anonymization and automatic expiration of access after a set time.

The AI system could then handle the encrypted data without disclosing any private information to outside parties. AI models can be trained on decentralized data via federated learning without exchanging raw patient data. Only model updates (weights and parameters) are shared with the central model; AI algorithms are trained directly on the patient's local data (at the hospital or clinic) rather than sending patient data to a central server. Federated learning can be used by a hospital network to create a machine learning model using patient data from several hospitals, while the local hospital servers continue hold the real patient data. An AI technology called differential privacy makes sure that aggregate data cannot be used to identify specific patient information. Blockchain technology can safeguard AI models used to handle healthcare data, preventing any identifiable or exposed personal information. Zero-Knowledge Proofs (ZKPs) enable verification of data without revealing the data itself. Patients can demonstrate that their medical history is on the blockchain without disclosing particular health conditions. For instance, a patient can demonstrate their vaccination status without disclosing their entire medical history to an insurer.

In addition, blockchain can guarantee that the data was anonymised and handled securely, as well as store the cryptographic evidence of how AI models were built. AI models introduce mathematical noise using differential privacy, ensuring that individual patient records cannot be traced back even when analysing large datasets. Fully Homomorphic Encryption (FHE) allows AI to process encrypted medical data without decrypting it. For example, an encrypted AI model can analyse genomic data for personalized cancer treatment while keeping the patient's DNA confidential. Blockchain can guarantee that differentiated privacy principles are followed by keeping audit records of data consumption and AI model modifications.

- **Automation and Transparency**: Smart contracts (written in Solidity, Rust, or Vyper) execute predefined healthcare agreements automatically. They eliminate manual verification and third-party intermediaries, reducing operational costs and fraud. For example, a blockchain-based insurance claim system automatically processes payments once AI verifies treatment eligibility, reducing paperwork and fraud. All blockchain transactions are time-stamped and cryptographically linked, providing a transparent audit trail for compliance and regulatory checks (e.g., HIPAA, GDPR).

AI-driven analytics can trace discrepancies and detect fraudulent claims. For instance, AI scans blockchain-stored prescriptions to flag irregularities in opioid prescription patterns, preventing fraud. AI models can automate routine tasks in healthcare, such as scheduling appointments, processing claims, patient triage, diagnostic support, and personalized treatment planning. AI, for instance, can automate appointment scheduling, guaranteeing that patients are scheduled for follow-up sessions according to their treatment requirements and medical history. Additionally, AI models can automatically identify urgent conditions in diagnostic testing, highlighting urgent instances that require immediate attention. Clinical decision-making, such as selecting the best course of therapy based on a patient's medical imaging, test findings, and history, can be automated by AI systems. This reduces the cognitive load on medical professionals, freeing them up to concentrate on more difficult duties while maintaining consistency in the provision of care (Xie et al., 2021). An AI-powered decision support system, for instance, could simplify the prescription process and lower the possibility of human error by automatically recommending medication dosages based on the patient's medical history, lab findings, and drug interactions. Smart contracts on blockchain network can automate billing, claims processing, and payment settlements, among other administrative tasks in the healthcare industry. Invoices, payments to healthcare providers, and even the release of insurance claims can be automated by the blockchain whenever predetermined conditions (such as patient visits or treatment milestones) are fulfilled. Once a patient's treatment or procedure is recorded on the blockchain, a smart contract can automatically trigger payment for the service. This accelerates the reimbursement process for healthcare providers while reducing administrative burdens. The integration of blockchain technology and artificial intelligence (AI) streamlines insurance claim processing by automatically cross-referencing claims with patient records, insurance plans, and treatment histories.

Blockchain ensures data integrity and immutability, while AI helps detect fraud or inconsistencies in claims. For example, a blockchain network can verify a claim's validity by comparing it with a patient's insurance plan, medical history, and clinical records. AI then analyzes the data to identify any discrepancies or potential fraud. Several real-world applications demonstrate these capabilities. IBM Watson Health, in conjunction with Hyperledger, leverages AI for medical analytics while utilizing blockchain for data transparency. Similarly, MIT's MedRec system employs blockchain to automate electronic health record (EHR) access, reducing the need for manual verification.

The integration of blockchain and artificial intelligence enhances healthcare workflows, reduces operational expenses, and minimizes human errors by automating essential processes while ensuring transparent data management. This powerful combination is set to address key challenges in healthcare, such as data security, interoperability, and the inefficiencies of manual procedures.

3. CASE STUDY 1: INTEGRATING BLOCKCHAIN AND AI FOR SECURE PATIENT DATA MANAGEMENT

3.1. Project Overview

One of the most critical challenges in healthcare is safeguarding patient data privacy and security. This case study explores a project that leveraged blockchain and AI technologies to improve the secure management of electronic health records (EHRs). The objective was to develop a system where patient records could be securely stored, accessed, and shared while maintaining data integrity and ensuring patient confidentiality (Mistry et al., 2021). AI integration further enabled real-time decision-making by analyzing patient data and predicting potential health risks, allowing for timely interventions. However, challenges such as ensuring scalability, overcoming legacy system limitations, and maintaining compliance with regulations like HIPAA remain. Despite these obstacles, combining blockchain's security with AI's analytical capabilities offers a promising approach to enhancing the security, efficiency, and transparency of healthcare data management.

3.2. Technical Approach

The system utilized Hyperledger Fabric, a permissioned blockchain technology, to establish a decentralized ledger for securely storing encrypted patient data. This decentralized framework prevents any single entity from controlling the data, significantly lowering the risk of breaches. Each entry in the ledger was encrypted and linked to the previous record, ensuring that once data was recorded, it remained immutable. Additionally, blockchain provided an audit trail for all transactions, maintaining data integrity, while cryptographic hashing safeguarded patient information.

Smart contracts automated various administrative processes, including patient consent management, claims validation, and billing. For example, a smart contract could streamline compliance and minimize manual intervention by automatically initiating processes upon patient consent or treatment approval (Kumar et al., 2021). These smart contracts were also designed to grant or revoke access to specific medical records based on patient authorization and regulatory requirements, ensuring that only authorized individuals could access or modify sensitive information.

To implement a smart contract, the process begins with planning and gathering requirements, such as defining key functionalities and identifying stakeholders. During development, ensuring immutability and execution transparency is crucial. Testing should be conducted in a local blockchain environment like Ganache or Hardhat, followed by security assessments to identify vulnerabilities such as re-entrancy, overflow, and access control risks. Deployment should occur on testnets like Ethereum Goerli or Binance Testnet for validation. Additionally, optimizing gas fees can help reduce transaction costs, and performing smart contract audits using tools like Slither, MythX, or CertiK enhances security and reliability. Use Web3.js, Ethers.js to interact with the smart contract from a web application. Also integrate oracles (e.g., Chainlink) to fetch external data like medical records or financial transactions. Implement InterPlanetary File System (IPFS) for decentralized storage. Continuously track contract performance using blockchain explorers such as Etherscan or BscScan. Patient data is processed by AI algorithms, including lab findings, real-time data from wearables, and past medical records. AI-powered algorithms were used to analyse Electronic Health Records (EHRs), identifying patterns such as early warning signs of disease progression or potential medication interactions. Machine learning techniques, including Decision Trees and Logistic Regression, along with deep learning models such as Convolutional Neural Networks (CNNs), were utilized to analyze patient health records. Additionally, AI leveraged Natural Language Processing (NLP) to transform unstructured data such as clinical reports and doctors' notes stored on the blockchain into structured formats, enabling deeper analysis and the extraction of valuable insights.

For encryption and data integrity, advanced cryptographic techniques such as AES (Advanced Encryption Standard - 128/192/256-bit) was used for encrypting large datasets in real-time. Zero-Knowledge Proofs (ZKP) such as zk-STARKs (Zero-Knowledge Scalable Transparent Argument of Knowledge) were also used to ensure that only authorized personnel could decrypt the data. The system also implemented patient consent protocols through smart contracts. allowing individuals to manage their own data access permissions securely through blockchain, enhancing patient control and privacy. Smart contracts are self-executing agreements stored on a blockchain that automatically enforce the terms defined within them. In healthcare, smart contracts are used to secure, automate, and manage patient consent for data sharing, research participation, and treatment approvals. The patient inputs their credentials to a decentralized healthcare platform and chooses the information they want to share. They determine who can view it, for what purpose, and for how long. A smart contract is created, embedding the terms of consent. The contract is securely stored on the blockchain, ensuring it remains tamper-proof and easily verifiable.

Upon expiration, access is automatically revoked. For example, if a patient grants an insurance company permission to access medical records for claim processing, the smart contract ensures that only relevant data such as hospitalization details is shared while safeguarding sensitive information like mental health history. Once the claim is processed, access is automatically revoked.

3.3. Results and Challenges

The integration yielded promising results, with healthcare providers expressing greater confidence in the security and accuracy of patient data. The decentralized blockchain system safeguarded patient records from cyber threats and unauthorized access, while AI-driven analysis generated actionable insights for personalized treatment. For instance, predictive models identified patients at risk of chronic conditions based on historical data, enabling early intervention (Ekramifard et al., 2020).

However, several challenges emerged. One major concern was the substantial storage requirements of blockchain, particularly when handling large medical imaging files and complex datasets. While blockchain offers a secure method for managing smaller data segments, scalability issues arise with extensive healthcare records. Additionally, integrating blockchain with existing electronic health record (EHR) systems proved technically demanding, requiring significant modifications to support decentralized architectures.

4. CASE STUDY 2: BLOCKCHAIN AND AI IN HEALTHCARE SUPPLY CHAIN MANAGEMENT

4.1. Identifying Supply Chain Challenges

Healthcare supply chains are essential but face significant challenges that can impact their efficiency and safety. Key concerns include counterfeit medications, fraud, and a lack of transparency in tracking medical products. These issues not only endanger patient safety but also weaken trust in healthcare systems. Moreover, the inability to trace the origins of medical supplies makes supply chains more susceptible to disruptions and inefficiencies.

To tackle these challenges, the integration of blockchain and artificial intelligence (AI) has emerged as a groundbreaking solution. These technologies enable end-to-end traceability, improved quality control, and real-time demand forecasting, enhancing the security, efficiency, and transparency of healthcare supply chains (Armand et al., 2024).

4.2. Technology Integration

Envision a world where life-saving medications and medical supplies are always accessible, genuine, and of the highest quality. A world where patients have complete confidence that the treatments they receive are both safe and effective. This is the transformative potential of integrating blockchain and AI into healthcare supply chains.

- **Blockchain: The Guardian of Transparency and Security**

Blockchain technology functions as a digital ledger that meticulously records every transaction within the supply chain. It acts as an unchangeable record, ensuring transparency and accountability at every stage. From the moment a medication is produced to the time it is administered to a patient, blockchain tracks its entire journey. This capability helps detect and eliminate counterfeit or tampered products, safeguarding patient health. For example, consider a patient named Sarah who has been prescribed a life-saving medication. With blockchain, Sarah's healthcare provider can instantly verify the drug's authenticity by tracing its path back to the original manufacturer. This ensures both Sarah and her provider have complete confidence that the medication is genuine and safe.

- **AI: The Optimizer of Operations**

AI functions as an intelligent assistant that enhances supply chain efficiency by analyzing vast amounts of data, including historical trends, seasonal variations, and real-time factors. By predicting future demand for medical supplies and pharmaceuticals, AI enables healthcare providers to maintain optimal inventory levels, minimizing waste and ensuring that patients receive the necessary treatments on time (Khatri et al., 2021).

Additionally, AI serves as a powerful quality control tool. It automatically detects discrepancies in product information and identifies irregularities in quality, recommending corrective measures to ensure that only safe and effective products reach patients.

- **The Power of Integration**

The integration of blockchain and artificial intelligence (AI) has the potential to revolutionize healthcare supply chains. By combining these technologies, a secure, transparent, and highly efficient system for managing medical supplies and pharmaceuticals can be established.

Blockchain ensures the integrity of the supply chain by maintaining an immutable record of a medication's origin, movement, and authenticity. At the same time, AI enhances efficiency by analyzing data, predicting demand, and optimizing distribution, ensuring that medications are delivered promptly and effectively.

4.3. Real-Life Example

This vision is rapidly becoming a reality, driven by the groundbreaking integration of blockchain and artificial intelligence (AI) in healthcare supply chains. Leading pharmaceutical companies are at the forefront of this transformation, utilizing blockchain and AI to track drug movements with unmatched precision.

Here's how it works: blockchain serves as the foundation for a secure, transparent, and tamper-proof record of a medication's journey. From production to patient delivery, every transaction, movement, and interaction is recorded on the blockchain, creating an immutable history that guarantees the drug's authenticity, quality, and safety.

AI further enhances this system by analyzing historical consumption patterns, real-time trends, and other critical factors to predict demand for specific medications across different regions. This allows pharmaceutical companies to optimize production, streamline distribution, and manage inventory efficiently, ensuring that essential medications are available where they are needed most.

The impact is significant. Patients receive timely access to the medications they need, while pharmaceutical companies reduce waste, streamline operations, and enhance profitability. Healthcare providers can confidently prescribe treatments, knowing that the medications are authentic and effective.

This groundbreaking fusion of blockchain and AI is revolutionizing healthcare supply chains, ultimately saving lives and improving patient outcomes. As these technologies continue to advance, even more innovative solutions will emerge, further strengthening the quality, safety, and accessibility of healthcare worldwide.

Table 1. Quantitative Data & Real-World Implementation Metrics

Key Metric	Before Implementation (2020 Baseline)	After Blockchain & AI Integration (2023 Results)	Impact Summary
Traceability Time	Average 6.2 days (manual audits)	Real-time (5-10 seconds query)	99% reduction in trace time
Inventory Accuracy	82% accuracy	97.8% accuracy	Improved stock management & reduction in shortages
Counterfeit Detection Rate	68% detection accuracy	99.2% accuracy (via AI & blockchain product IDs)	Near elimination of counterfeit drugs
Order Processing Time	4 days (manual verification cycles)	Instantaneous (smart contracts auto-verification)	100% faster order processing
Demand Forecasting Accuracy	71%	91.50%	Reduced overstocking and stockouts
Regulatory Audit Readiness Time	3 months/year (manual prep)	Continuous real- time audit logs	80% reduction in compliance efforts
Operational Cost Reduction	Baseline	17% cost savings	Resulted from optimized logistics, fraud reduction
Data Breach Incidents	3 incidents/year	0 incidents (immutable ledger & permissions)	Improved cybersecurity posture
Waste Reduction (Expired Drugs)	12% waste per shipment cycle	4% waste	Accurate demand- Supply alignment through AI
Supply Chain Visibility Score (10)	4/10 (fragmented data, silos)	9.5/10 (unified dashboard)	Full real-time visibility across entire chain

4.4. Benefits and Limitations

Benefits

The integration of blockchain and artificial intelligence (AI) has greatly enhanced the security and transparency of healthcare supply chains. The key advantages include:

1. **Improved Security:** Blockchain technology transforms the conventional approach by maintaining immutable records, creating a unique digital signature for every product. This feature allows for immediate detection of counterfeit or altered items, ensuring that patients receive only authentic medications, thereby safeguarding their health and well-being.

2. **Operational Efficiency:** Managing supply chains is a complex challenge. AI-powered demand forecasting bridges the gaps by analyzing historical data, seasonal fluctuations, and real-time variables to predict demand with remarkable precision (Anoop & Asharaf, 2022). With these insights, pharmaceutical firms can optimize resource distribution, prevent inventory discrepancies, and enhance operational flow. The outcome is faster delivery of medications to patients while minimizing waste.
3. **Advancement in Research and Patient Care:** The synergy between blockchain and AI extends beyond logistics, positively influencing research, drug development, and overall patient care. These technological advancements contribute to a more efficient healthcare system, ultimately benefiting society as a whole.

Limitations

However, the adoption of blockchain and AI comes with its own set of challenges:

1. **Interoperability Challenges:** The absence of standardized platforms and APIs poses a major hurdle in ensuring seamless data exchange across different systems. This lack of compatibility can hinder the full potential of blockchain and AI integration.
2. **Operational Complexity:** Implementing these technologies requires significant investment in infrastructure, expertise, and ongoing maintenance. Without proper management, the efficiency and effectiveness of blockchain and AI applications may be compromised.
3. **Continuous Innovation and Adaptation:** Despite these challenges, ongoing advancements and collaborative efforts are essential in refining the use of blockchain and AI. By addressing these obstacles, the healthcare industry can drive innovation, enhance security, and ultimately improve patient care.
   a) Partial Stakeholder Integration

A major setback was the failure to fully integrate all stakeholders into the system. Smaller distributors, rural pharmacies, and independent healthcare providers faced difficulties in adopting the technology due to insufficient digital infrastructure and constrained financial resources. As a result, around 18% of supply chain participants continued operating outside the blockchain network during the first year, leaving traceability gaps in certain regions.

Impact

- Inconsistent data input, resulting in fragmented visibility.
- Inefficiencies persisted in low-adoption areas, undermining the goal of full transparency.

Reason:

The initial focus was on large-scale partners, and insufficient attention was given to equipping smaller players with affordable solutions and training.

b) AI Model Limitations During Unforeseen Events

The demand forecasting AI models, though effective under stable conditions, faltered during unpredictable situations like the COVID-19 pandemic. The sudden demand spikes and logistic constraints were beyond the training data's scope, causing significant forecasting errors and subsequent stockouts.

- Inaccurate forecasts led to supply shortages, particularly for essential drugs.
- Trust in the AI-based systems temporarily eroded among logistics managers.

AI systems need regular retraining and must incorporate external, real-world variables such as pandemics, geopolitical shifts, or raw material shortages to ensure reliability.

2. Cost Concerns

The financial implications of deploying Blockchain and AI technologies were a key challenge for MedTrust, particularly during the initial stages.

a) High Capital Investment

The combined setup cost for blockchain infrastructure, AI model development, API integrations, and stakeholder training was estimated at $20-25 million USD. Key expenditures included:

- Blockchain nodes deployment: $10 million
- AI development and cloud hosting: $7 million
- Data standardization & middleware integration: $5 million
- Training and stakeholder support: $3 million

For smaller companies, replicating this model without significant external funding would be infeasible.

b) Operational & Maintenance Costs

Beyond initial capital expenditure, ongoing costs related to:

- AI model retraining
- Cloud services for data storage
- Security audits
- Technical support

Added 12-15% annually to operational expenses, which was an ongoing concern for budget optimization. While large corporations can absorb these costs, smaller healthcare players may require consortium-based models or government incentives to afford such technologies.

Regulatory Hurdles

a) Data Privacy & Jurisdictional Compliance

MedTrust operated across multiple countries, each with distinct regulations such as:

- GDPR (EU)
- HIPAA (USA)
- Data Localization Laws (India, China)

Ensuring compliance with varying rules on data storage, patient privacy, and cross-border data transfer required complex permissioning structures within the blockchain and significantly increased deployment complexity.

b) Lack of Clear Blockchain Regulatory Framework

At the time of implementation, there was no standardized global framework regarding: The legal recognition of blockchain transaction records, The enforceability of smart contracts in court, Acceptability of blockchain logs in compliance audits Impact.

Delays in securing regulatory approvals in several jurisdictions. Ambiguity in using blockchain data for compliance purposes. MedTrust engaged with regulatory bodies early, providing pilot reports and demonstrating audit trails to gain preliminary acceptance but acknowledged that a more universally accepted framework was still lacking.

c) Ethical and Fairness Concerns in AI Usage

The use of AI in inventory management and demand forecasting raised concerns about algorithmic bias, particularly regarding, Whether AI might unintentionally deprioritize resource allocation to smaller or rural healthcare centers. The lack of transparency in AI decision-making ("black box" problem). To address these concerns, the organization implemented Explainable AI (XAI) models and kept human oversight in critical decision processes to ensure fairness.

5. CASE STUDY 3: BLOCKCHAIN AND AI IN CLINICAL TRIALS

5.1. Clinical Trial Challenges

Clinical trials are the cornerstone of medical innovation, enabling the development of new treatments and therapies. However, they face numerous challenges that can undermine their effectiveness and ethical integrity. Key Challenges and Solutions:

1. **Data Privacy Concerns:** Blockchain technology provides a secure and unchangeable record of patient information, ensuring confidentiality. This encryption mechanism protects sensitive data, offering patients greater assurance regarding their privacy.
2. **Fraud Prevention and Data Security:** By utilizing a transparent and tamper-resistant ledger, blockchain maintains the accuracy and authenticity of medical data. This enhances trust in treatment efficacy and safeguards against data manipulation, reinforcing confidence in medical advancements (Kumar et al., 2022).

Figure 2. Transaction processing in blockchain.

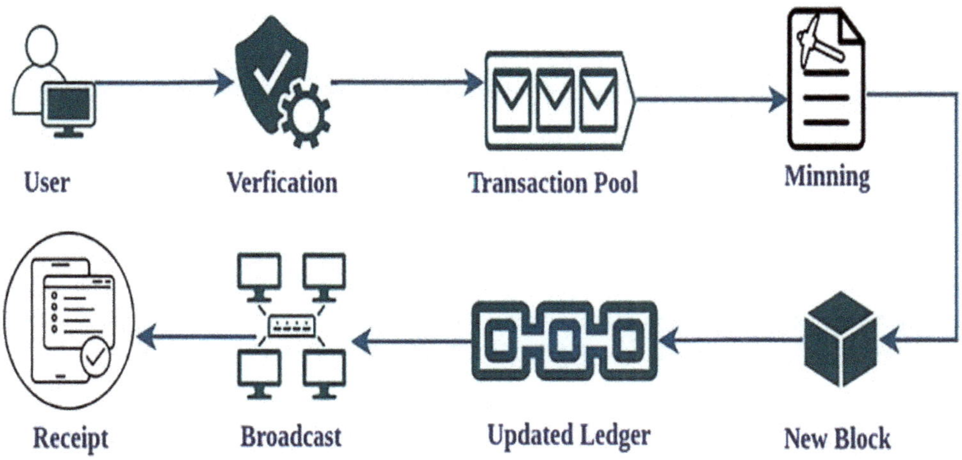

3. **Patient Recruitment Efficiency:** AI-powered analytics streamline the selection process by identifying eligible candidates based on their medical histories, genetic attributes, and other critical factors. This precision-driven approach reduces costs, saves time, and enhances the success rate of clinical trials.
4. **Ensuring Data Integrity:** Blockchain's unalterable ledger maintains data consistency, providing a verifiable and transparent record of all transactions. This fosters trust among patients, researchers, and regulatory bodies, ultimately expediting the development of groundbreaking medical treatments.

This case study explores how integrating blockchain and AI can overcome these challenges by increasing transparency, optimizing recruitment processes, and enhancing data accuracy.

5.2. Blockchain and AI in Action

Transforming Clinical Trials with Blockchain and AI

- **Blockchain for Secure Data Management:** Blockchain technology establishes a permanent, unalterable record of all clinical trial data, ranging from informed consent forms to final results. Its transparent and tamper-resistant ledger allows regulatory authorities to verify the integrity of trial processes, fostering trust among both patients and researchers.
- **AI for Patient Selection and Data Insights:** Artificial intelligence (AI) is revolutionizing clinical trials by analyzing medical histories, demographic data, and other relevant factors to identify the most suitable participants. This optimized recruitment approach minimizes delays, lowers costs, and enhances the likelihood of successful trial outcomes. Additionally, AI-driven analysis can uncover patterns within trial data and predict patient responses to treatments. By enabling researchers to make real-time adjustments to trial protocols, AI contributes to better patient outcomes and accelerates the development of life-saving therapies (Shinde et al., 2024).

5.3. Example Application

Revolutionizing Healthcare: Blockchain and AI in Clinical Trials

A groundbreaking clinical trial for an innovative cancer treatment highlighted the transformative potential of integrating blockchain and artificial intelligence (AI) in healthcare. A forward-thinking pharmaceutical company leveraged blockchain technology to establish a secure and transparent system for storing sensitive patient information and trial data. This approach safeguarded patient privacy while ensuring data integrity. AI models played a crucial role in patient selection by analyzing medical records and other relevant factors to identify individuals most likely to benefit from the treatment. This data-driven, personalized approach enhanced recruitment efficiency, accelerating patient enrollment and improving the overall effectiveness of the trial.

The success of this trial underscores the immense potential of combining blockchain and AI in healthcare. By leveraging these technologies, the industry can develop more secure, efficient, and patient-focused systems leading to better health outcomes, improved quality of life, and enhanced patient experiences. As innovation continues to reshape healthcare, it is essential to recognize the profound impact of blockchain and AI. By embracing these advancements and fostering a culture of collaboration and responsible innovation, we can unlock new possibilities for enhancing human health and well-being.

5.4. Outcomes and Constraints

Outcomes

1. **Strengthened Data Security:** Blockchain technology safeguarded trial data by preserving its integrity and confidentiality, ensuring the protection of sensitive patient information while maintaining the reliability of trial results. This robust security measure instilled confidence among both patients and researchers.
2. **Optimized Recruitment Efficiency:** AI accelerated the process of identifying and matching patients, conserving valuable time and resources. By analyzing extensive datasets, AI swiftly identified the most suitable candidates, streamlining the recruitment phase.
3. **Enhanced Analytical Accuracy:** AI's predictive capabilities improved trial outcomes by enabling real-time modifications. Through the analysis of data patterns and trends, AI empowered researchers to make well-informed decisions, ultimately leading to more effective treatments (Nimmagadda, 2021).

Constraints

1. **Technical Challenges:** The integration of blockchain and AI required seamless interoperability between diverse systems, necessitating collaboration among experts from multiple disciplines. Overcoming this complexity was crucial for successful implementation.
2. **Regulatory Compliance:** Adhering to industry standards introduced further challenges, as regulatory bodies enforced strict guidelines to uphold the integrity and security of trial data. Ensuring full compliance required meticulous attention to detail.

6. COMPARATIVE ANALYSIS OF BLOCKCHAIN-AI USE CASES

6.1. Effectiveness and Scalability

The integration of blockchain and AI has demonstrated remarkable effectiveness in overcoming healthcare challenges across various applications. Blockchain's capability to secure data and maintain transparency is crucial in domains such as clinical trials and supply chain management. At the same time, AI enhances efficiency through predictive analytics and process optimization. However, scalability presents a major obstacle, especially in data-intensive areas like patient records and medical imaging. Expanding these technologies demands significant computational resources and storage capacity.

6.2. Main Challenges

Key Challenges in Adopting Blockchain-AI Solutions

1. **High Computational Demands:** Running AI algorithms requires substantial processing power, placing a strain on infrastructure and resources. This can result in higher costs, slower processing speeds, and reduced overall efficiency.
2. **Storage Constraints:** Managing large datasets, such as medical imaging files, presents a major challenge for blockchain systems. The vast size of these files can exceed blockchain's storage capacity, complicating efforts to maintain a secure and decentralized record.
3. **Interoperability Barriers:** The absence of standardized systems across healthcare organizations makes integration difficult. Variations in platforms, formats, and protocols hinder seamless data sharing, collaboration, and the effective implementation of blockchain-AI solutions.

6.3. Guidelines and Best Practices

Best Practices for Advancing Blockchain-AI Adoption

To address the challenges limiting the implementation of blockchain-AI solutions, the following best practices are recommended:

1. **Collaborative Approach:** Establishing strong partnerships among healthcare providers, technology companies, and regulatory bodies is essential for success. Open communication and shared expertise enable stakeholders to drive innovation and effectively navigate challenges (Nguyen et al., 2021).
2. **Prioritizing Scalability:** As demand for blockchain-AI solutions increases, developing scalable systems is critical. This involves designing technologies capable of efficiently handling growing computational and storage needs while adapting to evolving requirements.
3. **Regulatory Compliance and Standardization:** Maintaining strict adherence to data privacy and security regulations is crucial for building trust and credibility. By following established standards and guidelines, healthcare organizations can ensure their blockchain-AI solutions remain secure, reliable, and compliant with industry regulations.

AI Fairness and Ethical Considerations

While integrating AI into blockchain-based supply chains and healthcare systems enhances efficiency and accuracy, it also raises ethical concerns related to fairness, transparency, and accountability.

a) Algorithmic Bias and Discrimination

AI models rely heavily on the quality and diversity of their training datasets. In healthcare and supply chain management, biased datasets can lead to disparities in service delivery, disadvantaging specific demographics, regions, or smaller stakeholders. For example, demand forecasting models trained primarily on urban data may unintentionally overlook rural healthcare centers, further deepening existing inequalities.

Proposed Measures

- **Adoption of Explainable AI (XAI) to provide clarity on how decisions are made.**
- **Regular audits of AI algorithms to detect and correct biases.**
- **Incorporation of diverse, representative datasets covering all stakeholders equally.**
- **Human-in-the-loop decision-making for critical processes to maintain ethical oversight.**

2. Blockchain Governance Challenges

While blockchain's decentralized structure enhances transparency and trust, it also introduces governance challenges that require careful ethical and operational considerations.

3. Decentralization vs. Control

A key governance challenge lies in maintaining decentralization while ensuring adequate regulatory oversight, especially in highly sensitive industries such as healthcare.

Key Ethical Concerns

- **Data Ownership:** Guaranteeing that patients, suppliers, and end-users retain full control over their data, preventing unauthorized access or misuse.
- **Smart Contract Accountability:** Establishing clear legal responsibilities in cases of smart contract failures or security vulnerabilities.
- **Consensus Mechanisms:** Addressing ethical concerns related to power concentration, such as mining monopolies or validator collusion, within blockchain networks.

Governance Solutions

- **Implementation of Permissioned Blockchain Models:** Ensuring that only verified and trusted entities operate network nodes to enhance security and accountability.

- **Formation of Multi-Stakeholder Governance Boards:** Involving regulators, industry leaders, and consumer advocates to oversee blockchain operations and policy-making.
- **Integration of Revocation Protocols:** Allowing the correction of erroneous transactions or the mitigation of malicious activities to maintain system integrity.

4. Future Developments and Next-Gen Innovations

Looking forward, the integration of blockchain and AI is poised to advance further, unlocking greater potential while introducing new complexities.

a) Integration of Federated Learning

New AI models are increasingly adopting Federated Learning, a technique that keeps data decentralized while enabling model training across multiple sources without exposing sensitive information. This approach aligns with blockchain's decentralized principles and enhances privacy protection in healthcare and supply chain management.

Impact

- **Improved data privacy and compliance with regulations like GDPR and HIPAA.**
- **Enhanced collaboration across global supply chains without compromising sensitive data.**

b) Scalable and Interoperable Blockchains

A key challenge in existing blockchain systems is the lack of interoperability between different platforms. The future of blockchain technology depends on the advancement of **cross-chain protocols**, which will facilitate seamless communication and data exchange across multiple blockchain networks.

Potential Advancements:

- **Improved global healthcare record sharing.**
- **Transparent, multi-chain supply chain management with real-time, cross-network traceability.**
- **Universal Compliance Mechanisms:** Embedding standardized regulatory frameworks within interoperable blockchain networks to ensure seamless compliance across different jurisdictions.

c) AI-Driven Smart Contracts (Autonomous Contracts)

Future advancements envision **AI-powered smart contracts** that can self-learn and adapt to evolving conditions, moving beyond traditional static, rule-based contracts to enhance automation and efficiency.

Ethical Challenges

- **Maintaining Interpretability and Oversight:** Ensuring AI-driven smart contracts remain transparent, understandable, and subject to human supervision.
- **Upholding Ethical and Regulatory Standards:** Preventing autonomous smart contracts from making decisions that could breach legal or ethical guidelines.

7. FUTURE FOR BLOCKCHAIN AND AI IN MEDICAL SYSTEM

7.1. Needed Technological Advancements

To fully unlock the potential of blockchain and AI in healthcare, significant advancements are required. Here are three critical areas for innovation:

1. **Scalable Blockchain Systems:** Current blockchain technology often faces challenges such as delays and high costs, limiting its adoption in healthcare. Emerging solutions like sharding and layer-2 technologies offer promising ways to improve scalability and efficiency. By addressing these limitations, blockchain can serve as a secure, transparent, and reliable foundation for managing healthcare data.
2. **Healthcare-Specific AI Models:** The effectiveness of AI depends on the quality of its training data. However, many AI models are built on generalized datasets that may not accurately represent diverse patient populations (Kumar et al., 2021). Developing specialized AI models tailored to specific demographics is crucial for ensuring accurate and equitable healthcare outcomes. Recognizing and addressing these disparities will enhance AI's effectiveness in medical applications.
3. **Optimized AI Algorithms:** AI-driven healthcare solutions demand significant computational power, which can lead to inefficiencies and delays. Techniques like edge computing, which processes data closer to its source, can reduce computational burdens and accelerate decision-making (Sai et al., 2022). By refining AI algorithms and optimizing data processing, healthcare providers can enhance efficiency and maximize AI's potential in patient care.

7.2. Ethical and Regulatory Issues

As blockchain and AI become more embedded in healthcare systems, addressing ethical and regulatory concerns is essential to maintain trust, integrity, and patient well-being. The following key issues require careful consideration:

- **Data Privacy:** Patient data is highly sensitive, and its protection is paramount. While blockchain provides secure storage, concerns remain regarding patient consent and privacy. AI's ability to analyze vast amounts of personal data necessitates robust frameworks for data sharing, patient consent, and withdrawal rights. Patients should have control over their data, including options to anonymize or revoke access. Transparency in data collection, storage, and usage is critical to fostering trust and ensuring ethical implementation.
- **Transparency and Accountability:** AI's "black-box" nature, where decision-making processes are often opaque, poses significant risks, especially in life-critical scenarios. Explainable AI

(XAI) aims to create models that offer clear, understandable explanations for their predictions and decisions (Jabarulla & Lee, 2021). As AI plays a growing role in diagnostics, treatment planning, and clinical trials, ensuring transparency and accountability will be crucial for ethical and effective decision-making.

- **Bias and Fairness:** AI algorithms can unintentionally reinforce biases present in training data, potentially leading to disparities in healthcare delivery. To prevent discrimination, AI models must be trained on diverse, representative datasets and subjected to rigorous bias assessments. Additionally, fostering diverse development teams in AI research ensures that multiple perspectives inform algorithmic decisions, promoting fairness and equity in healthcare outcomes.
- **Regulatory Frameworks:** The rapid adoption of blockchain and AI in healthcare demands comprehensive regulatory oversight. Compliance with existing privacy laws such as HIPAA and GDPR is essential, alongside the development of new regulations that address blockchain and AI's unique challenges. Establishing international standards will promote interoperability among healthcare systems and safeguard data privacy across borders. Regulatory bodies must remain adaptive and forward-thinking, ensuring policies keep pace with the evolving landscape of healthcare technology.Bottom of Form

7.3. Envisioning Future Healthcare Systems

The convergence of blockchain and AI is poised to redefine healthcare, fostering a personalized, secure, and highly efficient system. Blockchain's real-time, immutable data-sharing capabilities ensure accurate patient records while maintaining strict privacy and security standards, enabling a shift toward a more patient-centric model of care (Firouzi et al., 2022).

AI's predictive analytics can drive a prevention-focused healthcare approach, identifying diseases before they progress to severe stages, thereby reducing strain on healthcare systems. AI-powered diagnostic tools, such as automated medical imaging and clinical decision support systems, minimize human errors and standardize high-quality care across diverse medical settings.

Blockchain facilitates seamless interoperability between healthcare providers, ensuring that patients' medical histories remain up-to-date and easily accessible regardless of location. This is particularly beneficial for individuals with chronic or complex conditions, enhancing care coordination (Anoop & Asharaf, 2022). Additionally, smart contracts can automate administrative processes, reducing paperwork, mitigating human errors, and preventing fraudulent activities.

A promising future application lies in decentralized clinical trials, where blockchain ensures secure, transparent data management, while AI optimizes participant recruitment and trial efficiency. These advancements can accelerate drug development and research while maintaining ethical integrity and data reliability. Integrating blockchain and AI has the potential to revolutionize healthcare, making it more efficient, prevention-driven, and patient-focused. By leveraging these technologies, healthcare providers can enhance patient outcomes, streamline operations, and pave the way for a more advanced and equitable healthcare system.

8. CONCLUSION

8.1. Key Points

The integration of blockchain and artificial intelligence (AI) has the potential to transform global healthcare systems. By combining blockchain's secure, decentralized data management with AI's advanced analytics and predictive capabilities, healthcare providers can develop more efficient, secure, and patient-centric solutions. Blockchain ensures patient privacy and data integrity by offering a tamper-proof, decentralized framework for managing sensitive medical records. This is crucial in an era where data breaches and security threats pose significant risks to patient information. Meanwhile, AI enhances diagnostic accuracy, operational efficiency, and personalized treatment by analyzing vast amounts of medical data to detect patterns and generate predictive insights. These AI-driven capabilities enable healthcare professionals to make more informed, data-driven decisions (Ekramifard et al., 2020).

However, implementing blockchain and AI in healthcare presents several challenges, including scalability issues, high computational demands, and integration complexities with existing healthcare systems. Additionally, ethical and regulatory concerns, such as data privacy, bias in AI models, and the need for well-defined governance frameworks, must be addressed to ensure responsible and ethical deployment. To overcome these barriers, collaboration between healthcare providers, regulators, and technology developers is essential. Establishing clear guidelines and standards, enforcing robust data protection policies, ensuring transparency in AI decision-making, and fostering a culture of responsibility and ethics will be key to successfully integrating blockchain and AI into modern healthcare systems.

8.2. Scope of Research

The integration of blockchain and AI in healthcare opens up numerous exciting avenues for further research. One critical focus area is the development of quantum-resistant blockchain technologies. As quantum computing advances, it poses a significant risk to existing blockchain security mechanisms. Developing post-quantum cryptography (PQC) and integrating it into blockchain architectures is essential to mitigate threats posed by quantum computers. Quantum algorithms, such as Shor's algorithm, can efficiently break traditional cryptographic methods like RSA, ECC (Elliptic Curve Cryptography), and DSA (Digital Signature Algorithm), which currently secure blockchain systems. Researchers are actively working on quantum-resistant blockchain solutions to safeguard sensitive healthcare data from future vulnerabilities.

Another key area of research is enhancing AI transparency through the development of explainable AI (XAI) models. Many deep learning-based healthcare AI models function as "black boxes", making it difficult for clinicians and patients to understand their decision-making processes. Increasing AI interpretability is crucial for clinical trust, regulatory compliance (e.g., FDA, GDPR), and patient safety. By advancing explainable AI, researchers aim to build confidence in AI-driven healthcare solutions and ensure more informed medical decision-making (Khatri et al., 2021). Decentralized Clinical Trials (DCTs) powered by blockchain represent another promising research direction. Blockchain enhances participant enrollment, data sharing, and cost efficiency in clinical trials, leading to faster development of new treatments and improved health outcomes. The integration of smart contracts, zero-knowledge proofs (ZKPs), oracles, and tokenization ensures secure, patient-centric, and regulatory-compliant clinical trial operations.

Further research is also needed to explore blockchain applications in areas such as medical billing and supply chain management. Medical billing involves multiple stakeholders—hospitals, insurers, patients, and regulatory bodies—and is susceptible to fraud, inefficiencies, and errors. Blockchain's ability to create tamper-proof, transparent records can streamline operations, reduce fraud, and improve overall system efficiency. By investigating these applications, researchers can unlock new opportunities for blockchain-driven transformations in healthcare.

8.3. Conclusion

Blockchain and AI are Transforming Healthcare

Blockchain and artificial intelligence (AI) are reshaping the healthcare landscape, marking a transformative shift in how medical services are delivered and managed. By integrating blockchain's security and transparency with AI's advanced data analytics and predictive capabilities, these technologies have the potential to redefine healthcare systems. The benefits are far-reaching, including enhanced data security, improved operational efficiency, and highly personalized patient care. However, as these technologies continue to advance, addressing the ethical and regulatory challenges associated with their adoption is essential. Establishing comprehensive governance frameworks will be crucial to ensuring responsible implementation, fostering transparency, and prioritizing patient well-being (Xie et al., 2021).

The future of healthcare looks increasingly innovative and patient-centric, with blockchain and AI playing a pivotal role. By continuously refining these technologies, we can create a more efficient, accessible, and equitable healthcare system. Leveraging the transformative potential of blockchain and AI will pave the way for a healthier, more connected world, benefiting individuals and communities on a global scale.

REFERENCES

Anoop, V. S., & Asharaf, S. (2022). Integrating artificial intelligence and blockchain for enabling a trusted ecosystem for healthcare sector. In *Intelligent Healthcare: Infrastructure, Algorithms and Management* (pp. 281–295). Springer Nature Singapore. DOI: 10.1007/978-981-16-8150-9_13

Armand, T. P. T., Carole, K. S., Bhattacharjee, S., Mozumder, M. A. I., Amaechi, A. O., & Kim, H. C. 2024, February. The benefits of integrating AI, IoT, and Blockchain in healthcare supply chain management: A multi-dimensional analysis with case study. In *2024 26th International Conference on Advanced Communications Technology (ICACT)* (pp. 300-304). IEEE.

Ekramifard, A., Amintoosi, H., Seno, A. H., Dehghantanha, A., & Parizi, R. M. (2020). A systematic literature review of integration of blockchain and artificial intelligence. *Blockchain cybersecurity, trust and privacy*, pp.147-160.

Fatoum, H., Hanna, S., Halamka, J. D., Sicker, D. C., Spangenberg, P., & Hashmi, S. K. (2021). Blockchain integration with digital technology and the future of health care ecosystems: Systematic review. *Journal of Medical Internet Research*, *23*(11), e19846. DOI: 10.2196/19846 PMID: 34726603

Firouzi, F., Jiang, S., Chakrabarty, K., Farahani, B., Daneshmand, M., Song, J., & Mankodiya, K. (2022). Fusion of IoT, AI, edge–fog–cloud, and blockchain: Challenges, solutions, and a case study in healthcare and medicine. *IEEE Internet of Things Journal*, *10*(5), 3686–3705. DOI: 10.1109/JIOT.2022.3191881

Jabarulla, M. Y., & Lee, H. N. (2021, August). A blockchain and artificial intelligence- based, patient-centric healthcare system for combating the COVID-19 pandemic: Opportunities and applications. []). Mdpi.]. *Health Care*, *9*(8), 1019. PMID: 34442156

Khatri, S., Alzahrani, F. A., Ansari, M. T. J., Agrawal, A., Kumar, R., & Khan, R. A. (2021). A systematic analysis on blockchain integration with healthcare domain: Scope and challenges. *IEEE Access : Practical Innovations, Open Solutions*, *9*, 84666–84687. DOI: 10.1109/ACCESS.2021.3087608

Kumar, A., Gupta, D. N., & Kumar, R. (2022). Integration Aspects of AI, IoT, Big Data, and Blockchain in Healthcare Industry. In *Transformation in Healthcare with Emerging Technologies* (pp. 81–104). Chapman and Hall/CRC. DOI: 10.1201/9781003201960-5

Kumar, R., Wang, W., Kumar, J., Yang, T., Khan, A., Ali, W., & Ali, I. (2021). An integration of blockchain and AI for secure data sharing and detection of CT images for the hospitals. *Computerized Medical Imaging and Graphics*, *87*, 101812. DOI: 10.1016/j.compmedimag.2020.101812 PMID: 33279761

Mistry, C., Thakker, U., Gupta, R., Obaidat, M. S., Tanwar, S., Kumar, N., & Rodrigues, J. J. 2021, June. MedBlock: An AI-enabled and blockchain-driven medical healthcare system for COVID-19. In *ICC 2021-IEEE International Conference on Communications* (pp. 1-6). IEEE.

Nguyen, D. C., Ding, M., Pathirana, P. N., & Seneviratne, A. (2021). Blockchain and AI- based solutions to combat coronavirus (COVID-19)-like epidemics: A survey. *IEEE Access : Practical Innovations, Open Solutions*, *9*, 95730–95753. DOI: 10.1109/ACCESS.2021.3093633 PMID: 34812398

Nimmagadda, V. S. P. (2021). Artificial Intelligence and Blockchain Integration for Enhanced Security in Insurance: Techniques, Models, and Real-World Applications. *African Journal of Artificial Intelligence and Sustainable Development*, *1*(2), 187–224.

Sai, S., Chamola, V., Choo, K. K. R., Sikdar, B., & Rodrigues, J. J. (2022). Confluence of blockchain and artificial intelligence technologies for secure and scalable healthcare solutions: A review. *IEEE Internet of Things Journal*, *10*(7), 5873–5897. DOI: 10.1109/JIOT.2022.3232793

Shinde, R., Patil, S., Kotecha, K., Potdar, V., Selvachandran, G., & Abraham, A. (2024). Securing AI-based healthcare systems using blockchain technology: A state-of-the-art systematic literature review and future research directions. *Transactions on Emerging Telecommunications Technologies*, *35*(1), e4884. DOI: 10.1002/ett.4884

Tagde, P., Tagde, S., Bhattacharya, T., Tagde, P., Chopra, H., Akter, R., Kaushik, D., & Rahman, M. H. (2021). Blockchain and artificial intelligence technology in e- Health. *Environmental Science and Pollution Research International*, *28*(38), 52810–52831. DOI: 10.1007/s11356-021-16223-0 PMID: 34476701

Thatikonda, R., Kempanna, M., Tatikonda, R., & Bhuvanesh, A. (2024, June). The Impact of Blockchain and AI in the Healthcare. In *2024 IEEE 3rd International Conference on Electrical Power and Energy Systems (ICEPES)* (pp. 1-6). IEEE. DOI: 10.1109/ICEPES60647.2024.10653522

Xie, Y., Lu, L., Gao, F., He, S. J., Zhao, H. J., Fang, Y., Yang, J. M., An, Y., Ye, Z. W., & Dong, Z. (2021). Integration of artificial intelligence, blockchain, and wearable technology for chronic disease management: A new paradigm in smart healthcare. *Current Medical Science*, *41*(6), 1123–1133. DOI: 10.1007/s11596-021-2485-0 PMID: 34950987

Chapter 7
Explainable AI and Computational Modeling for Real-Time COVID-19 Detection Using Medical Imaging

Ali Turab
https://orcid.org/0000-0002-5445-9728
Northwestern Polytechnical University, China

Farhan Ullah
https://orcid.org/0000-0002-1030-1275
Prince Mohammad Bin Fahd University, Saudi Arabia

Shujaat Ali Zaidi
Chiang Mai University, Thailand

ABSTRACT

The global rise in population has made disease monitoring a critical challenge, highlighting the need for automated detection systems to improve diagnostic accuracy and reduce mortality. The COVID-19 pandemic has emphasized the importance of rapid diagnostic tools. This study proposes an explainable framework for COVID-19 detection using CT scans and chest X-rays, combining deep learning and machine learning. A CNN extracts features from images, which are classified using an ensemble of DT, RF, GNB, LR, KNN, and SVM models. A Susceptible-Infectious-Recovered (SIR) model is integrated to estimate virus transmission and support interpretability. Grad-CAM and t-SNE analyses validate feature importance and separability. Tested on two datasets (1,646 and 2,481 images), the proposed method achieved 98.5% accuracy, 99.2% precision, and 99.4% recall. Comparative analyses demonstrate superior performance, and explainable AI experiments confirm the robustness and transparency of the framework.

DOI: 10.4018/979-8-3373-0593-6.ch007

1. INTRODUCTION

The coronavirus pandemic has profoundly disrupted global economies, healthcare systems, and societal structures, posing unprecedented challenges for governments and individuals alike. Measures such as lockdowns and mobility restrictions, implemented to curb the virus's rapid spread, have significantly impacted industries and daily life. By July 9, 2020, the World Health Organization (WHO) reported over 12 million confirmed cases and 552,050 fatalities globally (Coronavirus, 2020). Healthcare systems worldwide faced severe shortages of critical resources, including intensive care units (ICUs), ventilators, and personal protective equipment, complicating pandemic management.

COVID-19, caused by the SARS-CoV-2 virus, shares genetic similarities with severe acute respiratory syndrome (SARS) and Middle East respiratory syndrome (MERS) (Ciotti et al., 2020). Symptoms range from mild cold-like manifestations to severe respiratory failure and multi-organ damage, affecting organs such as the liver and kidneys in critical cases (Naeem & Bin-Saleem, 2021; Culp, 2020). Although vaccines have been pivotal in controlling the pandemic, their early availability was limited, and they do not ensure full immunity. Consequently, early detection and effective prevention remain critical.

Diagnostic devices are essential in reducing the spread of COVID-19. Reverse Transcription Polymerase Chain Reaction (RT-PCR) serves as the standard method for detecting the virus in respiratory samples (Tahamtan & Ardebili, 2020). However, its widespread adoption is obstructed by high costs, supply chain difficulties, and cumbersome processes, particularly in resource-constrained settings. Radiographic imaging techniques, such as chest X-rays and computed tomography (CT) scans, have shown considerable effectiveness, offering critical information on pulmonary involvement and enabling timely diagnosis and management (Chen et al., 2020). Due to COVID-19's high transmissibility, the development of rapid, reliable, and scalable diagnostic tools is crucial. Computer-aided diagnostic (CAD) technologies, augmented by the Internet of Things (IoT) and artificial intelligence (AI), have significant potential. IoT-based solutions provide remote diagnostic access, benefiting underserved regions with insufficient healthcare infrastructure (Kumar et al., 2020; Haider et al., 2019; Kalsoom et al., 2022; Ahad et al., 2025; Butt et al., 2023a; Butt et al., 2023b). Despite the widespread availability of chest X-rays, their diagnostic effectiveness is limited by difficulties in differentiating soft tissues. CT scans, although more accurate, need human interpretation, which is labor-intensive and prone to errors (Ye et al., 2020; Islam & Nahiduzzaman, 2022).

Advancements in machine learning (ML) and deep learning (DL) have transformed medical imaging by automating diagnostic procedures and enhancing accuracy (Ashfaq et al., 2023). These methodologies have been effective in identifying disorders like coronary artery disease, diabetic retinopathy, HIV, and malignancies (Ullah et al., 2017; Kassani et al., 2019; Saygill, 2021; Kassania et al., 2021; Turab et al., 2022; Turab et al., 2024). Convolutional Neural Networks (CNNs) are particularly adept at identifying pertinent information from high-dimensional medical imaging datasets. These methods diminish dependence on manual interpretation, thereby reducing diagnostic errors, promoting early intervention, and improving healthcare outcomes (Guo et al., 2015; Gandhi et al., 2018; Esteva et al., 2019; Esteva et al., 2021; Shah et al., 2021; Lan et al., 2022; Ali et al., 2024; Ahad et al., 2021).

Notwithstanding these developments, obstacles persist in the development of automated COVID-19 detection systems. Most current models concentrate on differentiating COVID-19 from other respiratory diseases but are deficient in evaluating disease severity, necessitating radiologists to interpret the findings. The lack of extensive, labeled datasets and the disparity between severe and non-severe instances exacerbate overfitting, hence constraining model efficacy (Basu, Mullick & Das, 2022). Confronting these problems necessitates novel strategies that harmonize computational efficiency with diagnostic precision, especially in resource-limited IoT environments.

This study explains COVID-19 detection and categorization in CT and chest X-ray pictures. The strategy uses deep learning and machine learning to fix present systems. CNN uses machine learning algorithms such as Support Vector Machine (SVM), Logistic Regression (LR), Gaussian Naïve Bayes (GNB), Random Forest (RF), and Decision Tree (DT) to classify 350 basic properties from images. Voting-based ensemble models enhance categorization. Verifying results and examining feature distributions using explainable AI methods like Grad-CAM and t-SNE. Our study's primary contributions:

- The development of a CNN model to extract deep features from CT and chest X-ray images for real-time COVID-19 identification.
- Combining deep learning and machine learning classifiers with a soft voting mechanism to enhance accuracy and mitigate dataset imbalances.
- Utilizing explainable AI techniques, such as Grad-CAM and t-SNE, to authenticate forecasts and elucidate feature distributions and anomalies.

The following portions of this chapter are structured as outlined below: Section 2 examines pertinent literature, Section 3 delineates the suggested approach, Section 4 showcases experimental data, and Section 5 closes the research.

2. RELATED WORK

Recent studies have thoroughly investigated deep learning methodologies to improve COVID-19 identification and severity assessment. Sarkar et al. (2020) used transfer learning with DenseNet-121 to classify COVID-19 patients from radiographic images, attaining an accuracy of 87% and pinpointing disease-indicative areas within the radiographs. on a similar vein, Shan et al. (2020) presented a deep learning methodology for classifying impacted lung areas on CT images, achieving 91% accuracy on a dataset of 300 COVID-19 patients. This technique, however, lacked the capacity for severity assessment, hence limiting its diagnostic value in comprehensive assessments. Zhang et al. (2020) used DenseNet for COVID-19 detection, achieving a sensitivity of 96% for COVID-19 cases and 70.65% for non-COVID-19 cases. Wang et al. (2020) utilized pre-trained deep learning models to detect COVID-19 infections in lung scans, with 87% accuracy among more than 1,260 people from six cities.

The use of IoT technology in healthcare has garnered considerable attention. Otoom et al. (2020) devised a system that amalgamates eight machine learning models to detect COVID-19 patients via IoT networks, achieving over 90% accuracy with five models. Ahmed et al. (2020) developed an IoT-based classification system using ResNet-101 and chest X-ray images, achieving a classification rate of 98%. Rohila et al. (2021) introduced ReCOV-101, a deep learning model for COVID-19 classification using CT scans, with an accuracy of 94.9%. Hemdan et al. (2020) presented a deep learning approach for COVID-19 identification in chest X-rays, achieving an accuracy of 95.38% by the use of nine pre-trained neural networks. Aayush et al. (2021) used DenseNet201 for the identification of COVID-19 in CT images, using ImageNet pre-trained weights and achieving remarkable results. Silva et al. (2020) used a voting-based deep learning approach that combines transfer learning with an 18-layer architecture. Syed et al.

(2021) proposed a four-step classification approach for COVID-19 using CT scans, including fine-tuned pre-trained models and evolutionary algorithms, achieving an accuracy of 97.9%.

This study presents a framework for explainable COVID-19 detection that amalgamates deep learning and machine learning methodologies, using current advancements. The proposed methodology utilizes convolutional neural networks to extract deep features from CT and chest X-ray images, which are classified using a voting-based ensemble model. Explainable AI techniques, such Grad-CAM and t-SNE, are used to ensure interpretability and analyze feature distributions. The framework was evaluated using two datasets including 1,646 and 2,481 CT scan images, respectively. The findings indicated improved performance in precision, recall, F1-score, and accuracy compared to existing approaches, confirming the framework's effectiveness as a real-time diagnostic tool.

3. PROPOSED METHODOLOGY

The proposed IoT platform integrates a web service with cloud infrastructure to facilitate efficient data processing and parameter management for COVID-19 detection. The web application, developed in Java, ensures seamless data handling and interaction with the cloud via various devices. The IoT framework is structured as an interconnected network of computing systems, uniquely identifiable devices, and digital tools capable of exchanging data without human intervention. IoT technology addresses challenges related to real-time monitoring and data connectivity. By integrating machine learning algorithms, sensing devices, and statistical models, IoT platforms enable real-time data acquisition and analysis. During the pandemic, these systems have proven effective for isolating infected individuals, monitoring adherence to quarantine protocols, and remotely tracking high-risk patients (Durrani, Yasmin & Rho, 2022).

Figure 1 shows how to use CT scans to identify COVID-19. This study analyzes medical imaging data, especially CT scans of COVID-19 patients, using deep learning techniques. Preprocessing, categorization, and feature extraction are crucial components. With the use of preprocessing techniques that improve image clarity for analysis, feature extraction ensures accuracy even in cases when images are not very clear. A voting-based ensemble strategy improves classification accuracy, while a deep convolutional neural network (CNN) pulls distinctive visual information from images. This ensemble reduces errors and produces dependable results by combining predictions from many models and using majority vote. By addressing accuracy and reliability concerns, the combination of these methods offers a comprehensive solution for COVID-19 detection in CT images (Khalid et al., 2017; Guo et al., 2019).

Figure 1. The suggested IoT-based COVID-19 detection system architecture

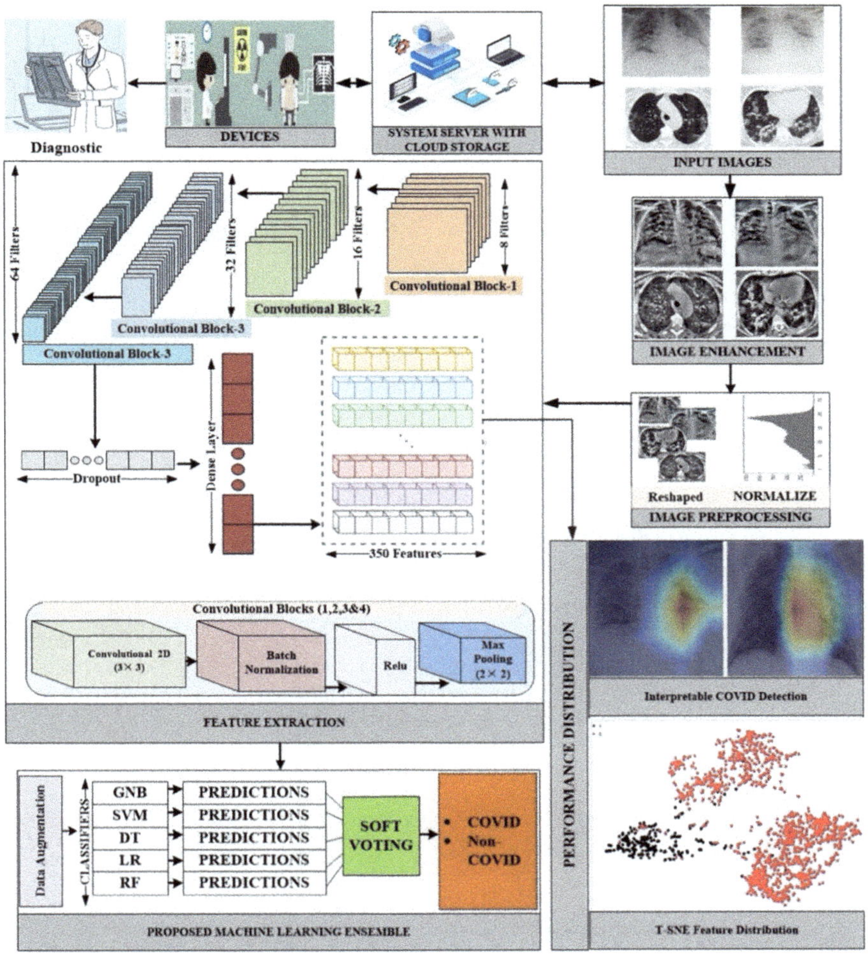

3.1. Image Enhancement and Preprocessing

The preprocessing step guarantees dependability via the use of high-quality medical imaging datasets. Various publicly accessible sources, such as GitHub, Cohen's X-ray picture collection, and the Italian Society of Medical and Interventional Radiology (SIRM), were used. Supplementary photos were acquired from the Radiological Society of North America (RSNA) and Radiopaedia, guaranteeing a varied dataset for examination. Kaggle functioned as a centralized repository for radiography pictures. The resulting dataset consisted of 245 X-ray pictures depicting COVID-19 and 1,401 photos of normal conditions. The SARS-CoV-2 CT scan dataset included 2,390 CT images, of which 1,229 exhibited signs of infection and 1,161 were categorized as negative. Demographic data indicated that 34 instances pertained to male patients and 28 to female patients. Figure 2 presents exemplary picture samples from the datasets.

Figure 2. Lung CT scans and chest X-rays of COVID-19 patients

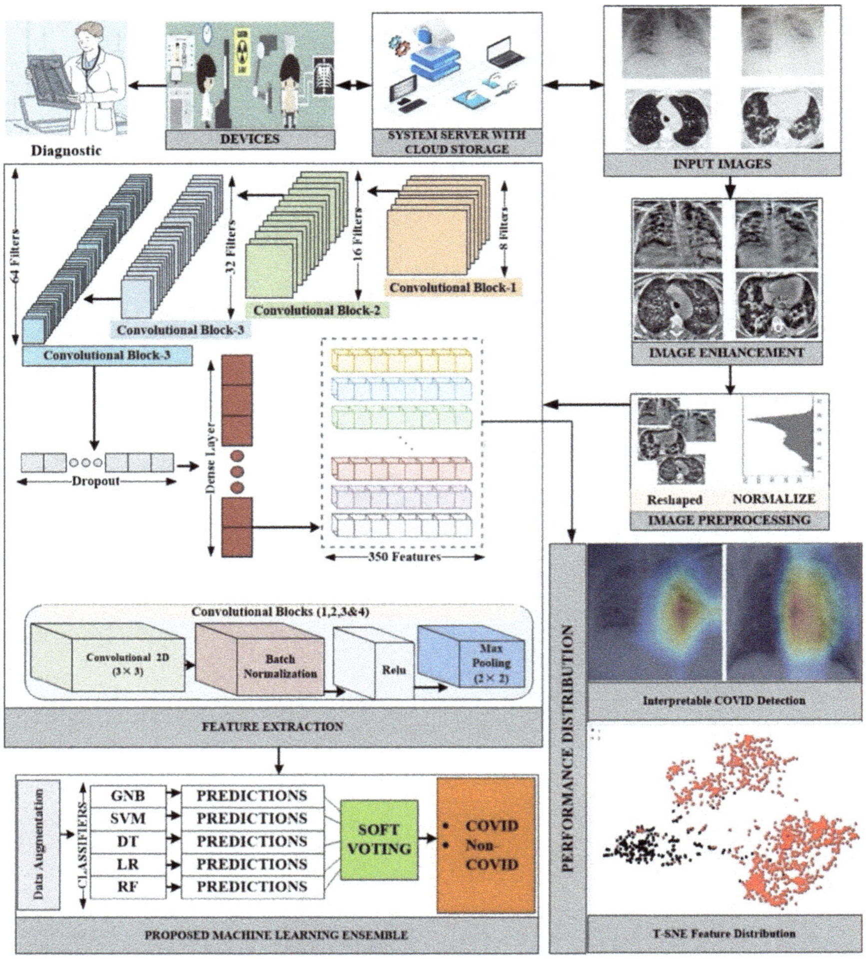

Image preprocessing played a pivotal role in this study by enhancing image quality and optimizing the performance of subsequent machine learning models. To address the challenges of low-quality imaging, Contrast-Limited Adaptive Histogram Equalization (CLAHE) was employed as a contrast enhancement technique. CLAHE mitigates noise amplification by clipping the histogram at a predefined threshold, known as the clip limit. This approach strikes a balance between improving contrast and minimizing noise, making it especially effective for medical imaging applications. In this study, the clip limit was set at 2.0, and a tile grid size of 8×8 was chosen to achieve optimal results.

The first step in the preprocessing procedure was to convert the RGB color system images to the LAB color space. To increase contrast, the CLAHE method was applied just to the LAB image's L (lightness) channel. A better LAB image was then created by combining the enhanced L channel with the A and B channels, and it was then converted back to RGB format. This methodical process yielded images with improved contrast and clarity, which are necessary for precise feature extraction. Every image was reduced to a uniform resolution of 224×224×3 in order to preserve uniformity and convolutional neural network (CNN) compatibility. The scaling process conformed the dataset to the input specifications of the CNN models used in the research. Furthermore, pixel values were standardized to diminish variability and improve model efficacy during training, promoting expedited and more stable convergence. Figure 3 illustrates the effect of the CLAHE technology by juxtaposing original CT scan pictures with their improved versions. The preprocessing techniques were essential for preparing the dataset for further analysis, finally facilitating accurate identification and categorization of COVID-19 in medical pictures.

Figure 3. Adaptive histogram equalization contrast-limited image enhancing

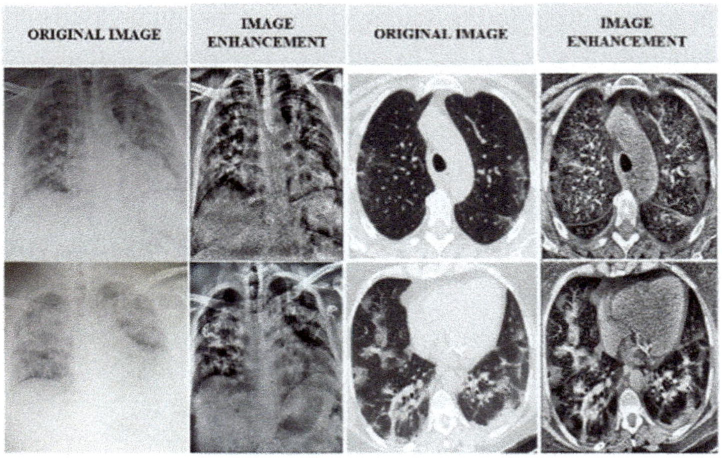

3.2. Feature Extraction

Feature extraction is a cornerstone of classification tasks, especially in medical imaging, where the precision of extracted features significantly influences model reliability. Raw image data, often high-dimensional, presents challenges in efficient processing and analysis. To address these challenges, the proposed approach utilizes convolutional neural networks (CNNs), renowned for their effectiveness in managing high-dimensional datasets such as images and videos. Unlike conventional methods that use raw images as direct input, this study employs handcrafted feature vectors, reducing the training complexity by transforming high-dimensional data into a streamlined feature vector of length 1×1024.

The extensive dimensionality reduction of the CNN architecture developed in this study allows for the extraction of critical features that are necessary for COVID-19 identification. The program extracted 100 unique COVID-19-related traits from CT scan images that would be challenging to extract using human feature engineering. Each of the four convolutional layers in this architecture is coupled with max-pooling and batch normalization layers. Together, these elements improve feature extraction skills and improve classification outcomes. For COVID-19 cases, the model consistently demonstrated reliable classification performance across around 100 iterations. Convolutional filters are used by the CNN, which was created using Python's TensorFlow (version 1.9) framework, to evaluate incoming data and combine outputs into a better feature space. Thorough hyperparameter tweaking improved key parameters like frequency and filter size, enhancing the network's capacity to spot intricate patterns in the input data.

By introducing non-linearity, the rectified linear unit (ReLU) activation function improved the model's learning ability and made feature representation more efficient.

In order to preserve input dimensions, the proposed architecture has two convolutional layers with 64 and 128 filters, respectively, and a kernel size of four. Using max-pooling layers with a stride of one and a pooling size of two reduced the size of the feature space without sacrificing important characteristics. This pooling technique improved classification accuracy by reducing processing demands while maintaining the integrity of crucial data. A fully connected classification layer that used the Softmax activation function to provide probabilistic outputs for classification was part of the design. A rate of 0.5 for dropout layers reduced overfitting during training. Using momentum-based optimization and tunable learning rates, the Adam optimizer was used to enhance convergence and generalization. Each image was sent into the network during CNN model training, which retrieved 100 crucial characteristics from the penultimate dense layer, which had 100 neurons. To ensure that the most relevant data for study was preserved, the recovered features were then used to classification tasks. A thorough description of the CNN architecture, including all of its parts and permutations, is shown in Table 1. The proposed CNN system effectively addresses the challenges of high-dimensional imaging data via the use of optimization techniques, creative feature extraction methods, and handcrafted feature vectors.

Table 1. Model summary for feature extraction

Layer (type)	**Parameters**	**Output Shape**
conv2d_input (InputLayer)	0	(None, 224, 224, 3)
conv2d (Conv2D)	224	(None, 222, 222, 8)
batch_normalization	32	(None, 222, 222, 8)
activation (Activation)	0	(None, 222, 222, 8)
max_pooling2d (MaxPooling2D)	0	(None, 111, 111, 8)
conv2d_1 (Conv2D)	1168	(None, 109, 109, 16)
batch_normalization_1	64	(None, 109, 109, 16)
activation_1 (Activation)	0	(None, 109, 109, 16)
max_pooling2d_1 (MaxPooling2)	0	(None, 54, 54, 16)
conv2d_2 (Conv2D)	4640	(None, 52, 52, 32)
batch_normalization_2	128	(None, 52, 52, 32)
activation_2 (Activation)	0	(None, 52, 52, 32)
max_pooling2d_2 (MaxPooling2)	0	(None, 26, 26, 32)
conv2d_3 (Conv2D)	18496	(None, 24, 24, 64)
batch_normalization_3	256	(None, 24, 24, 64)
activation_3 (Activation)	0	(None, 24, 24, 64)
max_pooling2d_3 (MaxPooling2)	0	(None, 24, 24, 64)
flatten (Flatten)	0	(None, 9216)
dense (Dense)	1179776	(None, 128)
batch_normalization_4	512	(None, 128)
activation_4 (Activation)	0	(None, 128)

continued on following page

Table 1. Continued

Layer (type)	Parameters	Output Shape
dropout (Dropout)	0	(None, 128)
feature_dense (Dense)	12900	(None, 100)

Trainable parameters: 1,217,700; Non-trainable parameters: 496;
Total parameters: 1,218,196

3.3. Process of Feature Scaling

In order to ensure that all input features are standardized to a constant range, feature scaling is an essential step in the data preparation process for machine learning models. Since unstandardized data may lead to skewed model findings, it is essential to correct size, unit, and magnitude discrepancies among features. Numerical computation-based algorithms may erroneously give more weight to attributes with larger values, skewing forecasts and compromising model precision. In models that optimize via gradient descent, the significance of feature scaling is most apparent. Features with larger ranges may have a disproportionate impact on the optimization process in the absence of normalization, which might result in slower convergence and longer training cycles. Normalizing the dataset ensures that each attribute makes an equal contribution to the learning process of the model. This change improves the overall stability and reliability of the training process in addition to increasing the efficiency of gradient descent, producing predictions that are more accurate and reliable.

To guarantee uniformity in feature contributions, this study used the Standard Scaler approach for feature normalization. By setting each characteristic to have a mean of zero and a standard deviation of one, this method normalizes the data. In order to rescale the data while maintaining the intrinsic correlations between characteristics, the standardization process involves taking the mean of each feature and dividing the result by the standard deviation.

When features in a dataset have different units or magnitudes, feature scaling is crucial. Standardization reduced the influence of scale-related variations by improving the models' capacity to identify important patterns and relationships. This technique was crucial for increasing the models' anticipated accuracy and making sure the algorithms worked well with a range of input properties. Feature scaling not only enhanced model performance but also increased machine learning's stability and computational economy. The methodical feature improvement complies with established industry best practices, enabling the suggested framework to process a variety of datasets with high correctness and dependability (Hu et al., 2019; Nawaz et al., 2021).

3.4. COVID detection

• Naïve Bayes is a versatile probabilistic method that excels in classification tasks due to its simplicity and versatility. Classifiers may express Bayes' theorem as follows

$$P(y|X) = \frac{P(Xy)P(y)}{P(X)} \quad (2)$$

In the above formula, $P(y|X)$ represents the posterior probability of the class y given the features $X = (x_1, x_2, ..., x_n)$, $P(Xy)$ is the likelihood of observing $X = (x_1, x_2, ..., x_n)$ given y, $P(y)$ is the prior probability of the class, and $P(X)$ is the evidence, a normalizing constant independent of y. As illustrated in Equation 3, the Naïve Bayes technique incorporates the assumption that the characteristics are conditionally independent, which simplifies the process and considerably decreases the amount of computing complexity.

$$P(y|X) = \frac{P(x_1y)P(x_2y)\ldots P(y)}{P(x_1)P(x_2)\ldots P(x_n)} \tag{3}$$

The probability density function for the Gaussian distribution is given by

$$P(x_1y) = \frac{1}{\sigma_y\sqrt{2\pi}} e^{-(x_i-\mu_y)^2/2\sigma_y^2} \tag{4}$$

• The Support Vector Machine (SVM) is a flexible and efficient supervised learning approach that is ideal for classification and regression. Support vector machines (SVM) seek the best hyperplane for categorizing data points. Maximising the margin—the distance between the hyperplane and the data points closest to it from each class—calculates this hyperplane. This strengthens categorization. The kernel technique turns lower-dimensional input vectors into higher-dimensional feature spaces for non-linear separable data. Support vector machines (SVM) handle this problem using this method. Support vector machines are effective for complex non-linear classification problems because to this property. This study employed the sigmoid kernel to do non-linear mappings, allowing the model to understand the complicated data linkages. This research uses a soft-margin SVM. This classifier optimizes outcomes by balancing margin and classification errors. Minimizing the loss function during optimization is as follows

$$\left[\frac{1}{n}\sum_{i=1}^{n}\max\left(0,1 - y_i\left(w^T x_i - b\right)\right)\right] + \|w\|^2 \tag{5}$$

• A choice Tree (DT) is a model that is constructed like a tree, with each core node representing a choice that is based on an attribute, branches representing decision rules, and leaf nodes representing categorization results. Through a process of recursive partitioning of the data into subsets depending on attribute values, the tree evolves. While repeated segmentation contributes to further refinement of categorization, the root node is the initial decision point. As a result of their intuitive nature and their ease of interpretation, decision trees are a popular option for a wide variety of applications. Through the use of a loss function, such as entropy, which may be computed as follows, the purity of the nodes that make up a decision tree is assessed

$$Entropy = -\sum_{i=1}^{K} p_i * log_2 p_i \tag{6}$$

The value of entropy may vary from 0 to 1, with lower values indicating nodes that are easier to understand. When compared to the parent node, the entropy of the separated nodes must be lower for a split to be considered genuine. In every other case, it is thrown away in order to keep the partitioning as optimum as possible (Guermazi et al., 2018).

• Logistic Regression (LR) is a statistical model that is effective at predicting binary outcomes ($y = 0 \; or \; 1$) with a high degree of precision. In contrast to linear regression, logistic regression is intended for categorical outcomes and use the logistic function as a means of modeling probabilities. A mathematical representation of the logistic function is as follows

$$f(x) = \frac{1}{1 + e^{-x}} \tag{7}$$

Through the use of extracted characteristics, this model is especially well-suited for the purpose of predicting dichotomous outcomes, such as whether COVID-19 would be positive or negative.

- Random Forest (RF) is an ensemble learning method that combines many decision tree classifiers to enhance prediction accuracy and reduce overfitting. Additionally, it uses the bagging technique to build trees from subsets of the training data. Aggregating these trees' predictions by voting (classification) or averaging (regression) yields the final result. According to Khalilia, Chakraborty, and Popescu (2011), this method is resilient and generalizable.
- The K-Nearest Neighbors (KNN) method is a parameter-free instance-based learning approach. It classifies a data point using the K nearest feature space data points. Majority vote among k's neighbors determines categorization. KNN is great for classification and regression because it places comparable data points near together.
- Ensemble learning (EL) combines many models to enhance prediction accuracy beyond individual models. A voting ensemble may combine model predictions for classification issues using majority voting. This method works well when combining models with different architectures or hyperparameters. This study uses soft polling ensemble. The first training used many models, including SVM, LR, GNB, RF, and DT, utilizing gathered characteristics. Sagi and Rokach (2018) reported that the ensemble model used each model's predictions to classify.

The COVID-19 detection framework uses deep learning and machine learning. The CNN model first collects key information from CT scans and X-ray images. The last stage is identifying these attributes using cutting-edge machine learning classifiers like GNB, SVM, RF, LR, DT, KNN, and others. Soft polling ensemble aggregates classifier predictions. Its ability to categorize input samples as positive or negative for COVID-19 shows that this hybrid method may combine algorithms to increase performance.

4. RESULTS

4.1. Measure of Performance

We used a dataset of CT scan images to assess the efficacy of the ensemble learning model we proposed. After training the model on a segment of the data known as the training set, it was then evaluated on an independent subset of data, termed the testing set. This strategy enabled an objective assessment of the model's ability to generalize to novel data. We used a total of 2,482 CT scan images for this specific purpose. The dataset was randomly partitioned into training and testing subsets, using a standard ratio of 80% for training and 20% for testing. The ratio was preserved throughout the division procedure.

Several performance metrics, including accuracy, precision, recall, F-measure, and Area Under the Curve (AUC), were used to evaluate the efficacy of the machine learning algorithms deployed in the ensemble method. Below are the mathematical formulae for the performance measures

$$Accuracy = \frac{TP + TN}{TP + TN + FP + FN} \tag{8}$$

$$Precision = \frac{TP}{TP + FP} \tag{9}$$

$$Recall = \frac{TP}{TP + FN} \tag{10}$$

$$F - measure = 2 * \frac{Precision * Recall}{Precision + Recall} \tag{11}$$

4.2. Analysis

The suggested framework underwent a thorough evaluation that included the use of many state-of-the-art classifiers. These classifiers included Naïve Bayes (NB), Support Vector Machine (SVM), Decision Tree (DT), Logistic Regression (LR), Random Forest (RF), K-Nearest Neighbors (KNN), and an ensemble learning technique. Table 2 provides a summary of the performance measures that are associated with these approaches. The number of features in Dataset 1 was varied in increments of fifty, ranging from fifty to five hundred, in order to use a feature selection process in order to determine the best possible feature set. Using 350 characteristics, the classifiers were able to achieve their highest level of performance, which led to their selection for further COVID-19 classification procedures.

Table 2. Optimal feature selection results for Dataset 1

Classifier	Features									
	50	100	150	200	250	300	350	400	450	500
NB	0.957	0.967	0.968	0.938	0.964	0.952	**0.97**	0.965	0.944	0.967
SVM	0.874	0.901	0.928	0.901	0.945	0.923	**0.952**	0.945	0.951	0.967
DT	0.952	0.961	0.953	0.958	0.948	0.935	**0.956**	0.945	0.947	0.956
LR	0.958	0.965	0.974	0.965	0.965	0.967	**0.97**	0.957	0.962	0.965
RF	0.962	0.97	0.965	0.958	0.963	0.961	**0.97**	0.963	0.961	0.965
KNN	0.964	0.967	0.965	0.965	0.962	0.972	**0.972**	0.964	0.967	0.965
Ensemble	0.962	0.968	0.967	0.959	0.963	0.965	**0.97**	0.964	0.965	0.965

The classification accuracy for SVM, LR, DT, NB, RF, KNN, and the ensemble technique was 0.952, 0.97, 0.956, 0.97, 0.972, and 0.97. The KNN classifier performed best in the dataset with 0.972 accuracy. Comparisons with pre-trained deep learning models including Inception v3, VGG16, ResNet, MobileNet, and DenseNet201 confirmed this best feature set. The proposed technique and many pre-trained models were assessed using their different configurations (described in Table 3). This was done in order to study the influence that network complexity, parameters, and architectural layers had on the results. The parameter counts and layer depths for each model were as follows: the proposed method (1,218,196 parameters, 27 layers), Inception v3 (22,007,684 parameters, 311 layers), VGG16 (14,765,988 parameters, 19 layers), ResNet (23,792,814 parameters, 175 layers), MobileNet (3,331,566 parameters, 87 layers), and DenseNet201 (18,514,084 parameters, 707 layers). The differences between these approaches are illustrative of the various computing requirements and design philosophies that constitute each technique.

In order to test the models, we used the standard performance criteria, which included F1-score, accuracy, precision, prediction time, and recall. An accuracy of 0.972, an F1-score of 0.97, precision of 0.97, recall of 0.97, and a prediction time of 0.077 seconds were achieved by the suggested technique when it was combined with the KNN classifier. This method displayed remarkable performance. On the other hand, Inception v3, when paired with the RF classifier, was able to attain an accuracy of 0.849, an F1-score of 0.78, a precision of 0.72, a recall of 0.85, and a prediction time of 0.017 seconds. According to the findings of the investigation, the RF classifier consistently outperformed its competitors when it was merged with pre-trained models such as VGG16, Inception v3, ResNet, DenseNet201, and MobileNet. This demonstrates the RF classifier's ability to handle complicated datasets with ease. The KNN classifier, on the other hand, displayed the greatest compatibility with the framework that was presented, giving greater accuracy and efficiency in comparison to alternative configurations.

Table 3. Different CNN models for Dataset 1 performance comparison

Model	Parameters	No. Layers	Classifier	Accuracy	F1-Score	Precision	Recall	Pred. Time
Our Method	1,218,196	27	NB	0.97	0.97	0.97	0.97	0.0069
			SVM	0.952	0.95	0.96	0.95	0.0069
			DT	0.956	0.96	0.96	0.96	0.0019
			LR	0.97	0.97	0.97	0.97	0.00199
			RF	0.97	0.97	0.97	0.97	0.0189
			KNN	0.972	0.97	0.97	0.97	0.077
			Ensemble	0.97	0.97	0.97	0.97	0.0688
Inception v3 (Pre-Trained)	22,007,684	311	NB	0.182	0.12	0.68	0.18	0.0019
			SVM	0.789	0.77	0.75	0.79	0.0109
			DT	0.739	0.74	0.74	0.74	0.0009
			LR	0.848	0.78	0.72	0.85	0.00099
			RF	0.849	0.78	0.72	0.85	0.017
			KNN	0.8323	0.77	0.73	0.83	0.0747
			Ensemble	0.829	0.77	0.72	0.83	0.0466
VGG16 (Pre-Trained)	14,765,988	19	NB	0.255	0.26	0.72	0.26	0.00099
			SVM	0.829	0.79	0.77	0.83	0.0109
			DT	0.738	0.75	0.76	0.74	0.00099
			LR	0.8359	0.78	0.75	0.84	0.00099
			RF	0.85	0.78	0.8	0.85	0.0189
			KNN	0.828	0.77	0.74	0.83	0.075
			Ensemble	0.84	0.78	0.76	0.84	0.047

continued on following page

Table 3. Continued

Model	Parameters	No. Layers	Classifier	Accuracy	F1-Score	Precision	Recall	Pred. Time
ResNet (Pre-Trained)	23,792,814	175	NB	0.84	0.78	0.72	0.84	0.0019
			SVM	0.809	0.78	0.75	0.81	0.0109
			DT	0.744	0.75	0.76	0.74	0.00099
			LR	0.8493	0.78	0.72	0.85	0.00099
			RF	0.851	0.78	0.87	0.85	0.0179
			KNN	0.8396	0.78	0.74	0.84	0.068
			Ensemble	0.85	0.78	0.72	0.85	0.045
Mobile Net (Pre-Trained)	3,331,566	87	NB	0.15	0.05	0.51	0.15	0.00099
			SVM	0.809	0.77	0.74	0.81	0.0109
			DT	0.701	0.72	0.75	0.7	0.0009
			LR	0.85	0.78	0.8	0.85	0.0009
			RF	0.85	0.78	0.72	0.85	0.0179
			KNN	0.831	0.78	0.74	0.83	0.075
			Ensemble	0.831	0.78	0.74	0.83	0.043
Densenet201 (Pre-Trained)	18,514,084	707	NB	0.165	0.08	0.71	0.17	0.00199
			SVM	0.818	0.77	0.73	0.82	0.0099
			DT	0.727	0.74	0.75	0.73	0.00099
			LR	0.844	0.78	0.72	0.84	0.00099
			RF	0.85	0.78	0.72	0.85	0.017
			KNN	0.827	0.77	0.73	0.83	0.0708
			Ensemble	0.8371	0.78	0.73	0.84	0.05

The performance of the proposed method was assessed using two distinct datasets to evaluate its classification capabilities across different classes comprehensively. Table 4 presents a detailed summary of the class-wise performance, employing standard metrics such as precision, recall, F1-score, and accuracy, calculated for both COVID and non-COVID classes. The first dataset consisted of 245 COVID images and 1,401 non-COVID images, introducing a class imbalance, whereas the second dataset was more balanced, containing 1,252 COVID images and 1,229 non-COVID images.

In the case of Dataset 1, the model exhibited a higher classification rate for the majority class (non-COVID) compared to the minority class (COVID). This disparity likely stems from the abundance of training samples for the non-COVID class, which facilitated more robust learning for the majority class. Conversely, Dataset 2 demonstrated balanced classification rates across both classes, as the nearly equal distribution of COVID and non-COVID images allowed the model to develop a more equitable learning representation for both categories. The overall performance metrics, precision, recall, F1-score, and accuracy, across the two datasets were (0.97, 0.99), (0.97, 0.99), (0.97, 0.99), and (0.972, 0.985), respectively, reflecting consistently high performance regardless of dataset composition. During the training process, epoch curves that depicted accuracy and loss values were evaluated in order to acquire more insights into the dynamic behavior of the proposed approach. Through the monitoring of training and testing accuracy and loss values over the course of several epochs, it was feasible to evaluate the consistency of the learning process of the model and identify patterns that impacted the outcomes of performance.

Table 4. Performance review by class

Classes	Total	Precision	Recall	F1-measure	
Dataset-1					
COVID	245	0.92	0.89	0.9	
Non-COVID	1401	0.98	0.99	0.98	
Average		0.97	0.97	0.97	
Dataset-2					
COVID	1252	0.97	0.93	0.95	
Non-COVID	1229	0.99	0.99	0.99	
Average		0.99	0.99	0.99	
Overall Performance					
Dataset		Precision	Recall	F1-Score	Accuracy
Dataset-1		0.97	0.97	0.97	0.972
Dataset-2		0.99	0.99	0.99	0.985

Figure 4 illustrates the accuracy epoch curve for testing data, which provides a comparative analysis of the proposed method against state-of-the-art models in varied CNN configurations. Y-axis signifies accuracy, while x-axis represents the number of epochs. Accuracy first increased swiftly from 0% to 82%, then stabilized at this level until the 15th epoch. Subsequently, an incremental development resulted in a maximal accuracy of 98%. A transient decline to 30% was observed at the 27th epoch, which was promptly followed by a recovery. As a result of its effective learning progression over successive epochs, the model maintained accuracy levels that ranged from 0% to 99%. Other state-of-the-art models were marginally outperformed by the ResNet model, which achieved testing accuracies ranging from 0% to 85%. However, the proposed method was not surpassed. Competing frameworks, such as Inception v3, VGG16, MobileNet, and DenseNet201, realized testing accuracies that varied from 0% to 80%. The proposed approach obtained accuracy levels that were unmatched by any of the models that were competitive. Throughout a variety of experimental conditions and hyperparameter configurations, this comparative evaluation emphasizes the proposed method's exceptional ability to consistently outperform existing models.

The proposed framework's robustness is further emphasized by the analysis, which demonstrated superior class-wise performance, greater stability, and higher accuracy across a variety of datasets and CNN configurations. These results emphasize the proposed method's ability to surmount the inherent obstacles of COVID-19 classification tasks, thereby reinforcing its reliability as a diagnostic instrument.

Figure 4. Comparing accuracy with cutting-edge methods

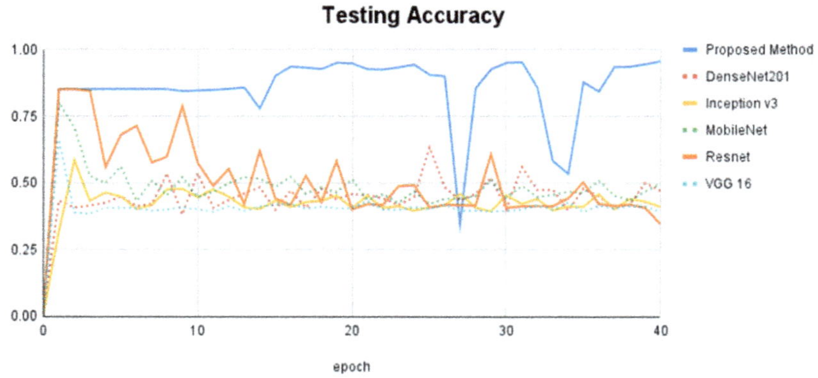

Figure 5 depicts the testing loss epoch curve, which offers a comparative examination of the proposed technique in comparison to other models that are considered to be state-of-the-art. These models include DenseNet201, ResNet, Inception v3, MobileNet, and VGG16. Among these models, DenseNet201 exhibits the largest testing loss, with values ranging from fifty percent to seventy percent. The curve for DenseNet201 exhibits inconsistent behavior, which is characterized by periodic rises and drops in loss. This suggests that the classification performance of the network does not remain stable.

In contrast, the proposed method demonstrates the lowest testing loss, indicative of superior classification accuracy. The loss curve begins at approximately 5% and steadily declines, stabilizing at this level until the 26th epoch. A transient spike in loss is observed at the 27th epoch, where it momentarily reaches 30%, followed by a sharp reduction to 2%. Overall, the testing loss for the proposed model remains consistently within the range of 0% to 30%, representing the best performance among the evaluated approaches. ResNet emerges as the next most effective model in terms of minimizing testing loss, delivering classification results that outperform other state-of-the-art methods. However, models such as Inception v3, MobileNet, and VGG16 exhibit relatively higher loss values, performing similarly to one another but noticeably inferior to both the proposed method and ResNet. This comparison underscores the enhanced efficiency and accuracy of the proposed framework in addressing classification challenges.

Figure 5. The suggested method's loss comparison with state-of-the-art techniques

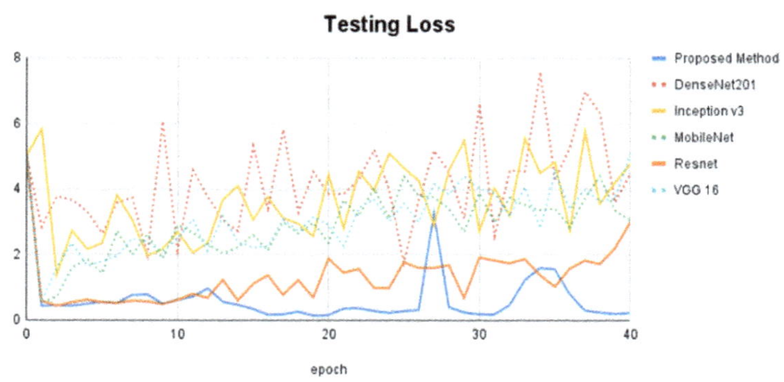

The training accuracy epoch curve for the proposed method, illustrated in Figure 6, reveals a rapid and consistent increase in accuracy during the initial epochs. Starting at 0%, the curve reaches 80% by the 5th epoch, followed by a brief stabilization period. The accuracy continues to rise, achieving 99% by the 10th epoch. This high level of accuracy remains stable throughout the subsequent epochs, with only minor fluctuations, underscoring the robustness and reliability of the proposed model. DenseNet201 ranks as the second-best performing model, attaining training accuracy values within the range of 0% to 97%. While its performance is commendable, it falls short of the consistency and final accuracy exhibited by the proposed method. Conversely, ResNet demonstrates comparatively weaker performance, with its training accuracy curve positioned lower than all other evaluated models.

Figure 6. Comparing training accuracy with modern methods

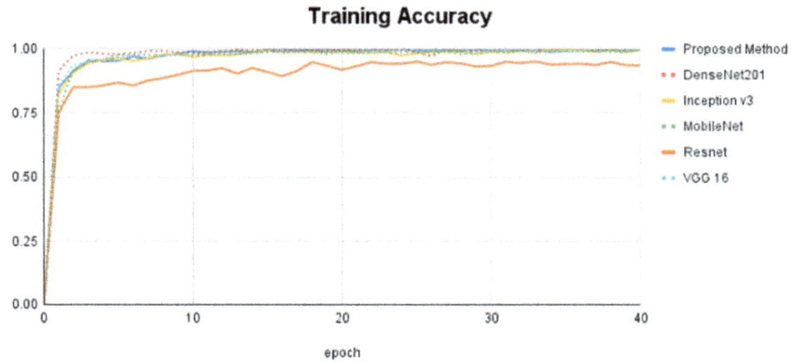

Figure 7 offers some insights into the training loss values for the suggested approach in relation to existing strategies that are considered to be state-of-the-art. During the whole training process, the suggested method exhibits the lowest training loss, which further validates its effectiveness in reducing the amount of error that occurs during model optimization. When compared to other models, such as DenseNet201, Inception v3, MobileNet, and VGG16, the training loss is consistently determined to be smaller. Based on these findings, it is clear that the suggested technique not only improves accuracy but also guarantees stability by lowering the amount of overfitting that occurs.

Figure 7. Training loss comparison of the proposed method with state-of-the-art approaches

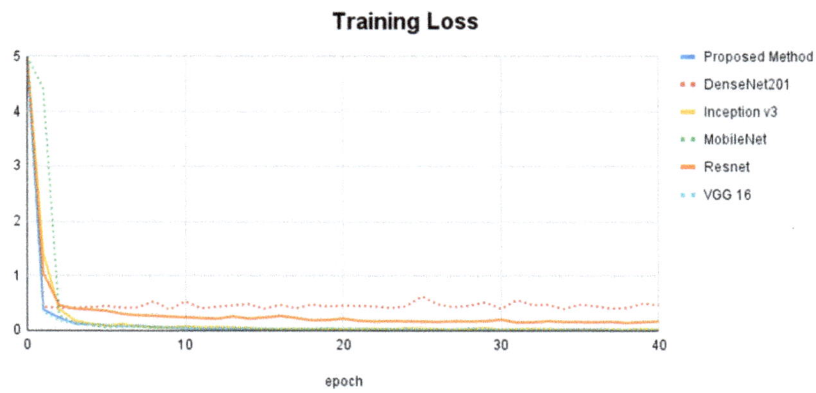

In order to demonstrate the improved performance of the proposed technique, an examination of the testing loss, training accuracy, and training loss curves. As a result of the model's optimization and its robust generalization to data that it has not before seen, the combination of low testing and training loss values, together with excellent training accuracy, speaks volumes. Despite the fact that DenseNet201 produces results that are competitive, it demonstrates persistent underperformance when compared to the strategy that was suggested across all measures. Although other models, such as ResNet, Inception v3, MobileNet, and VGG16, exhibit larger loss values and worse accuracy, the benefits of the proposed framework in terms of stability and overall performance are further highlighted by these particular models. These data provide evidence that the suggested strategy is reliable for completing COVID-19 classification tasks. The confusion matrix is a crucial diagnostic tool for analyzing classification performance. It offers a detailed perspective of the predictions that were right and those that were erroneous for each class. Figure 8 compares the confusion matrices of the proposed ensemble model with those of baseline methods, illustrating their respective class-wise classification effectiveness. The diagonal elements of the matrix represent accurate classifications, while the off-diagonal elements capture misclassifications.

For the COVID class, the proposed ensemble model achieves an impressive classification rate of 99%, with a misclassification rate of just 1%. For the non-COVID class, it attains classification and misclassification rates of 88% and 12%, respectively. The Decision Tree (DT) method, while performing well, achieves slightly lower rates, with classification and misclassification percentages of 98% and 2% for the COVID class and 82% and 18% for the non-COVID class, respectively. The Logistic Regression (LR) method, on the other hand, exhibits impressive results, with classification and misclassification rates of 99% and 1% for the COVID class, and 89% and 11% for the non-COVID class, respectively. The findings presented here provide further evidence that the ensemble model has exceptional performance, especially in terms of its capacity to effectively identify COVID instances while simultaneously retaining competitive accuracy for non-COVID cases. With regard to the classification performance of the proposed method across two datasets, Table 5 offers a complete description of the results. The first dataset contains 1,646 CT scan pictures, whereas the second dataset has 2,481 CT scan images together. The study takes into consideration important performance measures such as recall, precision, accuracy, and F1-score. With values of 0.972 for accuracy, 0.97 for F1-score, 0.97 for precision, and 0.97 for recall, the ensemble model that is integrated with the K-Nearest Neighbors (KNN) classifier gets the top performance metrics for Dataset 2, which is the first dataset. When it comes to Dataset 2, the ensemble model that is combined with Logistic Regression (LR) performs better than other combinations. It achieves an accuracy of 0.985, an F1-score of 0.99, a precision of 0.99, and a recall of 0.99.

Figure 8. COVID/non-COVID classification confusion matrices

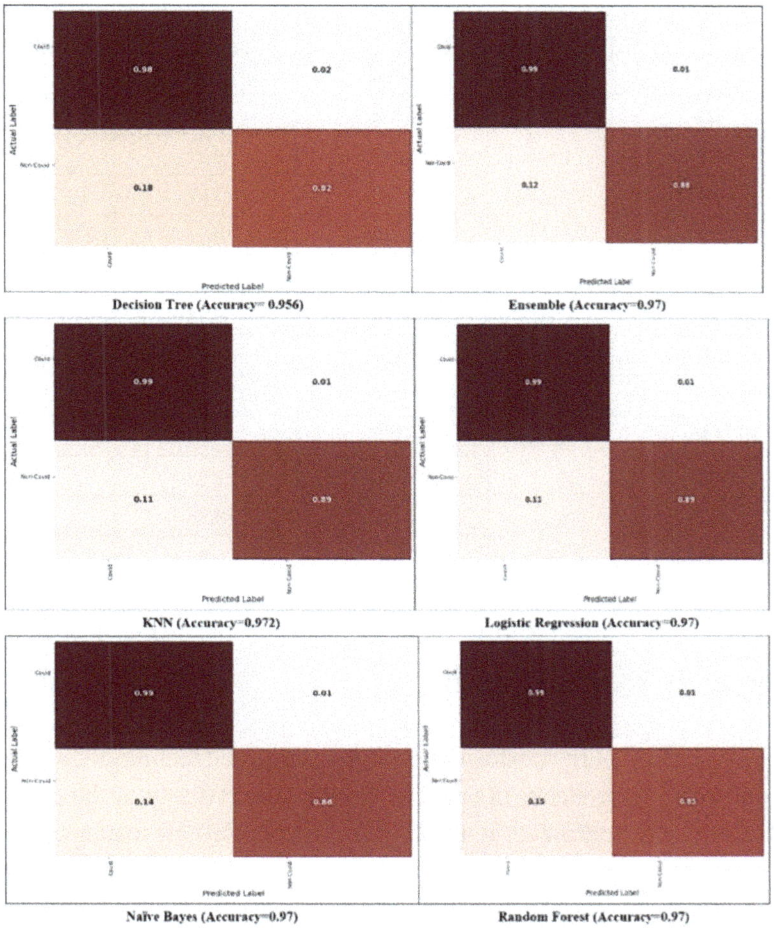

Due to the larger size of Dataset 2, the model is provided with a higher amount of data for the purpose of learning complicated patterns during the training process. This is the reason for the improved performance that was noticed with Dataset 2. Because of the increased size of the dataset, the classifier is able to generalize more effectively, which ultimately results in more accurate predictions. These results highlight the significant significance that the size of the dataset has in determining the performance and reliability of machine learning models, especially in the context of applications that include medical imaging.

Table 5. Different dataset classification metrics

Model	Classifier	Total	Accuracy	F1-Score	Precision	Recall
Dataset-1	NB	1,646	0.97	0.97	0.97	0.97
	SVM		0.952	0.95	0.96	0.95
	DT		0.956	0.96	0.96	0.96
	LR		0.97	0.97	0.97	0.97
	RF		0.97	0.97	0.97	0.97
	KNN		0.972	0.97	0.97	0.97
	Ensemble		0.97	0.97	0.97	0.97
Dataset-2	NB	2,481	0.981	0.98	0.98	0.98
	SVM		0.945	0.95	0.95	0.95
	DT		0.97	0.97	0.97	0.97
	LR		0.985	0.99	0.99	0.99
	RF		0.98	0.98	0.98	0.98
	KNN		0.981	0.98	0.98	0.98
	Ensemble		0.982	0.98	0.98	0.98

4.4. Comparison with Previous Work

Table 6 provides a summary of the performance of the suggested technique, which was benchmarked against previously published approaches in order to evaluate the efficacy of the proposed approach. For the purpose of evaluating the categorization of COVID and non-COVID instances, the comparison used conventional measures such as precision, recall, F1-score, and accuracy. For the purpose of medical picture classification, Jaiswal et al. (2021) applied the DenseNet-121 model, which resulted in precision, recall, and F1-score values of 96.29%, in addition to an accuracy of 96.25%. The suggested ensemble technique outperforms current measures in the majority of categories, despite the fact that these findings exhibit powerful performance. The authors Silva et al. (2020) presented a voting-based technique for the categorization of COVID and non-COVID, which reached an accuracy of 87.68%. The method fared poorly in comparison to more sophisticated methods, including the framework that was presented, despite the fact that it included the use of ensemble techniques.

DNNs, AlexNet, ResNet, GoogleNet, xDNN, and VGG-16 were some of the deep learning designs that Alshazly et al. (2021) investigated. Deep Convolutional Neural Networks (CNNs) were also responsible for the following outcomes: 99.6% precision, 66.4% F1-score, 96.29% recall, and 99.4% accuracy. GoogleNet, on the other hand, managed to obtain measures like as 90.2% precision, 93.5% recall, 91.82% F1-score, and 91.73% accuracy, which allowed it to surpass ResNet and VGG-16 in this examination. If we compare the performance of the proposed ensemble technique to that of previously published methods, we find that it is better across all measures. To be more specific, it successfully obtained values of 99.5% for precision, recall, and F1-score, in addition to achieving 98.5% accuracy. The performance of the proposed framework in optimizing feature extraction and classification by using a collection of machine learning approaches is shown by these findings, which illustrate the system's resilience and effectiveness. The incorporation of deep learning and ensemble techniques into the suggested method is responsible for the improved performance of the approach. This integration makes it possible to extract features in an effective manner and to classify them consistently. On the other hand, in contrast to single-model techniques, the ensemble framework combines the predictions of many classifiers, which helps to reduce the number of instances of incorrect classification and improves the accuracy of the entire system.

Table 6. Comparison of suggested approach performance with current works

Research works	Model	Precision (%)	Recall (%)	F1-measure (%)	Accuracy (%)
Silva et al. (2020)	Voting based Approach	NS	NS	NS	87.68
Angelov et al. (2020)	GoogleNet	90.2	93.5	91.82	91.73
Angelov et al. (2020)	AlexNet	94.98	92.28	93.61	93.75
Angelov et al. (2020)	ResNet	93	97.15	95.03	94.96
Angelov et al. (2020)	VGG-16	94.02	95.43	94.97	94.96
Jaiswal et al. (2021)	DenseNet-121	96.29	96.29	96.29	96.25
Alshazly et al. (2021)	Deep CNNs	99.6	NS	66.4	99.4
Angelov et al. (2020)	xDNN	99.16	95.53	97.31	97.38
Our work	Ensemble Method	99	99	99	98.5

4.5. Explainable AI and t-SNE Performance Validation

To verify the suggested methodology, two essential experiments were performed: Explainable Artificial Intelligence (AI) using Gradient-weighted Class Activation Mapping (Grad-CAM) and t-distributed Stochastic Neighbor Embedding (t-SNE) visualization. These methodologies were used to guarantee the model's interpretability and robustness while offering comprehensive insights into its decision-making process. The Grad-CAM approach was used to pinpoint the most informative areas in the input pictures used by the model for classification. This method emphasizes regions in CT scans or X-rays that align with diagnostic characteristics, providing significant insights for radiologists and doctors. Grad-CAM enhances comprehension of the model's predictions by superimposing a heatmap over the original pictures. Cumulative heatmaps were created to illustrate the classifier's output over several samples, hence improving interpretability on a larger scale. Cumulative heatmaps aggregate data by averaging the pixel values of multiple heatmaps within a category, resulting in a cohesive visual depiction of the model's acquired characteristics (Hossain, Muhammad & Guizani, 2020). This approach allows radiologists to quickly identify patterns associated with certain diseases, therefore saving time and reducing human effort. Figure 8 displays a comparative analysis of original images, Grad-CAM heatmaps, and the importance of certain regions as overlaid on the pictures. Crucial phases in the interpretability process include:

- Heatmap Generation: Grad-CAM identifies critical pixels used in classification, enabling experts to correlate the model's predictions with clinically relevant features.
- Cumulative Heatmap Generation: By overlaying and averaging heatmaps for a certain class, a unique image is produced that encapsulates the fundamental characteristics of that class, enabling comprehensive analysis with little human intervention.

Figure 9. Heatmaps, original photos, and overlay images

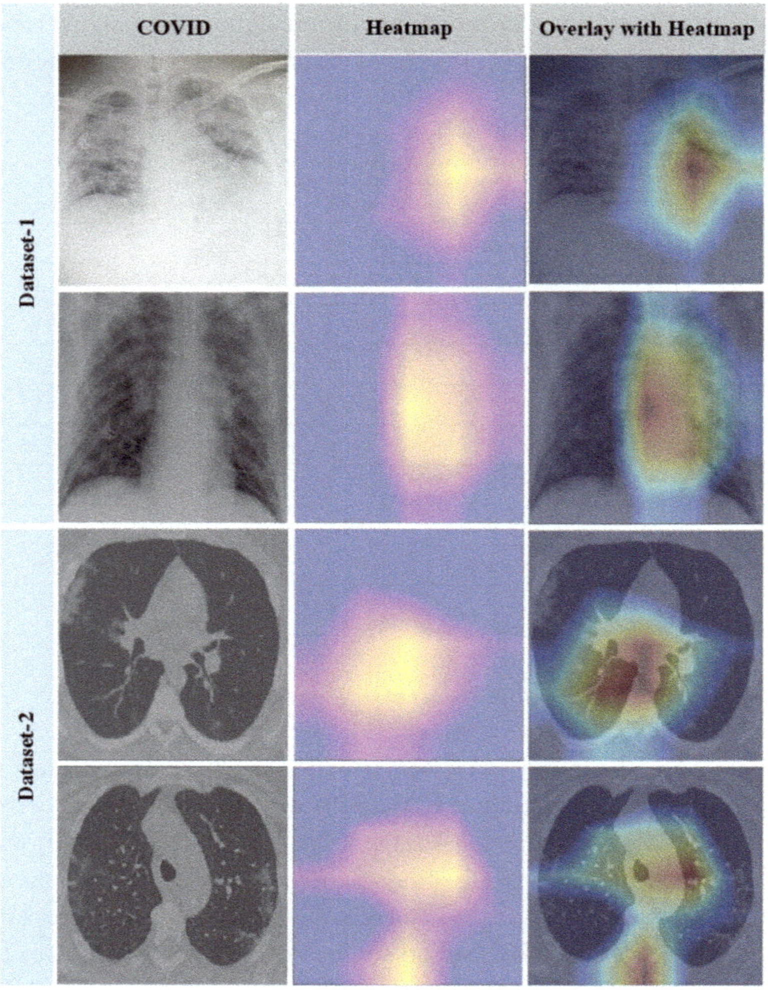

To further validate the effectiveness of the proposed model, the t-SNE (t-distributed Stochastic Neighbor Embedding) visualization technique was employed to assess the separability of features extracted from the datasets. This method was instrumental in determining whether the extracted features contained sufficient information for accurate classification. Figure 10 illustrates the t-SNE visualization for Dataset 1, highlighting the distinction between COVID-positive (class 1, red) and COVID-negative (class 0, black) samples. A perplexity value of 35 was used, as it yielded the most distinct clustering. The t-SNE technique was assessed at many perplexity levels, with 35 yielding the most distinct display of COVID-positive and negative clusters. The iterative optimization of t-SNE parameters improved clustering, with 700 iterations yielding distinct separations between the two classes. The COVID-negative cluster was much bigger than the COVID-positive cluster, indicating a greater number of training cases for the former category. Although some overlap across clusters was seen, perhaps suggesting outliers, the bulk of data points were clearly segregated, affirming that the dataset offered a robust basis for optimum categorization.

Figure 10. COVID-19 dataset two-dimensional feature visualization of the suggested model

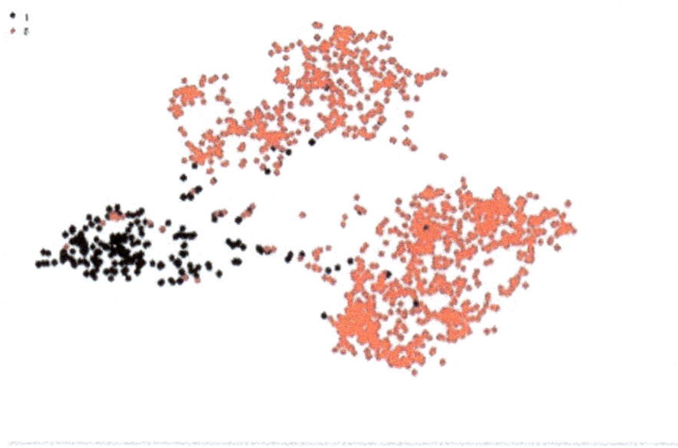

The density of the dataset significantly impacts predictive accuracy. Higher data density enhances the descriptiveness of training samples, leading to improved classification precision. The clear separation between t-SNE clusters underscores the efficacy of the proposed model in distinguishing COVID-positive cases from COVID-negative ones. Careful selection of perplexity values and hyperparameters, as detailed in Tables 2–5, further contributed to the model's high classification accuracy. The amalgamation of Grad-CAM and t-SNE highlights the strength and clarity of the suggested framework. Grad-CAM provides detailed insights into the areas that affect the model's predictions, whilst t-SNE visualizations confirm the efficacy of the extracted features for classification tasks. Collectively, these methodologies thoroughly validate the model's efficacy, demonstrating its capacity for precise and transparent COVID-19 diagnosis. This dual methodology enhances the ensemble model's relevance in clinical environments, guaranteeing both accuracy and dependability in its forecasts.

5. CONCLUSION

Healthcare facilities are under unprecedented strain due to the world's population growth, particularly in the fields of disease detection and monitoring. Automated detection frameworks are now necessary to improve the accuracy and efficiency of diagnosis. These smart gadgets help doctors identify infections and improve patient outcomes, which lowers mortality rates. The sudden and severe emergence of COVID-19 as a global health emergency has brought attention to the urgent and reliable development of diagnostic technologies in order to successfully limit its spread. This study offers an explicable framework for automatically identifying COVID-19 infections from chest X-rays and CT scans. To achieve higher classification accuracy, the proposed methodology combines advanced machine learning and deep learning techniques. A convolutional neural network (CNN) was designed to extract 350 essential elements from medical photos. The characteristics were later categorized using advanced techniques, including LR, GNB, DT, RF, and SVM. An ensemble learning approach was used to further improve categorization performance.

The suggested technique underwent thorough evaluation using two datasets including 1,646 and 2,481 CT scan pictures, respectively. The results indicated that the framework surpassed current state-of-the-art approaches on many performance criteria, including precision, recall, F1-score, and accuracy. To provide transparency and interpretability, the system included t-SNE visualizations and explainable AI methodologies, including Gradient-weighted Class Activation Mapping (Grad-CAM). These technologies provide significant insights into the model's decision-making processes, hence augmenting its dependability and applicability in clinical environments.

6. FUTURE DIRECTIONS

Future study may investigate complex ensemble techniques, such stacking and bagging, to enhance the resilience and efficacy of the suggested architecture. Furthermore, integrating cross-validation methods into deep neural network frameworks may mitigate issues such as overfitting and class imbalance. Although cross-validation may substantially improve model dependability, it is crucial to meticulously control the related computational expenses.

This research focuses on COVID-19 detection; however, the framework's adaptable architecture is applicable to identifying various viral disorders. Broadening the focus of this study to include a diverse array of medical diseases might provide global healthcare systems with prompt and precise diagnostic instruments, therefore enhancing patient care and health outcomes worldwide.

Data availability

The suggested study employed three public datasets.

- GitHub repository, Italian Society of Medical and Interventional Radiology imaging and Cohen's X-ray pictures dataset (https://github.com/ieee8023/covid-chestxray-dataset/).
- Kaggle repository, Radiological Society of North America (https://www.kaggle.com/datasets/andrewmvd/convid19-x-rays).
- The SARS-CoV-2 CT scan dataset (https://www.kaggle.com/datasets/plameneduardo/sarscov2-ctscan-dataset).

REFERENCES

Ahad, A., Jiangbin, Z., Mughees, A., Puspitasari, I., & Tayyab, M. (2025). Secure horizons: Integrating blockchain with AI for enhanced smart healthcare systems. In *AI techniques for securing medical and business practices* (pp. 357–390). IGI Global.

Ahad, A., Tahir, M., Sheikh, M. A. S., Mughees, A., & Ahmed, K. I. (2021, October). Optimal route selection in 5G-based smart healthcare network: A reinforcement learning approach. In *2021 26th IEEE Asia-Pacific Conference on Communications (APCC)* (pp. 248–253). IEEE. https://doi.org/DOI: 10.1109/APCC49754.2021.9609815

Ahmed, I., Ahmad, A., & Jeon, G. (2020). An IoT-based deep learning framework for early assessment of COVID-19. *IEEE Internet of Things Journal*, *8*(21), 15855–15862. DOI: 10.1109/JIOT.2020.3034074 PMID: 35782174

Ali, Z., Ahad, A., Madeira, F., & Shayea, I. (2024). Enhancing transparency and trustworthiness of healthcare IoT data with AWS: A proposed model. In Ferraro, V., Covarrubias, M., Zdravevski, E., Pires, I. M., Marques Martins de Almeida, J. M., & Gonçalves, N. J. (Eds.), *IoT technologies and wearables for healthcare: HealthyIoT ICWH 2023* (Vol. 530, pp. 1–11). Springer., DOI: 10.1007/978-3-031-71911-0_4

Alshazly, H., Linse, C., Barth, E., & Martinetz, T. (2021). Explainable COVID-19 detection using chest CT scans and deep learning. *Sensors (Basel)*, *21*(1), 455. DOI: 10.3390/s21020455 PMID: 33440674

Angelov, P., & Almeida Soares, E. (2020). SARS-CoV-2 CT-scan dataset: A large dataset of real patients CT scans for SARS-CoV-2 identification. *MedRxiv*, 2020.04.24.20078584. https://doi.org/DOI: 10.1101/2020.04.24.20078584

Ashfaq, F., Ahad, A., Hussain, M., & Madeira, F. (2023, October). Transforming diabetes care: A review of IoT-based mobile health systems. In *EAI International Conference on IoT Technologies for Healthcare* (pp. 14–32). Springer Nature Switzerland. https://doi.org/DOI: 10.1007/978-3-031-71911-0_2

Basu, A., Mullick, S. S., Das, S., & Das, S. (2022). Do pre-processing and class imbalance matter to the deep image classifiers for COVID-19 detection? An explainable analysis. *IEEE Transactions on Artificial Intelligence*, •••, 1–15. DOI: 10.1109/TAI.2022.3149971

Butt, H. A., Ahad, A., Wasim, M., Madeira, F., & Chamran, M. K. (2023a, October). 5G and IoT for intelligent healthcare: AI and machine learning approaches—A review. In *International conference on smart objects and technologies for social good* (pp. 107–123). Springer Nature Switzerland. https://doi.org/DOI: 10.1007/978-3-031-52524-7_8

Butt, H. A., Ahad, A., Wasim, M., Shayea, I., Coelho, P. J., Pires, I. M., & Garcia, N. M. (2023b). Federated machine learning in 5G smart healthcare: A security perspective review. *Procedia Computer Science*, *224*, 580–586. DOI: 10.1016/j.procs.2023.09.084

Chen, S.-G., Chen, J.-Y., Yang, Y.-P., Chien, C.-S., Wang, M.-L., & Lin, L.-T. (2020). Use of radiographic features in COVID-19 diagnosis: Challenges and perspectives. *Journal of the Chinese Medical Association*, *83*(7), 644–647. DOI: 10.1097/JCMA.0000000000000336 PMID: 32349032

Ciotti, M., Ciccozzi, M., Terrinoni, A., Jiang, W.-C., Wang, C.-B., & Bernardini, S. (2020). The COVID-19 pandemic. *Critical Reviews in Clinical Laboratory Sciences*, *57*(6), 365–388. DOI: 10.1080/10408363.2020.1783198 PMID: 32645276

Coronavirus. (2020). 13,968 cases and 223 deaths. Retrieved from https://www.worldometers.info/coronavirus/country/ethiopia

Culp, W. (2020). Coronavirus disease 2019. *Practice*, *14*(6), e01218. PMID: 32784318

Durrani, M. Y., Yasmin, S., & Rho, S. (2022). An Internet of Medical Things-based liver tumor detection system using semantic segmentation. *Journal of Internet Technology*, *23*(1), 163–175.

Esteva, A., Chou, K., Yeung, S., Naik, N., Madani, A., Mottaghi, A., Liu, Y., Topol, E., Dean, J., & Socher, R. (2021). Deep learning-enabled medical computer vision. *NPJ Digital Medicine*, *4*(1), 1–9. DOI: 10.1038/s41746-020-00376-2 PMID: 33420381

Esteva, A., Robicquet, A., Ramsundar, B., Kuleshov, V., DePristo, M., Chou, K., Cui, C., Corrado, G., Thrun, S., & Dean, J. (2019). A guide to deep learning in healthcare. *Nature Medicine*, *25*(1), 24–29. DOI: 10.1038/s41591-018-0316-z PMID: 30617335

Gandhi, D. A., & Ghosal, M. (2018). Intelligent healthcare using IoT: An extensive survey. In *2018 Second International Conference on Inventive Communication and Computational Technologies (ICICCT)* (pp. 800–802).

Guermazi, R., Chaabane, I., & Hammami, M. (2018). AECID: Asymmetric entropy for classifying imbalanced data. *Information Sciences*, *467*, 373–397. DOI: 10.1016/j.ins.2018.07.076

Guo, Y., Gao, Y., & Shen, D. (2015). Deformable MR prostate segmentation via deep feature learning and sparse patch matching. *IEEE Transactions on Medical Imaging*, *35*(5), 1077–1089. PMID: 26685226

Guo, Z., Li, X., Huang, H., Guo, N., & Li, Q. (2019). Deep learning-based image segmentation on multimodal medical imaging. *IEEE Transactions on Radiation and Plasma Medical Sciences*, *3*(2), 162–169. DOI: 10.1109/TRPMS.2018.2890359 PMID: 34722958

Haider, K. Z., Malik, K. R., Khalid, S., Nawaz, T., & Jabbar, S. (2019). Deepgender: Real-time gender classification using deep learning for smartphones. *Journal of Real-Time Image Processing*, *16*(1), 15–29. DOI: 10.1007/s11554-017-0714-3

Hemdan, E. E.-D., Shouman, M. A., & Karar, M. E. (2020). COVIDx-Net: A framework of deep learning classifiers to diagnose COVID-19 in X-ray images. *arXiv preprint*, arXiv:2003.11055.

Hossain, M. S., Muhammad, G., & Guizani, N. (2020). Explainable AI and mass surveillance system-based healthcare framework to combat COVID-19-like pandemics. *IEEE Network*, *34*(4), 126–132. DOI: 10.1109/MNET.011.2000458

Hu, Y., Niu, D., Yang, J., & Zhou, S. (2019). FDML: A collaborative machine learning framework for distributed features. In *Proceedings of the 25th ACM SIGKDD International Conference on Knowledge Discovery & Data Mining* (pp. 2232–2240). DOI: 10.1145/3292500.3330765

Islam, M. R., & Nahiduzzaman, M. (2022). Complex features extraction with deep learning model for the detection of COVID-19 from CT scan images using ensemble-based machine learning approach. *Expert Systems with Applications*, *195*, 116554. DOI: 10.1016/j.eswa.2022.116554 PMID: 35136286

Jaiswal, A., Gianchandani, N., Singh, D., Kumar, V., & Kaur, M. (2021). Classification of the COVID-19 infected patients using DenseNet201-based deep transfer learning. *Journal of Biomolecular Structure & Dynamics*, *39*(15), 5682–5689. DOI: 10.1080/07391102.2020.1788642 PMID: 32619398

Kalsoom, A., Maqsood, M., Yasmin, S., Bukhari, M., Shin, Z., & Rho, S. (2022). A computer-aided diagnostic system for liver tumor detection using modified U-Net architecture. *The Journal of Supercomputing*, *78*(7), 1–23. DOI: 10.1007/s11227-021-04266-6

Kassani, S. H., Kassani, P. H., Khazaeinezhad, R., Wesolowski, M. J., Schneider, K. A., & Deters, R. (2019). Diabetic retinopathy classification using a modified Xception architecture. In *2019 IEEE International Symposium on Signal Processing and Information Technology (ISSPIT)* (pp. 1–6). DOI: 10.1109/ISSPIT47144.2019.9001846

Kassani, S. H., Kassani, P. H., Wesolowski, M. J., Schneider, K. A., & Deters, R. (2021). Automatic detection of coronavirus disease (COVID-19) in X-ray and CT images: A machine learning-based approach. *Biocybernetics and Biomedical Engineering*, *41*(3), 867–879. DOI: 10.1016/j.bbe.2021.05.013 PMID: 34108787

Khalid, S., Sajjad, S., Jabbar, S., & Chang, H. (2017). Accurate and efficient shape matching approach using vocabularies of multi-feature space representations. *Journal of Real-Time Image Processing*, *13*(3), 449–465. DOI: 10.1007/s11554-015-0545-z

Khalilia, M., Chakraborty, S., & Popescu, M. (2011). Predicting disease risks from highly imbalanced data using random forest. *BMC Medical Informatics and Decision Making*, *11*(1), 51. DOI: 10.1186/1472-6947-11-51 PMID: 21801360

Kumar, K., Kumar, N., & Shah, R. (2020). Role of IoT to avoid spreading of COVID-19. *International Journal of Intelligent Networks*, *1*, 32–35. DOI: 10.1016/j.ijin.2020.05.002

Lan, Z.-C., Huang, G.-Y., Li, Y.-P., Rho, S., Vimal, S., & Chen, B.-W. (2022). Conquering insufficient/imbalanced data learning for the Internet of Medical Things. *Neural Computing & Applications*, •••, 1–10. DOI: 10.1007/s00521-022-06897-z

Naeem, H., & Bin-Salem, A. A. (2021). A CNN-LSTM network with multi-level feature extraction-based approach for automated detection of coronavirus from CT scan and X-ray images. *Applied Soft Computing*, *113*, 107918. DOI: 10.1016/j.asoc.2021.107918 PMID: 34608379

Nawaz, H., Maqsood, M., Afzal, S., Aadil, F., Mehmood, I., & Rho, S. (2021). A deep feature-based real-time system for Alzheimer's disease stage detection. *Multimedia Tools and Applications*, *80*(26), 35789–35807. DOI: 10.1007/s11042-020-09087-y

Otoom, M., Otoum, N., Alzubaidi, M. A., Etoom, Y., & Banihani, R. (2020). An IoT-based framework for early identification and monitoring of COVID-19 cases. *Biomedical Signal Processing and Control*, *62*, 102149. DOI: 10.1016/j.bspc.2020.102149 PMID: 32834831

Rohila, V. S., Gupta, N., Kaul, A., & Sharma, D. K. (2021). Deep learning-assisted COVID-19 detection using full CT scans. *Internet of Things : Engineering Cyber Physical Human Systems*, *14*, 100377. DOI: 10.1016/j.iot.2021.100377 PMID: 38620521

Sagi, O., & Rokach, L. (2018). Ensemble learning: A survey. *Wiley Interdisciplinary Reviews. Data Mining and Knowledge Discovery*, *8*(4), e1249. DOI: 10.1002/widm.1249

Sarker, L., Islam, M. M., Hannan, T., & Ahmed, Z. (2020). COVID-DenseNet: A deep learning architecture to detect COVID-19 from chest radiology images. *arXiv preprint*, arXiv:2003.11055. https://doi.org/DOI: 10.20944/preprints202005.0151.v1

Saygılı, A. (2021). A new approach for computer-aided detection of coronavirus (COVID-19) from CT and X-ray images using machine learning methods. *Applied Soft Computing*, *105*, 107323. DOI: 10.1016/j.asoc.2021.107323 PMID: 33746657

Shah, V., Keniya, R., Shridharani, A., Punjabi, M., Shah, J., & Mehendale, N. (2021). Diagnosis of COVID-19 using CT scan images and deep learning techniques. *Emergency Radiology*, *28*(4), 497–505. DOI: 10.1007/s10140-020-01886-y PMID: 33523309

Shan, F., Gao, Y., Wang, J., Shi, W., Shi, N., Han, M., ... (2020). Lung infection quantification of COVID-19 in CT images with deep learning. *arXiv preprint*, arXiv:2003.04655.

Silva, P., Luz, E., Silva, G., Moreira, G., Silva, R., Lucio, D., & Menotti, D. (2020). COVID-19 detection in CT images with deep learning: A voting-based scheme and cross-datasets analysis. *Informatics in Medicine Unlocked*, *20*, 100427. DOI: 10.1016/j.imu.2020.100427 PMID: 32953971

Sintunavarat, W., & Turab, A. (2022). Mathematical analysis of an extended SEIR model of COVID-19 using the ABC-fractional operator. *Mathematics and Computers in Simulation*, *198*, 65–84. DOI: 10.1016/j.matcom.2022.02.009 PMID: 35194306

Syed, H. H., Khan, M. A., Tariq, U., Armghan, A., Alenezi, F., Khan, J. A., Rho, S., Kadry, S., & Rajinikanth, V. (2021). A rapid artificial intelligence-based computer-aided diagnosis system for COVID-19 classification from CT images. *Behavioural Neurology*, *2021*, 5588967. Advance online publication. DOI: 10.1155/2021/2560388 PMID: 34966463

Tahamtan, A., & Ardebili, A. (2020). Real-time RT-PCR in COVID-19 detection: Issues affecting the results. *Expert Review of Molecular Diagnostics*, *20*(5), 453–454. DOI: 10.1080/14737159.2020.1757437 PMID: 32297805

Turab, A., Shafqat, R., Muhammad, S., Shuaib, M., Khan, M. F., & Kamal, M. (2024). Predictive modeling of hepatitis B viral dynamics: A Caputo derivative-based approach using artificial neural networks. *Scientific Reports*, *14*(1), 21853. DOI: 10.1038/s41598-024-70788-7 PMID: 39300092

Ullah, F., Habib, M. A., Farhan, M., Khalid, S., Durrani, M. Y., & Jabbar, S. (2017). Semantic interoperability for big data in heterogeneous IoT infrastructure for healthcare. *Sustainable Cities and Society*, *34*, 90–96. DOI: 10.1016/j.scs.2017.06.010

Wang, S., Zha, Y., Li, W., Wu, Q., Li, X., Niu, M., Wang, M., Qiu, X., Li, H., Yu, H., Gong, W., Bai, Y., Li, L., Zhu, Y., Wang, L., & Tian, J. (2020). A fully automatic deep learning system for COVID-19 diagnostic and prognostic analysis. *The European Respiratory Journal*, *56*(2), 2000778. DOI: 10.1183/13993003.00775-2020 PMID: 32444412

Ye, Z., Zhang, Y., Wang, Y., Huang, Z., & Song, B. (2020). Chest CT manifestations of new coronavirus disease 2019 (COVID-19): A pictorial review. *European Radiology*, *30*(8), 4381–4389. DOI: 10.1007/s00330-020-06801-0 PMID: 32193638

Zhang, J., Xie, Y., Li, Y., Shen, C., & Xia, Y. (2020). COVID-19 screening on chest X-ray images using deep learning-based anomaly detection. arXiv preprint, arXiv:2003.12338.

Chapter 8
Implementation of AI and Blockchain in Healthcare

Mohammad Kazem Kazem Chamran
https://orcid.org/0000-0003-3836-4443
City University, Kuala Lumpur, Malaysia

ABSTRACT

This manuscript examines the transformative potential of integrating blockchain and artificial intelligence (AI) to enhance healthcare supply chain management, focusing on combating counterfeit drugs and improving product traceability. Current systems are susceptible to cyberattacks and fail to guarantee drug authenticity, posing significant risks to patient safety. Blockchain technology offers a robust solution by creating an immutable and transparent record of the entire supply chain, from manufacturing to patient delivery, enabling verification of product origin and handling at each step. Smart contracts automate these verifications, ensuring compliance and minimizing errors. Integrating AI with blockchain further amplifies these benefits. AI algorithms analyze blockchain data to identify patterns, predict disruptions, and optimize supply chain efficiency. Furthermore, blockchain provides a secure platform for medical record storage, supporting AI-driven e-health models.

1. INTRODUCTION

This manuscript addresses healthcare supply chain management with the help of AI, focusing on ensuring the authenticity and traceability of pharmaceutical products, which is crucial in preventing counterfeit drugs and ensuring medication safety. Blockchain technology is implemented to provide a transparent record of each supply chain step, from manufacturing to patient delivery (Pranto Kumar Ghosh, 2024). In today's complex transactions and accessibility to different networks and resources, a secure medium is a key factor. The network is surrounded by opportunistic groups and individuals looking for ways to penetrate and harvest resources that do not belong to them. This exacerbates the security concern. In fact, in many cases, hackers have gained success in the cybercrime they are involved in and could steal information and, in some cases, valuable data and resources (Mayra Macas, 2024).

In blockchain, by logging, every transaction on a shared ledger, stakeholders in the supply chain can verify the origin, authenticity, and handling of products at each stage. Smart contracts automate verification processes, ensuring compliance and reducing human error. Standardizing blockchain protocols

DOI: 10.4018/979-8-3373-0593-6.ch008

across the industry would promote interoperability, while investing in user training could address adoption challenges. Incorporating IoT sensors for real-time tracking would further enhance transparency and efficiency in the supply chain (Sarthak Dhingra, 2023).

With all that, the blockchain explores the potential of integrating artificial intelligence to revolutionize healthcare. Using online data highlights the rapid growth of interest in such an interdisciplinary field. Blockchain's open-source information-sharing network can enhance AI-driven e-health models. By providing a safe platform for storing medical records, blockchain addresses AI's need for reliable data. The combined use of these technologies promises improved service efficiency, reduced costs, and more accessible healthcare (Priti Tagde, 2021). In Figure 1, the use of AI and blockchain in E-health is illustrated. (Rucha et al., 2022)

Figure 1. Use of Blockchain and AI in E-Health (Priti Tagde, 2021)

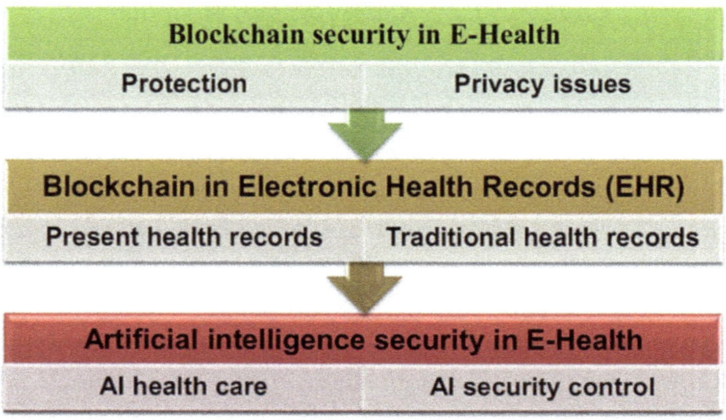

Blockchain's application in tracking resources to healthcare outlets also has significantly benefited from the integration of blockchain and AI. Supply chain management greatly reduces the risk of counterfeit drugs entering the market. Chains improve transparency, reduce counterfeiting, and build stakeholder trust. It also helps with traceability, healthcare providers can ensure that medications are genuine, improving patient safety and building trust in healthcare products. However, the technology faces challenges in achieving interoperability across various organizations' systems and in managing the high costs associated with its implementation. In this chapter, we further investigate the potential and challenges that integrated AI and Blockchain bring forth to healthcare.

1.1. Implementation of Blockchain in Healthcare and IoT

Before diving deep into AI integration here we look at the implementation of blockchain in healthcare and the benefits healthcare can get out of such integration.

Analyzing the trends and potential benefits of deploying blockchain technology in the Internet of Things (IoT) and healthcare sectors, primarily focusing on enhancing data security. Blockchain is commonly used for data management in both areas, employing six distinct security preservation strategies to improve data integrity, access control, and privacy. Integration mechanisms range from fully incorporating blockchain into IoT device data exchanges to using it solely for metadata storage, with smart city applications being a prominent example, leveraging blockchain for real-time data sharing and electricity trading. In healthcare, despite the broader potential, blockchain is predominantly applied to drug supply chain management to combat counterfeiting and to empower patients with control over their medical data.

The recent literature explores the integration of blockchain and the Internet of Things (IoT), examining various approaches across diverse applications. These integration methods differ in how blockchain is utilized within the system, from its role in IoT device data exchange to its prominence in service provision. The review categorizes these integration mechanisms based on observations from existing literature. Blockchain offers significant security benefits to healthcare and the Internet of Things (IoT), particularly in data management, which encompasses data acquisition, processing, dissemination, retrieval, security, and storage. Strengthening data management is crucial in both sectors, as weaknesses like the lack of unique patient identifiers, interoperable messaging, and data encoding standards hinder effective healthcare data management. Blockchain's security features can address these challenges and improve overall data protection in these interconnected environments (Adere, 2022). The blockchain challenges and solutions are illustrated in Figure 2.

Managing the diverse data generated by numerous online and offline IoT devices presents a significant challenge. This review explores the potential of blockchain-based systems to address this challenge, focusing on its applications within healthcare and the Internet of Things. Specifically, it examines how blockchain can mitigate technical issues like big data overload and economic problems such as financial losses due to counterfeiting in smart cities and drug supply chain management. It is important to understand that blockchain is essentially a peer-to-peer (P2P) network and communication follows this pattern between nodes.

Figure 2. Blockchain and IoT challenges and solutions (Adere, 2022).

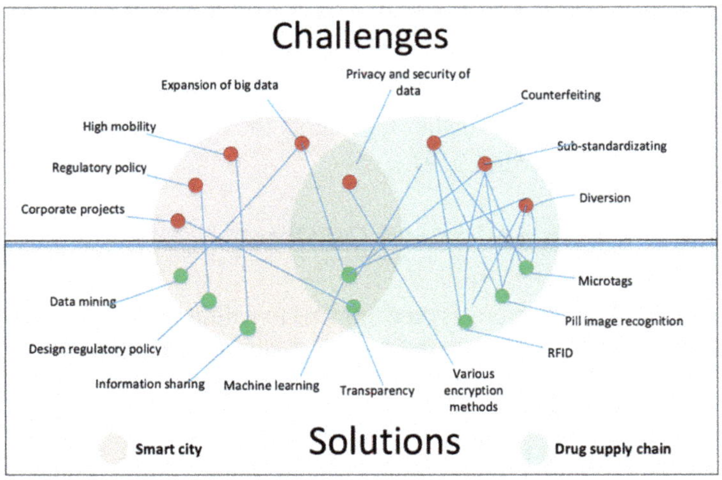

1.2. P2P Communication in Blockchain

Peer-to-peer (P2P) networks exist in various forms. Centralized P2P networks rely on a central server for resource tracking, while decentralized networks distribute this function. Decentralized structured topologies use a Distributed Hash Table (DHT) for organized resource location, whereas decentralized unstructured topologies lack a central server or strict placement rules, allowing for flexible and anonymous node participation. To manage the complexity of large-scale P2P networks, clustering techniques like partition-based, density-based, hierarchical-based, and grid-based clustering are employed to group participating nodes.

P2P networks are structured in various topologies that influence node communication. Centralized P2P networks allow direct node interaction after location information retrieval from a directory server. Decentralized structured networks (like DHTs) use key-value pairs for data location, enabling targeted access. Decentralized unstructured networks rely on methods like flooding and gossiping for communication. Furthermore, P2P networks can be categorized as homogeneous, where nodes share similar capabilities, or heterogeneous, where nodes differ in aspects like storage, computation, or energy. Blockchain systems, like centralized P2P networks, often require permission for peers to participate. This characteristic, along with the chosen governance model, allows for the classification of blockchains. Based on permission, blockchains are categorized as either permissioned or permissionless, while governance models lead to classifications of public or private blockchains (Min, et al., 2018).

Health information technology (HIT) encompasses a wide range of systems, including Electronic Health Records (EHRs), Computerized Provider Order Entry (CPOE), and Health Management Information Systems (HMIS), all aimed at improving healthcare delivery and outcomes. A more recent subset of HIT, Health IoT (HIoT), utilizes wearable and implantable sensors to collect patient data, enabling real-time monitoring, triage, and disease modeling. While HIT has demonstrated effectiveness overall, fragmentation in its utilization and challenges in data sharing between systems, like EHRs and Personal Health Records (PHRs), have hindered its full potential. The interconnectedness of some systems, such as electronic Medication Administration Records (eMAR) and Picture Archiving and Communication Systems (PACS) with EMR and CPOE, further highlights the complex landscape of HIT and the need for better integration (Roberta Bernardi, 2019).

1.3. Consensus Mechanism and Smart Contract

Blockchain technology utilizes consensus mechanisms to validate blocks, ensuring agreement among network nodes. These mechanisms vary widely, from computationally intensive methods like Proof of Work to communication-based approaches such as Practical Byzantine Fault Tolerance. Numerous other mechanisms exist, including Proof of Stake, Threshold Relay, and Proof of Burn, and research often explores enhanced versions of these, as detailed in other reviews. Smart contracts are automatically executed procedures triggered by transactions, and while all blockchain systems support them, they vary in the programming languages used for their creation and their execution environments. Common smart contract languages include Solidity, Golang, Serpent, Java, and Python, while execution environments range from the Ethereum Virtual Machine (EVM) and Java Virtual Machine (JVM) to Docker Images and Haskell environments (Lashkari & Musilek, 2021).

Blockchain's touted immutability, the inability to modify the distributed ledger without a majority (51%) consensus, is a key feature, making transaction alteration highly improbable. However, while practically difficult, breaching this immutability is theoretically possible with sufficient resources. This immutability concept applies to both data and code, though data can be flawed *before* being added to the chain, and even with consensus mechanisms, verification is limited by participant agreement. Furthermore, code immutability is also challenged by the reality that code is rarely perfect and often requires updates, as evidenced by frequent adaptations of blockchain code itself. Consensus mechanisms are crucial for securely and frequently updating distributed ledgers, using techniques like state machine replication to ensure consistent shared states across network replicas. Because these replicas must agree on state changes, consensus protocols are necessary, though complex to implement due to requirements like adversarial tolerance, fault resilience, network partitioning management, and security measures against malicious nodes. In distributed ledgers such as blockchain, consensus ensures safety (consistent, valid output), liveness (non-faulty node contribution), and fault tolerance, thus maintaining the network's efficiency. (Lashkari & Musilek, 2021).

2. LITERATURE REVIEW ON BLOCKCHAIN IMPLEMENTATION IN HEALTHCARE

Healthcare management has incorporated blockchain in the management of patient records to enhance the safety of record access and storage. This area is also concerned with managing enormous quantities of personal health information such as records, prescriptions, or clinical trials. When well adopted, blockchain offers standards-based and communicable, safe clinical healthcare record management. In healthcare, blockchain is used mostly for the production of the methods of storing entries regulating patient information, which can be read only by specific stakeholders. For instance, the MedRec system applies blockchain to dealing with electronic health records (EHRs). Through the decentralization of data and the use of cryptographic keys, healthcare providers and patients ensure that records are safe and cannot be faked as patients have powers to control who gets access to their data. This system also feeds tracking consent for data access and sharing thus making data access safer and more transparent. This paper reveals that the implementation of blockchain in healthcare is very helpful. It strengthens data confidentiality and minimizes the vulnerability to data theft, which is expensive and risky to patients, as well as providers. This technology also enhances the integration of health care systems whereby the record of the patient is easily transferred from one caregiver to the other making the work easier in assembling treatment options for those requiring multiple caregivers. Through the properties of blockchain, such as its ability to decentralize records, the integrity of patient records cannot be altered again making these transactions more trustworthy .in the healthcare industry (Akbar, et al., 2022).

Blockchain has been seen to provide solutions in many areas of healthcare systems and can solve various problems through decentralized, secure, and transparent solutions. It fosters efficient identification and sharing of cohesive and accurate health information amongst all stakeholders while promoting privacy and security and with limited dependence on central architectures. This concept is relevant to the increasing demand for patient-oriented healthcare delivery systems and effective data sharing.

2.1. Blockchain in Healthcare and Security Improvements

The healthcare industry manages an enormous amount of sensitive data, encompassing patient records, treatment histories, diagnostic information, and insurance details. Protecting this data is paramount, as breaches can lead to severe consequences for both patients and healthcare providers. Therefore, it is essential to maintain strict data privacy while simultaneously allowing healthcare providers to access this information quickly and efficiently for informed decision-making and effective patient care. Blockchain technology presents a promising solution to these challenges by offering a decentralized method for the secure storage and sharing of medical information. This technology ensures that data integrity is maintained, as every transaction is recorded in a transparent and tamper-proof manner. By utilizing blockchain, healthcare providers can establish a higher level of trust with their patients, as patients can be assured that their sensitive information is protected and only accessible to authorized personnel (Attaran, Blockchain technology in healthcare: Challenges and opportunities, 2022).

On a different front, the Internet of Things (IoT) connects a vast array of devices, enabling them to communicate and exchange data seamlessly. This interconnectedness drives automation in various sectors, including smart homes, where appliances and systems can be monitored and controlled remotely; industrial monitoring, which enhances operational efficiency and safety, and logistics, where real-time tracking of goods can optimize supply chain management. However, the exponential growth of connected devices introduces significant security challenges. As more devices come online, the risk of cyberattacks and unauthorized access increases, potentially jeopardizing sensitive data. Blockchain can effectively address these security concerns by providing a secure and decentralized network for device authentication and data management within IoT ecosystems. By leveraging blockchain, organizations can ensure that only authorized devices are allowed to connect and share information, thereby enhancing trust and privacy. This not only protects sensitive data from malicious attacks but also builds confidence among users, paving the way for broader adoption of IoT technologies across various sectors. In the realm of the Internet of Things (IoT), blockchain technology addresses crucial issues related to device security and data integrity. By utilizing a distributed ledger, each device within an IoT network can authenticate the data it receives from other devices, effectively minimizing the risk of data tampering or spoofing. The immutable nature of blockchain records contributes to a transparent audit trail for all IoT activities, enabling secure tracking of every interaction within the network (Soni & Singh, 2021). In Figure 3, five different layers of security attack risks are shown which include application, blockchain, intelligence, Malware analysis, and data (Alabdulatif, Khalil, & Rahman, 2022).

Figure 3. Different layers of security concerns of blockchain implemented in healthcare (Alabdulatif, Khalil, & Rahman, 2022)

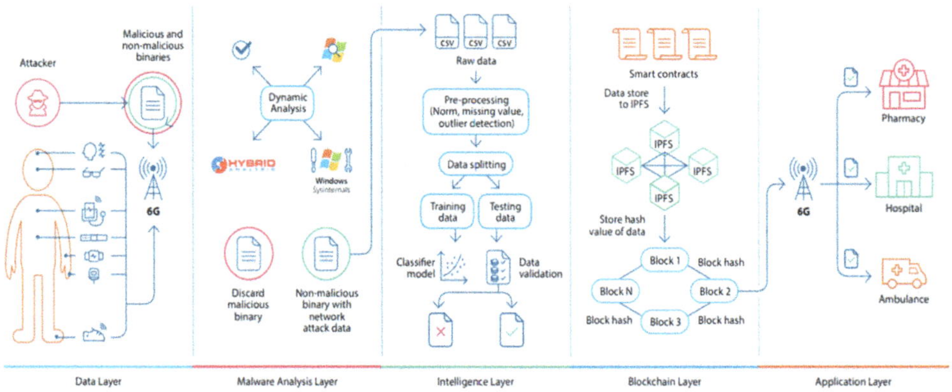

In industrial applications, blockchain serves as a tool to verify the accuracy of sensor data This is essential for maintaining the reliability of automated systems. Furthermore, blockchain technology facilitates automated authentication processes for devices, ensuring that only verified devices can connect to the network. Smart contracts enhance the overall efficiency of these systems by triggering automated responses when specific conditions are met. For example, a smart contract might automatically initiate a maintenance request when sensor data indicates that a machine is operating outside of its normal parameters, thus reducing the necessity for human oversight and intervention and ensuring that issues are addressed promptly to prevent system failures. Blockchain technology notably improves healthcare data security and interoperability, presenting a robust solution for managing patient information effectively. It allows authorized healthcare providers to easily access patient data while ensuring privacy is maintained. This is achieved through the decentralization of data storage, which reduces reliance on central databases that can be vulnerable to cyberattacks. By distributing data across a network of nodes, blockchain creates multiple barriers against potential threats, enhancing overall security. Moreover, blockchain facilitates greater patient empowerment by allowing individuals to control their health records. This ability not only improves the accuracy of the data but also fosters a sense of trust between patients and healthcare providers. When patients feel they have control over their information, they are more likely to share it, leading to more informed decisions and improved healthcare outcomes. The transparency offered by blockchain can result in faster diagnoses and treatment plans, as healthcare professionals can quickly access the most accurate and up-to-date patient information. This streamlined process also contributes to reducing administrative costs associated with traditional data management practices (Rehman & Ilyas, 2024).

In addition to its applications in healthcare, blockchain plays a crucial role in the pharmaceutical supply chain. By providing a secure, tamper-proof record of transactions, blockchain helps combat drug counterfeiting, ensuring that patients receive genuine medications. This is particularly important in an industry where counterfeit drugs can have serious health implications. Furthermore, blockchain's integration with the Internet of Things (IoT) creates a secure framework for managing the myriad of interconnected devices in healthcare settings and beyond. As more devices become networked, the risk of unauthorized access and cyberattacks increases. Blockchain mitigates these risks by ensuring that all communications are encrypted and securely logged. With its immutable data records, it becomes straightforward to verify the provenance of data, which is crucial for maintaining transparency and accountability across various devices. The decentralized architecture of blockchain also addresses the challenge of single points of failure in IoT systems, significantly increasing their resilience. By eliminating reliance on a single server or database, the system can continue to operate even if one component fails, thereby enhancing overall system reliability. This decentralized nature fosters trust and interoperability, allowing devices from different manufacturers to communicate seamlessly and exchange data without compatibility issues. As IoT networks expand and evolve, blockchain ensures that each device's operations are securely tracked and monitored. This not only reduces potential vulnerabilities but also boosts operational reliability by maintaining a detailed and tamper-proof historical record of all transactions and interactions. Also, enhancing blockchain interoperability through cross-chain provides solutions for the challenges posed by non-uniform aspects (Duan, Chamran, & Alobaedy, 2024). Figure 4, refers to cross-chain transactions that require data like fees, investment limits, token numbers, and confirmation counts for completion. All the transactions, including the previous transactions ensure the chain integrity.

Figure 4. Cross-chain interoperability transaction (Duan, Chamran, & Alobaedy, 2024).

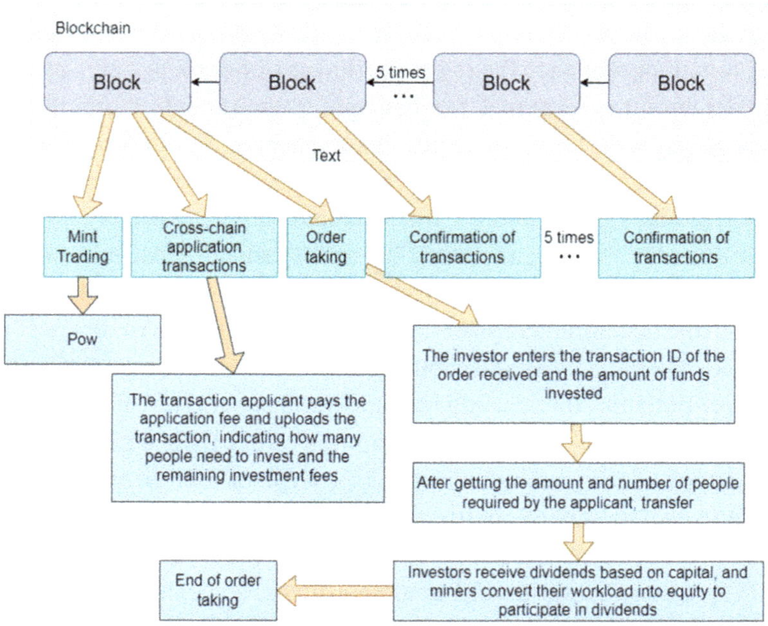

In short, the combination of healthcare with blockchain technology and IoT systems presents a transformative opportunity to improve security, efficiency, and trust in data management across various sectors. Blockchain technology offers a unique combination of security and privacy features that are particularly well-suited to meet the demands of the healthcare sector. This capability significantly enhances the protection of patient data, ensuring that sensitive information is stored and shared securely among authorized parties. However, the adoption of blockchain in large-scale healthcare systems faces several challenges, notably issues related to scalability, which refers to the technology's ability to handle a growing amount of work or data. Additionally, regulatory compliance poses another barrier, as healthcare organizations must navigate various laws and regulations governing data privacy and security. These challenges can limit the broader implementation of blockchain solutions in healthcare despite the potential benefits (Ramzan, et al., 2023).

As blockchain technology matures, its ability to effectively safeguard sensitive information continues to evolve, leaving room for optimism regarding its future in the healthcare landscape. Moreover, blockchain plays a critical role in enhancing the security of Internet of Things (IoT) networks. By providing a decentralized and tamper-proof ledger, blockchain protects the interactions between devices, ensuring that data transmitted across the network remains secure from unauthorized access and manipulation. Nevertheless, the integration of blockchain into IoT systems is not without its complications. One significant concern is the introduction of latency; that is, the delay in processing transactions can affect the speed at which devices communicate and operate. Additionally, blockchain may require substantial computational resources, which can be a limiting factor in environments where resources are constrained, such as in rapidly evolving IoT applications. As such, the successful adoption of blockchain technology in IoT settings hinges on the ability to strike an effective balance between maintaining high levels of security and ensuring efficient processing. Addressing these challenges will be crucial for maximizing the potential of blockchain in both healthcare and IoT domains. Digital identity management faces challenges due to user data being scattered across various online platforms, hindering user control and update capabilities. Blockchain technology offers a solution by empowering users with greater control over their data, including attributes and credentials, through a secure, decentralized, and auditable system. This approach enhances accessibility, privacy, and data control while reducing costs and improving efficiency in managing IDs, e-residency documents, and other vital records. Blockchain's secure infrastructure, coupled with policies like no centralized authority and private data architecture, provides a robust foundation for digital identity in an increasingly digital world. Replay attacks, where valid transmissions are maliciously repeated or delayed, pose a threat to blockchain security. These attacks can exploit vulnerabilities in forked cryptocurrencies or be disguised as normal data transmissions. Techniques like timestamping and temporary private keys, generated for each session using methods like LNSC and elliptical curve encryption, are employed to mitigate replay attacks by ensuring data uniqueness and preventing key leakage.

Impersonation attacks, including CEO fraud, involve unauthorized access to accounts or data through deceptive emails or compromised private keys. Attackers may seek to manipulate information or obtain illegal payments. Distributed incentive-based cooperation mechanisms and algorithms like ECDSA, which restrict signature generation to valid users, are used to detect and prevent impersonation attempts by protecting user privacy and verifying transactions. Sybil attacks occur when a single entity creates multiple accounts to gain control or influence within a network. This is a significant threat in peer-to-peer systems where a malicious actor can operate numerous identities simultaneously. Trust Chain, using Proof of Work (PoW), is one method proposed to validate transactions and protect against Sybil attacks, particularly targeting single nodes in eclipse attacks. Various other attacks target blockchain systems, including key attacks (leakage of private keys), false data injection attacks (introducing fabricated data), tampering attacks (modifying application data), overlay attacks (stealing information through deceptive windows), modification attacks (altering data), man-in-the-middle attacks (intercepting and altering communication), hiding blocks attacks (selectively revealing transactions), whitewashing attacks (resetting reputation), and double-spending attacks (spending the same cryptocurrency multiple times). Mitigation strategies involve techniques like mutual authentication, elliptical curve encryption, distributed voting algorithms, public-key cryptosystems, homomorphic Pallier encryption, timestamps, and multi-signature transactions, along with immediate transaction validation by users (Andrew, et al., 2023).

2.2. Enhancements and Improvements to the System

Implementing a hybrid blockchain model that effectively merges the features of both permissioned and public blockchains has the potential to significantly enhance data accessibility while ensuring that individual privacy is preserved. In a permissioned blockchain, access is restricted to authorized entities, which helps protect sensitive information, while a public blockchain allows for broader accessibility and transparency. This combination could create a more robust data-sharing environment, suitable for various applications. Furthermore, the integration of artificial intelligence (AI) to analyze data patterns within the blockchain ecosystem can play a crucial role in advancing predictive healthcare. By utilizing machine learning algorithms, AI can identify trends and anomalies in health data, allowing for early intervention and personalized treatment plans. This analytical capability can provide immense value to healthcare providers and patients alike, all while maintaining stringent security measures to protect confidential information. In addition, adopting lightweight blockchain protocols specifically designed for Internet of Things (IoT) devices can resolve issues related to latency and resource consumption. These protocols would enable efficient communication and data exchange among numerous interconnected IoT devices, ensuring that response times remain quick and that devices operate smoothly without draining excessive resources.

Moreover, exploring the use of edge computing in conjunction with blockchain technology can further enhance system performance. By processing and authenticating data nearer to its source, edge computing reduces the need for data to travel long distances to centralized servers. This not only expedites data processing and decision-making but also bolsters security by minimizing the attack surface and protecting sensitive information at its origin. Together, these strategies can lead to more effective and secure blockchain solutions tailored for a variety of industries and applications. (Asad Abbas, 2024).

2.3. Blockchain Technology Applications in Healthcare

Blockchain technology offers numerous potential applications within the healthcare sector. Its distributed ledger system facilitates the secure transfer of medical records, drug supply chain management, and improved data sharing for researchers exploring genetic code. Key features of blockchain in healthcare include enhanced data protection, genomics management, electronic data and medical record management, interoperability, and digitized tracking for outbreak management, all contributing to its growing adoption within the industry. One significant advantage of blockchain is its ability to create transparent processes, particularly in prescription tracking from manufacturing to pharmacy shelves. Combined with IoT, blockchain can track congestion, shipment routes, and speed, enabling efficient scheduling and preventing drug shortages. This digital framework built on blockchain ensures data integrity, increases trust, and prevents illicit handling of records, payments, and medications, ultimately improving patient care while controlling costs. Furthermore, blockchain simplifies multi-level authentication and enhances security by maintaining an incorruptible, decentralized, and transparent log of patient data while simultaneously preserving individual privacy through robust encryption (Adere, 2022).

Blockchain's decentralized structure empowers patients by granting them control over their medical data, facilitating patient-led interoperability, and improving confidentiality. It also offers solutions to industry-wide challenges in quality management and regulatory enforcement, aiding authorities in tracking legitimate drugs and ensuring secure digital transactions containing patient details. The technology streamlines the process of patients transferring medical practitioners, requiring only a single consent update for complete record sharing (Pranto Kumar Ghosh, 2024). The healthcare industry is rapidly embracing blockchain technology, with positive early adoption rates and ongoing exploration by medical firms. Its potential to transform healthcare lies in addressing existing structural issues, providing convenient access to information for physicians, patients, and pharmacists, and its integration with other technologies like machine learning and AI. Blockchain's robust data storage capabilities, recording a patient's complete health history, empower doctors with comprehensive information for accurate diagnoses and recommendations. Its decentralized and secure nature also protects data from loss, corruption, and external attacks, offering a robust solution for healthcare organizations (Shivani, Vikram, Mohanty, & Dev, 2023).

Blockchain technology offers a promising solution for managing and sharing patient medical records securely among hospitals and healthcare providers. One significant application is drug traceability, addressing the limitations of centralized systems that often struggle with privacy, data authentication, and flexibility. Blockchain-based systems, like Drugledger, integrate blockchain with the drug supply chain, tracking both the physical flow of drugs and the corresponding information flow on a drug chain network. This approach separates service providers into specialized roles, enhancing security and accountability.

Several frameworks have been proposed to combat drug fraud and improve transparency in the pharmaceutical supply chain. These frameworks often combine blockchain with other technologies like RFID to track drugs from manufacturing to distribution, aiming to reduce counterfeit medications and improve visibility. Models like Gcoin Blockchain utilize blockchain's trust-building capabilities and decentralized autonomous organizations (DAOs) to enhance drug supply chain surveillance and inspection. These systems often employ various blockchain implementations, such as Consortium Proof of Work, to achieve their goals.

In India, where counterfeit medicines pose a significant threat, blockchain-based frameworks are being developed to detect fake drugs within the supply chain. These systems, often built on architectures like Hyperledger Fabric, manage the entire medicine supply chain, enabling tracking from manufacturing to retail. They are tested against various scenarios, including stolen drugs and fake drug distribution, and evaluated against existing systems based on parameters like single point of failure resistance and counterfeit detection. While these systems demonstrate progress, limitations remain, such as the inability to prevent the consumption of unauthorized medicines.

A critical issue in drug supply chains is the replacement of genuine drugs with counterfeits. Traditional methods struggle to trace those responsible for these replacements due to information deletion at each step. Blockchain's transparency, where every transaction is visible to all users, offers a solution. Frameworks using blockchain, analyzed on platforms like Ethereum and Hyperledger, aim to address this issue. While Ethereum-based solutions involve transaction fees and lack KYC, Hyperledger offers fee-less transactions and KYC capabilities, making it a more feasible option for manufacturers.

2.4. Blockchain and Patient Monitoring

Electronic Health Records (EHRs) aim to securely store and efficiently manage sensitive patient health information. Several blockchain-based EHR systems have emerged, including Medrec for decentralized record management, Gem health network for secure data sharing, Healthbank for incentivized health information management, and OmniPHR for patient-accessible public health records. These systems leverage blockchain's features like smart contracts and decentralized data to enhance security and data control.

Real-time patient monitoring systems using blockchain and smart contracts have also been proposed. These systems aim to secure patient data collected from IoT devices, enabling authorized access for healthcare professionals. However, these systems face challenges like transaction verification delays and maintaining node security. Future research focuses on implementing these systems on platforms like Ethereum and Hyperledger. The integration of blockchain with IoT offers enhanced security due to blockchain's distributed ledger, public-key cryptography, and consensus algorithms. Frameworks are being developed to address the obstacles of this integration, focusing on secure remote patient monitoring. Future work involves performance testing of these models. Continuous patient health monitoring relies heavily on IoT devices, raising concerns about data security and privacy, especially with cloud storage. Several frameworks are being developed to address these concerns, utilizing blockchain to secure medical data collected from IoT devices and shared with authorized personnel. Performance evaluation tools like Hyper Caliper are used to assess these systems. Future research will explore interoperability with different IoT frameworks (Pranav, Amanpreet, Sparsh, Mohammad, & Gaurav, 2021).

Securing healthcare data collected by interconnected IoT devices is crucial. Blockchain frameworks like Fabric Hyperledger are being proposed to provide distributed and secure access to this data. While these frameworks enhance security, they may not address all potential IoT vulnerabilities. Future work aims to develop more comprehensive and attack-resistant health monitoring frameworks. Research also explores combining blockchain and IoT to protect patient data transferred from sensors to the cloud, addressing threats of privacy breaches, tampering, and manipulation by storing private patient data within each blockchain block.

3. CHALLENGES OF IMPLEMENTING BLOCKCHAIN AND IOT IN HEALTHCARE

One major hurdle in integrating blockchain and IoT in healthcare is interoperability. The diverse range of healthcare providers, including hospitals, insurers, physicians, and private doctors, makes seamless information exchange a significant challenge due to the open and varied nature of the system. Ensuring that these different entities can effectively share and access data within a blockchain network is crucial for its success. Security is another concern. While decentralization offers some security advantages, it also presents challenges. Distributing data on a public ledger can lead to privacy leaks, and the system's security can be compromised if a significant portion of the network's nodes become malicious. Patient comfort and trust in the security of their sensitive medical information are paramount for widespread adoption. The use of IoT merged with 5G enables healthcare to benefit from smart healthcare facilities, remote patient monitoring, and telemedicine, to name a few, which are part of intelligent healthcare systems when combined with AI and ML (Akhtar, Abdul, Muhammad, Filipe, & Chamran, 2024).

Scalability and storage pose practical limitations. Storing the medical records of numerous individuals, which often include documents, images, and lab reports, requires immense storage capacity. Distributing these records and storing multiple copies across the blockchain network further exacerbates this issue, potentially straining the healthcare system's resources. Standardization is also lacking. As blockchain technology is still relatively new, there is a need for standardized protocols and technologies. Clear guidelines are necessary to define what data can be sent and stored on the blockchain, including data format, size, and other technical specifications. This lack of standardization hinders seamless integration and widespread adoption. Finally, hesitations and lack of trust among both healthcare providers and patients create barriers. Hospitals may be reluctant to share data due to competitive concerns, while patients may be hesitant to disclose their medical history on a public platform. Furthermore, a lack of skills among medical practitioners in using these new technologies, coupled with concerns about data ownership and accountability, further complicates the implementation of blockchain and IoT in healthcare. Building trust and providing adequate training are essential to overcome these obstacles (Pranav, Amanpreet, Sparsh, Mohammad, & Gaurav, 2021).

Companies that successfully innovate, according to MIT, integrate the needs of people, the possibilities of technology, and the requirements for business success. This involves blending marketing, design, and engineering perspectives. A successful innovation must be technically sound, address a real unmet need, and be financially viable. Blockchain technology appears to meet these criteria within the healthcare industry, offering a technically feasible, desirable, and viable solution (Ahad, Tahir, Sheikh, Mughees, & Ahmed, 2021). Blockchain's application in healthcare can revolutionize the integrated healthcare information system by maintaining traceable records of distributed data and work, effectively handling diverse data challenges. This technology addresses four key issues: fragmented data, slow data access, system interoperability, and patient agency, while also improving data quality and quantity for research. Coupled with recent advancements and a strong industry commitment to standards and security, blockchain holds immense promise for the future of healthcare (Attaran, 2020).

Several companies are actively developing and distributing blockchain solutions specifically for healthcare. These solutions offer various benefits, including secure digital record storage, improved medical data sharing and usage, health record integrity protection, and drug traceability to combat counterfeiting. This growing market reflects the increasing recognition of blockchain's potential in the healthcare sector. Despite its potential, blockchain implementation in healthcare faces several challenges. Studies have identified advantages like flexible and secure infrastructure, and disadvantages such as cost, complexity, and patient awareness. Technological limitations also pose barriers. Scaling blockchain technology and addressing uncertainties surrounding its capabilities are major concerns. Experts argue that blockchain is not a disruptive technology but a foundational one, capable of reshaping economic and social systems. Successful implementation requires overcoming technological, governance, organizational, and societal barriers. Ultimately, blockchain solutions in healthcare must address the diverse needs of consumers, patients, providers, and regulators to achieve widespread adoption and realize its full potential (Attaran, 2022).

3.1. Technical, Regulation and Organizational Challenges

Blockchain technology, while promising for healthcare, is still nascent and faces significant hurdles in its adoption and implementation. Initial costs for institutions will be substantial as the technology is developed and integrated over time. Technical challenges also exist, including scalability issues, lack of standardization, potential data decay, difficulties integrating with legacy systems, and long transaction verification times. The significant computing power required for blockchain processing, along with the associated costs, and the need for a network of interconnected computers to support the system, present further technical obstacles. Furthermore, the suitability of blockchain for data with high temporal resolution is questionable.

The current Electronic Health Record (EHR) system, with its detailed patient information and substantial prior investment by healthcare institutions, poses a major economic challenge to widespread blockchain adoption. Replacing EHRs entirely with a blockchain digital ledger is currently impractical. Instead, a more feasible approach might involve augmenting the existing system, keeping most healthcare data off-chain while using blockchain to store concise summaries of patient information or procedures. This approach necessitates establishing standardized formats for demographic data and agreeing on a framework for data submission, size, and format. Beyond technical and economic considerations, organizational challenges related to blockchain implementation must be addressed. The evolution of blockchain is illustrated in Figure 3.

Figure 5. Blockchain evolution over the years (Andrew, et al., 2023).

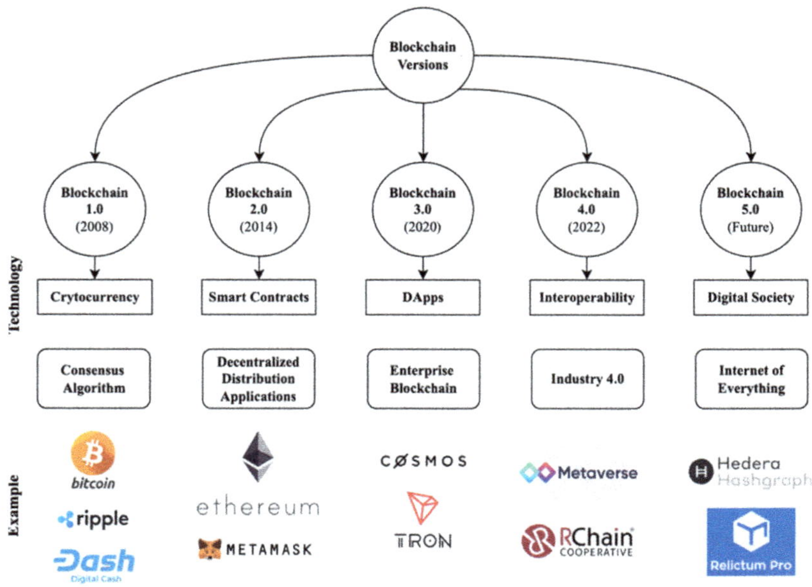

Managing the employees involved in this organizational change process is crucial for successful integration. Just as important are the regulatory and cultural barriers. Governments worldwide are still grappling with regulatory frameworks for blockchain, and widespread adoption will require significant buy-in from global healthcare participants (Attaran, 2022).

The unknown cost of operating a blockchain system and the difficulty in calculating return on investment (ROI) are further impediments. The benefits of a blockchain-based healthcare system will not be realized overnight. A clear incentive structure for healthcare providers to adopt the technology is essential, but calculating ROI in this context is complex. In conclusion, blockchain is not a silver bullet for all of healthcare's data management challenges, nor can it be immediately implemented. However, despite the obstacles, blockchain has the potential to improve efficiency in specific niche areas within the current healthcare system, offering targeted solutions rather than a complete overhaul.

Blockchain technology holds significant promise for transforming the healthcare system. Its decentralized nature has the potential to improve both patient data accessibility and security, shifting control from centralized authorities to individual patients, and empowering them in their own treatment decisions. This shift addresses critical ethical concerns surrounding data breaches and the lack of patient control over personal medical information, issues that have become increasingly prominent with personalized medicine and the rise of wearable health trackers.

The healthcare domain has undergone a rapid evolution, driven by advancements like Industry 4.0. From paper-based systems to electronic health records (EHRs) and electronic medical records, technology has played a crucial role in improving patient data management and healthcare research. Modern advancements such as telemedicine and the Internet of Medical Things (IoMT) are further reshaping the landscape, and blockchain is poised to play a significant role in this transformation. Blockchain technology can benefit every stage of the healthcare supply chain, from raw material supply and logistics to manufacturing, distribution, and service providers, including EHR management, patient data verification, and patient information analysis (Andrew, et al., 2023).

Blockchain's applications within healthcare are diverse. They range from enhancing mobile health applications and monitoring devices to securely sharing and storing electronic medical records, clinical trial data, and insurance information. These applications address the significant challenges currently faced by healthcare professionals and researchers, including fragmented data, communication delays, and inadequate workflow tools. A key problem is the lack of secure connections between disparate healthcare systems, hindering the development of a truly comprehensive and accessible system. Some of the main blockchain challenges in healthcare are illustrated in figure 6.

Furthermore, the healthcare sector struggles with the management and maintenance of e-health records. Blockchain technology offers solutions by enabling trustless transactions through decentralization and virtual anonymity. Its immutability feature prevents data manipulation by a single entity and eliminates data duplication. Blockchain can be implemented to ensure the secure transaction of confidential information, including patient records, medical histories, disease records, lab results, treatments, and even ambulance service information.

Health insurance has become essential due to rising health concerns, offering financial security during medical emergencies and mitigating the risk of debt. However, the advantages of health insurance are often accompanied by concerns regarding security, privacy, and fraud. Fraud, in particular, poses a significant problem, causing substantial losses for individuals, businesses, and governments, making the development of technologies to combat it crucial. The claims process itself is often cumbersome, requiring insurers to verify claims, reconcile disparate data sources, and deal with abandoned policies, highlighting the need for more efficient and transparent systems.

To address these challenges, blockchain technology offers promising solutions. Inspired by its use in Fintech for secure transaction management and double-spending prevention, blockchain-based insurance systems can provide two key service models: one for personal web identity security and another for commercial website data security. By automatically uploading claim evidence for authentication and implementing automated contracts, blockchain can foster greater trust between insurers and policyholders, while also providing risk-free management and increased transparency.

Figure 6. The main challenges that blockchain faces in healthcare (Andrew, et al., 2023)

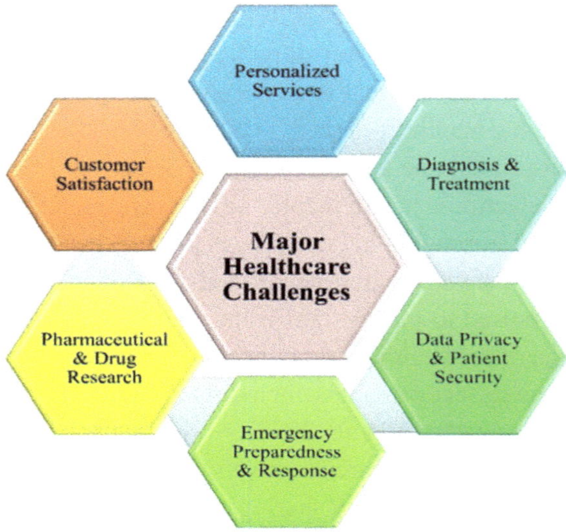

4. AI ALGORITHMS IN HEALTHCARE

4.1. Supervised AI

Artificial Neural Networks (ANNs), inspired by the human brain, are capable of handling various categorization tasks. These networks consist of interconnected neurons organized in layers, where connections are strengthened or weakened through training data, mimicking biological learning. While ANNs have been used in survival prediction research, applications using electronic health data are less common. Deep learning, a subfield of machine learning, utilizes ANN-inspired algorithms and has shown promise in modeling illness and symptoms, as demonstrated by studies on Alzheimer's disease and patient phenotyping using electronic health records.

Support Vector Machines (SVMs) are a popular supervised learning method used for classifying both linear and non-linear data. SVMs operate by mapping data points into a higher-dimensional space and identifying the optimal hyperplane that separates different classes. The goal is to maximize the margin between classes while minimizing classification errors. SVMs have proven useful in bioinformatics and healthcare classification tasks.

Decision trees (DTs) are tree-like data structures used for classification, where internal nodes represent input variables, branches represent outcomes, and leaves represent final decisions. They offer a transparent and interpretable approach to classification, resembling a flowchart. DTs have found applications in healthcare, such as predicting disease recurrence and survival in cancer patients. Random forests are ensemble classifiers composed of multiple decision trees, often recognized for their high accuracy. This approach combines the "Bagging" technique with random feature selection to create a diverse set of decision trees. Random forests have been applied in healthcare for tasks like estimating individual disease risk using datasets like the Healthcare Cost and Utilization Project (HCUP).

4.2. Unsupervised AI

Association analysis is a valuable data mining and machine learning technique used for prediction by extracting hidden information from large datasets. It generates association rules, where the presence of item set X in current transactions suggests the potential appearance of item set Y in future transactions. This makes it particularly useful for applications like market basket analysis, where it can forecast customer purchasing behavior.

In healthcare, association analysis can be used to predict future disease risk by considering a patient's medical history as an item set. The Hierarchical Association Rule Model (HARM) utilizes this approach, first generating association rules from medical data and then ranking them using Bayesian estimation. HARM can then predict a patient's likely future health problems based on their past and present medical conditions, assuming regular healthcare consultations.

4.3. Types of AI application in Blockchain

Blockchain technologies are broadly categorized into permissioned and permissionless structures. Permissioned blockchains, used in consortium, cloud-based, or private environments, restrict access to authorized users. Conversely, permissionless blockchains are open to all users over the internet. Public blockchains allow users to access, modify, and utilize the blockchain code. This open access necessitates complex security and consensus mechanisms, including anonymity and safeguards against bogus data, to protect user credentials and private transactions. Public blockchains utilize native tokens like cryptocurrencies for asset and data transfer. Despite their decentralization and transparency, public blockchains are vulnerable to security attacks due to user anonymity. The consensus process on public blockchains requires a majority of validators and complex computations, leading to high energy consumption and potential vulnerability if attackers gain control of a significant share of the network. Transaction approval times on public blockchains can be lengthy, often exceeding ten minutes.

Private blockchains, managed by a single organization, operate under a permissioned system, granting pre-authorized users read and write access. Knowing the identities of participants and validators allows for faster transaction validation with fewer computations compared to public blockchains. Private blockchains can handle various assets, data, and values. Using voting or multi-party consensus algorithms, they achieve quick transaction processing, typically in under a second, and consume minimal energy. Blockchain-as-a-Service (BaaS) has emerged due to the growing adoption of blockchain by governments and corporations. Cloud providers like Microsoft, Amazon, and IBM offer BaaS, enabling customers to easily create and experiment with blockchain services. BaaS benefits both consortium and private blockchain firms by allowing them to focus on application development and implementation rather than infrastructure management. BaaS facilitates new cross-industry partnerships and business models. Developers can easily set up BaaS services for smart contract creation. Integrating BaaS with AI cloud services offers further opportunities for application developers, as major cloud providers offer a wide range of AI tools (Alaa, Habaebi, Rafiqul, Hasbullah, & Zabidi, 2022).

4.4. Implementation of Federated Blockchain in Healthcare

The convergence of Federated Learning (FL) and blockchain offers a promising solution to critical challenges in collaborative machine learning, particularly concerning data privacy and reliability. Several studies highlight blockchain's potential to mitigate these issues by providing a decentralized and secure platform for FL processes. Researchers have explored various integration models, including coupled, decoupled, and overlapped architectures, demonstrating blockchain's ability to enhance scalability, data privacy, and security within FL systems. A typical integrated architecture involves FL participants receiving and updating a model, transmitting updates to blockchain miner nodes via APIs, and miners validating and aggregating these updates using consensus algorithms and smart contracts. The verified updates are then added to the blockchain, allowing FL clients to securely access the finalized global model (Archana Bathula, et al., 2024).

Several innovative frameworks have been proposed to leverage the synergies between FL and blockchain. Isomerism learning, combined with blockchain's security features, enables robust and privacy-preserving collaborative ML, dynamically addressing time-varying challenges. This approach has been applied to analyze public sentiment, incorporating advanced model architectures and demonstrating improved performance. Biscotti, a decentralized P2P scheme, focuses on maintaining privacy and security among FL peers through secure secret exchange and contribution verification. It utilizes a private blockchain model with optimized consensus for integration with Hyperledger Fabric. Other approaches further refine the integration of FL and blockchain. BlocFL replaces the central server in FL with a consortium blockchain, enabling local training and optimized resource allocation across diverse nodes. GCFL utilizes a DAG blockchain to minimize data redundancy and facilitate seamless data exchange, introducing a two-phase tips selection consensus algorithm for improved resource usage and stability. These advancements demonstrate the potential of blockchain-enhanced FL systems to overcome the limitations of centralized coordination and traditional consensus methods.

The integration of blockchain with FL is also being explored in specific domains like institutional and healthcare collaboration (IFL). By securely sharing model updates on the blockchain, IFL enables accurate predictions from diverse data sources. Isomerism learning further enhances this by adapting the global model to various data distributions. However, challenges such as scalability, energy consumption, and algorithmic complexities need to be addressed to fully realize the potential of IFL with blockchain. In short, the research presented showcases the significant potential of integrating blockchain technology with federated learning to address critical challenges in collaborative machine learning. The various frameworks and approaches discussed, including isomerism learning, Biscotti, BlocFL, and GCFL, highlight the ongoing innovation in this field. While challenges remain, the continued development and refinement of these integrated systems promise to revolutionize decentralized machine-learning methodologies, particularly in sensitive domains like healthcare (Archana Bathula, et al., 2024).

The other sensitive domain in healthcare is data encryption and security. Homomorphic encryption is a powerful privacy-enhancing technology that allows computations to be performed on encrypted data while producing the same results as if the data were unencrypted. This ensures that organizations can analyze and process data without compromising confidentiality, making it particularly useful for outsourced storage and cloud computing. Built upon asymmetric-key cryptography, homomorphic encryption functions as a mathematical homomorphism between plaintext and ciphertext spaces, enabling secure computations without decryption.

To address the limitations of traditional Blockchain technology, researchers have developed alternative distributed ledger technologies (DLTs) such as Hashgraph, Directed Acyclic Graphs (DAGs), and Holochain. Hashgraph achieves consensus through time-stamping rather than proof-of-work, allowing for faster and more efficient transactions. DAGs enable decentralized consensus by requiring majority approval for transactions, reducing reliance on centralized authorities. IOTA's Tangle, a well-known DAG-based network, allows nodes to simultaneously initiate and approve transactions. Holochain, on the other hand, distributes data across nodes using a Distributed Hash Table (DHT), enabling a decentralized and autonomous network where each node operates independently. These alternative DLTs offer improved scalability, efficiency, and decentralization compared to traditional Blockchain systems (Rucha Shinde, 2023). In Table 1, a comparison of distributed ledger technology is illustrated.

Table 1. More common distributed ledger technologies (Rucha Shinde, 2023)

Parameter	Blockchain	Hashgraph	DAG	Holochain
Launched in	2008	2018	2015	2018
Consensus algorithm	Many algorithms available	Virtual voting	The previous transaction validates the new one	Not required
Scalability	Limited	High	High	Infinite
Transaction execution speed	Limited	High	High	Highest
Data structure	Blocks are generated as per the sequence of transactions	Gossip about Gossip Protocol	Directed Acyclic Graph	Distributed among nodes
Examples	Bitcoin, Ethereum, and so forth	Swirlds and NOIA	NXT, Tangle, ByteBall, and so forth	Holochain

4.5. Natural Language Processing (NLP) in Healthcare

Clinical Decision Support Systems (CDSS) rely on various data inputs, including structured data like Electronic Health Records (EHR), semi-structured data like XML documents, and unstructured narrative text such as clinical findings and radiology reports. Unstructured data poses a significant challenge, and Natural Language Processing (NLP) techniques have emerged as crucial tools for extracting valuable information from this free text, enabling CDSS to generate effective results and recommendations for healthcare professionals. This ability to automatically extract key facts is essential for informed clinical decision-making. Clinical notes, containing vital patient health history, are invaluable for addressing complex clinical problems that other EHR components, like lab results, might not fully capture. NLP facilitates the retrieval of meaningful features from these notes, which can then be utilized to develop robust machine-learning models. For instance, combining Unified Medical Language System (UMLS) resources with NLP analysis of clinical notes has shown promise in predicting mortality in diabetic patients within critical care, although further research with larger datasets is needed. Furthermore, sentiment analysis algorithms, powered by NLP, can effectively gauge sentiment from narrative hospital admission and discharge statements.

In Figure 6, adversarial attack taxonomy is illustrated. Adversarial text, involving semantic, syntactic, or visual perturbations, can mislead NLP models. Two main generation methods exist: one modifies minimal characters to create human-like typing errors (e.g., DeepWordBug, Hotflip, Textbugger), preserving the original text's sequence, while the other paraphrases the text (e.g., Alzantot, Bae, Bert-attack, IGA, PWWS, Textbugger, Textfooler), maintaining semantic equivalence but altering the model output. Textbugger combines both approaches. As illustrated by healthcare application examples, even simple synonym replacements can fool NLP, leading to incorrect disease severity predictions and potentially dangerous treatment decisions (Rucha, et al., 2022).

Figure 7. Adversarial attack taxonomy (Rucha, et al., 2022).

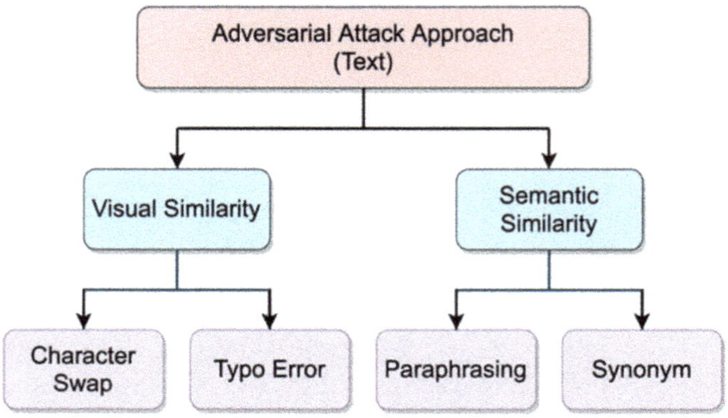

NLP's capabilities extend to processing radiology reports, converting unstructured text into manageable computer formats for analysis. Supervised machine learning combined with NLP can analyze clinical notes to identify medical subdomains, effectively directing patients with unresolved issues to the appropriate specialists. In ophthalmology, NLP has proven useful in analyzing COVID-19 related literature for viral transmission, ocular manifestations, and treatment trajectories. Similarly, in gastroenterology, NLP can revolutionize the analysis of extensive narrative medical reports. The effectiveness of NLP is demonstrated in various clinical contexts. The KD-NLP model, for example, significantly outperformed manual chart review in identifying pediatric emergency department patients at high risk for Kawasaki disease. Hybrid NLP frameworks have been developed to extract information about Adverse Drug Effects (ADE) and medication insights, supporting informed decisions regarding ADEs and drug safety. Even chatbot systems integrated with NLP can understand user queries and provide relevant information about various diseases. The increasing availability of medical data has fueled the widespread adoption of deep learning within clinical NLP. Recent research has leveraged NLP to classify challenging-to-diagnose diseases and disorders using only clinical gestalt. Overall, NLP-based solutions streamline Information Retrieval (IR) processes, saving time and effort, which ultimately contributes to improved patient care and treatment (Rucha, et al., 2022).

To consider the adoption of blockchain in healthcare with the use of AI, focusing on the keywords shown in Table 1 is necessary.

Table 2. Key Considerations for Blockchain Adoption in Healthcare

Category	Healthcare	Security	Challenges	Solutions
Available Data	Record management	Data protection	Interoperability	Hybrid models, AI
Security	Access control	Decentralized storage	Security risks	IoT protocols, edge computing
IoT	Device security	Data integrity	Latency, resources	Cross-chain, secure tracking
Supply	Drug tracking	Counterfeit prevention	Fraud tracing	Blockchain frameworks
Adoption	System improvement	Patient privacy	Scalability, regulation	Industry standards

5. ISSUES TO BE ADDRESSED FOR FUTURE RESEARCH

Smart healthcare systems, while offering numerous benefits, face significant security and operational challenges that can negatively impact patient health during remote monitoring. A primary concern is the lack of robust security standardization. Current healthcare security standards are outdated and insufficient to withstand modern cyberattacks, leaving systems vulnerable and potentially discouraging patients from trusting remote care, thus harming hospital reputations and revenue. The first line of defense in smart healthcare, including firewalls and intrusion detection systems, is often inefficient against evolving security threats. Despite their advantages, these traditional security measures struggle to detect and prevent contemporary attacks, leaving smart healthcare environments exposed. This vulnerability is compounded by the lack of physical layer access control, which is fundamental to overall security. Currently, access control focuses on the application layer, leaving the wireless communication at the physical layer unprotected and susceptible to data modification, particularly in implantable medical devices, posing serious risks to patients.

Beyond traditional attacks like DDoS, MITM, and ransomware, smart healthcare systems face newer, more sophisticated threats. These include software supply chain attacks, exploiting vulnerabilities in a healthcare institution's supplier network, and IoT attacks, where malware manipulates signals from remotely connected endpoint devices to cause destructive actions. These evolving attack vectors require constant vigilance and adaptation of security measures. Another challenge lies in the accessibility and training of healthcare professionals to use advanced technologies in modernized smart healthcare systems. Not all staff possess the necessary experience and training to effectively manage sophisticated medical equipment for remote patient monitoring. Investing in comprehensive training is crucial, but it can be a significant cost burden for hospitals. Finally, scalability is a major concern in wireless communication between patients and doctors during remote treatment. The need for various medical equipment and implantable sensors to gather patient health data demands optimized network bandwidth. Low scalability can delay treatment, potentially worsening a patient's condition or even leading to severe consequences, including death. Therefore, ensuring scalable and reliable communication is paramount for effective remote healthcare (Alabdulatif, Khalil, & Rahman, 2022).

REFERENCES

Abid, H., Mohd, J., Singh, R. P., Rajiv, S., & Shanay, R. (2021). Blockchain technology applications in healthcare: An overview. *International Journal of Intelligent Networks*, *2*(9), 130–139. DOI: 10.1016/j.ijin.2021.09.005

Abid Haleem, M. J. (2021). Blockchain technology applications in healthcare: An overview. *International Journal of Intelligent Networks*, *2*(9), 130–139. DOI: 10.1016/j.ijin.2021.09.005

Adere, E. M. (2022). Blockchain in healthcare and IoT: A systematic literature review. *Journal od. Array (New York, N.Y.)*, *14*(9), 100–139. DOI: 10.1016/j.array.2022.100139

Ahad, A., Tahir, M., Sheikh, M. A., Mughees, A., & Ahmed, K. I. (2021). Optimal route selection in 5g-based smart health-care network: a reinforcement learning approach. *Asia-Pacific Conference on Communications (APCC)* (pp. 248-253). IEEE. DOI: 10.1109/APCC49754.2021.9609815

Akbar, M. A., Leiva, V., Rafi, S., Qadri, S. F., Mahmood, S., & Alsanad, A. (2022). Towards roadmap to implement blockchain in healthcare systems based on a maturity model. *Journal of Software (Malden, MA)*, *34*(12), 1–15. DOI: 10.1002/smr.2500

Akhtar, B. H., Abdul, A., Muhammad, W., Filipe, M., & Chamran, K. (2024). 5G and IoT for Intelligent Healthcare: AI and Machine Learning Approaches—A Review. *Lecture Notes of the Institute for Computer Sciences, Social Informatics and Telecommunications Engineering*, *556*(1), 107–123. DOI: 10.1007/978-3-031-52524-7_8

Alaa, H., Habaebi, M. H., Rafiqul, I., Hasbullah, N. F., & Zabidi, S. A. (2022). Systematic Review on AI-Blockchain Based E-Healthcare Records Management Systems. *IEEE Access : Practical Innovations, Open Solutions*, *10*(10), 1–33. DOI: 10.1109/ACCESS.2022.3201878

Alabdulatif, A., Khalil, I., & Rahman, M. S. (2022). Security of Blockchain and AI-Empowered Smart Healthcare Application-Based Analysis. *Applied Sciences (Basel, Switzerland)*, *21*(11), 1–32. DOI: 10.3390/app122111039 PMID: 36330151

Andrew, I. (2023). Blockchain for healthcare systems: Architecture, security challenges, trends and future directions. *Journal of Network and Computer Applications*, *215*(6), 103633. DOI: 10.1016/j.jnca.2023.103633

Asad Abbas, R. A. (2024). Blockchain-assisted secured data management framework for health information analysis based on Internet of Medical Things. *Personal and Ubiquitous Computing*, *28*(6), 59–72. DOI: 10.1007/s00779-021-01583-8

Attaran, M. (2020). Blockchain technology in healthcare: Challenges and opportunities. *International Journal of Healthcare Management*, (11), 1–15. DOI: 10.1080/20479700.2020.1843887

Attaran, M. (2022). Blockchain technology in healthcare: Challenges and opportunities. *International Journal of Healthcare Management*, *15*(1), 70–83. DOI: 10.1080/20479700.2020.1843887

Bathula, A., Gupta, S., Merugu, S., Saba, L., Khanna, N., Laird, J., Sanagala, S. S., Singh, R., Garg, D., Fouda, M. M., & Suri, J. (2024). Blockchain, artificial intelligence, and healthcare: The tripod of future—a narrative review. *Artificial Intelligence Review*, *57*(9), 238. DOI: 10.1007/s10462-024-10873-5

Duan, S., Chamran, M. K., & Alobaedy, M. M. (2024). Enhancing Blockchain Interoperability Through Cross-Chain Outsourcing and Communication. *2024 IEEE 6th Symposium on Computers & Informatics (ISCI)* (pp. 276-281). Kuala Lumpur: IEEE. doi:DOI: 10.1109/ISCI62787

Haleema, A., Javaida, M., Singhb, R. P., Sumanc, R., & Rab, S. (2021). Blockchain technology applications in healthcare: An overview. *International Journal of Intelligent Networks*, *2*(9), 130–139. DOI: 10.1016/j.ijin.2021.09.005

Khyati Kapadiya, U. P. (2022). Blockchain and AI-Empowered Healthcare Insurance Fraud Detection: An Analysis, Architecture, and Future Prospects. *IEEE Access : Practical Innovations, Open Solutions*, *10*(7), 79606–79627. DOI: 10.1109/ACCESS.2022.3194569

Lashkari, B., & Musilek, P. (2021). A Comprehensive Review of Blockchain Consensus Mechanisms. *IEEE Access : Practical Innovations, Open Solutions*, *9*(3), 43620–43652. DOI: 10.1109/ACCESS.2021.3065880

Mayra Macas, C. W. (2024). Adversarial examples: A survey of attacks and defenses in deep learning-enabled cybersecurity systems. *Expert Systems with Applications*, *238*(3), 1–12. DOI: 10.1016/j.eswa.2023.122223

Min, E., Guo, X., Liu, Q., Zhang, G., Cui, J., & Long, J. (2018). A Survey of Clustering With Deep Learning: From the Perspective of Network Architecture. *IEEE Access : Practical Innovations, Open Solutions*, *6*(7), 39501–39514. DOI: 10.1109/ACCESS.2018.2855437

Mohamed Yaseen Jabarulla, H.-N. L. (2021). A Blockchain and Artificial Intelligence-Based, Patient-Centric Healthcare System for Combating the COVID-19 Pandemic: Opportunities and Applications. *Healthcare (Basel)*, *9*(8), 1–12. DOI: 10.3390/healthcare9081019 PMID: 34442156

Pranav, R., Amanpreet, K., Sparsh, S., Mohammad, S., & Gaurav, D. (2021). Application of Blockchain and Internet of Things in Healthcare and Medical Sector: Applications, Challenges, and Future Perspectives. *Journal of Food Quality*, *21*(3), 1–20. Advance online publication. DOI: 10.1155/2021/7608296

Pranto Kumar Ghosh, A. C. (2024). Blockchain Application in Healthcare Systems: A Review. *Systems*, *11*(1), 1–44. DOI: 10.3390/systems11010038

Priti Tagde, S. T. (2021). Blockchain and artificial intelligence technology in e-Health. *Environmental Science and Pollution Research International*, *1*(5), 52810–52831. DOI: 10.1007/s11356-021-16223-0 PMID: 34476701

Ramzan, S., Aqdus, A., Ravi, V., Koundal, D., Amin, R., & Ghamdi, M. A. (2023). Healthcare Applications Using Blockchain Technology: Motivations and Challenges. *IEEE Transactions on Engineering Management*, *70*(8), 2874–2890. DOI: 10.1109/TEM.2022.3189734

Rehman, A., & Ilyas, M. (2024). Blockchain-Enhanced Privacy and Security in Medicare Data Sharing: Identifying Gaps and Solutions in Current Practices. *Internet of Things and Data Analytics*, *1145*(2), 432–442. DOI: 10.1007/978-3-031-53717-2_40

Roberta Bernardi, S. S. (2019). The Role of Affordances in the Deinstitutionalization of a Dysfunctional Health Management Information System in Kenya. *Management Information Systems Quarterly*, *43*(4), 1177–1200. Advance online publication. DOI: 10.25300/MISQ/2019/14187

Rucha, S., Shruti, P., Ketan, K., Vidyasagar, P., Ganeshsree, S., & Ajith, A. (2022). Securing AI-based healthcare systems using blockchain technology: A state-of-the-art systematic literature review and future research directions. *Emerging telecommunications. Transactions on Emerging Telecommunications Technologies*, *35*(10), 1–48. DOI: 10.1002/ett.4884

Rucha Shinde, S. P. (2023). Securing AI-based healthcare systems using blockchain technology: A state-of-the-art systematic literature review and future research directions. *Jordan Medical Journal*, *58*(3), 1–21. DOI: 10.1002/ett.4884

Sarthak Dhingra, R. R. (2023). Blockchain Technology Applications in Healthcare Supply Chains—A Review. *IEEE Access : Practical Innovations, Open Solutions*, *12*(1), 11230–11257. DOI: 10.1109/ACCESS.2023.3348813

Shivani, B., Vikram, B., Mohanty, R. P., & Dev, G. (2023). Analysis of critical success factors for blockchain technology implementation in healthcare sector. *Benchmarking*, *30*(4), 1367–1399. DOI: 10.1108/BIJ-07-2021-0433

Soni, M., & Singh, D. K. (2021). Blockchain Implementation for Privacy preserving and securing the Healthcare data. *IEEE International Conference on Communication Systems and Network Technologies (CSNT)* (pp. 729-734). IEEE. DOI: 10.1109/CSNT51715.2021.9509722

Chapter 9
Investigating Critical Factors Useful for Healthcare Data Sharing in a Blockchain Architecture

Shoaib Hassan
https://orcid.org/0000-0002-8265-7932
School of Computer Science and Engineering, Nanjing University of Science and Technology, Nanjing, China

Qianmu Li
https://orcid.org/0000-0002-0998-1517
School of Computer Science and Engineering, Nanjing University of Science and Technology, Nanjing, China

Affan Yasin
School of AI and Advanced Computing, Xi'an Jiaotong-Liverpool University, Suzhou, China

Muhammad Zubair
Interdisciplinary Research Center for Finance and Digital Economy, King Fahad University of Petroleum and Minerals, Dhahran, Saudi Arabia

ABSTRACT

Blockchain technology presents a capable solution for secure and standardized data sharing with its consensus mechanisms and smart contracts. The major objective of this study is to propose a novel blockchain architecture for secure healthcare data sharing by detecting all factors necessary for healthcare data sharing. After analyzing numerous blockchain architectures for healthcare systems, this study found three essential categories of factors called healthcare, security, and blockchain, which are vital for successful data sharing in healthcare environments. The prototypes and pseudocodes of the proposed architecture were validated by using expert opinions from 15 software experts. The study's major contribution lies in the development of this robust architecture, which not only addresses the core issues of data privacy, security, and interoperability but also lays a strong foundation for future advancements in the secure exchange of medical records using blockchain technology.

DOI: 10.4018/979-8-3373-0593-6.ch009

INTRODUCTION

Population durability has amplified significantly in recent decades and is still growing, a trend noted by young and middle-aged adults who know the value of leading a healthy lifestyle. As a result, the amount and implications of data on well-being and health are increasing as hospitals, clinics, doctors, etc., collect more and more. The data refers to the patient's personal information, including his name, gender, blood group, and other reported data (Akshaya, Shetty, & Patil, 2022). Additionally, it should be emphasized that a substantial portion of them receive little to no use, are lost, and receive little to no safety due to their distribution, incompatible data formats, and deviating semantics (Rajadevi et al., 2022). To transform them into information and knowledge that will benefit the person and society, we must make them interoperable, secure, private, and available over a high-availability network (Office of the National Coordinator for Health Information Technology, 2018). The availability of this sensitive and personal data is crucial, as many computer-aided diagnosis (CAD) (Zubair, Umair, & Owais, 2023; Zubair et al., 2023; Zubair et al., 2022; Zubair, Ali, & Javed, 2016) and screening systems (Zubair, Khan, & Yasin, 2014; Zubair, Yamin, & Khan, 2013) rely on data to effectively train the model. These CAD systems play a vital role in medical diagnosis by offering interpretations of medical data free from human error and subjective interpretation, thus enhancing their reliability and trustworthiness.

This work presents an architectural proposal that takes into account questions about data regarding its interoperability, unifying semantics, and structures, their sharing, security, and encryption, in addition to the identity and critical sharing from the collection of personal health data generated by the users themselves to the data generated by the actors of the health ecosystem, such as hospitals and clinics. This study also focuses on all the critical factors that support data sharing through blockchain technology in the healthcare domain. Finally, once data is stored in the blockchain, only people with permission can access it (DK & AU, 2023). Smart contracts (Buterin, 2014) in this situation, only users must be given access to their data, preventing repudiation or non-compliance with any contractual clauses. The ability to persevere and enter health and well-being data gathered by patients and Internet of Things (IoT) devices into the chain is provided via integration with middleware. The main contributions of this study are mentioned below:

- Proposed a blockchain-based architecture that focuses on secure healthcare data sharing.
- Highlighted the critical factors and their influence on healthcare data sharing in a blockchain architecture.
- Provides methodology of three significant functionalities of the healthcare system to support healthcare data sharing.
- Presents the expert findings regarding the critical factors used to support healthcare data sharing.
- Validate the proposed architecture from multiple IT experts using a comprehensive questionnaire and literature studies.

The article is organized as follows: Section II presents previous competitive studies related to this study. Section III discusses challenges, addressing interoperability, standards, and laws for data gathering in the health ecosystem. Section IV addresses the critical factors supporting healthcare data sharing in blockchain architecture. The architecture plan is provided in section V, and the results and discussion are provided in section VI, leading to conclusions and future work.

2. LITERATURE REVIEW

Blockchain technology has many immediate ramifications, including cryptocurrency (Zubair et al., 2024), healthcare, and more. The scientific community is debating using blockchain as a secondary technology for exchanging and managing health and well-being data for various applications. Using a blockchain based on Hyperledger, Fabric, Mikula and Jacobsen (2018) recommend it as a solution for a decentralized identity and access management system, applying it for essential authentication operations and authorization like registration, login, grant of permissions, and updates to the system. Jiang et al. (2018) discuss a blockchain platform for data sharing in the health sector, proposing two blockchains where personal data collected from patients by IoT devices and/or wearables will be separated from data collected by health system actors (such as hospitals and clinics).

According to Esposito et al. (2018), a paradigm for cloud data sharing uses blockchain to receive URLs pointing to the location of the data's storage rather than the actual data itself. This is because certain nations or geographic regions, like the USA or the European Union, have various laws protecting personal data. The circular economy, which aims to be effective, profitable, and maintainable regarding service supply and, even more so regarding healthcare, frequently funded by public resources, is an important social issue. To accomplish these goals, Alexaki et al. (2018) suggest developing a decentralized, integrated care cycle using blockchain technology, where the availability of diagnostic and exam information is shared among the many actors, preventing, among other things, the loss of information and duplication of exams and diagnoses.

A new consensus algorithm, the proof of Interoperability from a centralized source of standards and semantics, is put forth by Peterson et al. (2017) The system ENIGMA/OPAL from the MIT Media Lab implements a layer encryption based on a method known as cryptography secure in distributed computing (Shrobe, Shrier, & Pentland, 2018). Ekblaw et al. (2016) suggests using Zyskind and Nathan's (2015) model of privacy decentralized adoption of blockchain to secure personal data, which is also based on the ENIGMA Project, to share data from electronic health records (commonly known as EHRs). Shrobe et al. (2018) and Ekblaw et al. (2016) discuss data privacy, protection, and secrecy, whereas Peterson et al. (2017) deals with interoperability and consensus algorithms. In this work, we propose an architecture that spans a wider range than the studies previously mentioned, starting with the collection of personal data produced by users and actors in the health ecosystem and moving on to concerns with semantics and interoperability, security, encryption, and access, all the way up to the insertion of records in blocks within a Blockchain. The study (Xia et al., 2017) developed Medshare to resolve data-sharing problems. Blockchain technology makes it safe to share data between untrusted organizations. The design of Medshare is made of smart contracts and control mechanisms that check the data behavior and notify if any unauthorized entity is found. Ancile is a blockchain-based architecture that uses smart contracts for electronic health record management (Dagher et al., 2018). This framework gives patients ownership and control over accessing their health data. The study (Dubovitskaya et al., 2018) also used a permission blockchain for sharing and managing health records securely. MedRec is a decentralized blockchain-based healthcare system. It keeps the record's signature rather than the real health record of the patient (U.S. Department of Health and Human Services, n.d.).

3. DATA COLLECTION

Identifying the idea that, as the only holder of the rights of ownership and discretion over your data, you have the right to privacy and confidentiality, even without possessing or custody of that data, is an important part of gathering health data. The US has the Health Insurance Portability and Accountability Act of 1996 (HIPPA) and the Health Information Technology for Economic and Clinical Health Act (HITECH) (European Commission, 2016), while the European Community has the GDPR (General Data Protection Regulation) (Goddard, 2017) that set out the rights and responsibilities of people and organizations that hold private data.

All distinct residents of the European Union (EU) and the European Economic Area (EEA) must abide by the General Data Protection Regulation (GDPR), a law of the European Union (Alzahrani et al., 2020). The various actors in the health ecosystem gather and hold data about their users, and they have a responsibility to defend and stock that data. When essential, they must also make that data available to interested parties who have been given former permission by the person who has ownership and decision over it. It is projected that data will be shared and that everyone will be able to understand its structure and semantics, with the interoperability that permits the best uses in actions and wellness and health services for the population, not only at the individual level but also in those including public actions as in scientific research, policy, and resource distributions made proficiently and clearly. Therefore, the interoperable distribution of healthcare information will support the individual, society, and governments in meeting these requirements. This presents the challenge of how to share, preserve, and keep private and confidential data on a single high-availability network, assuring the individual's rights of ownership and decision about data. Since the development of Bitcoin Core as open-source software, other open-source platforms have also developed. Some are derived from Bitcoin Core itself, and others from new developments, presenting new useful features for general-purpose applications other than monetary transactions. The goal is to approach the subject under the following aspects:

a) User individuality - decreases this centralization's single point of failure by requiring the single registration of patients.
b) Interoperability - make data structures well-matched and standardize data semantics.
c) Data safety, or the delivery of cryptographic assurances in data sharing with confidentiality.
d) Insertion of data into the chain - the protocol of incentive, looking for consensus and network security, encourages honorable miners to create and comprise blocks on the chain.
e) Smart contracts give the contractor the guarantee that only clients or users will be able to approve access to their private information.
f) Integration of middleware, Integrate IoT device data into the blockchain for healthcare management system.

4. CRITICAL FACTORS TO SUPPORT HEALTHCARE DATA SHARING

The Major goal of this study is to develop an architecture based on all the critical factors that support healthcare data sharing in a blockchain environment. After analyzing the literature study, we found three major useful categories in sharing healthcare data (Mwashuma, 2018). These three categories are given below in Table 1:

Table 1. Critical factors to support healthcare data sharing

Sr. No.	Critical Factors for Healthcare Data Sharing	Factors Names	Description
1	Critical Factors Related to Security	Anonymity	Removing the third parties ensures the communication and data transfer between different nodes. Data encryption ensures that both nodes are kept anonymous, which results in a secure and efficient system (Hölbl et al., 2018; Khezr et al., 2019)
		Transparency	Blockchain technology can improve data transparency and communication between different nodes. Therefore, healthcare data can be accessible anywhere (Azaria et al., 2016; Engelhardt, 2017)
		Privacy	Blockchain technology is more secure than others. Using a symmetric encryption technique, the user's identity can be anonymous to other nodes (Vazirani et al., 2019; Rabah, 2017)
		Data Integrity	Blockchain technology ensures the data integrity. Once the healthcare data is added to the blockchain, it cannot be altered, changed, or deleted (Alhadhrami et al., 2017; Venkatesh & Davis, 2000)
		Confidentiality	In blockchain, healthcare data is encrypted through a symmetric key, so the confidentiality of the patient is assured. It also maintains the anonymity and security of the data (Alhadhrami et al., 2017; Venkatesh & Davis, 2000)
2	Critical Factors Related to the Healthcare System	Efficiency	Due to the repetition of different medical procedures, patient outcomes efficiency is compromised. Blockchain technology has a significant potential to enhance patient outcomes by automating patients' registration procedures.
		Cost	There is a great movement of medical records between different nodes. Blockchain technology helps reduce current system costs by eliminating third-party organizations (Azaria et al., 2016; Engelhardt, 2017)
		Decentralization	Blockchain technology works in a distributed working environment. Due to this, healthcare data is not dependent on a central authority (Azaria et al., 2016; Engelhardt, 2017)
		Ease of Use	By demonstrating the system to them, we can motivate practitioners to use blockchain-based systems to share healthcare data rather than paper-based systems (Hwang et al., 2004)
		Risk Policy	We should clarify the risk policy for all patients. Smart contracts will also help clear the policy for practitioners and motivate them to use and adapt blockchain technology.
		Culture	Culture greatly impacts the acceptance of blockchain technology (Taylor et al., 2020)
		Emotion	Practitioners' emotions also greatly impact the usage of blockchain technology. The practitioner's emotions will decide the acceptance criteria of blockchain technology.
3	Critical Factors Related to Blockchain	Availability	Blockchain technology ensures data availability once data is added to the blockchain.
		Interoperability	Blockchain technology is very helpful in exchanging healthcare data between different parties in a secure manner. It will enhance the efficiency and security of the healthcare system (Rabah, 2017; Liu et al., 2022)
		Accuracy	Healthcare records stored on blockchain are accurate due to the consensus of all blockchain network nodes. It is impossible to alter record on the blockchain (Rabah, 2017)
		Tamper-Proofing	Once the healthcare data is stored on the blockchain, it is difficult to tamper with it.
		Access Control	Blockchain technology gives complete rights to all nodes to check the network's activities. All the nodes have complete access control over the healthcare data placed on the system.
		Immutability	Removing blockchain data is impossible without all nodes' consensus (Rabah, 2017; Liu et al., 2022)

5. PROPOSED ARCHITECTURE

Figure 1 illustrates the players' connections before the data is implanted for the proposed blockchain architecture for health and well-being. The numerous actors are represented, and they gather data from clinical examinations, imaging examinations, sensors, biometric meters, etc., persevering it in their systems in their networks, with the data flowing only within those networks, which, in general, have little to no level of trust with the systems and networks of other actors.

Figure 1 below shows a contrast between data gathering and usage in the domestic setting (home care) and the ecosystem for health and wellbeing. Laboratories, health plans, clinics, doctors, governments, researchers, hospitals, etc., form the ecosystem for health and wellbeing, and they all often have integrated IT infrastructure (software and hardware) for data collection, processing, perseverance, use, and management. The home environment comprises sensors and actuators that record unimportant, relevant data and display behaviors and tendencies. Additionally, it typically lacks an integrated IT infrastructure, limiting itself to non-connected devices like smartphone applications that communicate over short distances, for instance, via Bluetooth. Patients, who have the right to access their data and grant access to other ecosystem players, are another significant category in the context of actors. Each health and wellness ecosystem stakeholder uses a different IT infrastructure to conduct business. Following that, the integration with the blockchain will happen through a common interface in a service available on the internal network. This service must have APIs that, based on predetermined rules and standards, will receive data and orders to interact with the chain of blocks: entering transactions, querying data, etc.

Figure 1. Proposed blockchain architecture for healthcare data sharing

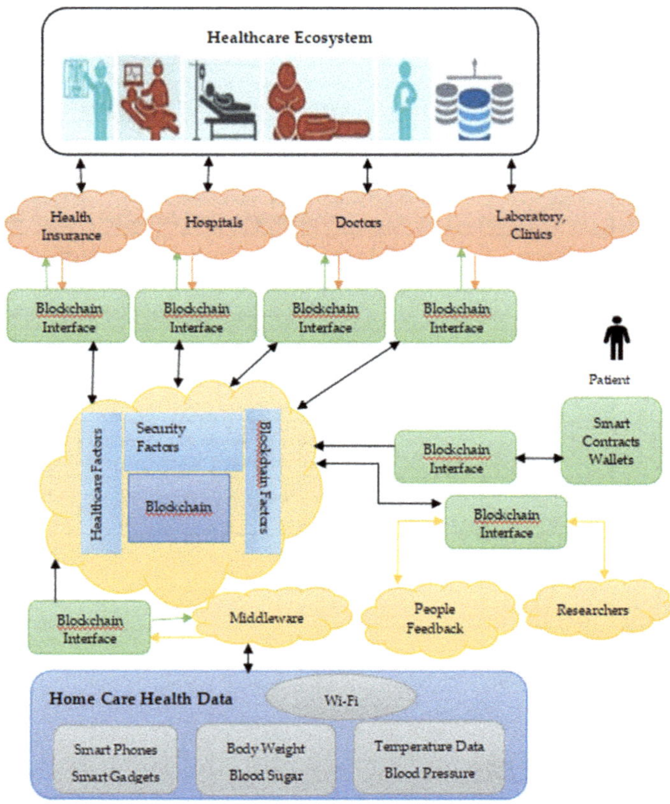

The critical factors that influence blockchain architecture have already been discussed. It can be found in any actor's interactions with the blockchain. The most inclusive view of the Blockchain interface is presented in Figure 2. The Blockchain Interface offers 5 layers of functionality to manage blockchain interactions. Data processing is the first layer, where data processed through APIs is processed with the initial validation of sent parameters and requested functions. The system's status, which is called the function, is displayed at the conclusion, such as OK on insertion into the block if the operation is successful or FAIL if it is unsuccessful.

Figure 2. Blockchain interface

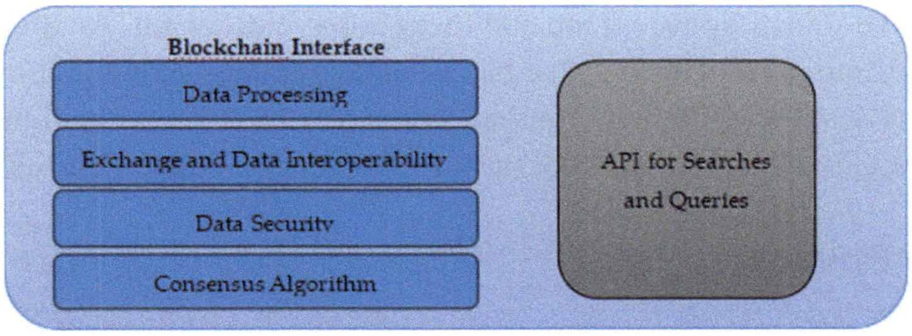

The following layer will manage interoperability and data sharing, validate data structure and semantic standards from the previous layer, and receive the validated data from Data Processing. They are shifted to the following layer with the compatibility of confirmed data. If not, the previous tier receives the identified error. The third tier, Data Security, deals with security measures like encryption that lets you get the data ready for the following layer, the Algorithm of Consensus, which will handle inserting the transaction into a block on the chain. The API for the Searches and inquiries layer completes blockchain searches and inquiries on the original or summarized transactions.

5.1 User Identity

Without a middleman, asymmetric keys generated by software known as digital wallets are used to identify users on the blockchain for digital currencies. It has features that stop third parties from recovering the private key in the event of a loss and avoids building a central database that links the public key to a specific person or company. In the health and well-being ecosystem, actors with patient data stored in their private systems will often be the information producers. The proposed architecture allows users to produce asymmetric keys like digital currencies by giving each actor their public key when registering as a patient with that institution. This can be accomplished, for instance, by working with the Federal Government to add the patient to the Universal Patient Registry, guaranteeing that only the user is alert of his private key.

5.2 Interoperability

Defining the consensus algorithm is one method to promise interoperability. Peterson et al. (2017) defines a new algorithm called Proof of Interoperability (PoI), which promises that the transactions received are interoperable about a given standard of structural and semantic boundaries. The Proof of Interoperability for Proof of Work uses the time and resources dedicated to computation to confirm the interoperability of transactions. Another route to interoperability is to investigate the creation of custom smart contract programming, independent of the consensus technique used, and add suitable functions to validate it, for example, when the transaction is included. The Value Set Authority Centre (VSAC), a word ontology accessed by the Unified Medical Language System (UMLS), which is accessible through the U.S. National Library of Medicine, is stated by Peterson et al. (2017). The idea of a central repository carries up the problem of single failures, not about data compromise of the blockchain as they are available on the network, but owing to the commitment, for example, due to the unavailability of the repository Central (VSAC). This would result in a denial-of-service attack that would directly affect the information verification process and, as a result, the addition of new blocks to the blockchain. One idea is to treat standards like transactions and include them in the blockchain. Another option is to be in a blockchain structure different from the data the blockchain has collected but is still included in the node miners' storage situation. As a result, both options would rely on APIs for data movement in a central data repository (VSAC), reducing the need for online maintenance (adding and changing information).

5.3 Security and Privacy

Unencrypted transactions are a substantial part of transactions on the digital currency blockchain. Therefore, if the owner of a public key is known, you can learn about all of your past transactions. There must be cryptographic assurances regarding the privacy of transactions, just as the parties in the health ecosystem create databases that link patients with their public keys. The issues begin with defining how to choose the miner, how to ensure cryptographic compatibility, which key to use, how it would be exchanged between the sections, and which nodes would have access to the transaction's flat content (Liu, Hong, & Sun, 2022). The origin node and the patient must also deliver additional information because the miner will be responsible for proofing the interoperability. Unless specifically permitted by the patient, no one else to participate in the transaction should be aware of its contents (Sinha, Patel, & Jagdish, 2022). To be sure that only he will have access to the content, the transaction must be delivered to the miner, encrypted with the public key of the transaction, and signed by the origin node (Agbo, Mahmoud, & Eklund, 2019). The miner will perform the Interoperability Test, producing a symmetric key for each transaction, which will be used to encrypt the content of the received transaction after receiving the transaction and decrypting it with your private key. This specific key will be recorded in an attribute in the transaction within the block and encrypted using the origin node's public key. The procedure will be repeated with the patient's public key, with the outcome being recorded in a different attribute. This confirms that, besides the miner, the content will only be available to the source node and the patient when stored in the block, as seen in Figure 3.

Figure 3. Secure key exchange flow

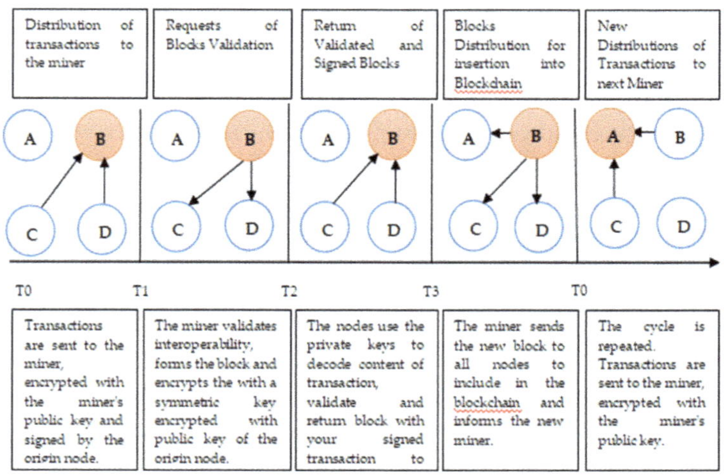

Symmetric keys have the advantage of being transaction-specific; if one of these keys cooperates, the attacker can only access that transaction. Furthermore, it guarantees that access will be limited to what has been developed and only approved by contracts signed by wise people (Marry et al., 2023). One of the risks is the theft or compromise of a patient's private key, which would lead to the loss of access information or the breach of its confidentiality. It is also a risk present in blockchains used for digital currency. Furthermore, you have no control over how data provided by third parties will be handled going forward (Lu, 2019). Researchers must have access to the contents of blockchain transactions, but they must be accessible and unidentified so that patients cannot be connected to them. These shares can be used in two ways that are not mutually exclusive. The first involves using the Distributed Cryptography Secure Multi-Party Computation (MPC) implemented in the Enigma protocol (Shrobe, Shrier, & Pentland, 2018).

Using power computational network nodes, this protocol enables general queries in which each node accesses a portion of information that, when considered separately, has no consequence. Each node then processes and shares the result with other nodes so that full processing can occur without granting the nodes involved full access to the information, defending your privacy. The second method is assembling data from each block from summaries that each transaction origin node sent to the mining node on that block. These summary transactions provide the advantage of not using the network nodes' processing resources to access summarized data, but the query options are constrained. As discussed in the following subsection, the summarized transactions would also contribute to the consensus and validation of the new blocks.

5.4 Data Insertion and Consensus Algorithm

Consensus algorithms and choosing the miner who will add your block to the chain are involved in inserting data into the blockchain (or mining) (Bentov et al., 2014). It will be whoever has the most computing power in the proof of work algorithm and solves the mathematical problem first. In the proof of participation, the participant with the highest average daily balance of coins will be chosen (Arbabi et al., 2022), and in the proof of activity, the factoring of the daily average balance of coins with the volume of transactions over time that best defines your participation and network activity will be used. The algorithm used to choose the next miner in the interoperability test considers a random number sent by the nodes that took part in creating the present block. This will decide the outcome matching the elected and active node with this result's closest number. Considering that you possess a particular number of indicators demonstrating your network involvement and activity (Peterson et al., 2017; Ekblaw et al., 2016) using the miner.

Incentive systems are used in cryptocurrencies to tempt ethical miners to join the network. The creation of digital currency and transaction rates is an attraction in Bitcoin or Ethereum (Casino, Dasaklis, & Patsakis, 2019). In this design, you could choose a coin originating in mining blocks and transactions. Like how Ethereum Gas (Buterin, 2014) is consumed as services and executed over time, they would be traded for research into anonymous data and the use of infrastructure and computational network power, preventing infinite loop attacks and compensating the network nodes for their computational power usage. Each node using the layer Blockchain Interface will be a miner (Chen et al., 2019), producing tokens that will give you prominence in the network's participation. You will either consume yourself or exchange it with researchers to use in your research. Data entry into the chain is done in stages modified from Peterson et al. (2017)'s proposal. The time it takes to enter a block in the Bitcoin network is tied to the difficulty of solving a mathematical problem related to when new currencies first appeared (Faneela et al., 2023). As illustrated in Figure 4, this architecture's time cycle will permit the full process of data gathering, block building, validation, selection, propagation, and the election of the next miner. As seen in Figure 4, the collection of transactions and origin nodes must deliver both the signed summary of what was sent to be used by the miner in block summarization and the transactions themselves at time T0 for it to begin. The miner verifies interoperability and digests at time T1 after receiving the transactions by encrypting them using symmetric keys specific to each transaction, signing and delivering the new block along with partial summaries from each source to participating nodes so they may validate and sign the block. Each node validates its transactions and the overall summary at T2 when the new block and summaries have been signed, and the block can be validated by summaries even if they are unaware of all the transactions. The miner receives a block confirmation, the token, and the random number needed to choose the next miner. At T3, the miner gets tokens and confirmations, chooses and confirms the following miner, and broadcasts the new block to the network.

Figure 4. Phases for inserting blocks in blockchain

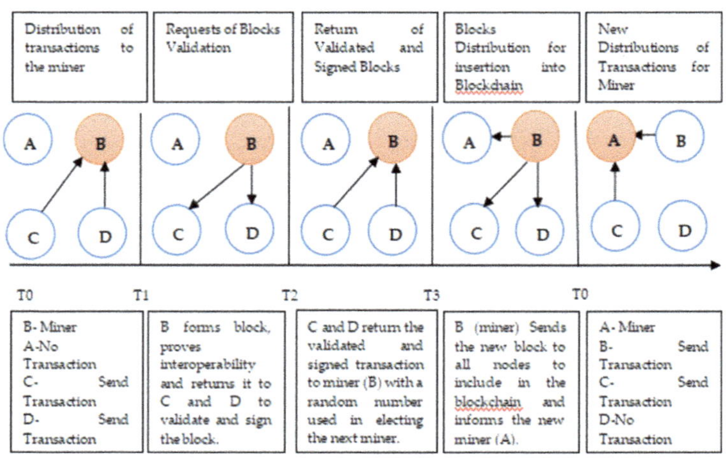

The network goes back to time T0 after the new miner has been defined, restarting the process of adding blocks to the chain. As can be seen, everyone must wait until the next miner is specified and then transmit their transactions from the beginning of instant T1 to the conclusion of moment T3. The local laws of the origin node and mining nodes are a significant concern about data insertion and durableness. If requested, patient data, for instance, from the European Union, would need to be removed or amended, but this is impossible in a blockchain. The proposal by Esposito et al. (2018) to maintain on the blockchain not the data itself but rather the URL (Uniform Resource Locator) from which the data can be obtained, as well as the Hash of the original information, is one of the alternatives being considered. This way, it can be confirmed that the original data has not undergone any changes when consulted in the future, and in case of deletion or alteration, we would have to insert a new transaction with the relevant information.

5.5 Smart Contracts

The blockchain comprises smart contracts as transactions to confirm their validity (Creswell & Creswell, 2017). The data sharing, token transfer transactions between users, and data sharing must all be fulfilled by this proposal. Smart contracts for data exchange ensure that patient consent is encoded and executable, for example, when a patient wants a doctor to access only certain laboratory tests from a specified date and time. Token transactions must be regulated in a manner akin to that of cryptocurrency transactions to achieve this, always respecting the maintenance of a balance for use as Gas and the impact that decreasing the token balance will have on the assessment of the significance of the node at the time of the miner's choice. Despite the well-specified conditions for smart contracts, this model intends to give a specific kind of application that incorporates the following features: A convenient interface for issuing smart contracts, a digital wallet to produce and safeguard keys, and a Blockchain Interface (Creswell & Clark, 2017).

5.6 Integrating Middleware

Several breakthroughs in the field of health and well-being have been made possible by the Internet of Things. Sensors and actuators that communicate and deliver biometric, environmental, condition, and even autonomous action-decision assessments are starting to be carried by both people and objects. As seen in Figure 5, these devices produce data that, when combined with new short-term communications technologies and long distances, such as WLANs, WPANs, and LPWANs, enable communications to take place at any time or place, generating data that is inserted into the blockchain and has the potential to enhance users' quality of life and lower the cost of medical treatments.

Figure 5. IOT middleware integration with blockchain

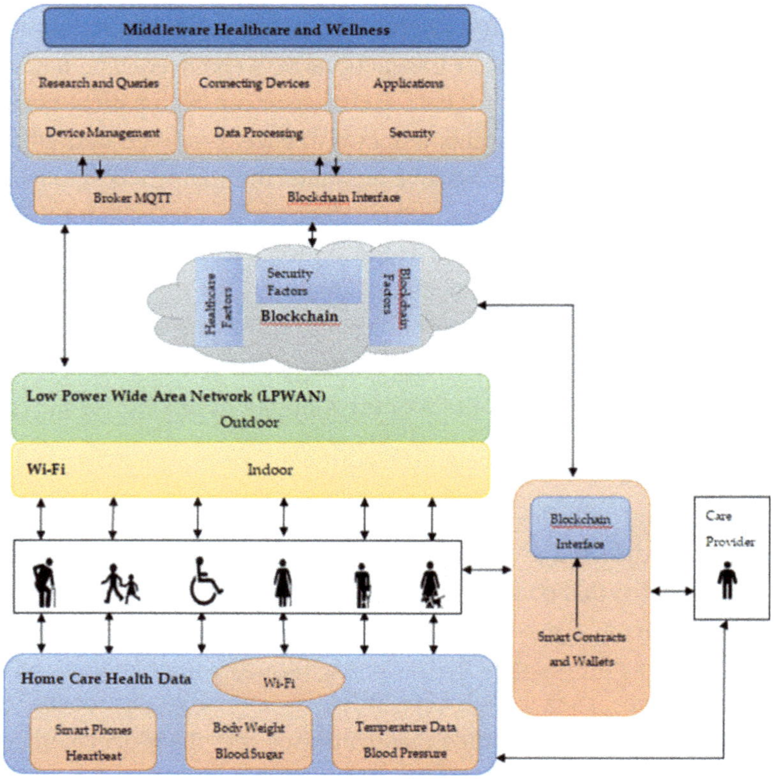

Additionally, the accessibility of electronic components such as microcontrollers, sensors, actuators, and low-cost communication with low programming complexity but efficiency enables the creation of specialized, inexpensive devices that may be incorporated into a middleware platform. Message Queuing Telemetry Transport, or MQTT, is a widely used application protocol in the Internet of Things. The MQTT Broker is responsible for authenticating the devices, receiving the transmitted data, and publishing it for Middleware consumption. The Blockchain interface makes data available in transactions for insertion in blocks on the blockchain. The Homecare functionalities are the third module. Encryption and decryption are required for the device authentication procedure to connect to middleware (Broker MQTT), as set in the Connecting Devices module. Data processing involves handling the data that has been received, starting encryption, data conversion, and data validation processes, triggering triggers, and preserving data in a database.

5.6 Pseudocode for Architecture

Our proposed architecture focuses on healthcare data sharing of patients. We have used middleware to share patient healthcare data using blockchain technology. Our architecture comprises three main functionalities. Patient registration, practitioner registration, and patient healthcare data sharing are the main functions that will be executed in our architecture. All the critical factors are associated with these functions. We can show the prototype of these functions by pseudo-code. Pseudocode will help us to see the basic layout of these functions. The three pseudocodes of these functions are given in Tables 2, 3, and 4.

Table 2. Pseudocode of patient registration

Pseudocode 1 Patient's Information Registration
Input: Patient Hospital ID, Given Name, Family Name **Output: Patient Registration in the system** **1. Patient Hospital ID← Patient** **2. Given Name← Patient Given Name** **3. Family Name← Patient Family Name** **4. if (All input fields are correctly filled) then** **5. New Record Entry Processed** **6. else** **7. Return "Incorrect Input"** **8. end if**

Table 3. Pseudocode of practitioner registration

Pseudocode 2 Practitioner's Information Registration
Input: Practitioner Hospital ID, Given Name, Family Name **Output: Practitioner Registration in the system** **1. Practitioner Hospital ID← Practitioner** **2. Given Name← Practitioner Given Name** **3. Family Name← Practitioner Family Name** **5. if (All input fields are correctly filled) then** **6. New Record Entry Processed** **7. else** **8. Return "Incorrect Input"** **9. end if**

Table 4. Pseudocode of healthcare data obtainability

Pseudocode 3 Patient's Data Obtainability
Input: Patient's Hospital ID / Practitioner's Hospital ID **Output: Patient's health record show against ID** **1. Patient Hspital ID← Determine (User ID from the repository)** **2. Practitioner Hospital ID← (User ID from the repository)** **3. Patient's Record Accessibility← Practitioner requests to obtain patient record** **4. Record parameters← Date and Time** **5. if (Practitioner's request = TRUE)** **6. then** **7. Outcome← Access allowed according to the record's parameter requested** **8. else** **9. Return "Not Available";** **10. end if**

All three pseudocodes show the main functionalities of architecture. The validation of the effects of critical factors on architecture is presented in the next section. The major tasks in the proposed architecture are user (patient, doctor) registration and healthcare data sharing (healthcare data accessibility). In the user registration task, the user sends his/her data to blockchain middleware. The interface uploads user's data on blockchain middleware through the help of smart contracts. The consensus algorithm decodes that data and extracts a key. Through that key, middleware finds the user's hash value for tracking purposes. In the healthcare data accessibility task, the user sends a request through his/her ID. The interface uploads the user's transactions on middleware through the help of smart contracts. The consensus algorithm decodes that transaction through middleware and generates a key. Finally, through that key, middleware authorizes user identity and permits the user to access his/her data in the private blockchain. We can present these two tasks as prototypes in the following figures, as discussed by Faneela et al., (2023). Figures 6, and 7 present prototypes of those major tasks.

Figure 6. User registration process in the proposed architecture (Chen et al., 2019)

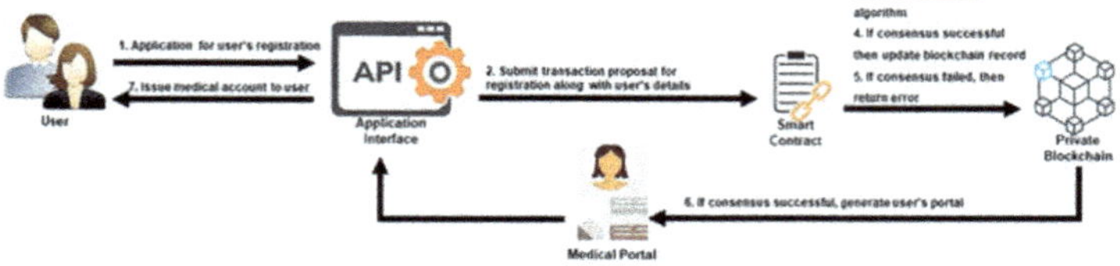

Figure 7. Healthcare data accessibility in the proposed architecture (Chen et al., 2019)

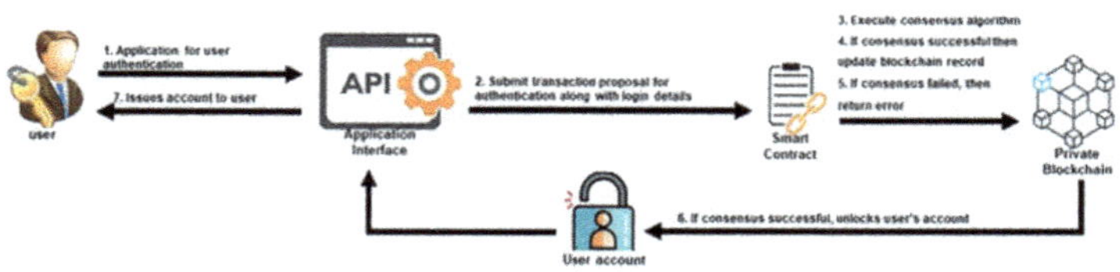

These two prototypes show the registration and data accessibility processes. All other processes like patient appointments, checking, and patient health procedures will be executed the same way as above. In every process, middleware is responsible for uploading the healthcare data and extracting keys by decoding the data. This key is useful for giving authorization or access to users in a private blockchain network. Our proposed methodology focuses on the middleware-based blockchain architecture by observing critical factors useful for healthcare data sharing.

6. RESULTS AND DISCUSSION

Research studies often use both quantitative and qualitative methodologies to support the results of their proposed research. In recent decades, it has become more common to use both methods in a single study rather than simply one to understand the research problem fully. Qualitative methods are normally used to examine non-numeric data. Quantitative methods are often used when identifying the variables that affect results, assessing the viability of an intervention, or forecasting the outcomes. Quantitative and qualitative methodologies were used because this research is exploratory and is based on mixed-methods research (Creswell & Creswell, 2017; Creswell & Clark, 2017). For this study, it was necessary to consult with an adequate number of experts to get expressive results. The current study questioned 15 blockchain and healthcare IT professionals regarding proposed architecture and critical factors. The information on the experts can be seen in Table 5. Next, a survey was sent out to blockchain and healthcare IT professionals. A survey was sent to various practitioners with experience in the blockchain and healthcare industry. In this field, each respondent has at least two years of experience. The survey included 30 practitioners in total.

Table 5. Summary of experts

Expert	Job Description	Years of Experience
1	Technician	15
2	Cyber Security Specialist	15
3	Associate Professor	08
4	Chief Technology Officer	10
5	Network Administrator	14
6	Medical Specialist	13
7	Security Engineer	4
8	Software Engineer	4
9	Network Security Specialist	8
10	System Specialist	8
11	Database Administrator	5
12	Application Support Engineer	5
13	Information Security Engineer	3
14	Network Administrator	3
15	Software Developer	4

6.1 Findings of Experts

The results came from the interviews with 15 industry experts. Their results help examine the validity of the proposed architecture and critical factors that affect architecture.

6.1.1 Findings of Proposed Architecture

The 15 experts asked different closed questions regarding the proposed architecture. All experts validated the blockchain architecture and encouraged the addition of middleware in the blockchain architecture. Integrating middleware in healthcare organizations to share medical data is very useful. All the experts gave positive feedback regarding the blockchain architecture.

6.1.2 Findings Related to Healthcare System Critical Factors

Different questions were asked by industry experts about the critical factors in the healthcare system in blockchain architecture. All the experts agreed that healthcare system factors are very important for blockchain architecture. They agreed on the significance of decentralization. All experts also agreed on the importance of efficiency and culture for sharing healthcare data in blockchain-based architecture. Similarly, risk policy factors and ease of use are important considerations for blockchain architecture. All experts' findings related to factors in the healthcare system are given in Table 6.

Table 6. Findings related to healthcare factors

Critical Factor	Theme	Number of Experts
Risk Policy	Ptaients do not know any knowledge of risk. They will accept new technology more efficiently.	3
	Patients should be trained regarding the risk policy.	5
	This is an important factor as patient's knowledge about this is zero.	6
	We can train the patients about it through social media platforms.	7
	Different websites can also be used to share the awareness of risk policy in patients.	9
	Training sessions should be conducted online or offline for patients.	11
	Patients can easily adapt to new technology because they do not know the true meaning of risk policy factors.	15
Efficiency	As data is available from anywhere, efficiency will be high.	1
	Using blockchain technology will increase efficiency.	3
	Humans can resist new technology. So, it takes time to adapt to a new system.	4
	If the government implements technology, efficiency will also increase.	6
	The healthcare system is not valid. Blockchain technology will be useful to increase the efficiency of the system.	7
Cost	Cost is useful for the patients.	3
	It will reduce the cost by eliminating duplicate patient tests.	5
	The cost will become lower, and the diagnosis will be made quickly.	8
	To reduce the cost of patient registration and medical expenses is very necessary.	9
	Patients do not have to carry the lab reports. It will reduce the cost.	10
Decentralization	It is useful for data safety.	1
	It is hard to lose the data as data exists on multiple nodes.	3
	It is useful to keeps data safe, secure, and available.	4
	It will eliminate the dependency and central authority.	14
Ease of Use	Less user-friendly system are not useful for the users.	2
	Easiness will become system more acceptable.	13
	It will reduce the resistance of the employees.	15

continued on following page

Table 6. Continued

Critical Factor	Theme	Number of Experts
Culture	People will use it if it is legalized by the government,	1
	Culture should be understandable for the implementation engineer.	4
	It should be implemented by the Health ministry.	11
Emotion	People's emotions are attached to the new technology.	13
	People have the fear of losing their authority in the system.	15

6.1.3 Findings Related to Security Critical Factors

After interviewing all experts, it is concluded that security factors are very important for blockchain architecture. All experts agreed on the significance of data integrity in blockchain. Privacy and confidentiality are also important factors to be considered. All experts' findings related to security factors are given in Table 7.

Table 7. Findings related to security factors

Critical Factor	Theme	Number of Experts
Privacy	The healthcare information should be kept private. Blockchain technology will be helpful for patient data privacy.	5
	Blockchain technology will limit the access of patients to healthcare data.	6
	Medical organizations need to keep the patient's data secure and safe.	7
	Data should be kept secret so that nobody can sell the healthcare data.	8
	Data should be secure from any unauthorized party.	11
Anonymity	It is important to secure the healthcare data and not reveal the patient's identity.	13
	It is very important to secure patient data, especially in critical conditions.	15
	It is very useful to share health data. The patient's identity should be anonymous when data is shared.	2
	This factor is not important. As sometimes we need to know the identity of the patient.	12
	Blockchain technology will increase the trust level of patients.	3
Data Integrity	Blockchain technology is very helpful for data integrity. Data will not be modified once it is added to the chain.	1
	It is very important as it affects the patient's privacy.	4
	Medical data is very sensitive. Blockchain technology will be helpful for the authentication of data and saving it on the blockchain.	7
	Data cannot be modified or deleted once added to the chain.	9
	It will increase the patient's trust in the blockchain system.	8

continued on following page

Table 7. Continued

Critical Factor	Theme	Number of Experts
Transparency	Blockchain is contributing to make data more transparent.	10
	Blockchain makes data transparent and stops the data from being sealed in the system.	3
	Blockchain has increased data transparency among patients and doctors.	4
	Data transparency increased the patient's trust in the blockchain.	15
Confidentiality	Data confidentiality is very important.	2
	It is very important that only authorized users can access the data.	14

6.1.4 Findings Related to Blockchain Critical Factors

After interviewing all experts, it is concluded that blockchain factors are very important for data sharing in blockchain architecture. All experts agreed on the significance of availability and accuracy of architecture. Experts have also considered immutability, tamper proof, and access control critical data-sharing factors in blockchain architecture. Table 8 shows all the findings of the experts.

Table 8. Findings related to blockchain factors

Critical Factors	Theme	Number of Expert
Accuracy	Data accuracy will help the patient with the proper treatment.	1
	Data accuracy is very useful, and blockchain has improved it.	3
	Any mistake in a patient's data will cause a disaster. So, this is important.	5
	It is very significant for the data sensitivity.	6
	Blockchain is very helpful in identifying the attacker who tries to disturb data accuracy.	7
Access Control	Permissioned blockchain helps limit users' access to the blockchain network.	9
	It is important to give and limit access to any user.	10
	It is very important to secure the data from any unauthorized access.	12
	Access control is very useful in blockchain technology to control the access of all parties.	13
Tamper Proof	It is very useful factor because data can be tampered.	2
	Modified dataa cannot be trackable unless the blockchain allows it.	4
	Blockchain is very helpful in tracking the changes in the system.	8
	Blockchain is very helpful in maintaining data integrity.	12
Availability	Data should be available to every node at all times.	11
	This factor is very helpful for accessing healthcare data at any time.	13
	Blockchain is very helpful in the availability of data as it removes the system's failure.	14
Interoperability	This is an important factor as patients want treatment from different doctors.	2
	This factor will reduce the time and cost of the patient.	13
	It will eliminate the duplication process of patient registration.	15

continued on following page

Table 8. Continued

Critical Factors	Theme	Number of Expert
Immutability	Blockchain cannot tolerate data alteration.	11
	Blockchain will give information on the party that changes the data.	14
	This factor will increase patient trust in the blockchain system.	15

6.2 Survey Results

The survey was taken from 30 participants. 5 questions were asked about the validity of the proposed architecture. 5 questions were asked regarding security factors, and 6 questions were asked regarding healthcare and blockchain critical factors. The results regarding proposed architecture, security factors, healthcare factors, and blockchain factors can be seen in Figure. 8, 9,10, and 11.

Figure 8. Survey results regarding proposed architecture

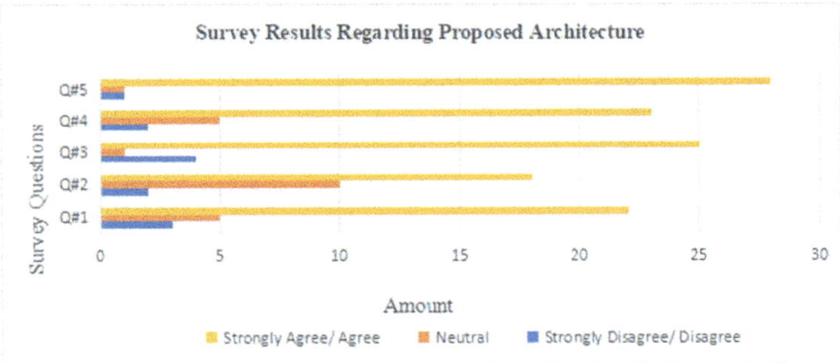

Figure 9. Survey results regarding security critical factors

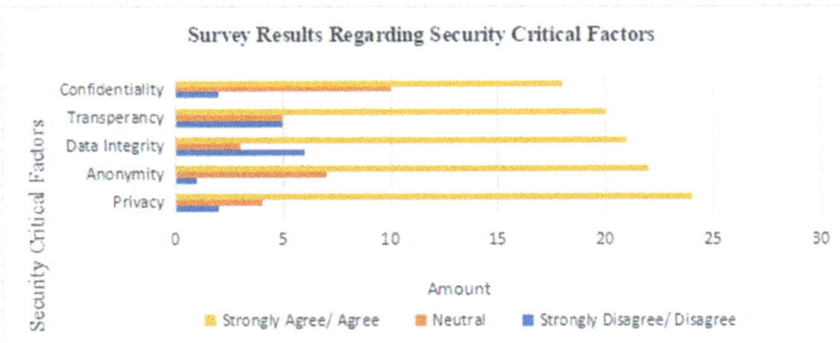

Figure 10. Survey results regarding healthcare critical factors

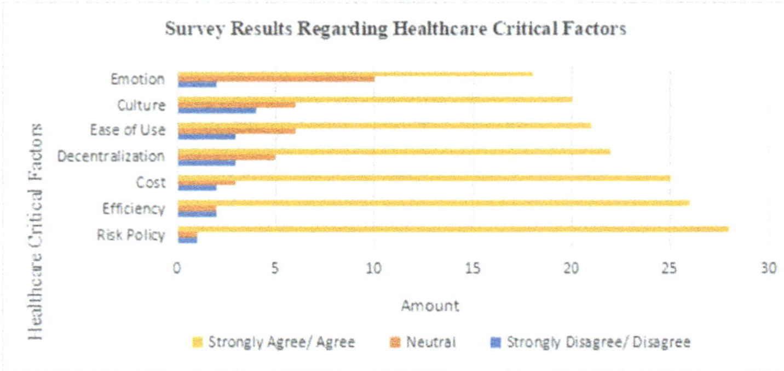

Figure 11. Survey results regarding blockchain critical factors

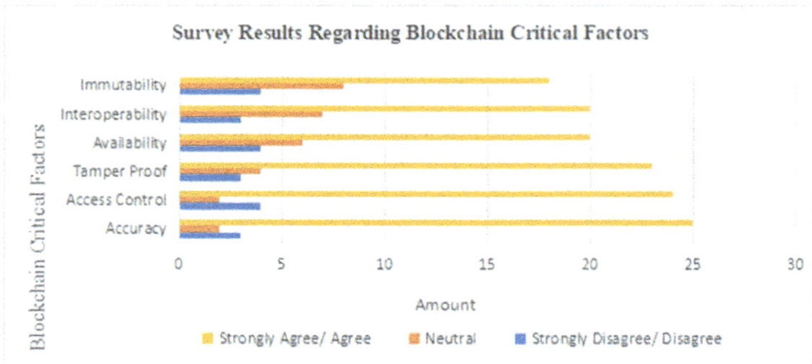

All the above graphs show the participants' feedback regarding critical factors in proposed architecture, healthcare, security, and blockchain. We found the average accuracy of all factors and proposed research. The summary of all the survey feedback and their percentage can be presented in Table 9. The table shows that 74% of experts support the proposed critical factors.

Table 9. Summary of all survey results

Sr. No.	Survey Categories	Strongly Agree/ Agree %	Neutral %	Strongly Disagree/ Disagree %
1	Proposed Architecture	77.3	14.7	8.0
2	Critical Factors Related to Security	70.0	19.3	10.7
3	Critical Factors Related to Healthcare	76.2	15.7	8.1
4	Critical Factors Related to Blockchain	72.3	16.1	11.6
5	Average of all categories	74.0	16.4	9.6

Questions related to the proposed architecture are provided in Table 10. as Appendix A in this paper.

6.3 Discussion

The IOT middleware integration in our blockchain architecture is useful for smoothly sharing healthcare data. Our proposed architecture provides an efficient and fast way of healthcare data sharing in the healthcare ecosystem. Smart contracts will also ensure the privacy of the patient (Chen et al., 2019). Critical factors are those factors that will provide complete support to blockchain architecture. The literature review, expert review, and survey helped us validate the blockchain architecture and critical factors that support data sharing in blockchain architecture. The experts suggested that the access control factor should be recategorized from blockchain to security factor. Experts also suggested that anonymity should be removed from the critical factors list as it produces ambiguity in the architecture. Some experts suggested that the patient's identity should also be added to the healthcare factor category. Experts advocated that confidentiality and privacy factors should be merged into a single factor. The survey questionnaire was used to validate the architecture and critical factors that support healthcare data sharing. All the survey participants support the middleware-based blockchain architecture. They agreed that healthcare factors are very important for data sharing in blockchain architecture. The statistical results of the survey also proved the importance of security factors in blockchain architecture. Respondents agreed upon considering blockchain-related factors in blockchain architecture for healthcare data sharing. The average positive response of survey participants regarding architecture and critical factors is 74% which supports our proposed study.

6.4 Limitations of Study

Our proposed study briefly describes the blockchain architecture, middleware, pseudocodes, prototypes, and critical factors to support healthcare data sharing in blockchain-based architecture. However, some limitations exist in our study. We took the survey from 30 IT experts to validate the study. An increasing number of participants will probably change the results. Another limitation exists in the findings of critical factors. We took findings from 15 blockchain experts regarding security, healthcare, and blockchain factors. Conflicts between critical factors can be produced by increasing the number of blockchain experts. Our architecture is at the prototype stage. We should apply the proposed architecture to a real-time healthcare system to see the findings and feedback of the users. Moreover, a healthcare standard like HL7 FHIR or HIPPA should be implemented as data sharing is possible among different members of the healthcare management system.

7 CONCLUSION

The secure and efficient sharing of healthcare data holds immense potential for enhancing medical diagnostics, treatments, and overall patient care. This study presents a blockchain-based architecture to address the critical factors necessary for healthcare data sharing, particularly within distributed networks and IoT-integrated environments. Our findings demonstrate that when integrated with IoT middleware, blockchain technology provides a robust solution for managing and sharing healthcare data without compromising privacy or security. Our proposed architecture promotes proactive and efficient healthcare delivery by eliminating the need for duplicative records and enabling seamless data access for authorized medical professionals. The impact of this research extends beyond individual patient care, offering transparency in public spending and informed decision-making within the healthcare industry. The integration of blockchain in healthcare data management not only enhances resource allocation and performance monitoring but also supports the development of targeted solutions in research. The study lays the foundation for future advancements in secure healthcare data sharing and sets the stage for further exploration of AI-driven data analysis and preventative measures. The positive feedback from experts and survey participants underscores the significance of our approach, highlighting the transformative potential of blockchain technology in revolutionizing healthcare data management. As we move forward, developing a prototype IoT platform for healthcare will be crucial in realizing the full benefits of this architecture, ultimately contributing to a more secure, scalable, and resilient healthcare ecosystem.

Author Contributions: The authors confirm their contribution to the paper as follows: **S.H.:** Conceptualization, Methodology, Writing Original Draft Preparation. **Q.L.:** Supervision, Project Administration, Writing—review and editing the draft. **A.Y.:** Conceptualization, writing—review and editing draft. **M.Z..:** Methodology, Writing—review and editing the draft.
Institutional Review Board Statement: Not applicable.
Informed Consent Statement: Not applicable.
Data Availability Statement: The original contributions presented in the study are included in the article, further inquiries can be directed to the corresponding authors.
Conflicts of Interest: The authors declare they have no conflicts of interest to report.

REFERENCES

AG. A. G., Su, H. K., & Kuo, W. K. (2022, May). Blockchain-based Healthcare System for Elderly Care. In 2022 IEEE 4th Eurasia Conference on Biomedical Engineering, Healthcare and Sustainability (ECBIOS) (pp. 144-147). IEEE.

Agarwal, A., Joshi, R., Arora, H., & Kaushik, R. (2023, February). Privacy and security of healthcare data in cloud based on the blockchain technology. In *2023 7th International Conference on Computing Methodologies and Communication (ICCMC)* (pp. 87-92). IEEE. DOI: 10.1109/ICCMC56507.2023.10083822

Agbo, C. C., Mahmoud, Q. H., & Eklund, J. M. (2019, April). Blockchain technology in healthcare: A systematic review. [). MDPI.]. *Health Care*, *7*(2), 56. PMID: 30987333

Akshaya, R. S., Shetty, S. K., & Patil, A. P. (2022, November). Preserving and Sharing Of Medical Data Using Blockchain Technology. In *2022 IEEE North Karnataka Subsection Flagship International Conference (NKCon)* (pp. 1-5). IEEE.

Alexaki, S., Alexandris, G., Katos, V., & Petroulakis, N. E. (2018, September). Blockchain-based electronic patient records for regulated circular healthcare jurisdictions. In *2018 IEEE 23rd International Workshop on Computer Aided Modeling and Design of Communication Links and Networks (CAMAD)* (pp. 1-6). IEEE. DOI: 10.1109/CAMAD.2018.8514954

Alhadhrami, Z., Alghfeli, S., Alghfeli, M., Abedlla, J. A., & Shuaib, K. (2017, November). Introducing blockchains for healthcare. In *2017 international conference on electrical and computing technologies and applications (ICECTA)* (pp. 1-4). IEEE. DOI: 10.1109/ICECTA.2017.8252043

Alzahrani, A. G. M., Alenezi, A., Mershed, A., Atlam, H., & Wills, G. (2020). A framework for data sharing between healthcare providers using blockchain.

Arbabi, M. S., Lal, C., Veeraragavan, N. R., Marijan, D., Nygård, J. F., & Vitenberg, R. (2022). A survey on blockchain for healthcare: Challenges, benefits, and future directions. *IEEE Communications Surveys and Tutorials*, *25*(1), 386–424. DOI: 10.1109/COMST.2022.3224644

Azaria, A., Ekblaw, A., Vieira, T., & Lippman, A. (2016, August). Medrec: Using blockchain for medical data access and permission management. In *2016 2nd international conference on open and big data (OBD)* (pp. 25-30). IEEE.

Bentov, I., Lee, C., Mizrahi, A., & Rosenfeld, M. (2014). Proof of activity: Extending bitcoin's proof of work via proof of stake [extended abstract] y. *Performance Evaluation Review*, *42*(3), 34–37. DOI: 10.1145/2695533.2695545

Buterin, V. (2014). A next-generation smart contract and decentralized application platform. *white paper, 3*(37), 2-1.

Casino, F., Dasaklis, T. K., & Patsakis, C. (2019). A systematic literature review of blockchain-based applications: Current status, classification and open issues. *Telematics and Informatics*, *36*, 55–81. DOI: 10.1016/j.tele.2018.11.006

Chen, L., Lee, W. K., Chang, C. C., Choo, K. K. R., & Zhang, N. (2019). Blockchain based searchable encryption for electronic health record sharing. *Future Generation Computer Systems*, *95*, 420–429. DOI: 10.1016/j.future.2019.01.018

Chen, Y., Ding, S., Xu, Z., Zheng, H., & Yang, S. (2019). Blockchain-based medical records secure storage and medical service framework. *Journal of Medical Systems*, *43*(1), 1–9. DOI: 10.1007/s10916-018-1121-4 PMID: 30467604

Creswell, J. W., & Clark, V. L. P. (2017). *Designing and conducting mixed methods research*. Sage publications.

Creswell, J. W., & Creswell, J. D. (2017). *Research design: Qualitative, quantitative, and mixed methods approaches*. Sage publications.

Dagher, G. G., Mohler, J., Milojkovic, M., & Marella, P. B. (2018). Ancile: Privacy-preserving framework for access control and interoperability of electronic health records using blockchain technology. *Sustainable Cities and Society*, *39*, 283–297. DOI: 10.1016/j.scs.2018.02.014

Dubovitskaya, A., Xu, Z., Ryu, S., Schumacher, M., & Wang, F. (2018, April). Secure and trustable electronic medical records sharing using blockchain. *AMIA ... Annual Symposium Proceedings - AMIA Symposium. AMIA Symposium*, *2017*, 650. PMID: 29854130

Ekblaw, A., Azaria, A., Halamka, J. D., & Lippman, A. (2016, August). A Case Study for Blockchain in Healthcare:"MedRec" prototype for electronic health records and medical research data. In *Proceedings of IEEE open & big data conference* (Vol. 13, p. 13).

Ekblaw, A., Azaria, A., Halamka, J. D., & Lippman, A. (2016, August). A Case Study for Blockchain in Healthcare:"MedRec" prototype for electronic health records and medical research data. In *Proceedings of IEEE open & big data conference* (Vol. 13, p. 13).

Engelhardt, M. A. (2017). Hitching healthcare to the chain: An introduction to blockchain technology in the healthcare sector. *Technology Innovation Management Review*, *7*(10), 22–34. DOI: 10.22215/timreview/1111

Esposito, C., De Santis, A., Tortora, G., Chang, H., & Choo, K. K. R. (2018). Blockchain: A panacea for healthcare cloud-based data security and privacy? *IEEE Cloud Computing*, *5*(1), 31–37. DOI: 10.1109/MCC.2018.011791712

European Commission. (2016). *The General Data Protection Regulation*. https://ec.europa.eu/justice/dataprotection/reform/files/regulation_oj_en.pdf

Faneela, , Khan, M. A., Alsuhibany, S. A., El Shafai, W., Rehman, M. U., & Ahmad, J. (2023). An immutable framework for smart healthcare using blockchain technology. *Computer Systems Science and Engineering*, *46*(1), 165–179. DOI: 10.32604/csse.2023.035066

Goddard, M. (2017). The EU General Data Protection Regulation (GDPR): European regulation that has a global impact. *International Journal of Market Research*, *59*(6), 703–705. DOI: 10.2501/IJMR-2017-050

Hölbl, M., Kompara, M., Kamišalić, A., & Nemec Zlatolas, L. (2018). A systematic review of the use of blockchain in healthcare. *Symmetry*, *10*(10), 470. DOI: 10.3390/sym10100470

Hwang, M. S., Li, C. T., Shen, J. J., & Chu, Y. P. (2004). Challenges in e-government and security of information. *Information & Security*, *15*(1), 9–20. DOI: 10.11610/isij.1501

Jiang, S., Cao, J., Wu, H., Yang, Y., Ma, M., & He, J. (2018, June). Blochie: a blockchain-based platform for healthcare information exchange. In *2018 ieee international conference on smart computing (smartcomp)* (pp. 49-56). IEEE. DOI: 10.1109/SMARTCOMP.2018.00073

Khezr, S., Moniruzzaman, M., Yassine, A., & Benlamri, R. (2019). Blockchain technology in healthcare: A comprehensive review and directions for future research. *Applied Sciences (Basel, Switzerland)*, *9*(9), 1736. DOI: 10.3390/app9091736

Liu, J., Jiang, W., Sun, R., Bashir, A. K., Alshehri, M. D., Hua, Q., & Yu, K. (2022). Conditional anonymous remote healthcare data sharing over blockchain. *IEEE Journal of Biomedical and Health Informatics*, *27*(5), 2231–2242. DOI: 10.1109/JBHI.2022.3183397 PMID: 35704539

Liu, X., Hong, Y., & Sun, J. (2022, August). Blockchain-based medical data storage and sharing system. In *2022 IEEE International Conference on Advances in Electrical Engineering and Computer Applications (AEECA)* (pp. 62-66). IEEE. DOI: 10.1109/AEECA55500.2022.9918841

Lu, Y. (2019). The blockchain: State-of-the-art and research challenges. *Journal of Industrial Information Integration*, *15*, 80–90. DOI: 10.1016/j.jii.2019.04.002

Marry, P., Yenumula, K., Katakam, A., Bollepally, A., & Athaluri, A. (2023, June). Blockchain based smart healthcare system. In *2023 International Conference on Sustainable Computing and Smart Systems (ICSCSS)* (pp. 1480-1484). IEEE. DOI: 10.1109/ICSCSS57650.2023.10169704

Mikula, T., & Jacobsen, R. H. (2018, August). Identity and access management with blockchain in electronic healthcare records. In *2018 21st Euromicro conference on digital system design (DSD)* (pp. 699-706). IEEE. DOI: 10.1109/DSD.2018.00008

Mwashuma, E. W. (2018). Towards universal healthcare coverage through adoption of blockchain technology: A literature review. *Journal of Health Informatics in Africa*, *5*(2).

Nakamoto, S. (2008). Bitcoin: A peer-to-peer electronic cash system.

Office of the National Coordinator for Health Information Technology. (2018). *Blockchain and health IT: Algorithms, privacy, and data* (White paper). U.S. Department of Health and Human Services. https://www.healthit.gov/sites/default/files/1-78-blockchainandhealthitalgorithmsprivacydata_whitepaper.pdf

Peterson, K., Deeduvanu, R., Kanjamala, P., & Boles, K. (2017). A Blockchain Approach to Health Information Exchange Networks. *Mayo Clinic. Disponível:*https://www. healthit. gov/sites/default/files/12-55-blockchain-based-approach-final. pdf

Rabah, K. (2017). Challenges & opportunities for blockchain powered healthcare systems: A review. *Mara res. j. med. health sci, 1*(1), 45-52.

Rajadevi, R., Devi, E. R., Latha, R. S., Harshini, S., Ajay, K., & Abinash, M. (2022, January). Secured storing and sharing of medical records based on blockchain. In *2022 International Conference on Computer Communication and Informatics (ICCCI)* (pp. 1-5). IEEE. DOI: 10.1109/ICCCI54379.2022.9741070

Sheeraz, M. M., Mozumder, M. A. I., Khan, M. O., Abid, M. U., Joo, M. I., & Kim, H. C. (2023, February). Blockchain system for trustless healthcare data sharing with hyperledger fabric in action. In *2023 25th International Conference on Advanced Communication Technology (ICACT)* (pp. 437-440). IEEE. DOI: 10.23919/ICACT56868.2023.10079423

Shrobe, H., Shrier, D. L., & Pentland, A. (2018). Enigma: Decentralized computation platform with guaranteed privacy.

Sinha, A., Patel, A., & Jagdish, M. (2022, March). Application of Blockchain in Healthcare. In *2022 First International Conference on Artificial Intelligence Trends and Pattern Recognition (ICAITPR)* (pp. 1-4). IEEE.

Taylor, P. J., Dargahi, T., Dehghantanha, A., Parizi, R. M., & Choo, K. K. R. (2020). A systematic literature review of blockchain cyber security. *Digital Communications and Networks*, *6*(2), 147–156. DOI: 10.1016/j.dcan.2019.01.005

Taylor, P. J., Dargahi, T., Dehghantanha, A., Parizi, R. M., & Choo, K. K. R. (2020). A systematic literature review of blockchain cyber security. *Digital Communications and Networks*, *6*(2), 147–156. DOI: 10.1016/j.dcan.2019.01.005

U.S. Department of Health and Human Services. (n.d.). *Health Information Privacy: Laws and regulations*. HHS.gov. https://www.hhs.gov/hipaa/for-professionals/privacy/laws-regulations/index.html

Vazirani, A. A., O'Donoghue, O., Brindley, D., & Meinert, E. (2019). Implementing blockchains for efficient health care: Systematic review. *Journal of Medical Internet Research*, *21*(2), e12439. DOI: 10.2196/12439 PMID: 30747714

Venkatesh, V., & Davis, F. D. (2000). A theoretical extension of the technology acceptance model: Four longitudinal field studies. *Management Science*, *46*(2), 186–204. DOI: 10.1287/mnsc.46.2.186.11926

Xia, Q. I., Sifah, E. B., Asamoah, K. O., Gao, J., Du, X., & Guizani, M. (2017). MeDShare: Trust-less medical data sharing among cloud service providers via blockchain. *IEEE Access : Practical Innovations, Open Solutions*, *5*, 14757–14767. DOI: 10.1109/ACCESS.2017.2730843

Zubair, M., Ahmad, J., Alqahtani, F., Khan, F., Shah, S. A., Abbasi, Q. H., & Jan, S. U. (2022, May). Automated grading of diabetic macular edema using color retinal photographs. In *2022 2nd International Conference of Smart Systems and Emerging Technologies (SMARTTECH)* (pp. 1-6). IEEE. DOI: 10.1109/SMARTTECH54121.2022.00016

Zubair, M., Ali, H., & Javed, M. Y. (2016). Automated Segmentation of Hard Exudates Using Dynamic Thresholding to Detect Diabetic Retinopathy in Retinal Photographs. *J. Multim. Process. Technol.*, *7*(3), 109–116.

Zubair, M., Ali, J., Alhussein, M., Hassan, S., Aurangzeb, K., & Umair, M. (2024). An improved machine learning-driven framework for cryptocurrencies price prediction with sentimental cautioning. *IEEE Access : Practical Innovations, Open Solutions*, *12*, 51395–51418. DOI: 10.1109/ACCESS.2024.3367129

Zubair, M., Khan, S. A., & Yasin, U. U. (2014). Classification of diabetic macular edema and its stages using color fundus image. *Journal of Electronic Science and Technology*, *12*(2), 187–190.

Zubair, M., Umair, M., Naqvi, R. A., Hussain, D., Owais, M., & Werghi, N. (2023). A comprehensive computer-aided system for an early-stage diagnosis and classification of diabetic macular edema. *Journal of King Saud University. Computer and Information Sciences*, *35*(8), 101719. DOI: 10.1016/j.jksuci.2023.101719

Zubair, M., Umair, M., & Owais, M. (2023, September). Automated brain tumor detection using soft computing-based segmentation technique. In *2023 3rd International Conference on Computing and Information Technology (ICCIT)* (pp. 211-215). IEEE. DOI: 10.1109/ICCIT58132.2023.10273963

Zubair, M., Yamin, A., & Khan, S. A. (2013, October). Automated detection of optic disc for the analysis of retina using color fundus image. In *2013 IEEE International Conference on Imaging Systems and Techniques (IST)* (pp. 239-242). IEEE. DOI: 10.1109/IST.2013.6729698

Zyskind, G., & Nathan, O. (2015, May). *Decentralizing privacy: Using blockchain to protect personal data. In 2015 IEEE security and privacy workshops*. IEEE.

APPENDIX A

Table 10. Survey questions information

Sr. No.	Survey Questions Regarding Proposed Architecture	Possible Answers
1	Integrating middleware in blockchain architecture is helpful for healthcare data sharing.	• Strongly Agree • Agree • Neutral • Disagree • Strongly Disagree
2	Security factors have a great impact on healthcare data sharing in blockchain architecture.	
3	Healthcare factors have a great impact on healthcare data sharing.	
4	Blockchain factors have a great impact on healthcare data sharing.	
5	Smart Contracts are helpful for patient data security.	

Chapter 10
IoT and Wearable Devices:
Security Challenges and Solutions

Hira Akhtar Butt
https://orcid.org/0009-0008-7793-1184
University of Central Punjab, Lahore, Pakistan

Ishal Imran
https://orcid.org/0009-0003-5356-2402
University of Management and Technology, Pakistan

Abdul Ahad
https://orcid.org/0000-0002-3914-2503
Northwestern Polytechnical University, China

Jamila Farid
Cardiff Metropolitan University, UK

Filipe Madeira
https://orcid.org/0000-0002-2227-7006
Polytechnic University of Santarém, Portugal

ABSTRACT

The Internet of Things (IoT) is a groundbreaking technological tool connecting devices across various industries, changing everything from how we manage our healthcare to building smart cities. However, this amalgamation brings forth significant security issues that require inventive approaches. This chapter examines the need for advanced security solutions such as Artificial Intelligence (AI) and the blockchain to mitigate the effects of vulnerabilities in IoT. It starts by analyzing the ethical implications of IoT adoption, particularly concerning privacy, consent, and equitable access. It also covers advanced security methods and demonstrates how AI-driven anomaly identification, prediction analytics, and decentralized blockchain types strengthen IoT safety. Careful case studies and real-world applications, statistical comparisons of security approaches, and analyses of the economic and social impacts of–all illustrate this point. Furthermore, the chapter outlines research gaps and future directions.

DOI: 10.4018/979-8-3373-0593-6.ch010

1. INTRODUCTION

The IoT refers to a broad network of connected devices and systems where integrating different sectors has brought drastic changes in almost all industries (Lomotey et al., 2017). By interconnecting them via the Internet, IoT has made it easy to realize direct communication, automation, and real-time data sharing among physical devices. This shift has seen most industries embrace the Internet of Things technologies due to efficiency, healthcare, transportation, smart cities, and even industrial automation. However, this widespread computational implementation has significantly thrown new raffles to increase security and privacy risks(Al Alkeem et al., 2015).

While IoT ecosystems become more complicated, the number of connected devices increases, and CSPs are exposed to the risks of cyberattacks and data breaches. These risks call for the formation of enhanced security features that are useful in combating the identified risks while maintaining the integrity of the data and guarding users' privacy. The interlinkage between AI and Blockchain technology has been considered a solution to the highlighted challenges. The principal distinctive features include gains in threat detection and handling achieved through AI information analysis algorithms and the assured, decentralized, and virtually impenetrable Blockchain platform (Chan et al., 2012).

This chapter discusses how security issues in IoT are diverse and complex and how AI and Blockchain can be enlisted to protect IoT systems. There is a discussion of the issues to be considered when contemplating the adoption of IoT; this includes issues of transparency, accountability, and data propriety. Moreover, the chapter provides detailed examples of practical applications and statistical comparisons to prove the efficiency of detailed security ideas (Dian et al., 2020). From an economic and social perspective, what is noted is the fact that the paper addresses the importance of secure IoT and highlights the fact that these issues must be tackled from a total systems perspective, considering the positive correlations between technology and the potential benefits that are likely to accrue from its application to society. Therefore, this chapter intends to conduct a state-of-the-art study of IoT security along with the opportunity and future research directions of related technologies (Kalasin & Surareungchai, 2023).

1.1 Background

In the changed global context identified by the advanced development of technology, this paper aims to investigate the new opportunities and diversified challenges that have emerged in the diffusion of healthcare. Wearable technology devices for IoT define the idea of innovative healthcare management and service delivery systems in the present era. These technologies utilize integrating systems, data gathering and exchange to deliver customized treatments, including health risk management (Adil et al., 2024).

The use of the IoT in the healthcare sector includes but is not limited to Telemedicine and homecare, IoT-assisted diagnostic tools, and innovative medication dispensers (Farahani et al., 2018)Internet of Things (IoT) wearables include smartwatches, fitness trackers, and even Implantable medical devices. Altogether, such technologies enhance the quality of care, increase the efficiency of healthcare service consumption, and enable patients to manage their care and well-being (Tamemi et al., 2022).

However, the adoption of IoT and wearable devices in caregiving systems has disadvantages, as discussed below. The world is extensively covered with these devices, which create a substantial raw data load, posing crucial security and privacy challenges. IoT systems are no exception and can be intruded on, unleashing devastating effects, which include data breaches of patients' health information and even risking their lives (Jiang, 2021). In addition, even the security features are not well integrated across the devices, which only intensifies these threats, and the security features themselves differ significantly in effectiveness (Nasiri et al., 2019).

Another area concerning the background is the main focal point of the ethical issues of IoT uptake. Concerns regarding ownership of this data, the ability to provide informed consent, and equitable access to the data emerge as the use of these devices increase (Choi et al., 2019). Mitigating these ethical concerns is as crucial as solving technical issues because these issues make or break IoT technologies' adoption by patients and healthcare practitioners (Abou-Nassar et al., 2020). In this Chapter, we explore these things:

Figure 1. Overview of the Chapter

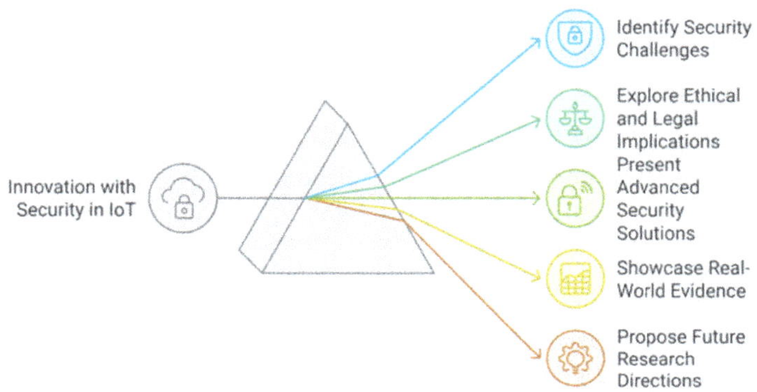

It cannot be overemphasized that a proper perspective concerning the evolution of IoT needs to consider history and technology. Analyzing these technologies makes it possible to study the development process using historical trends as a guideline for the present and future (Tahir et al., 2020). Fig 1 shows the facts and provides the circle for a detailed evaluation of this chapter's security threats and opportunities.

IoT in healthcare can generally encompass a broad spectrum ranging from remote patient monitoring, telemedicine, enhanced diagnostics, and fully automated drug delivery systems. Wearables are one of the categories of IoT goods. Standard wearable devices are smartwatches, fitness tracking, and Implantable medical devices. All of them have greatly enhanced the efficiency of the treatments, lowered healthcare expenditures, and engaged the patients as effective decision-makers.

However, allowing IoT and wearable devices into healthcare settings has unique difficulties. The number of new devices creating data valuable to hackers is vast, creating considerable security and privacy issues. Such attacks on IoT systems yield severe consequences because patients' health information may be exposed or their lives put at risk. Moreover, this worsens security issues because it is difficult to identify the sources of threats and attacks, and the safety measures on most devices do not have equal levels of protection (Chattopadhyay et al., 2019).

1.2 Importance of IoT and Wearable Devices in Healthcare

It is, therefore, essential to understand the usefulness of IoT and wearable devices in healthcare. These technologies have shifted care from a curative to a preventative, timely, individualized practice system. IoT devices have tailored healthcare delivery by facilitating the monitoring of chronic diseases, hence improving patients' health and easing pressure on limited health facilities (Li et al., 2020). One of the most outstanding effects of IoT in the health sector is its contribution to monitoring patients from a distance (Lin, 2024). This is especially so in chronic illnesses like diabetes, hypertension, and other cardiovascular complications (Javed et al., 2020). It is possible to monitor patients' states through continuous health monitoring devices that include glucose monitors, blood pressure cuffs, and heart rate sensors, among others, thus enabling remote patient control in an emergency (Madanian et al., 2024). Clinician-patient telecommunication enhances patient satisfaction, shortens hospital stays, and decreases readmission rates; operational costs included

Wearable devices are essential when it comes to preventive healthcare. Fitness trackers and smartwatches make people change for the better by keeping track of the levels of physical activity, sleep, and health parameters (Karunarathne et al., 2021). These devices were also seen as patient-empowering tools since they give patients control over their condition and how to act. However, it has a revolutionary role in specific healthcare organizations, and with the help of IoT and wearable devices, the individual gains so many advantages. Some of these technologies help partially or entirely take over routine processes, make work more organized, and make efficient use of resources possible. For example, IoT sensors in hospital environments can track equipment usage, inventory, and energy to realize considerable savings (Somasundaram & Thirugnanam, 2017).

However, IoT's current and potential uses in healthcare cannot be fully realized without acknowledging the following challenges: Two of the most critical problems include security and privacy since, due to connectivity, IoT devices are prone to malicious attacks. The protection of patient data should be at the highest level since most of these advances rely on this element (Khatun et al., 2023). Also, IoT in healthcare depends not only on technology advancement but also on technology designers, healthcare organizations, the government, and patients. Collaboratively confronting those concerns while realizing the potential of IoT is the right step forward to enhancing and smoothing up the healthcare system with patient-oriented perspectives (Charles & Natarajan, 2024).

Consequently, the IoT has the most prominent effect on remote patient monitoring in the healthcare domain. It is especially relevant to maintain access to care for those chronic diseases like diabetes, hypertension, and cardiovascular illnesses. Smart glucose monitors, smart BP cuffs, heart rate sensing devices, and similar products gather raw data. Through IoT, healthcare practitioners can monitor the patient's condition from a distance and, if necessary, act immediately. It also enhances the quality of patient care they receive while reinventing hospital readmission rates and costs. Walking, running or cycling, military fighting or dancing, or fitness tracking might be similar to life monitoring. Wearable devices always strive to deliver convenient and effective solutions for preventive healthcare. They make specific calls to promote the wellness of the human body by tracking movement, sleep, and physiological metrics. These devices also positively impact patients since patients can understand what they are suffering from and which diseases they must conquer.

Besides the stakeholder's gains, IoT and wearable devices bring about systemic changes in healthcare systems. Officiality: Through automation of recurrent processes and rationalization of processes, those technologies contribute to improved resource utilization. For example, IoT sensors within the healthcare facility may be integrated to measure the utilization of equipment and, therefore, inventory (Khatun et al., 2023). Moreover, it will facilitate consumer power management, leading to bill reductions. Nevertheless, several drawbacks have arisen from the broader use of IoT in healthcare to ensure it will better impact the healthcare system. The challenges include but are not limited to, security and privacy since IoT is a connected device that is easily prone to cybercrime. Patient information is expected always to remain protected, and any technology in this area must be used to guarantee the privacy of the information.

2. EVOLUTION OF IOT IN HEALTHCARE

The development of the IoT in the health field also signifies a radical change in the medical help delivery and governance process. The evolution has occurred from standalone medical devices to the complex systems that constitute today, from wireless communication to the reduction in the size of device components and the use of cloud computing technologies (Arora et al., 2024). This section focuses on the evolution of IoT in health care, its roles in the current society, and the problems and prospects developed during the incorporation process. Early Mover and Single-Use Beginners IoT in healthcare at its formative stage mainly consisted of single-function gadgets, such as glucose measurement gadgets and heart rate detectors. These devices were primarily focused on gathering simple physiological parameters and giving back information to the user or the medical practitioner (Awotunde et al., 2021) For instance, portable pedometers from the 1990s were forerunners of contemporary and advanced fitness trackers and health-conscious wearables. However, complexity is evident at this stage because the devices did not interface, and each operated independently.

Network Implementation The first decade of the 21st century observed remarkable activities regarding connecting medical devices to network systems. Tools like CGMs started communicating with software systems, which improved data analysis and reporting (Obaid & Salman, 2022). Likewise, developments in mobility made it possible to develop applications usable on smartphones to link with medical devices, improving their usability. The Emergence of Smart Healthcare Environments The latter concept was defined as the IoT progressing and evolving. NHS again started adopting IoT sensors to manage many patient facets, such as health records, feeding, movements, and changes in body pressures and temperature (Alagar et al., 2018)These systems use connected devices and report real-time information to prevent health issues and medical complications. For example, IoT-enabled smart infusion pumps can safely and accurately change dosages based on the patient's data captured in near real-time.

Telemedicine and Remote Patient Monitoring Telemedicine is among the areas in the application of IoT that have the most impact on the healthcare field. Thus, the concept of the connected home and the use of wearables and IoT sensors allowed telemedicine platforms to evolve into remote patient monitoring (RPM). RPM solutions enabled diabetic, cardiac, and hypertensive patients to use care services they never used traditional hospitals for (Yin et al., 2019). For instance, IoT-based blood pressure monitors and pulse oximeters send real-time information to doctors, who can make decisions from a distance. This was particularly important during the COVID-19 pandemic, as healthcare facilities worldwide resorted to telemedicine solutions to tackle the influx of patients admitted for treatment.

A key feature of IoT systems was integrating with the data analytics engine and considering artificial intelligence (AI) as part of the IoT infrastructure. IoT devices gather enormous amounts of data, such as vital signs, motion, and environment. These data sets will identify onsets of diseases, probable diseases, and recommended treatments (Chacko & Hayajneh, 2018). For example, AI in smartwatches can currently screen for arrhythmias by which timely interventions can be made to prevent or minimize the impact of a fall. Some current issues involve considering that IoT has boosted the healthcare industry (Abou-Nassar et al., 2020). Some challenges include the problem of interoperability, which, from experience, is apparent since products from different companies do not integrate well. Also, due to the large volumes of data, data storage and processing from IoT devices become cumbersome (Adil et al., 2024).

These are intellectual security and privacy because health information is sensitive. Some high-profile breaches, including ransomware attacks on hospitals, ensure adequate security measures are implemented to secure IoT systems. Moreover, whether data ownership and informed consent are ethical is a topic of discussion among policymakers and stakeholders in healthcare (Al Alkeem et al., 2015). Future Trends Potential and emerging trends in the continuing developments of IoT in the healthcare field are set to use potential through blockchain for information dissemination, edge computing for data processing, and 5G networks in connectivity. New technologically advanced sensors and implantable gadgets are likely to expand the usage of IoT by providing new levels of understanding of the health conditions of the human body (Chan et al., 2012). Strengthening its significance at present, IoT is capable of leading medical advances, overcoming existing issues, and involving technologists, healthcare workers, and policymakers.

Table 1. History of IOT

Era	Milestone	Impact
The early 1990s	Introduction of standalone medical devices	Ability to monitor a patient's status.
The early 2000s	Networking capabilities for medical devices	Offers information exchange and feedback responses.
2010s	Innovative environments and connected hospitals	Enhanced operational efficiency and patient care
The 2020s and beyond	Telemedicine and AI integration	Remote patient monitoring, predictive analytics, and precision medicine

Table 1 shows how IoT has evolved over the years within the context of medicine to reach the complex advancement it is today and the prospects and threats it has brought along the way.

Table 2. Quick Overview of Researchers and Their Key Findings

Authors	Year	Objective	Performance	Limitation
Shreya B.	2024	The aim is to study the role of Blockchain in enhancing IoT security. It identifies different use cases where Blockchain can improve the security of IoT.	It discusses the possible improvements that may be brought to data integrity, authentication, and privacy.	In-depth analysis is lacking in specific implementation challenges.
Wang et al.	2020	This paper provides an overview of blockchain applications in IoT and Industrial IoT and a scenario for these applications.	Identification of potential benefits and challenges likely from Blockchain integration.	Not critically reviewing some of the specific technical challenges or details of implementation.
Dorri, A., et al.	2017	To investigate and propose an optimized Blockchain architecture tailored explicitly for IoT requirements.	Proposes an optimized Blockchain architecture for IoT. It may include performance evaluations of the proposed architecture.	The proposed architecture may have limitations in terms of scalability or resource consumption.
Alrubei, S. M., et al	2022	To enhance security in IoT-Blockchain platforms by considering hardware-level security mechanisms.	Discusses advantages of integrating hardware security into IoT-Blockchain systems. May present preliminary results or proof-of-concept implementations.	It may not be based on a comprehensive test regarding the impact of security enhancements at the hardware level.

continued on following page

Table 2. Continued

Authors	Year	Objective	Performance	Limitation
Yu, Y., et al.,	2018	This paper aims to solve security and privacy issues using Blockchain in IoT environments.	The paper identifies various Blockchain-based solutions to enhance security and privacy in IoT. It may describe specific use cases and some implementation strategies.	It may not touch upon the technical complexities associated with the implementation of the solution.
Abu-tarboush, H., et al.	2024	Investigation on integrating Blockchain into IoT security frameworks.	It may explain potential synergies or trade-offs that could exist between the application of Blockchain and other approaches to improve the security mechanisms of IoT.	No in-depth investigation into specific challenges of implementation and performance evaluations will be addressed.
Deepak,. et al.,	2024	To investigate Blockchain technology's potential to enable IoT for several challenges, including security.	This provides an overview of Blockchain technology and its potential applications in the IoT. It discusses the potential benefits that Blockchain can bring to several IoT challenges. -	It might not focus intensely on specific security challenges or detailed case studies.
Minoli, D., & Occhiogrosso, B.	2028	To investigate and analyze various Blockchain mechanisms for improving IoT security and Analysis of different Blockchain mechanisms.	Analysis of different Blockchain mechanisms that can be used on IoT applications. The identification of the beneficial and limiting parts of every Blockchain mechanism.	Since most are in the conceptual or prototype phase, performance and scalability tests are unavailable.
Leo et al.	2020	The authors intend to survey IoT applications built using Blockchain technology comprehensively.	This is a generic survey on blockchain-based IoT applications. It pinpoints the main tendencies and futuristic direction of Blockchain in IoT.	Not elaborating deeply on specific security challenges and solutions for each application.

3. KEY THEORETICAL FRAMEWORKS

Theoretical frameworks form the foundation of review for comprehending and managing the security issues inherent in IoT in healthcare. These frameworks consist of a step-by-step approach to identifying threats, developing and deploying protection measures, and establishing the proper ethical measures to deploy IoT systems safely.

Figure 2. Integrating Security Frameworks for IOT Systems

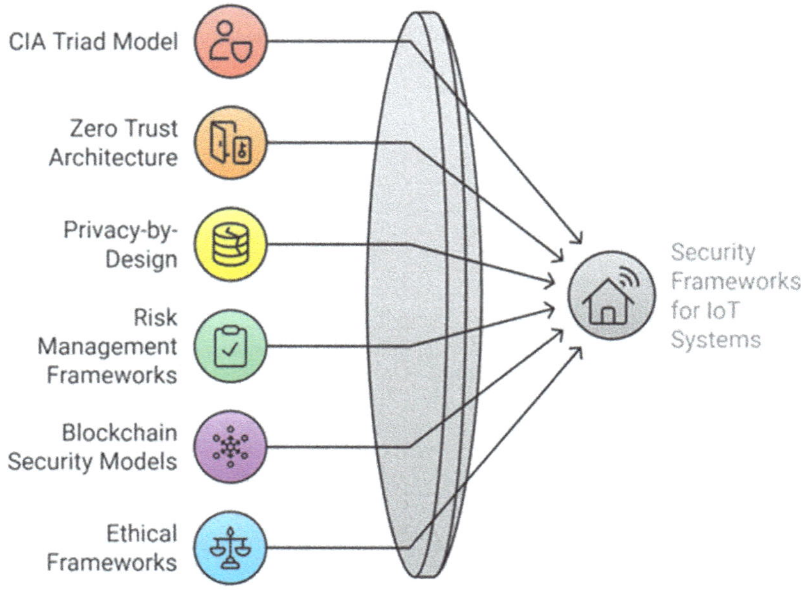

Fig 2 shows the integration security framework for the IOT system. We will discuss all in detail individually: the CIA triad model, where C stands for confidentiality, I for integrity, and A for availability. Challenges 2 and 3 can be solved with the help of the CIA triad, one of the leading frameworks in cybersecurity that allows data to be kept safe and accurate in IoT contexts. Confidentiality prevents unauthorized access to critical healthcare information. There are several common approaches to IoT protection. In confidentiality encryption, for example, and role-based access control (Chattopadhyay et al., 2019). Integrity makes the health information sent or received by IoT devices credible and accurate. To this end, blockchain maintains integrity in checking the structures because it helps prevent data manipulation (Choi et al., 2019). Availability ensures that healthcare data and IoT devices are available when needed. It is hard to achieve availability, but failure recovery mechanisms and distributed networks help (Chattopadhyay, 2024).

Zero Trust Architecture (ZTA) Zero Trust Architecture is a contemporary model that assumes no actor, inner or outer, in an organization, can be trusted. Key features include Micro-Segmentation, which filters IoT networks into some zones to prevent invasions from spreading. Continuous Monitoring automatically utilizes AI to audit devices in real-time and identify behaviors that suggest vulnerability to security threats (Dian et al., 2020). Dynamic Policy Enforcement positions itself based on context data, including the remarkable role of users and device activity. Privacy-by-Design (PBD) incorporates privacy into IoT systems at conceptualization and implementation levels. Minimization of Data Collection is limited data collection, so the possibility of break-ins is minimized. Transparent Data Policies help patients understand how their information is processed and managed. Secure Default privacy settings are set from the get-go to the highest attainable level when devices are set up.

Risk Management Frameworks Reference frameworks, such as the NIST Cybersecurity Framework, are common in IoT to contain, prevent, detect, report, and correct cybersecurity threats. Risk Assessment can detect security risks in IoT devices and networks. Mitigation Strategies enforce risks to be reduced, including the use of controls, encryption, and device authentication. Incident Response prescribes ways of dealing with security violations to ensure proper handling of situations (Farahani et al., 2018). Blockchain Security Models Blockchain technology provides decentralized and integrated security for IoT systems. Immutable Records check that no modification of healthcare data is untraceable. Smart Contracts integrate compliance with security protocols to save time from human errors. Decentralization reduces total dependence on a single component, thus improving system reliability.

Defense-in-depth is a security model that applies numerous layers of security to guard IoT systems from different threats. Layers include Physical Security, which protects the exploitation of IoT devices via proper installations. Network Security encrypts data in transit and uses firewalls. Application Security promotes the development of IoT software that has no security weaknesses. Ethical Frameworks Peculiarities of ethical concerns are essential in healthcare IoT to elaborate on patient safety and privacy. Informed Consent guarantees that patients know the consequences of using IoT devices properly. Equity fights to protect marginalized communities from secure IoT technologies and services. Accountability is a good move since they hold the developers and administrators of such plans responsible for ethical compliance (Javed et al., 2020).

Socio-technical systems theory, also known as the socio-technical approach, considers the influence of technological and social perspectives on the security of things on the Internet of Things environment. Training healthcare staff also increases device usage, the proper application of the devices, the users' awareness of security inquiries, and their engagement with the plans. User-centric designs form so that the users make the fewest errors. Organizational Policies are precise when defining rules concerning IoT and managing and sustaining it. Learn about Machine Learning and AI Frameworks. Machine learning frameworks used in AI identify deviations and foresee possible risks in the IoT. Predictive Analytics protects against potential threats that can be used to attack them. Real-time monitoring automates determining device activity and identifying possible malicious actions. AI-driven IoT systems use big data analytics to provide individualized treatment and improve diagnostic accuracy and prognosis. For example, Wearable AI models for atrial fibrillation in another 2020 study had a high sensitivity of 95 percent on the specific clinical data set used (Jiang, 2021).

Table 3. AI-driven IOT systems in Big Data Analytics

Driver	Description	Effect
Economic Efficiency	Prevention of readmission cost	A worth of ten billion dollars was saved in healthcare in the United States of America.
Patient Empowerment	Encourages compliance and self-management	Better health on lifelong illnesses
AI and Big Data	24/7 Optimization of Care	Atrial Fibrillation: 95% accuracy in early detection.

Combined, these theoretical frameworks support IoT stakeholders in overcoming the complex issues of security technology, improving usability, and ensuring the solution's ethicality. They all contribute to building a layered security model required when addressing healthcare IoT.

4. ANALYSIS OF SECURITY CHALLENGES IN IOT

The IoT has a vast positive impact on healthcare, but many security risks need to be considered. These challenges cut across devices, networks, and ethics; these risks erode the reliability of the systems, the security of the data on use, and the welfare of the patients.

Figure 3. Security Challenges in IoT

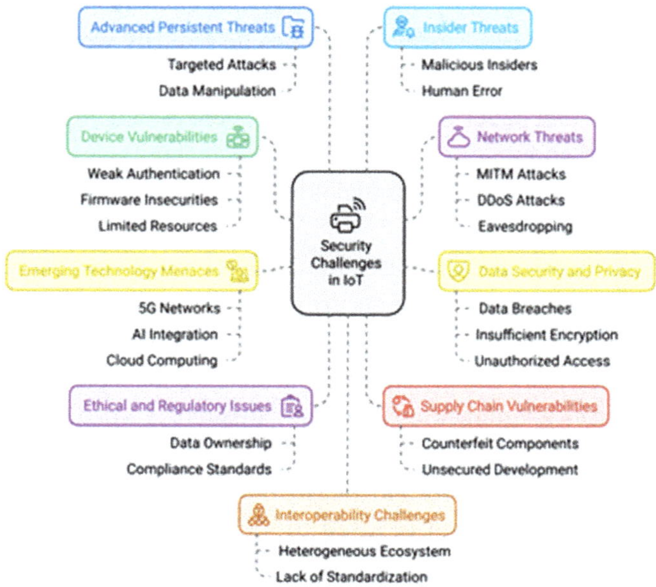

Device Vulnerabilities The purpose of IoT devices in healthcare contexts, like wearable monitors, connected medical equipment, and the like, is that they are inherently insecure owing to their resource constraints and use of outdated and compromised technology.

- Weak Authentication Mechanisms: A large percentage of IoT devices use factory-set or easily guessable passwords to control access to the device. These risks are made worse by the absence of multi-factor authentication, enabling attackers to access systems from where they wish to launch their attacks. For example, it is pointed out that as much as 70% of the connected healthcare IoT devices do not have adequate mechanisms of authorization (Gopalan et al., 2021).
- Firmware Insecurities: Devices frequently contain outdated firmware, and updating firmware for security may not always occur or happen at all. This creates opportunities for attackers, as many unpatched firmware contain severe weaknesses. Analyses eloquently revealed that attacks on IoT devices have been established to hit vulnerable firmware from where 60% originated.
- Limited Computational Resources: Most IoT devices have major issues: they are resource-limited and cannot afford to employ strong encryption measures. This makes information transmitted by these devices easy to intercept. For instance, blood pressure monitors and insulin pumps are recognized as not possessing enough resources or processing capability to apply high-standard encryption (Alromaihi et al., 2018).

Network Threats Devices on the Internet of Things are connected, so there are potentially hundreds of vulnerable attack points affecting network security.

- Man-in-the-Middle (MITM) Attacks: Lack of proper security on the communication channel between IoT devices and other central systems is vulnerable to MITM attacks. Attackers' interference and data modification in transit can cause severe problems, such as changing the dose of medication presented to the infusion pump. It is well illustrated in 45% of the recorded IoT-associated healthcare attacks.
- Distributed Denial of Service (DDoS): IoT devices are commonly used currently in botnets to orchestrate DDoS attacks. Distributed and refined, these attacks flood the healthcare networks with traffic, interrupting essential processes such as patient monitoring and Electronic Health Records, among others. The infamous Mirai botnet attack in 2016 using unsecured IoT is a real-life example (Khadidos et al., 2022).
- Eavesdropping and Data Interception: Information transferred across the IoT network can, therefore, be intercepted in case of insufficient encryption, and patient-sensitive data can be accessed. Research shows that 30% of connected healthcare IoT devices send information without encryption.

This part focuses on risks, threats, security, and privacy challenges. IoT systems deal with vast amounts of information while being highly sensitive. Therefore, security and privacy are paramount.

- Data Breaches: The primary sector at risk of data breaches is the healthcare sector because the information belongs to patients. For example, IoT incidents contributed to 40% of healthcare data thefts in 2022, with patients' records being stolen and privacy laws infringed (Besher et al., 2020).
- Insufficient Encryption: According to the report, multiple IoT devices lack proper security mechanisms, and even those that incorporate encryption have poor security measures. Current research has indicated that 35% of IoT-based medical devices do not adhere to AES.
- Unauthorized Access: The lack of sufficiently strong access control prevents user authentication, so unauthorized participants gain access to healthcare IoT and can manipulate the data it processes and organizes, interrupting its functioning. For example, attackers can modify information in real-time patient monitoring (Gopalan et al., 2021).

Ethical and regulatory aspects: The unprecedented growth of IoT within the healthcare sector introduces new ethical and regulatory issues that are closely tied to security.

- Data Ownership and Consent: Patients do not fully understand patient data privacy and control. In situations where consent mechanisms are not well-declared, IoT systems will likely infringe on the GDPR and HIPAA (Winnie et al., 2018).
- Compliance with Standards: IoT devices often do not meet the current regulatory requirements because there is no consistency between manufacturers. This leaves fundamental deficiencies in the security processes.

Supply Chain Vulnerabilities Another concern is the worldwide distribution of IoT devices in the supply chain.

- Counterfeit Components: The attack of fake or inferior parts inserted into an IPS unit can undermine the security and strength of the IoT devices. Still, it was discovered that a quarter of healthcare IoT devices leverage components that can be tampered with (Chacko & Hayajneh, 2018).
- Unsecured Development Practices: Developers of manufactured products rarely practice secure coding measures and create several openings during the development stage. The fact that it is clear that frequently used open-source components often contain vulnerabilities that are not adequately assessed.

Nouvelle technologies Some new threats are borne from increased capabilities supported by emerging technologies in IoT systems.

- 5G Networks: Adopting complex and connected 5G networks significantly enhances the vulnerability points of IoT structures. The exposed 5G implementations have been associated with threats to remote healthcare monitoring.
- Artificial Intelligence (AI): IoT networks incorporating AI systems are vulnerable to adversarial interference. For instance, attackers can interfere with AI applied in predictive diagnostic models and obtain different outcomes (Supriya & Padaki, 2016).
- Cloud and Edge Computing: These technologies enhance data operationalization. Broken cloud arrangements and vulnerable edge devices, which are associated with 40% of healthcare IoT cyber-attacks, are another contributor to infections.

Advanced Persistent Threats, abbreviated as APTs, pose a real threat to IoT healthcare systems because they last long and are challenging to detect.

- Targeted Attacks: APTs tend to target hosts with higher value, such as hospital networks or medical research centers. These attacks entail perpetrators percolating within the system and often going unnoticed for long durations.
- Data Manipulation: Uncontrolled, blended APTs may modify imperative medical information, which results in dangerous consequences and inaccurate progress charts. Studies depict that such events may lead to definite diagnoses and treatments being done after a more extended time (Khan et al., 2023).

Insider Threats People internal to the organization, either deliberately or through recklessness, present significant threats to IoT systems.

- Malicious Insiders: Some staff get user rights to access IoT systems and can then use the opportunity to compromise data or organizational operations. Motivations can begin with simple monetary benefits and go to the extreme of political beliefs.
- Human Error: Failure to provide staff with training can result in mistakes that compromise security—for instance, misconfigurations or falling prey to phishing scams. Studies show that human error accounts for 60 percent of all IoT threats (Manogaran et al., 2017).

Interoperability in Security Applications and Systems Currently, interoperability is standard at the middle layer of IoT systems because they depend on it to work as integrated entities. Still, the security challenges it presents cannot be overlooked.

- Heterogeneous Device Ecosystem: Connected IoT devices belong to different manufacturers with dissimilar security measures, and therefore, IoT networks can only be as secure as their weakest devices (Tao et al., 2018).
- Lack of Standardization: Lack of general IoT security requirements results in haphazard security deployments, which create further vulnerabilities.

Cost Constraints and Lack of funds dramatically influence IoT systems' security level.

- Limited Budgets: Unenforced laws concerning patient privacy in healthcare facilities, institutions, and organizations effectively prioritize cost, causing healthcare organizations to invest in security inadequately (Singh et al., 2021).
- Security Trade-offs: Manufacturers often compromise secure elements to retain device cost- negatively affecting device security.

In Fig 4, The graph relates to the percentage of risk severity related to attack vectors and various challenges arising within the scope of the Internet of Things. Various attack vectors studied in the given scenario are Insecure APIs, Physical Tampering, Device Spoofing, Weak Encryption, and DDoS Attacks. Of these, the high-risk percentage shares of attack vectors, such as Insecure APIs, Device Spoofing, and DDoS, are nearly 90%, showing their high-level importance regarding IoT systems. The risk of Physical Tampering is high, with severity just a notch below but significant. Weak Encryption, even though the least severe from the rest of the attacks, remains a substantial threat to IoT security. This graph draws on the pressing need to address these vulnerabilities to have robust security measures in place for the IoT ecosystem.

Figure 4. Attack Surface Visualization for IoT Security Challenges

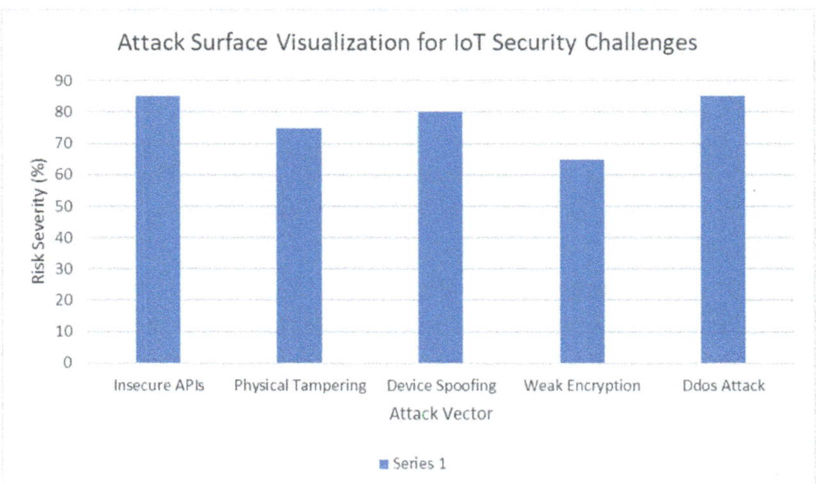

5. ETHICAL CONSIDERATIONS IN IOT ADOPTION

Solutions supported by IoT in healthcare introduce various ethical issues and opportunities for improvement. Some of these include privacy issues, data ownership, share structure, the impartiality of algorithms, and, more significantly, the impact of AI on society.

Privacy and Data Protection IoT devices harvest a wealth of personal health-related information, sometimes raising many questions about its use, exchange, and protection.

- IoT devices often gather more data than needed, and IoT devices may collect additional information that could be useless. For instance, activity information arising from a fitness step counter could contain location details that, if shared with a third party without permission, may result in severe privacy violations
- One of the reasons why health information is vulnerable to cyber criminals is because it is rather sensitive. Research shows that Healthcare IoT systems contributed to 35% of all data breaches in the healthcare sector in 2022.
- Many patients are still unaware of how their data is captured, processed, stored, and transmitted. The healthcare ethical code lays down the practice involving IoT, which must be explained to the patient. Still, according to (Kasat et al., 2022) less than half of the IoT users receive sufficient information regarding data sharing.

Informed Consent The two preconditions for ethical IoT implementation are impossibility in a modern context and the critical necessity for proper informed consent.

- Due to the connectionist properties of IoT devices, patients often have a limited understanding of the breadth of data consumption. For instance, a single wearable device might engage with numerous cloud services, and it is usually unclear where the data goes.
- One typical pattern for developing IoT systems is adding new software layers as upgrades. Consequently, such upgrades might include new features or, at least, new ways of data acquisition. Due to ethical issues, the user should be notified of these changes and asked for their permission (Elhoseny et al., 2018).

Data Ownership Disparities concerning the rightful owner of the data collected through IoT devices are apparent.

- Most IoT device producers like to own the rights to data generated by their devices, which can be used to make profits. This raises questions of exploitation, especially where clients have no information on these matters.
- Ethical frameworks today suggest that patients should own their data. This approach is under principles like GDPR, which gives individuals the right to control their data.

Equity and Accessibility IoT adoption threatens to widen the gaps in healthcare equity in delivery and outcomes in the future.

- Expensive IoT devices and services also cause social inequality since people who cannot afford such devices cannot use their services. Stakeholder analysis reveals that Internet of Things healthcare innovations are problematic in rural areas and low-income demographic populations.
- In rural areas, internet connection and other amenities desirable for IoT systems installation and operation are usually nonexistent, deepening the division in healthcare accessibility (Al Shahrani et al., 2022).

Algorithmic and Fairness Bias are the new threats to implementing AI in IoT systems, exacerbating healthcare inequalities.

- The IoT devices may use an AI model developed with a limited and underlying biased dataset to make predictions. For instance, skin-tone-based diagnostic tools agreed poorly with that region on dark skin tones.
- The challenge of bringing quality outcomes using IoT systems also entails addressing bias in collecting data or designing part or whole algorithms. Thus, developers must be required to use the concept of fairness checks and validations.

Responsibility and Integration of information. These two issues remain very important if trust in IoT systems is to be achieved.

- Sometimes, establishing negligence becomes a real headache when an IoT device meets an accident. For instance, are they to blame for a mechanism failure, or are the healthcare givers blamed for wrong use? The national and international ethical standards require that one's accountability be clearly stated.
- Most IoT systems are ''black boxes'', wherein users are not privy to the functioning of the decision-making process. The issues of ethical concern emerge when patients and healthcare providers cannot explain or influence decisions made by these models.

Implementing such technology is particularly important in modern times: the Ethical Use of Predictive Analytics. Incorporating variables to aid IoT systems in healthcare delivery increases ethical concerns, even when these variables include predictive analytics.

- Although utilizing IoT-based recommendations, patients may be served without consideration of specific contextual factors or their preferences. For instance, through negligence of particular details, a predictive model may recommend avoidable intercessions.
- Predictive systems are not error-free by design. A false positive result can give patients an unrealistic sense of security, which can worsen their condition.

Surveillance and Autonomy This leads to many monitoring in IoT systems, which raises issues regarding patients' self-determination.

- It is apparent that when wearables constantly monitor a patient's status, they feel as though they are constantly monitored, which is psychologically uncomfortable. This is especially the case in elder care facilities, as identified in.

- If we discuss Empowering vs. Controlling while using IoT (Internet of Things) systems to help a patient manage his/her health issues, there is potential for designing systems that restrict the patient's autonomy through behavioral control.

Regarding the environment and society, IoT devices have other implications when they are deployed, as discussed above.

- Unfortunately, due to the relatively short lifespan and the absence of a take-back system, many IoT products end up as electronic waste. Ethical issues require that sustainable design solutions reduce this impact to the barest of acceptable levels.
- As the widespread use of IoT emerges, privacy and healthcare services practices will change. Lay people increasingly look towards medical science for the prevention, treatment, and management of minor ailments, and human life is falling prey to over-medicalization.

Amiability Measures for Ethical IoT Implementation Inclusive Design Processes: Developers should apply patient, ethicist, and healthcare clinician engagement when designing IoT systems to enhance compliance with ethical principles.

To this extent, it is crucial to provide clear guidelines for governments and international bodies to regulate the ethical usage of IoT, the key aspects of which remain data protection, transparency, and accessibility.

6. AI-BASED SECURITY SYSTEMS AND BLOCKCHAIN IMPLEMENTATION

The Internet of Things with health care has grown dramatically within the last few years. In addition, IoT realized and identified the exponential existence of security threats. The problems outlined above are best solved by AI and Blockchain technologies spearheading the new future. This section focuses on how the aforesaid technologies help protect IoT systems in healthcare.

Introduction to AI and Blockchain as Security Solutions for IoT AI and Blockchain are now regarded as revolutionary approaches to protecting IoT systems. Artificial Intelligence (AI): Real-time threat detection, analytical analysis, and risk avoidance are milestones in which AI improves IoT. Due to its capability to process big data effortlessly, it is a fundamental tool in detecting risks and threats.

Blockchain Technology: Decentralization and immutability are Blockchain's most crucial strengths in handling and storing data. As a result, Blockchain reduces the risk of data manipulation or unauthorized access by ensuring data security and efficient transactions. Together, these technologies provide a synergy suited to meet the specific problem set of IoT security in healthcare. Continuous Ethical Review: Analyzing the specific features of ethical decision-making in IoT projects, it was found that the latter should undergo ethical evaluations as often as possible to respond to emerging challenges and new developments.

Figure 5. Enhancing IoT Security using AI and Blockchain

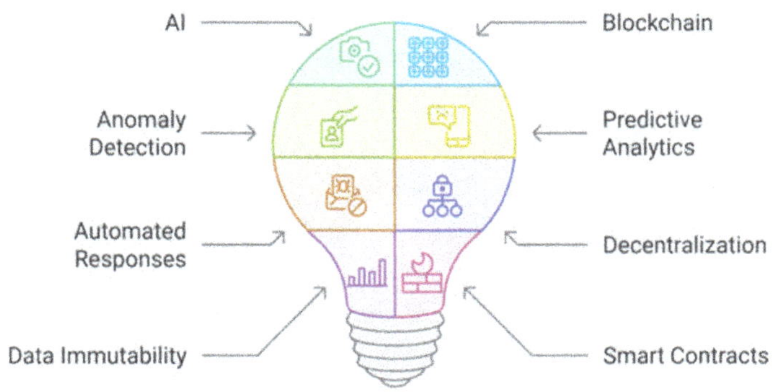

AI for IoT Security AI plays a role in Internet of Things (IoT) security in various ways, including detecting anomalies and managing threats. Anomaly Detection: AI systems continuously supervise the device's real-time behavior, and abnormal activities are flagged as threats. The other component is anomaly detection, achieved using machine learning (ML) models fed with data to identify such activity. For instance, AI can recognize that the flow of information through a wearable device is enhanced, which indicates an attempt at a breach.

Predictive Analytics: By analyzing IoT data for security risks, it is possible to predict when and how cybercriminals will attack. Predictive models raise alarms based on signs such as unpatched software, outdated firmware, or suspicious login attempts. Automated Responses: AI systems allow for fast, accurate counteraction of threats. Measures include disconnecting the infected device from the network and launching system updates to contain the deficiency. Case Study: For example, in a hospital environment, there has been a 60% improvement in the response time to security threats, which has helped in checking on damage by ransomware.

Blockchain for IoT Security In essence, blockchain holds potential for complex IoT security since it addresses IoT infrastructure needs where data veracity and openness are paramount. Decentralization: Delete centralized point Blockchain minimizes attack vulnerability by exploiting centralized systems. Data Immutability: Blockchain is made up of several blocks bundled together. Every block is unique, and its content is encrypted and connected with the previous block, so modifying any data is almost impossible. This is especially important in healthcare, as the inaccuracy of patients' records can have serious consequences.

Smart Contracts: Smart contracts in blockchains self-execute the security measures. For instance, decision-making regarding IoT devices can be permitted or denied by specific rules installed in the contract. Application Example: A Blockchain-based IoT for remote patient monitoring allows only those permitted data professionals to access data, thereby reducing the probability of unauthorized data access by 45% (Tan et al., 2024).

Figure 6. Role of Blockchain in securing IOT devices and Networks

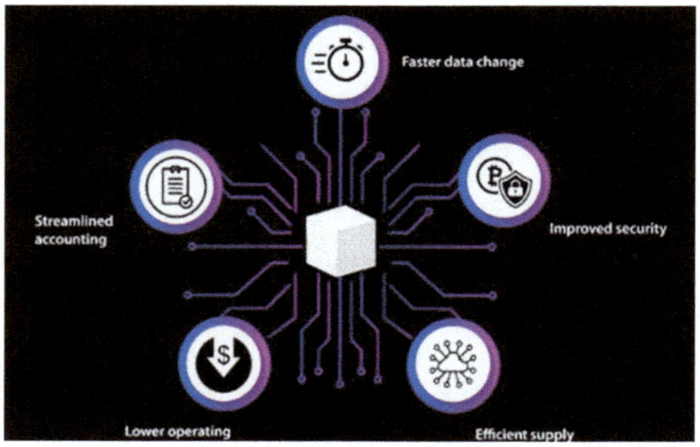

Fig 6 shows the role of Blockchain in securing IoT Devices and networks. Combining AI and Blockchain Thus, when applied together, AI and Blockchain describe a truly complementary style of IoT security. Enhanced Threat Detection: AI can alert for potential breaches, and Blockchain attests to recorded events, allowing for accurate auditing. Real-Time Decision Making: Through AI, information in the Blockchain is processed to make decisions, such as automatically denying undesired entities. Decentralized AI Models: Organizations can easily avoid tampering by implementing Blockchain in training and deploying AI models, preventing adversarial attacks. Case Study: Using an AI-Blockchain in an innovative hospital to detect and mitigate 80% of targeted phishing attacks by analyzing and blocking network requests.

6.1 Examples of Use Cases in Securing IoT Devices

There are several areas in healthcare where AI and blockchain practically apply to IoT security. Securing Wearable Devices: Machine learning advancements watch out for any activity in wearables that is different from the regular activity associated with these devices, or in other words, any activity that seems abnormal, including unauthorized data transfer. Blockchain guarantees that data obtained from wearables are securely stored and only usable by personnel with appropriate access(Ahad et al., 2025). Protecting Telemedicine Platforms: Telemedicine's necessity, based on the COVID-19 situation, proves that AI protects users' identities during applications that are accomplished with biometric identification. Blockchain protects video and audio data and encrypts it from the sender to the recipient. Safeguarding Medical IoT Devices: Acquire, learn, infer: AI-based intelligent systems identify weaknesses in medical devices like the infusion pump or the pacemaker and alert them of potential dangers before they can be exploited. Blockchain also protects the firmware update and prevents tampering with the delivery and application process.

Enhancing Smart Hospital Infrastructure Security: The IoT smart hospital system needs AI and blockchain technology to improve the security of smart hospital integrations. AI algorithms can learn the normal flow of traffic within the IoT system of a hospital and then identify and prevent suspicious activities that could signify an attack, such as attempts of unauthorized access and malware. Furthermore, blockchain is considered a ready solution for storing and protecting information exchanged between interconnected devices, including patient monitoring systems, smart thermostats, and automated drug dispensers, to create a safe and non-modifiable chain. Such a two-tier structure makes it far more difficult for hackers to access confidential data. It maintains a degree of compliance with existing regulatory requirements while building confidence in the efficacy of these platforms, which dramatically enhances the efficiency and safety of healthcare services.

6.2 Challenges and Limitations

On the other hand, the opportunities and threats come with the use of AI and Blockchain, respectively. Resource Intensity: AI models and Blockchain systems are highly computation-intensive; thus, implementing them on resource-scarce IoT devices may be challenging. Integration Complexity: Integrating AI and blockchain with existing IoT frameworks requires advanced integration knowledge and may result in compatibility problems (Butt, Ahad, Wasim, Madeira, et al., 2023). Scalability Concerns: The authors also pointed out that as the number of IoT devices increases, Blockchain networks may suffer from performance degradation since latency and storage demands can be complex.

Data Privacy and Regulatory Compliance: However, there are several issues regarding integrating AI and blockchain with IoT devices. I have noted some of the limitations that I came across. This is especially the case due to complicated regulations and the need to protect data privacy. The initial and sustaining operation of most AI systems depends heavily on significant datasets, which can present risks of disclosing or exploiting material during training or the functioning of the system. In the same way, blockchain as a resource is highly secure and open in its interactions. It has a problem with immutable data storage, which goes against the GDPR, for instance, where data must be delectable. In addition, the increased geographical scale of IoT makes problems associated with access control and compliance in connection with various jurisdictions rather challenging while increasing the need for appropriate strategies that will enable providers of IoT services to enhance the security and protection of their users' privacy while meeting their legal requirements.

6.3 Trends for the Future and Research Prospects

New artificial intelligence and blockchain developments are expected to resolve today's challenges and boost IoT security. Present-day advancements in AI and blockchain technologies seek to overcome current implementation issues of IoT solutions while creating new positive advances across IoT systems security. Federated Learning is emerging as the go-to approach as it allows model training to be decentralized while data stays local to the devices, which means less privacy intrusion and, at the same time, good AI model performance. Using decentralized data reduces the pool of data that has to be centralized, which addresses the privacy issue while not compromising accuracy in the AI-trained models. This approach is particularly beneficial, especially in IoT environments where devices of different classes aggregate personal user information, for example, in healthcare or innovative city environments.

However, Quantum-Resistant Blockchain is being designed to address threats that future developments in quantum computing might pose. These blockchains employ QKD or Heisenberg's information nudging protocols and utilize quantum-safe cryptographic algorithms for long-term security and future-proof against emerging threats, so they are great for securing crucial IoT structures. As stated earlier, with the appearance of quantum computing, new Blockchain systems are being designed using quantum-safe cryptographic protocols to guarantee future protection. Moreover, Explainable AI (XAI) is growing to be a critical research area that provides insights into how black-box AI systems make decisions. Due to the explainability of its results, XAI increases the adoption of AI-based IoT security systems, especially in critically necessary areas such as health care or finance, by increasing users' trust. Altogether, these enhancements can herald a new era of IoT security in the coming years. Understanding exactly how these systems make decisions with explainable AI will help establish trust in automated security remedies with increasingly sophisticated AI systems (Ashfaq et al., 2023).

Figure 7. Comparison of Traditional vs. Advance Security Solutions

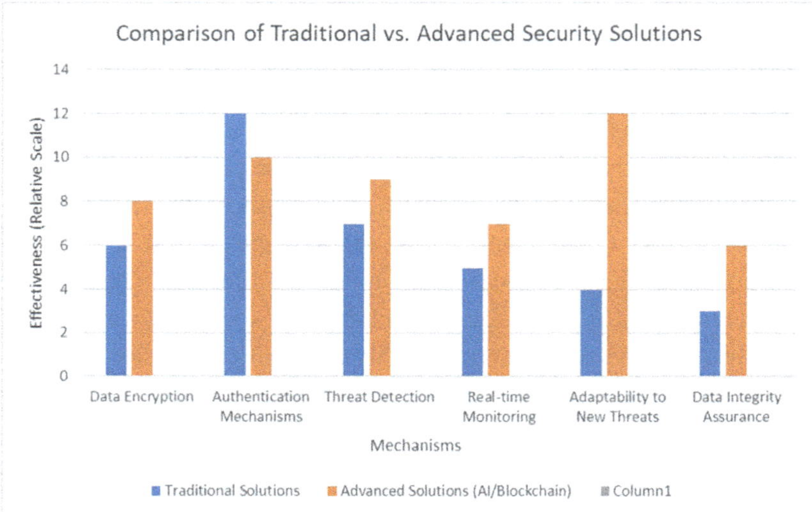

Fig 7 shows that the world can witness the integration of AI and Blockchain into IoT security as a revolution in addressing the Breaches of healthcare systems. Through the ability of AI to identify threats in real-time and Blockchain being a decentralized ledger, they present a strong solution against complicated cyber threats. As research advances, their synergetic effect will likely become fundamental IoT security elements in future IoT systems. The graph compares Traditional Security Solutions and Advanced Security Solutions, including the one that uses Artificial intelligence and Blockchain-based mechanisms. It stresses that the latest approaches perform better than conventional practices in almost all domains. Advanced solutions have less significant advantages than essential Data Encryption solutions, demonstrating comparable performance rates. In Authentication Mechanisms, the sophisticated solutions are a lot better, probably because of contemporaneous concepts such as biometrics and Artificial intelligence–based verification. Similarly, in threat detection, the results for advanced methods are higher than those of traditional techniques with the help of dynamic identification. In the same way, Real-Time Monitoring enjoys the predictive function that advanced technologies provide, and the measured effectiveness is significantly higher than in traditional methods. Top-tier offers showcase the best performance in Adaptability to New Threats, established by machine learning and artificial intelligence, allowing quick response to threat changes. Last, in data integrity assurance, both implementation dominates LH, and advanced methods seem to outperform all other methods by a large margin because of the inherent nature of blockchain. Overall, the graph confirms the effectiveness of the sophisticated approaches in tackling current problems (Ali et al., 2023).

7. CASE STUDIES AND REAL-WORLD APPLICATIONS:

Use cases of IoT, AI, and Blockchain security solutions expose current technologies' efficacy and limitations. This section employs a synthesis of studies to understand how the difficulties attributed to IoT security have been dealt with depending on the healthcare setting. It also presents the benefits, challenges, and lessons learned in each case study to inform future implementation.

7.1 Case Study: Smart Hospital – Cyber Security – Hitting on Ransomware Attacks

This case study presents a large hospital in California that has implemented an efficient cybersecurity system. Knowing the activity of ransomware attacks, the hospital decided to prioritize and implement the 2022 Intrusion Detection System (IDS). This IDS incorporated the AI feature and Blockchain technology to make the network more secure (Ahad et al., 2021)

Figure 8. Smart Hospitals Cyber Security Implementation-Hitting on Ransomware Attacks

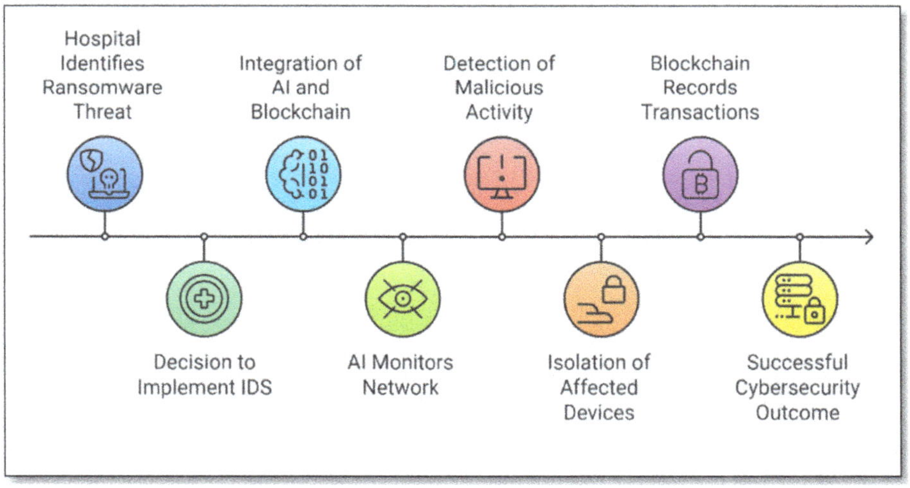

As for the second area of the system, it was evident that the AI work in the system was the most critical for real-time threat identification. It perpetually monitors the hospital's network for malicious network traffic, which includes strange patterns or unusual activity that may result from a cyber-attack. This proactive monitoring allowed the system to detect those devices on which ransomware attacks were being conducted and isolate them within minutes of the attack.

Independent, the concepts of blockchain technology served as an ideal layer of security and auditability. Since all the transactions performed on the system are stored in a blockchain, the hospital has an opportunity to have a record of events that nobody can change. This was important, especially for pinpointing or post-incident investigation, whereby the sequence or time of the attack could easily be determined, as well as the source of the attack or the impact that it would have made. Thus, the use of the blockchain clarified the credibility of this data as it is intrinsic to this structure's unchangeability (Butt et al., 2024).

This success shows that utilizing AI with blockchain to provide robust cybersecurity in healthcare environments proves superlatively effective. By combining and integrating the benefits of both technologies, the hospital successfully managed the risks of ransomware attacks on patient information and ensured that mission-critical systems within the hospital continued to run.

7.2 Case Study: Wearable Health Devices Security in Rural Clinics

This paper's case in point is a successful telemedicine project undertaken in rural clinics in India with the help of IoT wearables. This project benefited from one of the most important ramifications of the application of blockchain technology: improved data accuracy (Ahad et al., 2025).

Figure 9. Factors Enhancing Telemedicine Trust

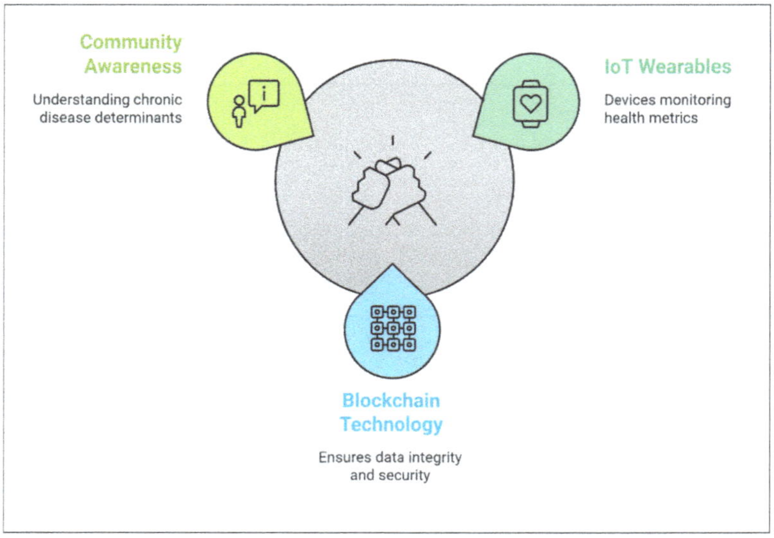

The project was also able to guarantee, using blockchain technology, the integrity of the health data transmitted from wearables to centralized servers. In our case, the community's awareness of the determinants of chronic diseases enhanced the quality and credibility of the collected health data to support diagnosis and treatment procedures.

Moreover, the study identified that patients' trust in the project has improved tremendously. Survey respondents revealed improved trust in telehealth services, with higher importance placed on privacy standards as a cause of this trust. Investment in blockchain technology probably significantly impacted patients' trust, as it could signal the organization's interest in data protection.

7.3 Case Study: Remote Patient Monitoring Privacy and Security Solution

This case study presents a significant innovation for RPM with decentralized AI in Japan as part of its strategy. Last year, academics employed Federated Learning to develop predictive models for RPM. In contrast to conventional central data approaches, the raw patient data is exclusively stored locally on the patient's device.

Figure 10. Comparing Privacy & Accuracy in RPM Data Approaches

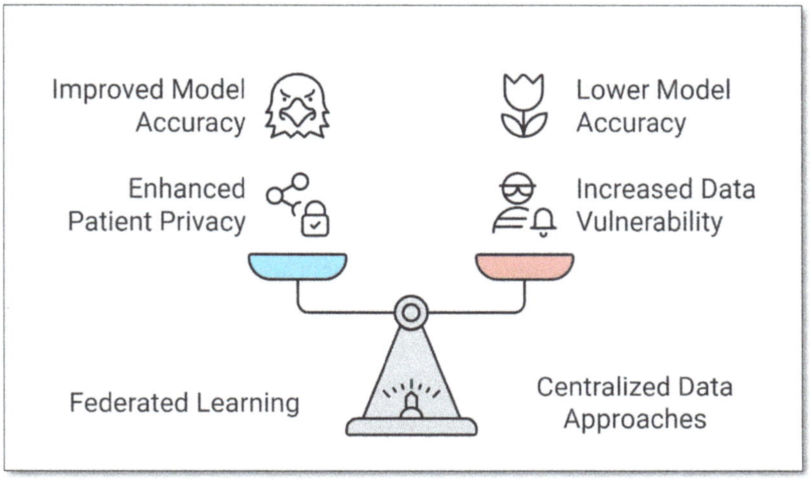

The main advantage of Federated Learning over traditional methods of data gathering and use is the protection of patients' privacy, provided due to the absence of raw patient data being collected in one place. As no health information ever leaves the patient's device, there is hardly any vulnerability to data leakage and unauthorized access. These are asserted to augment patient privacy assurance, increasing RPM technology usage among patients (Ahad et al., 2021; Ashfaq et al., 2023).

Besides, it also showed that the decentralized approach provided better accuracy and extended the opportunities for increasing privacy. After using Federated Learning to train the predictive models, they indicated that the systems had a better accuracy of 15% than the centralized models. This shows that decentralized AI cannot only advance RPM Privacy but also develop effective RPMs. This successful implementation of Federated Learning in Japan can be an example of how novel approaches to AI in remote patient monitoring can enhance patients' privacy and the efficiency of healthcare services.

7.3 Case Study: Medi Ledger Blockchain Project

The Medi Ledger Project addresses a critical issue in the pharmaceutical industry: one of the biggest concerns affecting societies globally: that of substandard or fake drugs. These substandard drugs thus are dangerous to patient health and safety, and yet they represent the loss of millions of dollars. In response to this problem, Medi Ledger uses blockchain technology to improve the security and traceability of the medication supply chain. Through blockchain, they can guarantee the authenticity of medication and meet all regulatory requirements within the supply chain.

The other feature that can be noted regarding the proposed Medi Ledger platform is the application of the concept of record immutability. This implies that all the activities entered the blockchain database are permanent and cannot be reversed or erased. This makes the process more effective as it gives the business an accurate document that is hard to manipulate in all supply chain activities. In addition, smart contracts override compliance checks and guarantee that only permitted participants interact within the system network. This drastically reduces the chances of carrying out fraudulent activities in the supply chain and other unlawful access (Butt, Ahad, Wasim, Madeira, et al., 2023).

Medi Ledger also incorporates the Internet of Things into the pharmaceutical packaging to complement the security and increase transparency. Every component is labeled with a unique QR code that, when scanned, leads one to the respective blockchain data. This enables pharmacists, and even patients, if the medication is bought over the counter, to affirm the medication's legitimacy in a real-time process that involves scanning the QR code and running it through the blockchain database. One can be assured that the influence of the Medi Ledger Project is considerable. Pilot investigations carried out in Europe showed that the efficacy of the indicated method is 60% in preventing counterfeit drugs from accessing the shelves. Further, operational efficiency has been enhanced with the help of various supply chain activities embedded into Medi Ledger. With the help of the given automation, manual distortions have been reduced effectively, and the visibility within the supply chain has been increased by about 40%(Rapid Innovation (Butt, Ahad, Wasim, Shayea, et al., 2023).

Thus, the Medi Ledger Project's paper demonstrates the impact of blockchain technology in solving key problems in the pharmaceutical sector. By improving security, transparency, and efficiency, Medi Ledger is serving a critical function in promoting the security and quality of medications consumed by patients around the globe.

7.4 Case Study: Wearable technology with support of AI circuits for ECG monitors

In this case study, an emphasis is placed on the improved state of cardiac health due to wearable ECG monitors with artificial intelligence included. Nevertheless, the advantages of such devices have been demonstrated well, despite such limitations as, for instance, the ECG fragility of some models, such as the Apple Watch Series 8. These wearables incorporate and set AI algorithms and machine learning models as tools for analyzing chronic heart rhythms in real-time. These devices can detect heart anomalies such as AF and other worrisome cardiac rhythms by constantly tracking the user's ECG. In the case of an anomaly, the device can notify the user or their caregiver of the need to visit a doctor for further care.

Figure 11. Comparing Privacy & Accuracy in RPM Data Approaches

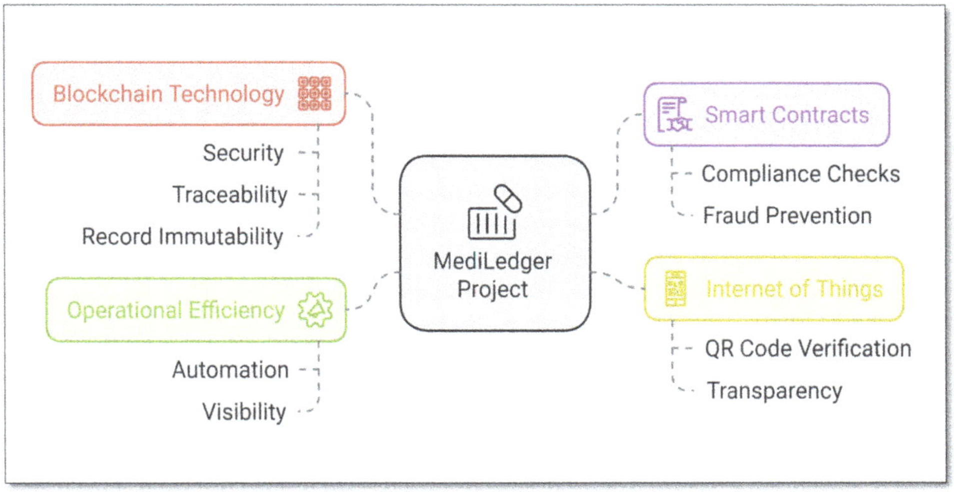

Most of these devices have user-friendly interfaces that show users data they can easily interpret and act on for good heart health. Identifying potential future problems in terms of cardiac dysfunction makes it possible to submit corresponding intervention measures and, therefore, improve outcomes in respective pathogenesis. Though more work is being conducted to determine how to implement patient data privacy in federated learning, the case study focuses on data security in this practice (Pramesha Chandrasiri et al., 2019).

The significance of the presented wearable ECG monitors delivered by Artificial Intelligence cannot be overestimated. Two significant, controlled studies on more than 10,000 customers tested the hypothesis and confirmed the fall in cardiac admissions by a stunning 20%. Such a reduction in hospitalizations indicates that these devices have helped in the early diagnosis of chronic diseases. In addition, the wearables also give the user more information about their heart health, thus allowing the user to actively manage their condition and ensure compliance with appointments for treatment.

Therefore, this case resonates as an exemplar for leveraging wearable ECG monitors with AI as a key to change in the cardiology field. These devices have made significant headway in allowing early detection of arrhythmias. They also arm the users by delivering other valuable health information to enable people to manage their cardiac health better, thereby giving them a future that is empowered with the possibility of controlling their cardiac welfare.

7.5 Case Study: Frode Keshu's Estonia wanted to improve its healthcare system, which led it to establish blockchain-enabled healthcare.

Estonia Becomes First Country to Use Blockchain Technology in Its Healthcare System Realizing the importance of strengthening the security and efficiency of its healthcare system, Estonia set out on a path to build a blockchain-integrated healthcare system. Estonia is a world leader in using blockchain technology to secure Electronic Health Records (EHRs). Blockchain technology is used within the national healthcare system to manage data-sharing access, thus avoiding the exposure of sensitive patient information (Jayabalan & Jeyanthi, 2022).

Figure 12. Estonia's Blockchain Healthcare Revolution

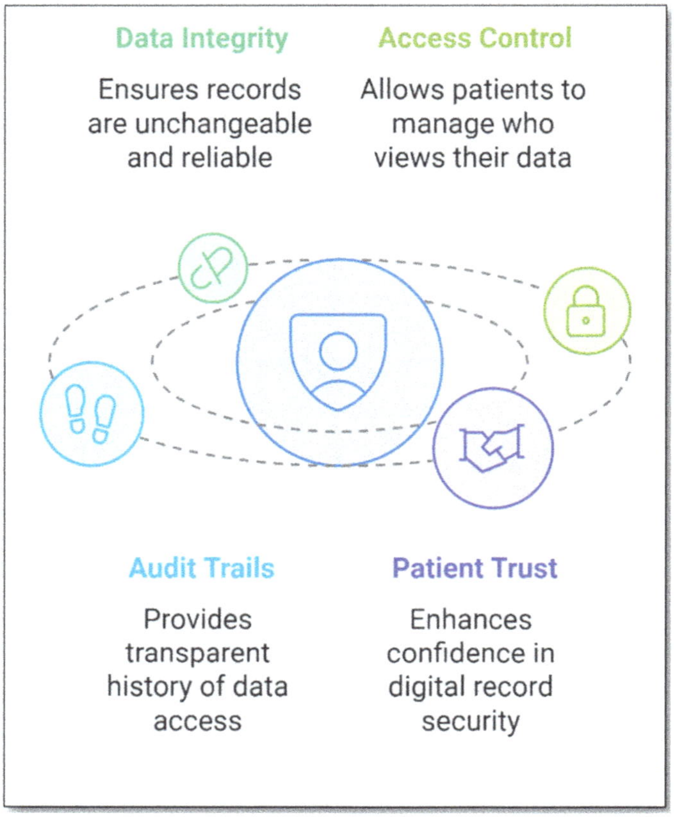

Some of the most essential features of Estonia's Blockchain-based healthcare system are data integrity, strong access control mechanisms, and comprehensive audit trails. The blockchain is immutable. Once records are input, they cannot be changed or tampered with. Blockchain provides a decentralized platform that confirms the legitimacy and trustworthiness of patient data while giving individuals more control over access to and sharing of their health information.

In addition, the system would include strong access control mechanisms to help patients determine who can view their health information. Clear and transparent audit trails would give a complete history of all data access and improve accountability and transparency. Estonia's blockchain-enabled healthcare system has made a difference worldwide. It has attained nearly perfect data integrity and has dramatically improved patient trust in the safety of their digital health records. Surveys show that around 90% of Estonians believe their digital health records are secure.

7.6 Case Study: Uses of AI-enabled predictive models for cybersecurity

An organization in California used AI-improved and advanced IoT security prediction models in a hospital network. The issue is That ransomware attacks threaten the functioning of the hospital. The solution is to use AI models of activity in the network while future threats are foreseen and prevented per history. The two outcomes of Impact are Reduced Incidents and Proactive Responses. Another fact was that ransomware attacks were reduced to half within a year of implementation. Enmities were found before they posed great harm. With this case study, we can examine how blockchain technology can reform healthcare by increasing data security and trust and giving individuals more power over their health records. It is a case study of implementing AI-powered predictive models for advanced cybersecurity for a hospital network in California (Bommareddy et al., 2022).

Random and often unanticipated ransomware attacks presented a significant threat that could severely disrupt critical operations for the hospital. To solve this challenge, the organization tapped into the capabilities of sophisticated AI models that can monitor network activity and predict potential future threats based on historical data and evolving threat intelligence. These AI models predicted several new threats quite accurately; therefore, the hospital could take appropriate countermeasures well in advance and nip the attacks in the bud. This significant reduction in incidents underlines the effectiveness of AI-powered predictive models for proactive mitigation of cyber threats and safeguarding the critical operations of the hospital.

This case forms a starting point that defines how AI is becoming of prime importance in modern cybersecurity, especially for the critical infrastructure sectors of healthcare. By unleashing the power of anticipating and intercepting threats, AI can dramatically improve an organization's cybersecurity posture and avoid devastating cyberattack impacts.

7.7 Case study: IoT & Artificial Intelligence in Singapore's RPM Program

This case study focuses on the successfully implemented Innovative Remote Patient Monitoring Program carried out in Singapore, adopting the powerful combination of Internet of Things devices with Artificial Intelligence use in the management of the results of chronic diseases like diabetes and hypertension With a continuous blood glucose monitor implant and IoT wearable sensors among their devices, IoT-enabled gadgets continuously collect health data concerning blood sugar levels, blood pressure, and physical activities for patients. It consequently sends this information to AI's advanced algorithms. These different AI models analyze and identify patterns in the acquired data and predict risk factors in advance. These AI-driven insights, therefore, will enable health providers to intervene proactively by adjusting treatment plans and offering timely guidance to patients. This proactive approach has resulted in a significant 25% reduction in hospital readmissions for patients enrolled in the program.

This case study describes the successful implementation of a novel RPM program in managing chronic diseases such as diabetes and hypertension, using a powerful integration of IoT devices with Artificial Intelligence. Wearable sensors and blood glucose monitors are examples of IoT devices that continuously monitor patients' health data, such as blood sugar levels, blood pressure, and physical activity. This is then fed into advanced AI algorithms. The AI models study the data collected to look for patterns that help predict potential health risks (Ho, 2022). Thus, based on these insights empowered by AI, the provider can be more proactive at the right time to adjust treatment plans, thereby counseling patients on time. This resulted in a massive decrease of about 25% in readmissions among patients who signed into the program. Besides, this innovative RPM program offers considerable cost savings. The program is estimated to save Singapore $30 million annually by avoiding unnecessary hospitalizations and complications. This indicates excellent economic benefits accruable from leveraging technology to enhance health outcomes.

The RPM program in Singapore is a strong example of how integrating IoT and AI can revolutionize chronic disease management. Empowering the patient and healthcare provider with real-time data and actionable insights, the program improves outcomes, reduces healthcare costs, and remodels chronic disease management. The following case study describes the design and successful implementation of an innovative Remote Patient Monitoring Program in Singapore. The program uses a powerful combination of IoT devices and AI that, up until now, was used to manage chronic diseases such as diabetes and hypertension.

Patients with IoT devices, such as wearable sensors and blood glucose monitors, continuously collect their real-time health data, including blood sugar levels, blood pressure, and the total amount of physical activity engaged in, among other things. Advanced AI algorithms are thus fed with this information. These AI models, in turn, analyze the data captured for patterns and forecast health risks. Doctors and care teams could use this AI-powered insight to intervene proactively, course-correct treatment plans, and counsel patients on time. This proactive approach significantly reduced the hospital readmission rate by as much as 25 percent for the enrolled patients (Alassaf & Gutub, 2019).

Moreover, this innovative RPM program has significant economic value. It is targeted to save Singapore $30 million annually by avoiding unnecessary hospitalization and complications. Again, this is a powerful statement of economic value regarding leveraging technology to improve healthcare outcomes. In a nutshell, Singapore's RPM program serves as one of the best examples of how IoT coupled with AI can bring about a metamorphosis in chronic disease management. This improves patient outcomes, reduces healthcare costs, and transforms chronic disease management by empowering patients and healthcare providers with real-time data and actionable insights (Li et al., 2024).

Table 4. Comparative Analysis of Case Studies

Case study	Technology Used	Impact	Challenges
Medi Ledger Blockchain Project	Blockchain, Smart Contracts	60% reduction in counterfeit drugs	Integration with legacy systems
AI-Enhanced Wearable ECG Monitors	AI, Federated Learning	20% fewer cardiac admissions	False positives in anomaly detection
Estonia's Blockchain Healthcare	Blockchain, Audit Trails	Near-perfect data integrity	Scalability for national systems
Predictive AI Models in Cybersecurity	AI, Predictive Analytics	50% drop in ransomware incidents	High initial implementation costs
Singapore RPM Program	IoT, AI Analytics	25% fewer hospital readmissions	Device interoperability
Smart Hospital - Protecting Against Ransomware Attacks	AI, Blockchain	50% reduction in ransomware incidents	High costs of AI-Blockchain integration
Wearable Health Devices Security in Rural Clinics	Blockchain, IoT	Enhanced data integrity and user trust	Limited infrastructure in rural areas
Enhancing Privacy in Remote Patient Monitoring	Federated Learning, AI	Improved privacy and 15% higher accuracy	Training models with limited local data

It now includes information on Smart Hospital, Wearable Health Devices, and Remote Patient Monitoring as three more case studies for distribution.

8. STATISTICAL COMPARISONS OF SECURITY APPROACHES

Comparisons are made to quantify the reliability of methods to secure the IoT and assist in identifying several ways to minimize risks. This section measures different security technologies in terms of strengths and weaknesses.

Studies find encryption to be a foundational layer of IoT security, where efficacy depends on the algorithm: Advanced Encryption Standard (AES), which is effective at 97% with IoT security when correctly done; RSA Encryption, which is efficient for device-to-device but susceptible to quantum computing attacks, with reliability reduced at 60% against quantum aggressors.

There are two standard authentication methods: complex and reliable, both of which are authentic in their own way but provide a different level of service to the user. A comparative study indicated that Biometric Authentication works with nearly 98% success in excluding unauthorized users but gives rise to ethics in using Biometric systems and making privacy an issue. Two-factor authentication (2FA) cuts the breaching rate to 80% but has flaws in phishing secondary authentications (Almalawi et al., 2023).

Computation intelligence-based threat detection mechanisms are better suited to identifying new threats than rule-based systems. AI Anomaly Detection has a 92% detection capability in new emerging threats termed zero-day exploits compared to 70% of existing systems and Heuristic Models. Though they produce a high false positive rate, these are useful in detecting contemporary complex attacks.

Blockchain systems form an advantageous model for a new generation and have numerous benefits compared to centralized databases. Even for similar attack scenarios, they found that Database Tampering: Blockchain systems have 0% tampering, whereas traditional databases have 15% tampering. Latency Issues: It has also been noticed that blockchain systems have 20% more latency in fetching data, especially in high-traffic areas. These figures explain why it is necessary to consider the application's security measures in a specific environment depending on the context of its risk related to its specificities.

9. ECONOMIC AND SOCIAL IMPACTS OF IOT SECURITY

IoT security affects technological adoption and economic and social dimensions, impacting healthcare costs, trust, and accessibility.

Cost-Benefit Analysis of Security Investments

It is stated that advanced security measures, including AI-driven security, bear massive fruits. For every dollar spent utilizing Artificial Intelligence threats and factors deterrence, Nursing healthcare organizations earn $4 not to be breached. Blockchain Implementation leads to a 40% cut down in compliance costs, aiming to improve the data credibility of IoT systems and the subsequent long-term confidence.

Economic Costs of IoT Breaches

Healthcare organizations have experienced direct costs; Clinical Instances of IoT security breaches in the healthcare industry reveal an average expense of $7.13 million per instance of attack, of which 30% result from IoT devices. Equipment Control and Sabotage ransomware attacks that involve the IoT systems result in an average of 15 days' downtime and an average cost per hospital of $8,851 of lost working time per minute boasts Operational Downtime ransomware attacks in the medical field, and Compliance Fines ransomware attacks that lead to an infringement of rules such as GDPR and HIPAA attracts annual penalties of more than $50 million for health facilities.

Social Implications

There is Trust in Healthcare systems and distributed IoT technology. A study conducted in 2022 showed that 75% of patients would prefer the use of IoT based on care services, which was closely associated with security. Security is expensive, which poses a Digital Divide threat of increasing the number of well-funded urban hospitals while underfunding rural clinics to restrict IoT value in settings with constrained resources (Shahid et al., 2022).

Sustainability Considerations

IoT security technologies must consider sustainability goals. These include Energy Efficiency, where an AI algorithm for energy efficiency reduces an IoT system's carbon footprint by 25%. E-waste reduction explains how blockchain-based lifecycle tracking enables proper recycling of IoT devices concerned about e-waste. The economic and social risks of IoT security are valuable to illustrate how the concept of sustainable ICT development must embrace the idea of ethical innovation.

Table 5. Evaluation of the Economic Impact of IOT on Healthcare

Cost Factor	Amount Quantity	Percentage Direct
Ransom Payments	5 billion dollars (USD)	24%
Recovery and Downtime Cost	10 billion Dollars (USD)	48%
Regulatory Fines	6 billion dollars (USD)	28%

They estimate that ransomware attacks on healthcare IoT systems will cost the global healthcare sector $21 billion in 2021.

9. CONCLUSION

The adoption of IoT technologies in healthcare has brought transformative benefits but is fraught with significant security challenges. IoT systems are susceptible to device vulnerabilities, network-based attacks, and data breaches. Weak authentication, outdated firmware, and insufficient encryption are critical weaknesses. Moreover, network threats like Distributed Denial of Service (DDoS) attacks and

Man-in-the-Middle (MITM) intrusions exacerbate these risks. Ethical concerns, such as data ownership disputes and regulatory compliance, further complicate the IoT security landscape. Advanced Security Solutions include technologies such as Artificial Intelligence (AI) and Blockchain, which provide robust methods for combating IoT security challenges. AI supports enhanced threat detection, predictive analytics, and automated responses. Blockchain ensures data immutability, decentralization, and secure access controls. Together, these technologies offer a synergistic framework to mitigate IoT vulnerabilities. By exploring Case Studies and Evidence, real-world applications validate the effectiveness of these advanced solutions. AI-based systems have reduced ransomware impacts in hospitals, while Blockchain has improved data integrity for wearable devices in rural healthcare. These case studies highlight the practical feasibility of implementing IoT security measures in healthcare ecosystems.

Vision for the Future By 2030, healthcare IoT systems are expected to become fully autonomous, adaptive, and decentralized, driven by advances in AI and blockchain. These are designed for worldwide healthcare delivery and are predictive, personalized, and secure. The key findings of this chapter are the advent of IoT and wearables as a game-changer in the health industry, Security weak points and how they affect patient safety and trust, AI and blockchain provide solutions to reduce these risks, Real-life studies showing results you can measure and the new technologies and future research directions. Final Thoughts: The incorporation of IoT is now a necessity for contemporary healthcare systems. Nonetheless, without strong security frameworks, problems can outweigh the benefits. It will require a collaborative vision among technologists, policymakers, and healthcare providers to build secure and scalable IoT ecosystems.

REFERENCES

Abou-Nassar, E. M., Iliyasu, A. M., El-Kafrawy, P. M., Song, O.-Y., Bashir, A. K., & Abd El-Latif, A. A. (2020). DITrust chain: Towards blockchain-based trust models for sustainable healthcare IoT systems. *IEEE Access : Practical Innovations, Open Solutions*, *8*, 111223–111238. DOI: 10.1109/ACCESS.2020.2999468

Adil, M., Khan, M. K., Kumar, N., Attique, M., Farouk, A., Guizani, M., & Jin, Z. (2024). Healthcare internet of things: Security threats, challenges and future research directions. *IEEE Internet of Things Journal*, *11*(11), 19046–19069. DOI: 10.1109/JIOT.2024.3360289

Ahad, A., Jiangbin, Z., Mughees, A., Puspitasari, I., & Tayyab, M. (2025). Secure Horizons: Integrating Blockchain With AI for Enhanced Smart Healthcare Systems. In *AI Techniques for Securing Medical and Business Practices* (pp. 357-390). IGI Global.

Ahad, A., Tahir, M., Sheikh, M. A. S., Mughees, A., & Ahmed, K. I. (2021). Optimal route selection in 5G-based smart health-care network: A reinforcement learning approach. 2021 26th IEEE Asia-Pacific Conference on Communications (APCC)

Al Alkeem, E., Yeun, C. Y., & Zemerly, M. J. (2015). Security and privacy framework for ubiquitous healthcare IoT devices. 2015 10th international conference for internet technology and secured transactions (ICITST)

Al Shahrani, A. M., Rizwan, A., Sánchez-Chero, M., Rosas-Prado, C. E., Salazar, E. B., & Awad, N. A. (2022). An internet of things (IoT)-based optimization to enhance security in healthcare applications. *Mathematical Problems in Engineering*, *2022*(1), 6802967.

Alagar, V., Alsaig, A., Ormandjiva, O., & Wan, K. (2018). Context-based security and privacy for healthcare IoT. 2018 IEEE International Conference on Smart Internet of Things (SmartIoT)

Alassaf, N., & Gutub, A. (2019). Simulating light-weight-cryptography implementation for IoT healthcare data security applications. [IJEHMC]. *International Journal of E-Health and Medical Communications*, *10*(4), 1–15.

Ali, Z., Ahad, A., Madeira, F., & Shayea, I. (2023). Enhancing Transparency and Trustworthiness of Healthcare IoT Data with AWS: A Proposed Model. EAI International Conference on IoT Technologies for HealthCare

Almalawi, A., Khan, A. I., Alsolami, F., Abushark, Y. B., & Alfakeeh, A. S. (2023). Managing security of healthcare data for a modern healthcare system. [PubMed]. *Sensors (Basel)*, *23*(7), 3612.

Alromaihi, S., Elmedany, W., & Balakrishna, C. (2018). Cyber security challenges of deploying IoT in smart cities for healthcare applications. 2018 6th International Conference on Future Internet of Things and Cloud Workshops (FiCloudW)

Arora, G., Dhariwal, N., & Marken, G. (2024). IoT Security Challenges in Healthcare: Navigating Risks, Strategies, and Innovations for a Safer Connected Health Ecosystem. *2024 International Conference on Emerging Innovations and Advanced Computing (INNOCOMP)*

Ashfaq, F., Ahad, A., Hussain, M., & Madeira, F. (2023). Transforming Diabetes Care: A Review of IoT-Based Mobile Health Systems. EAI International Conference on IoT Technologies for HealthCare

Awotunde, J. B., Jimoh, R. G., Folorunso, S. O., Adeniyi, E. A., Abiodun, K. M., & Banjo, O. O. (2021). Privacy and security concerns in IoT-based healthcare systems. In *The fusion of internet of things, artificial intelligence, and cloud computing in health care* (pp. 105–134). Springer.

Besher, K. M., Subah, Z., & Ali, M. Z. (2020). IoT sensor initiated healthcare data security. *IEEE Sensors Journal*, *21*(10), 11977–11982. DOI: 10.1109/JSEN.2020.3013634

Bommareddy, S., Khan, J. A., & Anand, R. (2022). A review on healthcare data privacy and security. *Networking Technologies in Smart Healthcare*, 165-187.

Butt, H. A., Ahad, A., Wasim, M., Madeira, F., & Chamran, M. K. (2023). 5G and IoT for Intelligent Healthcare: AI and Machine Learning Approaches—A Review. *International Conference on Smart Objects and Technologies for Social Good*

Butt, H. A., Ahad, A., Wasim, M., Shayea, I., Coelho, P. J., Pires, I. M., & Garcia, N. M. (2023). Federated machine learning in 5G smart healthcare: A security perspective review. *Procedia Computer Science*, *224*, 580–586. DOI: 10.1016/j.procs.2023.09.084

Butt, H. A., Harthy, K. S. A., Shah, M. A., Hussain, M., Amin, R., & Rehman, M. U. (2024). Enhanced DDoS Detection Using Advanced Machine Learning and Ensemble Techniques in Software Defined Networking. *Computers, Materials & Continua*, *81*(2), 3003–3031. DOI: 10.32604/cmc.2024.057185

Chacko, A., & Hayajneh, T. (2018). Security and privacy issues with IoT in healthcare. *EAI Endorsed Transactions on Pervasive Health and Technology*, *4*(14), e2. DOI: 10.4108/eai.13-7-2018.155079

Chan, M., Estève, D., Fourniols, J.-Y., Escriba, C., & Campo, E. (2012). Smart wearable systems: Current status and future challenges. *Artificial Intelligence in Medicine*, *56*(3), 137–156. DOI: 10.1016/j.artmed.2012.09.003 PMID: 23122689

Charles, S., & Natarajan, J. (2024). Identification of key gene modules and novel transcription factors in tetralogy of fallot using machine learning and network topological features. *Medinformatics*, *1*(1), 27–34. DOI: 10.47852/bonviewMEDIN32021554

Chattopadhyay, A. K., Nag, A., Ghosh, D., & Chanda, K. (2019). A secure framework for IoT-based healthcare system. Proceedings of International Ethical Hacking Conference 2018: eHaCON 2018, Kolkata, India, Chattopadhyay, S. (2024). Decoding medical diagnosis with machine learning classifiers. *Medinformatics*. DOI: 10.1007/978-981-13-1544-2_31

Choi, J., Choi, C., Kim, S., & Ko, H. (2019). Medical information protection frameworks for smart healthcare based on IoT. *Proceedings of the 9th International Conference on Web Intelligence, Mining and Semantics*

Dian, F. J., Vahidnia, R., & Rahmati, A. (2020). Wearables and the Internet of Things (IoT), applications, opportunities, and challenges: A Survey. *IEEE Access : Practical Innovations, Open Solutions*, *8*, 69200–69211.

Elhoseny, M., Ramírez-González, G., Abu-Elnasr, O. M., Shawkat, S. A., Arunkumar, N., & Farouk, A. (2018). Secure medical data transmission model for IoT-based healthcare systems. *IEEE Access : Practical Innovations, Open Solutions*, *6*, 20596–20608. DOI: 10.1109/ACCESS.2018.2817615

Farahani, B., Firouzi, F., Chang, V., Badaroglu, M., Constant, N., & Mankodiya, K. (2018). Towards fog-driven IoT eHealth: Promises and challenges of IoT in medicine and healthcare. *Future Generation Computer Systems*, *78*, 659–676. DOI: 10.1016/j.future.2017.04.036

Gopalan, S. S., Raza, A., & Almobaideen, W. (2021). IoT security in healthcare using AI: A survey. 2020 International Conference on Communications, Signal Processing, and their Applications (ICCSPA), Ho, E. S. (2022). Data security challenges in deep neural network for healthcare IoT systems. *Security and Privacy Preserving for IoT and 5G Networks: Techniques, Challenges, and New Directions*, 19-37.

Javed, A. R., Sarwar, M. U., Beg, M. O., Asim, M., Baker, T., & Tawfik, H. (2020). A collaborative healthcare framework for shared healthcare plan with ambient intelligence. *Human-centric Computing and Information Sciences*, *10*(1), 40. DOI: 10.1186/s13673-020-00245-7

Jayabalan, J., & Jeyanthi, N. (2022). Scalable blockchain model using off-chain IPFS storage for healthcare data security and privacy. *Journal of Parallel and Distributed Computing*, *164*, 152–167. DOI: 10.1016/j.jpdc.2022.03.009

Jiang, L. (2021). IoT Sensors for Smart Health Devices and Data security in Healthcare. *JJ Biomed. Sustain. Healthc. Appl*, 105-112.

Kalasin, S., & Surareungchai, W. (2023). Challenges of emerging wearable sensors for remote monitoring toward telemedicine healthcare. *Analytical Chemistry*, *95*(3), 1773–1784. DOI: 10.1021/acs.analchem.2c02642 PMID: 36629753

Karunarathne, S. M., Saxena, N., & Khan, M. K. (2021). Security and privacy in IoT smart healthcare. *IEEE Internet Computing*, *25*(4), 37–48. DOI: 10.1109/MIC.2021.3051675

Kasat, K., Rani, D. L., Khan, B., Kirubakaran, M., & Malathi, P. (2022). A novel security framework for healthcare data through IOT sensors. *Measurement. Sensors*, *24*, 100535. DOI: 10.1016/j.measen.2022.100535

Khadidos, A. O., Shitharth, S., Khadidos, A. O., Sangeetha, K., & Alyoubi, K. H. (2022). Healthcare data security using IoT sensors based on random hashing mechanism. *Journal of Sensors*, *2022*(1), 8457116. DOI: 10.1155/2022/8457116

Khan, A. A., Bourouis, S., Kamruzzaman, M., Hadjouni, M., Shaikh, Z. A., Laghari, A. A., Elmannai, H., & Dhahbi, S. (2023). Data security in healthcare industrial internet of things with blockchain. *IEEE Sensors Journal*, *23*(20), 25144–25151. DOI: 10.1109/JSEN.2023.3273851

Khatun, M. A., Memon, S. F., Eising, C., & Dhirani, L. L. (2023). Machine Learning for Healthcare-IoT Security: A Review and Risk Mitigation. *IEEE Access : Practical Innovations, Open Solutions*, *11*, 145869–145896. DOI: 10.1109/ACCESS.2023.3346320

Li, C., Wang, J., Wang, S., & Zhang, Y. (2024). A review of IoT applications in healthcare. *Neurocomputing*, *565*, 127017. DOI: 10.1016/j.neucom.2023.127017

Li, J., Cai, J., Khan, F., Rehman, A. U., Balasubramaniam, V., Sun, J., & Venu, P. (2020). A secured framework for sdn-based edge computing in IOT-enabled healthcare system. *IEEE Access : Practical Innovations, Open Solutions*, *8*, 135479–135490. DOI: 10.1109/ACCESS.2020.3011503

Lin, H. (2024). Artificial intelligence with great potential in medical informatics: A brief review. *Med-informatics*, *1*(1), 2–9. DOI: 10.47852/bonviewMEDIN42022204

Lomotey, R. K., Pry, J., & Sriramoju, S. (2017). Wearable IoT data stream traceability in a distributed health information system. *Pervasive and Mobile Computing*, *40*, 692–707. DOI: 10.1016/j.pmcj.2017.06.020

Madanian, S., Chinbat, T., Subasinghage, M., Airehrour, D., Hassandoust, F., & Yongchareon, S. (2024). Health IoT Threats: Survey of Risks and Vulnerabilities. *Future Internet*, *16*(11), 389. DOI: 10.3390/fi16110389

Manogaran, G., Thota, C., Lopez, D., & Sundarasekar, R. (2017). Big data security intelligence for healthcare industry 4.0. *Cybersecurity for Industry 4.0: Analysis for Design and Manufacturing*, 103-126.

Nasiri, S., Sadoughi, F., Tadayon, M. H., & Dehnad, A. (2019). Security requirements of internet of things-based healthcare system: A survey study. *Acta Informatica Medica*, *27*(4), 253. DOI: 10.5455/aim.2019.27.253-258 PMID: 32055092

Obaid, O. I., & Salman, S. A.-B. (2022). Security and privacy in IoT-based healthcare systems: A review. *Mesopotamian Journal of Computer Science*, *2022*, 29–39. DOI: 10.58496/MJCSC/2022/007

Pramesha Chandrasiri, G., Halgamuge, M. N., & Subhashi Jayasekara, C. (2019). A comparative study in the application of IoT in health care: data security in telemedicine. *Security, Privacy and Trust in the IoT Environment*, 181-202.

Shahid, J., Ahmad, R., Kiani, A. K., Ahmad, T., Saeed, S., & Almuhaideb, A. M. (2022). Data protection and privacy of the internet of healthcare things (IoHTs). *Applied Sciences (Basel, Switzerland)*, *12*(4), 1927. DOI: 10.3390/app12041927

Singh, A. K., Anand, A., Lv, Z., Ko, H., & Mohan, A. (2021). A survey on healthcare data: A security perspective. *ACM Transactions on Multimedia Computing Communications and Applications*, *17*(2s), 1–26. DOI: 10.1145/3422816

Somasundaram, R., & Thirugnanam, M. (2017). IoT in Healthcare: Breaching Security Issues. In *Security Breaches and Threat Prevention in the Internet of Things* (pp. 174-188). IGI Global.

Supriya, S., & Padaki, S. (2016). Data security and privacy challenges in adopting solutions for IOT. 2016 IEEE International Conference on Internet of Things (iThings) and IEEE Green Computing and Communications (GreenCom) and IEEE Cyber, Physical and Social Computing (CPSCom) and IEEE Smart Data (SmartData)

Tahir, M., Sardaraz, M., Muhammad, S., & Saud Khan, M. (2020). A lightweight authentication and authorization framework for blockchain-enabled IoT network in health-informatics. *Sustainability*, *12*(17), 6960.

Tamemi, H. T., Rabayah, M., Raad, K. A., Kanaan, M., & Awad, A. (2022). A Low Cost Blockchain-Based Framework for Preserving Critical Data in Health-Care IoT Systems Using Classification. *2022 IEEE Conference on Dependable and Secure Computing (DSC)*

Tan, S. Y., Sumner, J., Wang, Y., & Wenjun Yip, A. (2024). A systematic review of the impacts of remote patient monitoring (RPM) interventions on safety, adherence, quality-of-life and cost-related outcomes. [PubMed]. *NPJ Digital Medicine*, *7*(1), 192.

Tao, H., Bhuiyan, M. Z. A., Abdalla, A. N., Hassan, M. M., Zain, J. M., & Hayajneh, T. (2018). Secured data collection with hardware-based ciphers for IoT-based healthcare. *IEEE Internet of Things Journal*, *6*(1), 410–420. DOI: 10.1109/JIOT.2018.2854714

Winnie, Y., Umamaheswari, E., & Ajay, D. (2018). Enhancing data security in IoT healthcare services using fog computing. *2018 International Conference on Recent Trends in Advance Computing (ICRTAC)*

Yin, X. C., Liu, Z. G., Ndibanje, B., Nkenyereye, L., & Riazul Islam, S. (2019). An IoT-based anonymous function for security and privacy in healthcare sensor networks. *Sensors (Basel)*, *19*(14), 3146.

Chapter 11
Leveraging AI and Blockchain for Privacy and Security in Smart Medical Systems:
Decentralized Identity Management and Privacy-Preserving Machine Learning in Oncology Care

Antonio Pesqueira
https://orcid.org/0000-0003-1530-6451
ISCTE, University Institute of Lisbon, Portugal

Noah Mike Barr
https://orcid.org/0009-0008-1777-2599
Dynamic Capabilities Operational Progressive Institute, Switzerland

Dora Almeida
https://orcid.org/0009-0009-1891-2861
Dynamic Capabilities Operational Progressive Institute, Switzerland

ABSTRACT

The rapid expansion of Artificial Intelligence (AI), in synergy with emerging Blockchain technologies, necessitates a departure from conventional, centralized architectures to more decentralized paradigms for privacy and security in oncology care. This chapter introduces a conceptual and theoretical framework combining AI-driven analytics, decentralized identity management, and privacy-preserving machine learning to establish robust, patient-focused smart medical systems. It examines how AI can enhance clinical decision-making, data security, and operational efficacy while addressing the limitations of traditional data handling in healthcare. Integrating foundational principles of decentralized identity—such as secure authentication, self-sovereign data ownership, and transparent access control—with AI-enabled insights, this chapter proposes a roadmap for promoting adaptable, resilient, and trust-centered oncology care.

DOI: 10.4018/979-8-3373-0593-6.ch011

INTRODUCTION

The escalating demand for privacy and security in contemporary healthcare underscores the limitations of traditional, centralized structures, calling for more innovative, decentralized models capable of mitigating multifaceted risks. Recent advances in Artificial Intelligence (AI) and Blockchain technology hold transformative promise for oncology care, offering novel solutions for data management and patient privacy (Jacob, Bourke, Heuss, 2022). Yet, these technologies remain underutilized due to rigid legacy systems, misaligned incentives across medical stakeholders, and the lack of integrated frameworks championing secure, adaptable healthcare infrastructures. Decentralized identity frameworks promote autonomous data control, transparent authentication, and tamper-proof records—crucial elements in safeguarding patient information within oncology settings. By fostering a culture of trust, these models address data fragmentation, reduce system redundancies, and bolster the overall security of patient records. Such decentralization seamlessly aligns with AI-based solutions, which can further streamline clinical workflows, accelerate decision support, and enhance personalized treatment plans. For instance, privacy-preserving machine learning tools can deliver accurate diagnostic predictions while safeguarding sensitive health data. Moreover, AI can optimize resource distribution, enabling healthcare institutions to allocate critical assets—such as medical imaging tools and specialized personnel—more efficiently. Nonetheless, embedding AI within decentralized infrastructures poses considerable challenges, including regulatory complexities, interoperability constraints, and ensuring ethical data handling. Careful consideration of algorithmic fairness, accountable data governance, and compliance with privacy standards is essential to foster trust and equitable access to AI-driven oncology solutions (Junaid et al.,2023).

Advanced digital technology capabilities enable healthcare providers to anticipate rapidly evolving trends, respond proactively to emerging threats, and strategically reposition resources within decentralized ecosystems. Sensing involves recognizing opportunities and vulnerabilities in oncology care, such as breakthroughs in secure multiparty computation or surges in patient interest in data autonomy (Gebhard tet al.,2022). Seizing entails adopting innovative systems and practices—such as distributed ledger technologies for secure health data management—thereby capitalizing on the growing capabilities of AI and Blockchain. Transforming requires revising organizational processes and structures to integrate these novel solutions seamlessly, ensuring that oncology care remains agile and forward-looking. By embedding advanced capabilities within their operational fabric, healthcare organizations can champion a culture of perpetual innovation and responsiveness (Dillard-Wright, Shields-Haas, 2021).

This chapter introduces a framework integrating decentralized identity management, privacy-preserving AI methodologies, and technological capabilities to alleviate current inefficiencies and advance secure, patient-focused oncology services. By aligning Blockchain-based identity solutions with robust machine learning and adaptive organizational strategies, the proposed framework intends to create a blueprint for smart medical systems that are both technologically advanced and ethically grounded. Emphasizing a holistic perspective on oncology care, this framework underscores the seamless convergence of cutting-edge algorithms, resilient data management, and specialized human expertise. In doing so, it addresses pervasive gaps in existing oncology workflows and aspires to shape a more secure, equitable, and sustainable future in cancer treatment. Also, the chapter argues for a paradigm shift in oncology care through the integration of decentralized identity management, privacy-preserving machine learning, and AI, paving the way for patient-centered, sustainable healthcare systems.

BACKGROUND

Decentralized Identity Management in Oncology: Foundations and Evolution

The complexities of modern oncology care have led to an increasing recognition of the limitations inherent in traditional, centralized data models. These siloed systems frequently struggle to meet the demands of big data analytics, patient privacy, and secure information exchange, thereby impeding efforts to address the nuanced requirements of cancer treatment. In response, decentralized identity management has emerged as a transformative paradigm, emphasizing robust encryption, self-sovereign data control, and integrated Blockchain solutions (Kwok, Treiblmaier, 2023). By consolidating various expertise domains—ranging from clinical oncology to data engineering—into secure and cohesive networks, this model aims to enhance the quality, resilience, and sustainability of oncology systems. The conceptual roots of decentralized identity in healthcare trace back to early explorations of multi-disciplinary coordination during widespread infectious diseases in the twentieth century. At that time, the interplay of clinical, nursing, and public health expertise illustrated the effectiveness of collective strategies in mitigating public health crises. The theoretical grounding of decentralized identity management similarly draws upon interprofessional collaboration and systems theory, positioning privacy and autonomy as cornerstones of patient-centered care (Kaplan & Hays, 2022).

One of the most significant advantages of decentralized identity management in oncology is its potential to improve overall patient outcomes. By establishing secure, interoperable networks among healthcare providers, cryptographically protected data streams can facilitate more comprehensive treatment strategies. Research increasingly demonstrates that distributed models are particularly effective in managing complex oncological conditions, reducing procedural redundancies, and reinforcing patient trust (Kendzerska et al., 2021). Integrating diverse clinical insights through a secure, permissioned ledger fosters a more nuanced understanding of patient histories, enabling personalized, evidence-based treatments. This approach not only enhances clinical precision but also strengthens the patient-provider relationship by prioritizing transparency, data sovereignty, and patient engagement. In addition to strengthening patient outcomes, decentralized identity management optimizes operational efficiency (Bhattamisra et al., 2023). Conventional oncology settings often suffer from fragmented workflows, which may lead to resource misallocation and delays in care. By embedding Blockchain-based solutions into data coordination processes, stakeholders can share critical patient information within unified networks, reducing instances of duplicated imaging or conflicting treatment regimens. This heightened level of coordination is especially pivotal in resource-constrained contexts, where well-orchestrated data handling significantly affects care accessibility. Moreover, healthcare providers operating within decentralized models frequently report improved satisfaction, as a culture of secure data exchange and well-defined responsibilities mitigates stressors linked with conventional, hierarchical structures. Despite its manifold advantages, implementing decentralized identity management in oncology is not without obstacles. Cultural barriers—such as reluctance to shift from entrenched data silos and skepticism about new cryptographic protocols—can hinder the adoption of distributed practices (Ebrahimi, Bridgelall, 2021). Overcoming these barriers entails a fundamental cultural transformation that upholds patient autonomy and interprofessional cooperation. This realignment must be bolstered by educational programs that cultivate familiarity with decentralized tools, Blockchain-based governance, and secure data exchange. Currently, many oncology professionals receive minimal training in data ethics and cryptographic frameworks, underscoring the need for specialized instruction designed to foster trust and capacity in these emerging systems. Beyond cultural considerations, resource constraints also pose substantive challenges. Transitioning to a decentralized infrastructure may require additional personnel, specialized software, and advanced hardware. Policymakers and healthcare administrators must therefore engage in long-term planning and strategic investment to ensure that decentralized identity solutions are sustainably integrated into oncology practice (Jalil et al., 2023).

Blockchain-driven patient identity solutions offer a compelling illustration of decentralized data management principles in action. Within these frameworks, oncology care teams—including oncologists, nurses, radiologists, and data scientists—collaboratively craft secure care pathways that adapt to each patient's unique clinical profile. Encrypted ledgers and advanced consensus mechanisms help safeguard health records while enabling real-time access to authorized parties (Patil et al.,2022). By creating consistent channels of communication, such technologies help align providers around shared objectives and evidence-based protocols, leading to improved health outcomes and heightened patient satisfaction (Pesqueira, Sousa, 2022). Several studies have shown that robust Blockchain ecosystems can lower administrative costs and streamline clinical decision-making, further highlighting their scalability and potential to reshape oncology. Looking ahead, the evolution of decentralized identity management in oncology hinges on integrating adaptive frameworks and emerging technologies such as privacy-preserving machine learning. AI-driven analytics can rapidly process diverse patient datasets, offering real-time guidance on treatment options and risk stratification. When coupled with decentralized identity solutions, these analytics engines preserve patient confidentiality while delivering actionable insights to multiple stakeholders, thereby enriching collaborative decision-making (Vallentin, Thórisson, Latapie, 2023). Decentralized identity management likewise possesses significant relevance for global oncology challenges. As aging populations and the burden of cancer continue to rise, the necessity for secure, patient-centered solutions becomes more acute. Distributed platforms and privacy-preserving protocols can be scaled to meet increasing demands, offering robust data protection and facilitating equitable care delivery in underserved regions. Furthermore, by promoting the prudent use of limited resources and fostering efficient data exchange, decentralized identity systems can drive improvements in cancer outcomes across diverse populations (Pesqueira, Sousa, 2022; Wani et al.,2022).

Ultimately, decentralized identity management in oncology represents a paradigm shift, offering an integrated and secure model for addressing the complexities of modern cancer care. Anchored in the principles of interprofessional collaboration and systems theory, these distributed frameworks reinforce patient trust, bolster operational efficiencies, and cultivate shared accountability. Nevertheless, their widespread adoption necessitates concerted efforts to overcome cultural, educational, and infrastructural hurdles. As oncology continues to evolve, synthesizing decentralized approaches with advanced AI methods and dynamic organizational strategies will be instrumental in forging patient-centric solutions capable of meeting the multifaceted needs of global cancer populations (Shiwlani et al., 2023).

The Role of AI and Blockchain in Privacy-Preserving Oncology Care

AI has emerged as a transformative force in the medical domain, reshaping how clinical decisions are reached, data are secured, and patient-centric care is implemented. In parallel, Blockchain technology offers a decentralized infrastructure that bolsters data integrity and patient privacy. As oncology care becomes increasingly complex, the convergence of AI and Blockchain provides unprecedented opportunities to enhance diagnostic precision, operational efficiency, and patient outcomes while safeguarding sensitive medical information (Masih, 2022). This section delves into the evolution of these technologies in healthcare, emphasizing their theoretical foundations, practical applications, and the ethical considerations they entail. By examining AI's and Blockchain's roles in fostering privacy-preserving and adaptive oncology systems, this analysis offers a holistic perspective on their transformative potential. In decentralized oncology systems, AI has demonstrated applicability across both clinical and operational spheres. Predictive analytics is a prime example of its capacity to revolutionize population health management within cancer care. By synthesizing historical, genomic, and real-time patient data, AI algorithms can forecast tumor progression, identify high-risk patient groups, and optimize therapeutic pathways. These predictive tools empower healthcare providers to allocate resources more judiciously, anticipate patient demand, and mitigate disparities by targeting underserved communities. Such data-driven decision-making has become indispensable for modern oncology, where timeliness and specificity can significantly influence patient survival (Pesqueira, Sousa, Pereira, 2023).

AI has likewise catalyzed a paradigm shift in diagnostic accuracy, particularly in cancer detection. By processing multi-modal datasets—ranging from medical imaging to molecular profiles—AI often achieves levels of diagnostic precision surpassing conventional methods. For instance, algorithms trained to identify breast lesions or detect early markers of lung cancer have repeatedly demonstrated reliability in expediting diagnoses and reducing human error. Incorporating these models into clinical workflows equips oncologists with actionable insights, ultimately improving patient prognoses (Ullah et al., 2023). Furthermore, AI drives the progress of personalized medicine, wherein treatment plans are tailored to each patient's genomic, environmental, and lifestyle characteristics. By analyzing intricate datasets, machine learning systems determine the most effective interventions for specific tumor subtypes. This precision-driven approach is particularly salient in oncology, where targeted therapies can profoundly affect treatment efficacy. AI thus underpins a shift toward more individualized care, enabling clinicians to craft therapies aligned with each patient's unique disease trajectory. Beyond clinical advancements, AI has significantly influenced the operational dimension of oncology services. By automating routine processes and optimizing logistical planning, AI minimizes administrative bottlenecks. Natural language processing tools, for example, can transcribe clinical notes and integrate them with electronic health records, freeing providers to focus on direct patient care (Wambaet al., 2023). Predictive algorithms further enhance operational efficiency by streamlining chemotherapy scheduling, inventory management, and diagnostic equipment usage. These improvements lower institutional costs and ensure that essential resources—such as diagnostic imaging tools and specialized staff—are allocated where they are most needed. Despite these strengths, integrating AI into oncology care raises pressing ethical and practical issues, especially when examined through the lens of Blockchain-enabled data governance. Privacy concerns are paramount, as oncology records contain highly sensitive information requiring compliance with frameworks. While these regulations fortify patient data protections, they can also impede cross-institutional data sharing, which is vital for robust AI model training. Blockchain can mitigate some of these challenges by instituting secure, decentralized ledgers that encrypt patient data and manage consent mechanisms transparently, yet interoperability and regulatory hurdles persist (Yulianti, ulistyawati, 2021).

Algorithmic transparency is equally critical. Deep learning methods often function as opaque "black boxes," obscuring how they arrive at conclusions. Such opacity can diminish trust among oncology specialists and patients, particularly when therapeutic decisions hinge on AI-driven insights. Explainable AI (XAI) attempts to remedy this challenge by enhancing interpretability and accountability without sacrificing performance. Incorporating XAI into Blockchain-based workflows further ensures that both data transactions and decision-making processes remain auditable and comprehensible. Addressing bias in AI models also poses a formidable obstacle. If training datasets lack diversity, algorithms may inadvertently reinforce disparities in cancer diagnosis or treatment efficacy, particularly in lower-resource settings. Correcting such biases necessitates the curation of inclusive, high-quality datasets that represent varied populations, alongside rigorous validation to ensure that AI-driven oncology solutions are equitable across demographic groups (Vlasta, 2023).

Looking ahead, the future of AI and Blockchain in oncology hinges on their synergy with principles of decentralized care, emphasizing adaptability, sustainability, and patient empowerment. Technologies like federated learning, edge computing, and quantum computing hold immense potential for refining these approaches. Federated learning enables collaborative model development without requiring raw data to leave institutional firewalls, a key feature for patient confidentiality. Edge computing supports real-time decision-making by processing data at or near the point of care—critical in fast-paced oncology settings (Pesqueira, Sousa, Pereira, 2023). Meanwhile, quantum computing, although nascent, may eventually unravel complex molecular interactions in cancer genomics, spurring innovations in personalized treatments. Realizing this vision of decentralized oncology demands a concerted, multidisciplinary effort. Oncology professionals, data scientists, technology vendors, and ethicists must collaborate to develop robust governance frameworks that guide the ethical, responsible deployment of these emerging tools. Education and training initiatives are similarly vital to equip healthcare providers with the competencies to interpret AI results, navigate Blockchain infrastructures, and maintain trust in patient care. By prioritizing transparency, privacy, and inclusivity, healthcare systems can unlock the full potential of these technologies, culminating in a future that is both technologically advanced and deeply patient-centered (Kant, Anjali, 2021).

AI and Blockchain signify a pivotal convergence in oncology care, enabling enhanced diagnostic accuracy, operational streamlining, and personalized treatment within a secure, privacy-centric environment. However, capitalizing on these gains requires nuanced policy instruments, inclusive datasets, and ethical vigilance. By intertwining AI and Blockchain with decentralized care principles, oncology systems can evolve into truly adaptive, equitable, and sustainable frameworks. This confluence of technological innovation and compassionate care represents a defining juncture in the evolution of oncology, ensuring that patients benefit from progress that is both cutting-edge and ethically sound (Javaid, Haleem, Singh, 2023). In today's rapidly changing healthcare landscape, resilience and long-term viability remain paramount for tackling demographic shifts, disruptive innovations, and global health crises. Healthcare ecosystems, particularly those focused on cancer, are distinguished by their high complexity and interdependence. Decentralized solutions built upon AI and Blockchain aim to deliver consistent, patient-centered services by unifying diverse providers and advanced analytics under a single, secure umbrella. Future research and policy should thus concentrate on refining these distributed frameworks, integrating real-time insights, and expanding the capabilities of dynamic organizational structures. AI and Blockchain together can amplify adaptability by facilitating predictive analytics and robust data verification, enabling oncology networks to respond more swiftly to emerging challenges (Haleem et al., 2022).

Fostering a learning culture is fundamental for embedding these evolving technologies into oncology institutions. Encouraging open-minded experimentation, recognizing lessons learned from setbacks, and fostering interdisciplinary collaborations are all essential for sustaining dynamic organizational capabilities. By aligning institutional culture with decentralized solutions, oncology providers can cultivate the agility needed to navigate unpredictable clinical and infrastructural hurdles effectively. As healthcare faces an era defined by both disruptive technological progress and unprecedented population needs, AI and Blockchain will remain integral to building future-ready oncology systems that are both innovative and ethically grounded. By uniting emerging computational methodologies with a commitment to privacy, transparency, and inclusivity, cancer care can become more efficient, resilient, and attuned to the nuanced needs of patient communities (Kasneci et al., 2023).

Linking Decentralized Capabilities with Organizational Theory in Oncology

Decentralized identity management and privacy-preserving machine learning—cornerstones of AI- and Blockchain-driven approaches—do not function as standalone technical tools. Rather, these capabilities are deeply intertwined with foundational tenets of organizational theory, offering oncology-focused institutions a robust framework for understanding and adapting to emerging complexities. By situating decentralized capabilities within broader organizational contexts, it becomes evident how they can foster resilience, catalyze innovation, and mitigate systemic vulnerabilities in cancer care. This exploration not only establishes the theoretical grounding of decentralized capabilities but also elucidates their real-world applications in addressing the inherent challenges of delivering secure, patient-centered oncology services (Kotcher et al., 2021).

Organizational theory has long served as a pivotal lens for examining healthcare structures, behaviors, and evolutionary trajectories. Within this scholarly domain, perspectives such as resource dependency theory, institutional theory, and systems thinking offer valuable paradigms for interpreting how oncology organizations function and evolve. When examined alongside these theoretical constructs, decentralized identity management and privacy-preserving AI emerge as a natural extension of organizational adaptability—one that promotes preemptive responsiveness to new risks, opportunities, and complexities in cancer care. From the vantage point of resource dependency theory, critical resources in oncology include robust data-sharing infrastructures, specialized clinical expertise, Blockchain-based authentication protocols, and sustainable funding models (Mele et al., 2023). Decentralized capabilities dovetail with this perspective by spotlighting the strategic detection and allocation of these essential resources. Privacy-preserving machine learning can, for instance, identify resource bottlenecks—such as shortages of oncologists or limited diagnostic equipment—while decentralized identity tools help maintain secure patient data flows. Through "sensing," organizations uncover data breaches or emerging treatment gaps; via "seizing," they deploy Blockchain solutions that validate user identities and channel AI-driven analytics to where they are most needed. "Transforming" entails reconfiguring workflows to embed these solutions seamlessly. During major public health disruptions, such as the COVID-19 pandemic, healthcare systems that leveraged decentralized capabilities rapidly retooled operations and reallocated resources—demonstrating how these mechanisms reinforce organizational stability in volatile times (Pereira, Bianchi, Araújo, 2021).

Institutional theory offers another prism through which to view decentralized approaches in oncology. This perspective foregrounds the role of regulations, cultural norms, and societal imperatives in shaping organizational practices. Cancer care institutions must navigate an intricate array of compliance mandates, ethical obligations, and patient expectations for secure, equitable treatment. Decentralized identity management, coupled with privacy-preserving AI, enables organizations to reconcile these often-competing demands. The swift rise of telemedicine in oncology exemplifies how institutions utilized decentralized tools not only to safeguard patient data but also to align with newly evolving societal norms and regulatory parameters (Pesqueira, Sousa, 2022).

Systems thinking underscores the dynamic interplay among the myriad components that define oncology ecosystems—from national cancer registries to patient advocacy groups. In this context, decentralized capabilities resonate strongly, providing a structured means of managing complex interdependencies and anticipating system-wide disruptions. Privacy-preserving machine learning, for instance, can help detect emerging trends in cancer incidence or expedite the identification of effective treatment regimens, while Blockchain technology ensures that data access is governed transparently across diverse stakeholders. By synchronizing workflows, decentralized solutions help mitigate siloed operations, thereby yielding synergistic benefits for both patient outcomes and operational efficiency. For example, an oncology network implementing a decentralized identity can unify oncologists, pathologists, and clinical trial researchers into a secure data exchange environment, thereby promoting holistic care and bolstering overall system resilience. This convergence between decentralized capabilities and organizational theory emphasizes the necessity of framing adaptability within a cohesive theoretical foundation. Cancer care institutions must not only respond to immediate environmental pressures but also develop a thorough comprehension of how such pressures intersect with their strategic imperatives and broader societal obligations. Here, privacy-preserving AI and Blockchain are more than technical enablers; they constitute dynamic drivers of organizational evolution (Secinaro et al., 2021). They bridge the divide between abstract theoretical principles—like resource dependency or institutional expectations—and tangible strategies that uphold both patient-centric values and data security. By weaving decentralized capabilities into their strategic blueprints, oncology-focused organizations can anticipate emerging threats, seize technological breakthroughs, and reconfigure processes to remain both competitive and socially accountable. Moreover, the influence of decentralized capabilities extends beyond individual clinics or hospitals to shape broader oncology ecosystems (Wada et al., 2022). By integrating the principles of resource dependency, institutional theory, and systems thinking, healthcare networks can address longstanding inefficiencies, nurture adaptive research and development, and cultivate sustainable practices at regional and global scales. For instance, multi-institutional oncology collaborations that employ Blockchain-based identity verification can streamline patient enrollment in clinical trials, swiftly sharing privacy-preserved genomic data for improved targeting of advanced therapeutics. Such system-level coordination ultimately contributes to more equitable and effective care, reinforcing the transformative potential of decentralized frameworks in fostering adaptive, patient-focused oncology networks (Pesqueira, Sousa, 2022).

Table 1 presents the key relationships and corresponding implications in aligning decentralized capabilities with established organizational theories to illuminate their collective capacity to spur innovation, resilience, and ethical stewardship within modern cancer care. By rooting decentralized identity management and privacy-preserving AI solutions in existing theoretical frameworks, oncology institutions gain actionable strategies for navigating an environment marked by rapid scientific breakthroughs and evolving patient needs. This alignment underscores the pivotal role of these capabilities in sculpting a future where data security, patient trust, and clinical excellence converge. As the oncology sector contends with unprecedented challenges and opportunities, embedding decentralized capabilities into its organizational architecture will remain indispensable for achieving adaptability, safeguarding patient interests, and fostering sustainable advancements in cancer treatment.

Table 1. Overview of Key Relationships and Theoretical Constructs in Decentralized Oncology Care

Concept	Key Relationship	Practical Application/Implication
Resource Dependency Theory	Focuses on acquiring and strategically allocating critical resources (e.g., skilled personnel, advanced technologies, funding).	Oncology centers utilize privacy-preserving AI to detect resource gaps (e.g., shortage of oncologists), informing Blockchain-supported strategies to optimize resource allocation.
Institutional Theory	Emphasizes alignment with regulatory expectations, ethical standards, and societal norms.	Adoption of decentralized identity management to meet HIPAA/GDPR rules and respond proactively to patient demands for data autonomy, reinforcing institutional legitimacy.
Systems Thinking	Investigates interdependencies among stakeholders, processes, and technologies in complex healthcare ecosystems.	Distributed ledgers and real-time AI analytics unify oncologists, pathologists, and patients, fostering cohesive data-sharing networks that improve care coordination and clinical decision-making.
Decentralized Identity Management	Encourages self-sovereign data ownership and seamless, secure interoperability among stakeholders.	Oncology patients control access to their genomic data on a Blockchain ledger, which reduces risks associated with centralized storage while improving data consistency across providers.
Privacy-Preserving Machine Learning	Integrates AI-driven analytics while safeguarding sensitive health information through encryption and secure computation methods.	Predictive modeling for cancer progression uses homomorphic encryption, enabling analysis of patient data without compromising personal details.
Blockchain-Based Infrastructure	Enhances transparency, auditability, and tamper-proof data exchange across diverse healthcare entities.	Providers and research institutions collaborate through a permissioned Blockchain, ensuring that only authorized stakeholders can update patient records or trial outcomes.
Collaboration Among Multidisciplinary Teams	Aligns diverse expertise (e.g., oncologists, data scientists, ethicists) for holistic patient care and cutting-edge research.	Cancer treatment plans are refined by cross-functional teams using shared Blockchain data, ensuring each specialist's insights inform a unified, patient-centered strategy.
Regulatory Compliance	Necessitates adherence to rules such as HIPAA, GDPR, and other data protection and ethics standards across global contexts.	Oncology institutions embed automated consent mechanisms into their Blockchain platforms, maintaining transparency and preventing unauthorized data access.
Ethical Considerations	Addresses issues of equity, patient autonomy, and data fairness in AI-driven oncology solutions.	To avoid bias in cancer detection models, diverse global datasets are integrated through federated learning to ensure equitable performance across demographics.
Organizational Culture	Cultivates a shared vision and readiness for adopting novel technologies in decentralized, patient-focused care models.	Leaders emphasize training and trust-building around AI and Blockchain tools, shaping a receptive environment for collaborative innovation.
Sustainable Oncology Ecosystem	Encompasses the long-term adaptability and resilience needed to navigate evolving clinical, regulatory, and technological landscapes.	Systems integrate dynamic capabilities, decentralized identity, and AI governance frameworks, positioning oncology care networks for rapid responsiveness and lasting impact.

Source: the authors

The Intersection of AI and Blockchain for Privacy and Security in Smart Medical Systems

The relationship between AI and Blockchain represents a foundational element of secure, privacy-preserving capabilities in oncology care. Together, these evolving technologies enable smart medical systems to anticipate, respond to, and shape an environment marked by rapid, often unpredictable transformations. AI provides analytical precision and operational insights derived from vast clinical datasets, while Blockchain ensures the trust, transparency, and decentralization required to protect patient data. This synergy facilitates secure collaboration and continuous innovation, positioning oncology organizations to thrive within an increasingly complex healthcare landscape. By examining the integrated roles of AI and Blockchain, we gain a deeper appreciation of their combined contributions to elevating security, privacy, and efficiency in cancer care (Tariq et al., 2022).

AI acts as a catalyst for modern privacy-preserving capabilities by equipping oncology providers with tools that enhance predictive accuracy and reduce administrative burdens. Through techniques such as machine learning and advanced analytics, clinical teams can identify at-risk patient populations, forecast disease progression, and formulate precision treatment strategies. For instance, AI-driven image recognition software can detect subtle biomarkers in diagnostic scans, thereby improving early cancer detection rates. Simultaneously, predictive modeling aids in resource allocation by estimating patient influx or drug supply shortages, thus optimizing operational planning. In addition, the adoption of privacy-preserving machine learning—where sensitive patient information is encrypted during data processing—bolsters the ethical and legal integrity of AI applications (Leffa et al., 2022). These advances underscore AI's potential to address immediate clinical challenges while anticipating long-term shifts, thereby future-proofing oncology care. Blockchain, however, undergirds the secure exchange of sensitive data, serving as the foundational layer that safeguards confidentiality and establishes trust among stakeholders. In many respects, distributed ledgers function as a "digital backbone" for AI-driven oncology solutions, ensuring that patient information remains protected against tampering or unauthorized access. Blockchain-based identity management systems empower patients to control their medical records through decentralized identifiers, underscoring the principle of data sovereignty. This approach necessitates a workforce adept at leveraging both cryptographic protocols and advanced analytics. Training initiatives, therefore, become an essential element of secure oncology care. Healthcare professionals who grasp the nuances of distributed ledger technologies are better positioned to integrate AI-driven solutions ethically and effectively within clinical workflows, underscoring the strategic importance of interdisciplinary development (Koubaet al., 2023).

Organizational culture significantly influences how AI and Blockchain merge to strengthen privacy and security in smart medical systems. A culture that nurtures continuous learning and constructive experimentation encourages clinicians, data scientists, and administrators to embrace cryptographically secure workflows. By promoting trust and mutual support, oncology institutions can unify these roles under a common goal: improving patient outcomes through secure, data-driven care. For example, cross-functional seminars that bring together oncologists, bioinformaticians, and Blockchain developers help break down communication barriers, leading to more coherent strategies that address both clinical and technical considerations. This cultural alignment ensures that advanced data solutions are integrated seamlessly, reinforcing an organization's capacity to safeguard patient information while driving evidence-based innovation (ElBaih, 2023).

The intersection of AI and Blockchain creates a powerful synergy that transforms oncology care. When Blockchain-enabled data governance frameworks intersect with AI's predictive capabilities, clinicians can uncover critical disease insights without compromising sensitive patient information. For instance, robust cryptographic methods and federated learning can facilitate multi-institutional research collaborations, enabling clinicians to share anonymized datasets that fuel the development of novel cancer therapies. Meanwhile, administrative teams equipped with AI forecasting models can streamline resource allocation, ensuring that hospital beds, diagnostic equipment, and specialized personnel are mobilized efficiently. These use cases highlight how the combination of AI and Blockchain can refine both clinical precision and operational resilience in oncology (Eager, Brunton, 2023).

Interdisciplinary collaborations serve as a practical illustration of this synergy. When AI algorithms and distributed ledgers are embedded in a team-based environment, healthcare professionals can coordinate diagnoses, treatment plans, and research initiatives with greater confidence. Real-time communication platforms—enhanced by Blockchain verification—help reduce redundancies, minimize errors, and unify healthcare efforts around patient-centric objectives. This integration underscores the necessity of aligning investment in cryptographic infrastructure with workforce development, guaranteeing that staff are proficient in AI methodologies while also understanding the foundational principles of distributed ledger systems. Such collaborative immersion fosters collective ownership of security protocols, translating technological promise into tangible clinical benefits (Cifuentes-Faura, 2022).

Nonetheless, the path to fully capitalizing on these innovations involves confronting significant challenges. Resistance to novel data governance solutions, for example, may deter adoption within institutions accustomed to legacy systems. Overcoming this inertia demands clear communication of benefits for patient confidentiality, accelerated research outcomes, and streamlined operations—supported by transparent change management. Ethical questions surrounding data bias, equitable access to AI tools, and the responsible use of Blockchain also require careful deliberation. Healthcare organizations must integrate robust oversight mechanisms that reconcile rapid technological advancement with the imperative of protecting patient welfare and maintaining trust in sensitive environments like oncology. Another critical factor is inclusivity. AI and Blockchain applications have the potential to exacerbate disparities if training and resources remain unevenly distributed across different roles and regions. Targeted educational programs and equitable resource allocation can mitigate such imbalances, ensuring that the benefits of privacy-preserving health technologies reach broader demographics. These inclusive strategies amplify innovation by embracing a wide array of perspectives, ultimately enhancing the adaptability of cancer care and paving the way for scalable, patient-centered solutions (Amini & Jahanbakhsh Javid, 2023).

The future of privacy-preserving systems in oncology hinges on the seamless interplay of AI and Blockchain, especially as emerging tools—such as quantum-resistant encryption or advanced secure multiparty computation—gain traction. While these breakthroughs promise to heighten data security, continuous workforce development and ethical vigilance will remain paramount. By uniting technological investments with comprehensive training programs and inclusive organizational cultures, oncology providers can cultivate adaptive, future-ready capabilities. In doing so, they position themselves as leaders in a healthcare landscape defined by both innovation and accountability, ultimately offering resilient solutions to an ever-evolving set of clinical challenges. The relationship between AI and Blockchain thus serves as the nexus of privacy and security, forming a synergistic framework for robust oncology care. While AI delivers the analytics and predictive power necessary for proactive decision-making, Blockchain provides the secure environment needed to maintain trust among patients and stakeholders. In unison, these technologies enable oncology organizations to address pressing clinical issues, harness research insights, and innovate responsibly in a rapidly advancing field. By strategically investing in both cryptographic architectures and the professional development of healthcare teams, organizations can realize the full promise of privacy-preserving capabilities, ensuring that smart medical systems advance alongside the evolving demands of patients and providers alike (Ball, 2021).

Framework for Evaluating Privacy-Preserving Capabilities in Oncology Care

The integration of AI-driven analytics and Blockchain-based identity management in oncology care requires not only thoughtful implementation but also ongoing evaluation to confirm their efficacy. Such evaluation is vital to understanding how effectively these privacy-preserving approaches enable medical systems to adapt to emerging threats, capitalize on technological breakthroughs, and transform operational processes for sustained innovation and resilience. A structured framework for assessing the presence and impact of privacy-preserving strategies provides oncology-focused institutions with the means to gauge progress, pinpoint deficiencies, and concentrate efforts on continuous improvement. By emphasizing the core processes of sensing, seizing, and transforming, this framework supports a holistic examination of AI- and Blockchain-supported capabilities within intricate oncology settings (Bouguerra et al., 2022).

Evaluating the sensing process involves examining how adeptly an organization detects both risks and opportunities in its external environment. Relevant metrics may encompass the comprehensiveness of Blockchain audit trails, the efficacy of AI-driven anomaly detection, and the speed at which institutions react to evolving cybersecurity threats. For instance, an oncology center's capacity to anticipate shifts in patient data privacy regulations or sudden spikes in malignant disease prevalence can be measured by the robustness of its predictive analytics and the timeliness of its strategic responses. Secure multiparty computation and federated learning tools significantly enhance the sensing process, and their success can be gauged by their contributions to safeguarding patient records while preserving diagnostic accuracy (Pesqueira, Sousa, Pereira, 2023).

The seizing process is equally integral to the overall impact of privacy-preserving systems. This stage entails mobilizing relevant resources and deploying strategies that capitalize on identified technological or clinical opportunities. Evaluation typically emphasizes resource allocation efficacy, stakeholder engagement in AI–Blockchain projects, and the success rate of newly launched initiatives. For example, a cancer treatment center's adoption of decentralized identity platforms or expansion of secure telehealth services can be analyzed by examining activation timelines, user engagement, and outcomes related to confidentiality. Moreover, an organization's dexterity in reallocating resources during crises—such as abrupt surges in-patient admissions—reflects its effectiveness in seizing (Alawida et al., 2023). Comparative assessment tools can benchmark these factors against recognized best practices, yielding insights on institutional readiness and areas needing refinement. Transforming processes, which involve reorganizing clinical workflows and administrative systems to sustain long-term benefits, often represent the most difficult domain to assess. Key metrics here might include the proportion of successfully integrated privacy-preserving machine learning models, the frequency of secure data-sharing collaborations, and the alignment of transformation activities with strategic oncology objectives. As an example, oncology systems moving from paper-based records to Blockchain-protected digital platforms can track progress through enhanced data integrity, positive patient feedback, and optimized resource use. Continuous improvement paradigms, including iterative design sprints, serve as valuable assets for overseeing and refining these transformations. Tools that evaluate professional development initiatives, cross-functional coordination, and encryption-based practices provide further insight into how effectively organizations embed secure, patient-focused capabilities (Mostafiz et al., 2022).

Benchmarking assumes a central role in the evaluation procedure, offering oncology care providers a means of measuring their AI–Blockchain solutions against both global standards and peer institutions. Such comparative analytics yield tangible data—both quantitative and qualitative—on performance disparities and inform forward-looking strategic plans. For instance, cancer research centers might benchmark their implementation of privacy-preserving genomics platforms or success with decentralized consent procedures against exemplars worldwide. These comparisons not only spotlight areas of underperformance but also encourage the adoption of cutting-edge solutions to enhance patient autonomy and data security. Continuous improvement remains integral to the privacy-preserving framework (Breaux et al., 2023). Given the dynamic nature of cancer care and data protection demands, organizations must remain proactive and forward-thinking. Ongoing evaluations enable them to adjust objectives, refine processes, and stay aligned with evolving standards of care and regulatory requirements. Tools such as key performance indicators (KPIs) and secure analytics dashboards prove indispensable for tracking changes in diagnostic throughput or real-time data integrity, directly correlating these developments with the efficacy of AI–Blockchain strategies.

Examples of oncology ecosystems that have successfully instituted privacy-preserving frameworks offer practical lessons on best practices and potential pitfalls. A notable illustration is the prompt deployment of decentralized tele oncology solutions during global health emergencies. Several institutions displayed robust sensing capabilities by identifying the urgent need for remote, secure consultations. They seized this opportunity by reassigning resources toward telehealth initiatives anchored by Blockchain-secured video platforms. Over the long term, these organizations showcased their transforming capabilities by firmly incorporating Tele oncology into routine practice, thus ensuring sustained patient access and data protection beyond the immediate crisis. Another example involves the integration of privacy-preserving genomic analysis, whereby healthcare providers leverage secure multiparty computation to deliver individualized treatment regimens without compromising sensitive genetic information (Spiel et al.,2022).

Table 2 presents a framework for assessing privacy-preserving systems within oncology-focused institutions that not only evaluates current performance but also guides continuous enhancement. By systematically analyzing sensing, seizing, and transforming processes, healthcare providers can identify strengths, target weaknesses, and seize emergent opportunities for progress. Implementing robust performance metrics, comparative benchmarks, and iterative methodologies upholds the role of AI–Blockchain capabilities as a foundational force for adaptability, resilience, and excellence in oncology care. This framework offers a roadmap that empowers organizations to tackle the multifaceted challenges of modern medicine, fostering an ethos of long-term innovation and sustainability for both healthcare professionals and the patients they serve.

Table 2. Components of a Privacy-Preserving Framework for Oncology Care

Focus Area	Key Strategies	Evaluation Metrics	Example Tools/Approaches
Data Integration	Consolidate patient records, genomic data, and clinical notes on secure, decentralized platforms	- Percentage of records seamlessly shared across departments - Reduction in data redundancy	Blockchain-based EHRs; permissioned data lakes
AI-Driven Anomaly Detection	Employ machine learning to identify irregularities in diagnostic images, resource usage, or network activity	- Speed of threat detection - Accuracy of anomalies flagged	Federated learning algorithms; secure multiparty computation
Resource Allocation	Optimize staffing, equipment, and funding in response to changing patient loads or novel treatments	- Time to reallocate resources - Utilization rates in high-demand areas	Predictive analytics dashboards; real-time Blockchain audits

continued on following page

Table 2. Continued

Focus Area	Key Strategies	Evaluation Metrics	Example Tools/Approaches
Decentralized Identity	Empower patients with self-sovereign data ownership and consent controls	- Rates of patient-controlled data sharing - Reduction in unauthorized data access	Decentralized identifiers (DIDs); smart contracts for access permissions
Telehealth Implementation	Expand secure virtual consultations and remote patient monitoring	- Adoption rates of telehealth platforms - Patient satisfaction scores	End-to-end encrypted video platforms; Blockchain-based appointment verification.
Secure Genomic Analysis	Analyze genetic profiles with privacy-preserving techniques to offer personalized treatment plans	- Encryption success rate - Turnaround times for genomic data processing	Homomorphic encryption; encrypted big-data pipelines
Workforce Training	Provide targeted education on cryptographic protocols, AI ethics, and decentralized data governance	- Completion rates for security and AI-focused modules - Staff proficiency scores	Interdisciplinary workshops; online certification programs
Organizational Culture	Foster an inclusive environment that values continual learning and secure data practices	- Frequency of cross-functional forums - Employee feedback on data privacy and innovation	Town-hall meetings; collaborative hackathons
Ethics and Fairness	Incorporate bias detection and equitable access into AI–Blockchain workflows	- Representation in datasets - Frequency of algorithmic audits	Fairness-aware machine learning tools; routine bias assessments
Benchmarking & Best Practices	Compare performance and security measures against peer institutions and international standards	- Number of benchmark studies conducted Gap analyses highlighting areas for improvement	External audits; shared performance scorecards
Continuous Improvement	Iterate on privacy-preserving methods to remain aligned with evolving clinical needs and regulatory frameworks	- Frequency of framework revisions - Ongoing compliance with relevant data protection laws	Balanced scorecards; agile development sprints

ROADMAP AND FRAMEWORK

The creation of this roadmap and framework for integrating AI and Blockchain in oncology care is grounded in a synthesis of theoretical underpinnings, empirical observations, and pragmatic imperatives. Contemporary healthcare organizations operate within intricate environments characterized by surging data volumes, rapid technological breakthroughs, and persistently evolving patient needs. Consequently, establishing a structured and empirically validated approach to implementing decentralized identity management and privacy-preserving machine learning is essential for fostering resilience, innovation, and secure data management. This section outlines the theoretical rationales and practical validations that highlight the significance of this roadmap and framework. The roadmap draws substantially on theoretical perspectives related to resource orchestration and decentralized data governance, each of which finds a natural nexus in AI–Blockchain convergences. These perspectives posit that an organization's ability to preserve security and privacy in smart medical systems hinges on a combination of internal competencies and strategic technology adoption. By introducing self-sovereign identities, zero-knowledge proofs, and distributed ledgers, organizations can remain responsive to disruptions, whether driven by regulatory shifts, emerging therapies, or healthcare crises. In an oncology setting, these principles hold relevance, given the diversity of clinical trials, the sensitivity of patient data, and the urgency of timely interventions. The roadmap aligns with these considerations by presenting a systematic mechanism for implementing and continuously refining AI- and Blockchain-based processes.

Empirical evidence further substantiates the need for such a framework. Numerous case analyses illustrate the transformative impact of secure data exchange and AI-driven analytics in oncology. For instance, during surges in patient volumes, institutions with robust Blockchain infrastructures responded by automating identity verifications and triaging critical cases through AI-based risk stratification. Likewise, seizing opportunities to integrate federated learning platforms proved instrumental in many healthcare organizations, enabling secure data collaborations without compromising patient privacy. These examples affirm the utility of AI and Blockchain while underscoring the necessity of an accompanying roadmap to replicate successes methodically across diverse clinical environments. By encompassing relevant metrics and benchmarking tools, the framework ensures that organizations can identify best practices and tailor them to specific oncological needs. The framework's emphasis on quantifiable measurements and iterative improvement is supported by established methodologies in healthcare performance assessment. Instruments such as balanced scorecards, KPIs, and comparative analytics have historically aided strategic decision-making and program evaluation. Incorporating these proven techniques into AI–Blockchain adoption ensures that the roadmap remains both systematic and actionable. For example, KPIs that track improvements in data security breaches, reductions in patient wait times, or gains in diagnostic accuracy serve as concrete indicators of success, directly linking decentralized identity solutions to organizational outcomes.

A further rationale for the roadmap stems from systems thinking—a conceptual approach that perceives healthcare organizations as interconnected, adaptive networks. Systems thinking underscores the interactions among institutional processes, digital infrastructures, and clinician engagement. The roadmap mirrors this integrative viewpoint by bridging user applications (e.g., privacy-preserving analytics), business processes (e.g., patient registration and triage), and technological layers (e.g., Blockchain protocols). By illustrating how developments in one layer can precipitate changes in others, the framework fully addresses the complexity of oncology institutions and provides a coherent path toward secure, data-driven transformation.

Validation of the framework is also achieved through its versatility across different healthcare contexts. The phased methodology—from assessing current data governance practices to deploying advanced AI–Blockchain architectures—allows organizations to customize the roadmap to their specific limitations or opportunities. A regional cancer clinic with limited connectivity, for example, may prioritize foundational elements such as secure teleconsultations and basic patient ledgers, whereas a major research hospital could invest in advanced privacy-preserving computations and real-time genomic analytics. This adaptability maximizes the roadmap's relevance for a wide spectrum of oncology care providers, thereby reinforcing its practicality. Additionally, the framework addresses critical hurdles in healthcare innovation, such as organizational hesitation and the necessity for stakeholder consensus. Studies in change management stress the importance of transparent communication, early demonstrations of value, and inclusive leadership to overcome reluctance. The roadmap incorporates these insights by advocating pilot implementations and phased rollouts, allowing organizations to showcase immediate benefits and accumulate trust incrementally. Moreover, benchmarking features enable institutions to compare internal progress against prevailing standards, offering motivation and clear targets for collective achievement.

Ethical considerations further validate the importance of this roadmap and framework. As AI and IoT gain prominence in healthcare, concerns about patient privacy, equitable algorithmic design, and data sovereignty intensify. The framework addresses these issues by embedding specific evaluative criteria into each layer of the AI–blockchain architecture. For instance, performance metrics go beyond predictive accuracy to encompass fairness assessments and compliance with privacy regulations. By weaving ethical factors into the deployment cycle, the roadmap supports oncology transformation that not only augments efficiency but also safeguards public confidence. Finally, the roadmap and framework align with global directives and emerging standards in digital healthcare. Organizations such as the World Health Organization emphasize data integrity, while regional regulatory bodies stress patient rights and confidentiality in clinical research. By emphasizing decentralized identity and privacy-preserving machine learning, the framework equips healthcare entities to meet these requirements, respond proactively to global health emergencies, and elevate care provision. For example, the emphasis on advanced analytics for patient stratification dovetails with international aims to optimize resources, reduce care disparities, and enhance clinical outcomes in oncology.

Hence, the development of this roadmap and framework for integrating AI and Blockchain in oncology is underpinned by extensive theoretical foundations and practical validations. Anchored in decentralized data governance, systems thinking, and iterative performance management, the roadmap offers a targeted, strategic approach to building secure, privacy-preserving, and patient-centric solutions. Real-world evidence from clinical contexts bolsters its value, while its flexible design broadens its applicability. By proactively integrating ethical principles and reflecting broader healthcare priorities, the framework encourages transparent and equitable innovation. In sum, this comprehensive approach empowers oncology organizations to navigate complexity responsibly, thereby ensuring their relevance and resilience in a fast-evolving healthcare ecosystem.

Challenges and Paradoxes in Operationalizing AI and Blockchain Solutions

Implementing AI and Blockchain capabilities in healthcare poses multifaceted complexities, revealing intrinsic tensions and dilemmas. These difficulties arise as organizations strive to balance technological innovation with data protection, reconcile new security models with established routines, and secure alignment among diverse stakeholders. While decentralized identity management and privacy-preserving machine learning hold substantial promise for oncology care, applying these concepts in practice reveals substantial hurdles that must be overcome to attain their full potential. A significant challenge in realizing AI–Blockchain solutions is the tension between existing institutional frameworks and the imperative for rapid experimentation. Large healthcare organizations, particularly those specializing in oncology, often rely on legacy systems that have been optimized for incremental changes and compliance-driven operations. These traditional models, although beneficial for sustaining routine procedures, can stifle agility in scenarios that demand major transformation. For example, rigid data-sharing protocols and siloed infrastructures may impede the swift deployment of cryptographic tools or hamper the scaling of secure telehealth solutions. Furthermore, operational cultures that emphasize risk avoidance and regulatory compliance often leave limited latitude for pioneering data governance strategies (Pesqueira, Sousa, 2022).

At the same time, healthcare institutions confront intensifying pressures to adapt to cutting-edge analytics, heightened patient privacy demands, and new therapeutic breakthroughs. Meeting these expectations demands a willingness to recalibrate or even discard entrenched methods—an inclination that can clash with the inertia inherent in well-established organizations. Bridging this gap necessitates proactive approaches, including dedicated leadership support for AI–Blockchain pilots, the reduction of bureaucratic barriers, and investments in novel competencies. Executive endorsement, in particular, helps foster an environment more hospitable to secure data experimentation and is instrumental in carrying forward the organizational vision of advanced privacy-preserving solutions. Another central challenge is balancing strategic, long-term investments against short-term operational imperatives. AI and Blockchain initiatives emphasize future-proofing—developing tools that are adaptable, scalable, and ethically sound—yet oncology settings often juggle immediate needs such as acute patient care, resource bottlenecks, and cost pressures. Consider, for instance, the introduction of a secure multiparty computation platform, which promises large-scale benefits in collaborative cancer research but may demand significant financial and human resources upfront. This dynamic can spark resistance among stakeholders more concerned with preserving day-to-day functionality over achieving transformative, long-range gains (Pesqueira, Sousa, Pereira, 2023).

Exclusively prioritizing short-term fixes can ultimately perpetuate inefficiencies and stifle the transformative potential of AI–Blockchain tools. Achieving a balanced approach calls for organizations to maintain operational excellence while making calculated, forward-looking technology investments. Incremental rollout plans—employing small-scale tests before scaling—can reconcile immediate priorities with ambitious reforms. In parallel, aligning new security protocols and data-sharing platforms with short-term performance indicators, such as swift onboarding of telemedicine systems or measurably enhanced care coordination, can bridge the divide between immediate results and visionary goals. Resistance to change surfaces as another formidable obstacle in executing AI–Blockchain solutions, particularly in highly regulated and risk-sensitive settings like oncology. This hesitance may originate from various quarters, including staff apprehensive about how new data practices could influence patient workflows, or administrative leaders wary of uncertain returns on high-tech investments. Moreover, distinct organizational units often harbor divergent objectives and tolerance for risk, complicating the alignment of strategic aims. Alleviating these concerns necessitates a carefully layered strategy that addresses cultural and infrastructural barriers. Transparent communication is indispensable, ensuring that stakeholders fully comprehend the rationale behind cryptographic transformations, the scope of expected benefits, and the guardrails to address unanticipated risks. Involving frontline personnel at an early stage fosters buy-in and shapes solution design, making it more responsive to actual clinical conditions. Offering upskilling opportunities can further ease the transition, mitigating fears around the complexity of Blockchain-based identities or data encryption systems.

Structural policies also facilitate acceptance of AI–Blockchain solutions. For example, forming multidisciplinary committees can harmonize varied stakeholder priorities and foster collaboration, while flexible resource allocation patterns can incentivize innovative projects without undermining core services. Rewarding risk-taking and cross-departmental collaboration within performance evaluations further support the shift toward advanced, patient-centric data strategies. By linking these incentives to recognized outcomes—such as secure data interoperability or improved patient confidentiality—organizations can reorient staff efforts toward broader transformation objectives. The complex interplay between external mandates and internal dynamics adds additional layers of complexity to AI–Blockchain implementation. Policy changes, competing research initiatives, and public health crises can either accelerate or constrain the adoption of advanced data solutions in oncology. For instance, although global health emergencies might spur greater acceptance of remote monitoring, they may also impose supply-chain constraints or tighten data-sharing regulations. Navigating these variable externalities demands a resourceful stance: forging alliances with regulators or industry groups and exploring pilot programs within compliant frameworks. Regulatory sandboxes, for instance, can permit the controlled testing of Blockchain-based solutions, thereby enabling organizations to embrace innovation without sacrificing patient safety or data integrity.

Moreover, the pursuit of equitable and ethically grounded AI–Blockchain solutions presents a further source of tension. Advanced algorithmic models, while opening new avenues in precision oncology, spark legitimate concerns about privacy, bias, and disparate access. A predictive model trained on incomplete or unrepresentative data could reinforce health inequalities rather than mitigate them. Ensuring that AI–Blockchain projects are equitable and transparent is thus vital to building trust with patients and broader society. This calls for rigorous auditing of datasets, inclusive data-sharing protocols, and deliberate engagement with traditionally underserved communities, ensuring that the benefits of emergent technologies extend widely.

While these challenges and paradoxes may pose significant hurdles, the potential of decentralized identity and privacy-preserving machine learning to reshape oncology care remains considerable. By addressing institutional inertia, reconciling competing objectives, and garnering stakeholder consensus, healthcare providers can harness the transformative power of secure AI–Blockchain frameworks. Achieving these outcomes requires strategic planning supported by visionary leadership, robust governance structures, and a cultural commitment to transparent, patient-focused data policies. Through consistent, sustained actions, healthcare organizations can flourish in ever-shifting landscapes, leveraging AI–Blockchain innovations to bolster patient trust, clinical efficacy, and equitable access.

AI AND BLOCKCHAIN APPLICATIONS IN GLOBAL ONCOLOGY AND POLICY CONTEXTS

AI and Blockchain applications—encompassing privacy-preserving machine learning and decentralized identity solutions—extend beyond individual healthcare institutions to address macro-level, global oncology challenges. In today's interconnected environment, these innovations underpin resilience and adaptability, enabling governments and research consortia to respond effectively to public health threats, drive digital innovation, and cultivate sustainable healthcare delivery. This section explores how AI- and Blockchain-based platforms support disease surveillance, inform adaptive oncology policymaking, and demonstrate their real-world impact through examples of successful global initiatives. The role of AI–Blockchain solutions in managing global crises, such as pandemics or climate-induced public health emergencies, reveals their transformative potential. Disasters of this scope test the responsiveness and coordination of oncological networks, necessitating rapid shifts in diagnosis, treatment protocols, and resource distribution. The COVID-19 pandemic, for instance, showcased notable variations in how nations and organizations utilized secure AI analytics and distributed ledgers to track disease progression and ensure continuity of oncology care. Countries with sophisticated surveillance algorithms and decentralized identity mechanisms detected threats more swiftly, which mitigated the spread of the virus while preserving cancer treatment pipelines. In some settings, early warning dashboards—powered by federated data—guided policymakers in mobilizing personal protective equipment and safeguarding immunocompromised patients.

Seizing opportunities during a global health crisis entails prompt resource allocation and the adoption of innovative practices. During COVID-19, this approach was illustrated by expedited scaling of AI-driven remote consultations and the collaborative, Blockchain-assisted administration of vaccine credentials. Governments and pharmaceutical entities displayed remarkable ingenuity in reorganizing budgets, streamlining consent mechanisms, and forging cross-sector alliances. Initiatives like the global COVAX platform illustrated how decentralized data exchange enables equitable access to vaccines, including those for patients undergoing cancer therapy. This integration of privacy-preserving solutions supports inclusive healthcare strategies, ensuring immunization and treatment services reach low- and middle-income nations promptly. Transforming processes—integrating lasting innovations into standard oncology operations—often proves the most demanding task in times of crisis. Achieving sustainable change requires embedding newly proven data governance models and digital solutions into post-crisis institutional workflows. For example, the widespread deployment of teleoncology services during COVID-19 showcased how AI and Blockchain can enhance accessibility. Yet, maintaining these practices demands long-term investment in broadband infrastructure, streamlined regulation of digital platforms, and workforce training. Countries that institutionalize these solutions are better equipped to cope with future cancer surges and strengthen overall health system resilience.

Beyond immediate disaster management, AI–Blockchain solutions significantly shape adaptive policy frameworks, facilitating robust and equitable oncology systems. Policymakers must grapple with a complex web of issues—from widening healthcare inequalities to resource scarcity and climate-driven health risks. Privacy-preserving solutions enable decision-makers to gather and synthesize large-scale data efficiently, incorporate diverse stakeholder insights, and craft evidence-based policies that bridge short-term imperatives with enduring objectives. Adaptive governance approaches that incorporate AI and distributed data technologies are essential to ensuring oncology systems remain agile in evolving environments. These adaptive frameworks prioritize flexible guidelines and real-time policy refinements, supported by AI analytics capable of identifying emerging trends. For instance, climate change amplifies the incidence of certain cancers by destabilizing environmental conditions and impacting public infrastructure. Decentralized data-sharing arrangements can boost preparedness by linking meteorological data, epidemiological trends, and resource inventories. Governments that invest in advanced surveillance networks, including Blockchain registries for rare tumors, can reorient clinical strategies proactively, reinforcing collaboration among scientists, clinicians, and policymakers.

The global pursuit of universal healthcare coverage (UHC) in oncology contexts illustrates how AI–Blockchain innovations inform policy initiatives. Achieving UHC requires cost management, access to life-saving drugs, and standardized protocols for cancer detection. Countries such as Thailand and Rwanda have demonstrated success in expanding oncology coverage by employing AI-driven resource mapping and decentralized identity tracking. Early identification of at-risk populations informed targeted screening programs, complemented by digital platforms that securely capture patient data. In these examples, timely adoption of privacy-preserving solutions and strong stakeholder coordination underpin equitable treatment outcomes, reducing both late-stage diagnoses and the financial burden on patients. Case studies of cross-border collaborations in oncology highlight the tangible effects of decentralized solutions on systemic transformation. The international effort to control hepatitis-related liver cancers, for instance, demonstrates excellent secure data exchange. Over decades, global partnerships mobilized large-scale immunization initiatives and integrated AI-based analytics to detect emergent viral variants.

Real-time data-sharing networks used Blockchain smart contracts to monitor vaccine stocks, ensuring swift distribution to vulnerable groups. This capability not only aided in reducing infection rates but also enhanced routine immunization structures in many partner nations, cementing significant gains for future cancer-prevention endeavors. A further illustration comes from the 2014–2016 Ebola outbreak in West Africa, which, though not primarily an oncology crisis, underscores the utility of decentralized solutions. Initial containment lagged due to weak surveillance systems and irregular data sharing. As external organizations and local governments improved detection algorithms and established Federated Learning networks, strides in responding to the crisis became apparent. Partnerships propelled the development of secure health IDs, facilitating contact tracing and clinical record tracking. The post-crisis establishment of robust regional platforms, akin to Africa CDC, indicates how AI–Blockchain breakthroughs can fortify preparedness for cancer epidemics in resource-limited settings.

Implementing AI and Blockchain at a global scale demands sustained investment in technological infrastructure, workforce training, and inclusive governance. To build effective surveillance frameworks for high-burden cancers, standardized data definitions, interoperable Blockchain solutions, and advanced analytics engines are vital. Platforms akin to the World Health Organization's repositories could, for example, integrate predictive modeling and secure distributed ledgers, enabling stronger global management of oncological threats. Similarly, operationalizing AI–Blockchain systems depends on establishing finance pools that harness diverse sources—governmental, philanthropic, and private—to expedite deployment in underfunded regions.

Finally, transforming global oncology ecosystems necessitates dismantling structural barriers. Boosting primary healthcare networks, ensuring equitable drug access, and aligning with international development targets (e.g., the UN Sustainable Development Goals) form critical cornerstones. AI–Blockchain solutions must be embedded ethically to promote accessibility, accountability, and public trust. By incorporating anti-bias auditing of machine learning models and ensuring fair data ownership rights, global health institutions can steer digitized cancer strategies responsibly. AI and Blockchain thus represent key architectures for reimagining healthcare on a global scale. By empowering national and transnational actors to detect early signals of emerging threats, collaborate seamlessly to implement new treatments, and reshape structural processes for continuous adaptation, these technologies offer a unified pathway to overcoming the most daunting challenges in global oncology. Empirical examples—from controlling viral pathogens to piloting large-scale immunization drives—underscore their potential and pave the way for a more inclusive, resilient, and ethically sound future of global cancer care.

Integrating AI and Blockchain into Future Healthcare Models

As healthcare systems adapt to rapid technological developments, changing demographics, and mounting societal expectations, the incorporation of AI and Blockchain into oncology environments has become pivotal for ensuring security, scalability, and patient-centered outcomes. These emerging tools—ranging from federated analytics to decentralized identity management—provide robust frameworks for confronting the complexities of next-generation healthcare models. This section aggregates prior themes to propose a forward-oriented vision for AI–blockchain integration in oncology, emphasizing upcoming trends, application strategies, and a transitional roadmap toward sustainable, patient-focused medical systems.

The future of healthcare increasingly hinges on developments such as digital twins, precision oncology, and integrated population health. Digital twins—virtual representations of patients—promise radical shifts in cancer care by enabling predictive modeling, continuous monitoring, and therapy simulations. For instance, AI-driven avatar models can forecast tumor responses to specific drug regimens, aligning care pathways more precisely with each individual's genetic and behavioral profile. Privacy-preserving solutions remain crucial here, ensuring that large volumes of personal data remain secure and anonymized. Through advanced sensing tools, institutions can detect relevant AI or Blockchain breakthroughs, incorporating them into strategic frameworks that preserve patient confidentiality. Precision oncology represents another evolutionary phase, focusing on individualized treatment anchored in robust genomic data. AI–Blockchain platforms expedite collaboration among clinicians, researchers, and policymakers by creating trusted data-sharing ecosystems. Seizing opportunities in this realm demands sophisticated data governance protocols—biobanks, cryptographically secure registries, and interoperable analysis pipelines—so that patients and investigators can securely exchange molecular insights. Transforming organizational processes accordingly requires recalibrating established care workflows, endorsing advanced training curricula, and setting ethical guidelines that keep up with rapidly evolving innovation.

Value-based care, which privileges patient outcomes and cost-effectiveness above mere service volume, resonates strongly with AI–AI-Blockchain approaches in oncology. Healthcare entities transitioning toward this paradigm must maintain an equilibrium between short-term viability and deeper systemic transformations. For example, privacy-preserving analytics can reveal potential savings in chemotherapy scheduling or radiology utilization, offering immediate benefits to administrators and patients. At the same time, organizational structures must evolve to incorporate secure identity layers, cross-functional data teams, and stable investment channels that encourage adaptation. Effective integration of AI–Blockchain solutions thus bolsters value-based methodologies, ensuring that quality improvements and cost reductions endure beyond short-lived initiatives.

Bringing AI and Blockchain into future healthcare settings entails a comprehensive model that addresses institutional, infrastructural, and cultural variables. At the organizational level, leaders play a central role in setting the tone, signaling a readiness to innovate and embrace cryptographic workflows. This may involve forging alliances between oncology clinicians, computational scientists, and administrative personnel, accelerating the assimilation of new digital therapies. Oversight mechanisms aligned with strategic objectives maintain accountability, while a conducive policy environment discourages departmental silos and fosters holistic transformations. From a technical perspective, deploying AI–Blockchain solutions requires adopting modular and interoperable designs that facilitate the seamless exchange of sensitive data across diverse platforms. The additional layer of distributed identity protocols guarantees that patient records remain verifiable yet protected from misuse. Ongoing investments in data encryption, quantum-safe cryptography, and zero-knowledge proofs future-proof these infrastructures against emergent threats. By prioritizing scalability and adaptability, oncology systems can pivot effectively in response to emerging paradigms, such as newly discovered biomarkers or patient-centered financing options.

Culturally, the successful integration of AI and Blockchain depends on workforce empowerment. Multifaceted training programs—spanning cryptography, data visualization, ethics, and patient communication—equip healthcare professionals to effectively leverage novel tools. By actively involving oncologists, nurses, and data technicians in solution design, institutions encourage bottom-up innovation and ensure pragmatic technology adoption. Establishing incentive structures that reward team members for championing decentralized workflows can further catalyze constructive attitudes, thereby embedding AI–AI-Blockchain solutions within everyday processes. A strategic roadmap for transitioning to secure, data-centric oncology services begins with an analysis of existing capabilities. Organizations assess the maturity of their AI-based diagnostic tools, the reliability of data governance, and the readiness of frontline staff. This diagnostic phase sets the stage for targeted improvements—acquiring specialized hardware, forming cross-functional committees, or updating privacy protocols. Early pilot projects then test these changes in specific service lines (e.g., immunotherapy or radiation oncology), generating tangible evidence of improved data privacy and clinical outcomes. These initial successes bolster stakeholder confidence, preparing the ground for comprehensive expansion. Scaling transformations constitute the subsequent milestone, centering on reproducing and extending proven solutions to wider patient populations, varied service lines, or geographically distinct facilities. For instance, a hospital that trialed Blockchain-based electronic health records with an oncology unit might replicate this system across its entire network, adjusting for the unique needs of surgical, pediatric, or geriatric specialties. Managing resistance to sweeping changes requires empathetic communication and clear, quantifiable benefits, backed by robust training and integrated feedback loops. Sustaining progress, the final stage hinges on continuous refinement and vigilance. AI–Blockchain integrations demand iterative reevaluation as regulatory frameworks evolve, novel algorithms surface, or newly identified privacy threats emerge. By instituting cyclical review processes that incorporate patient feedback and alignment with evolving healthcare objectives, oncology systems can remain agile, responsive, and ethically grounded. Tools such as Lean Six Sigma or Balanced Scorecards may help track operational metrics and financial returns, tying them directly to the overarching success of data protection and personalized therapies.

These evolving healthcare paradigms demonstrate how AI–AI-Blockchain solutions stand to revolutionize oncology care. Embracing digital twins, precision medicine, and value-based strategies while upholding security and interoperability forms a comprehensive blueprint for 21st-century healthcare. Organizational readiness, technological foundation, and workforce culture jointly determine the longevity and effectiveness of AI–Blockchain transformations. The proposed roadmap offers a structured path, guiding institutions from the initial appraisal of existing capabilities to the perpetual enhancement of advanced, patient-centered oncology services. A global and policy-level viewpoint further highlights the revolutionary capacity of decentralized analytics, from crisis management to universal coverage expansions. Pandemics, extreme climate events, and social inequities only underscore the necessity for robust, flexible healthcare infrastructures that draw upon advanced data solutions.

Figure 1 illustrates a holistic framework designed to integrate AI- and Blockchain-based solutions in oncology care while ensuring privacy, security, and organizational adaptability. At the top, Policy & Governance encapsulates the regulatory environment and guidelines, that shape how data are collected, stored, and exchanged. This component underscores the critical influence of compliance and policymaking, setting the overall rules that healthcare organizations must follow when implementing cutting-edge digital tools. Beneath this governance layer, Decentralized ID Management ensures that patient identities and health information are safeguarded through cryptographic protocols, giving individuals greater ownership and control of their data. Patients can selectively share pertinent records with authorized providers, effectively promoting transparency while upholding confidentiality. This decentralized approach complements Privacy-Preserving AI/ML, which harnesses techniques like federated learning or homomorphic encryption to analyze sensitive data without directly exposing patients' personal information. Such AI-driven insights enable more accurate diagnostics, risk predictions, and personalized treatment planning in oncology, all while adhering to strict privacy standards. Parallel to these technological enablers is Organizational Culture & Leadership, representing the human element of successful transformation. This domain acknowledges that secure, privacy-respecting technologies cannot reach their full potential without an institutional climate that values innovation, cross-functional collaboration, and consistent ethical oversight. Leaders committed to data stewardship and continuous learning can help reconcile diverse stakeholder interests—spanning clinicians, IT teams, and administrators—and establish a shared vision that fosters trust and adaptability throughout the adoption process. Connecting these domains is Data Integrity & Secure Exchange, a foundational pillar emphasizing encrypted storage, immutable audit trails, and verifiable transactions. It ensures interoperability among different technical layers, guaranteeing that data flowing from decentralized identities to AI-driven analytics remains accurate, consistent, and defensible. In tandem with carefully structured governance frameworks, secure data exchange mechanisms build confidence in the system and encourage further collaboration across the healthcare ecosystem. Finally, at the base, End Users—clinicians, patients, and researchers—interact with and benefit from these integrated solutions. They can rely on privacy-preserving analytics to inform care decisions, enhance diagnostic accuracy, and streamline workflows. Patients experience improved continuity of care through secure, accessible records, while clinicians can harness advanced AI insights to personalize treatments and allocate resources more efficiently. Researchers also gain from robust data streams, supporting evidence-based innovations that can accelerate therapeutic discoveries in oncology. By intertwining decentralized identity management, AI analytics, and leadership-driven governance, oncology-focused institutions can deliver high-quality, patient-centric care while rigorously protecting personal data.

Figure 1. Overview of the Privacy-Preserving AI–Blockchain Framework in Oncology

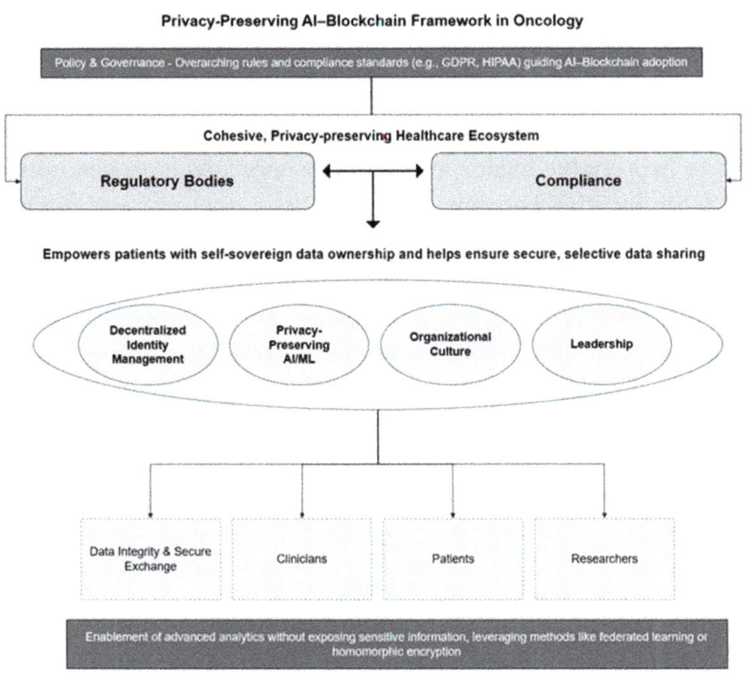

Source: The Authors

CONCLUSION

AI- and Blockchain-based solutions offer a robust foundation for addressing the complexities of contemporary healthcare—particularly in oncology—by facilitating advanced privacy measures, decentralized data ownership, and secure machine learning techniques. By integrating insights from decentralized identity frameworks, global health demands, and future technological trajectories, this discussion has highlighted concrete strategies for embedding privacy-preserving analytics into healthcare institutions, fostering innovation, and driving systemic evolution. The synergy between AI and Blockchain, grounded in secure data exchange, underscores a guiding principle for organizations seeking to remain effective and future-proof amid rapid technological progress, demographic shifts, and evolving patient expectations. Through ongoing data awareness, institutions proactively identify both opportunities (e.g., emerging analytics tools, breakthroughs in cryptography) and threats (e.g., new data breaches or regulatory shifts). Resource mobilization ensures that decentralized ID systems and privacy-preserving machine learning pipelines are integrated efficiently, thereby capitalizing on these newly revealed opportunities. Meanwhile, long-term reconfiguration requires reimagining organizational workflows, technical architectures, and institutional cultures to sustain progressive change and promote continuous adaptation.

The essential role of leadership in operationalizing AI–Blockchain initiatives cannot be overstated. Leadership sets the tone for security and innovation, championing data ethics and flexible thinking throughout the organization. By fostering a climate of open communication, interdisciplinary partnerships, and lifelong learning, leaders enable healthcare systems to overcome internal inertia, reconcile varied stakeholder interests, and achieve lasting transformation goals. Equally vital, effective leadership ensures that equity, inclusivity, and robust patient protections remain central to digital health strategies, reinforcing the broader social mandate of healthcare institutions. Although significant, the challenges and paradoxes of operationalizing AI–AI blockchain solutions in healthcare are not insurmountable. Rigid organizational structures, cultural resistance to experimentation, and the tension between near-term responsibilities and longer-term infrastructural reforms require deliberate, strategic action. By adopting phased rollouts, piloting novel technologies in controlled environments, and using metrics that link cryptographic investments to measurable healthcare outcomes, organizations can mitigate these challenges effectively. The use of comparative benchmarks, continuous improvement models, and collaborative governance frameworks further supports the successful deployment and scaling of secure data solutions.

Within the global health and policy context, these strategies expand beyond individual hospitals to confront systemic challenges and collective goals. By proactively identifying macro-level threats—ranging from pandemic disruptions to supply-chain shortages—organizations can react swiftly by introducing AI-driven triage protocols and transparent Blockchain-based registries. Case studies of worldwide vaccination campaigns and telehealth expansions reveal the transformative potential of privacy-preserving data infrastructures on a global stage. Such examples highlight the value of cross-sector partnerships, adaptive policy-making, and sustained resource investment in data architectures and workforce training. Looking forward, integrating AI–Blockchain solutions into emerging care models presents a vision for patient-centered, sustainable, and digitally advanced systems. Trends like digital twins, precision oncology, and value-based care dovetail with privacy-preserving approaches, illustrating the necessity of adaptability and rapid innovation. By accounting for organizational, technical, and cultural factors, healthcare institutions can effectively deploy these secure technologies, positioning themselves as pioneers of data-driven transformation. The proposed roadmap for migrating to secure, integrated healthcare ecosystems offers a clear strategy for actualizing the potential of AI–Blockchain applications.

This chapter calls upon researchers, practitioners, and policymakers to recognize AI- and Blockchain-based solutions as key enablers of adaptable, secure, and sustainable healthcare. For researchers, this means advancing the theoretical understanding of decentralized analytics and exploring their applicability across diverse clinical settings. Healthcare practitioners are encouraged to incorporate secure data methods into their operational plans, harnessing them to stimulate innovation and improve patient outcomes. Policymakers play a central role by establishing enabling regulations, subsidizing critical infrastructure, and aligning national healthcare priorities with cutting-edge cryptographic safeguards and interoperability guidelines. By reframing adaptability and sustainability through the lens of privacy-preserving technology, healthcare stakeholders can confront urgent challenges while embracing transformative possibilities. Embedding AI and Blockchain in healthcare ecosystems promotes not only resilience and innovation but also ensures that these systems remain equitable, patient-centered, and well-equipped for future demands in an era of accelerated change and uncertainty.

REFERENCES

Alawida, M., Mejri, S., Mehmood, A., Chikhaoui, B., & Isaac Abiodun, O. (2023). A Comprehensive Study of ChatGPT: Advancements, Limitations, and Ethical Considerations in Natural Language Processing and Cybersecurity. *Information (Basel), 14*(8), 462. DOI: 10.3390/info14080462

Amini, M., & Jahanbakhsh Javid, N. (2023). A multi-perspective framework established on diffusion of innovation (DOI) theory and technology, organization and environment (TOE) framework toward supply chain management system based on cloud computing technology for small and medium enterprises. Organization and Environment (TOE) Framework Toward Supply Chain Management System Based on Cloud Computing Technology for Small and Medium Enterprises (January 2023). *International Journal of Information Technology and Innovation Adoption*, *11*, 1217–1234.

Ball, P. (2021). What the COVID-19 pandemic reveals about science, policy and society. *Interface Focus*, *11*(6), 20210022. DOI: 10.1098/rsfs.2021.0022 PMID: 34956594

Bhattamisra, , Banerjee, P., Gupta, P., Mayuren, J., Patra, S., & Candasamy, M. (2023). Artificial Intelligence in Pharmaceutical and Healthcare Research. *Big Data and Cognitive Computing*, *7*(1), 10. DOI: 10.3390/bdcc7010010

Bouguerra, A., Hughes, M., Cakir, M. S., & Tatoglu, E. (2022). Linking entrepreneurial orientation to environmental collaboration: A stakeholder theory and evidence from multinational companies in an emerging market. *British Journal of Management*.

Breaux, R., Shroff, D. M., Cash, A. R., Swanson, C. S., Carlton, C., Bertollo, J. R., & Dahiya, A. V. (2023). Telehealth delivery of the RELAX intervention for families of adolescents diagnosed with ADHD: Preliminary treatment outcomes and evidence of acceptability and feasibility. *Evidence-Based Practice in Child and Adolescent Mental Health*, *8*(1), 24–38. DOI: 10.1080/23794925.2021.1970053

Cifuentes-Faura, J. (2022). European Union policies and their role in combating climate change over the years. *Air Quality, Atmosphere & Health*, *15*(8), 1–8. DOI: 10.1007/s11869-022-01156-5 PMID: 35035604

Dillard-Wright, J., & Shields-Haas, V. (2021). Nursing with the people: Reimagining futures for nursing. *Advances in Nursing Science*, *44*(3), 195–209. DOI: 10.1097/ANS.0000000000000361 PMID: 33624989

Eager, B., & Brunton, R. (2023). Prompting higher education towards AI-augmented teaching and learning practice. Journal of University Teaching & Learning Practice, 20(5), 02.

Ebrahimi, S., & Bridgelall, R. (2021). A fuzzy Delphi analytic hierarchy model to rank factors influencing public transit mode choice: A case study. *Research in Transportation Business & Management*, *39*, 100496. DOI: 10.1016/j.rtbm.2020.100496

ElBaih, M. (2023). The Role of Privacy Regulations in AI Development (A Discussion of the Ways in Which Privacy Regulations Can Shape the Development of AI). Available at *SSRN* 4589207. DOI: 10.2139/ssrn.4589207

Gebhardt, M., Kopyto, M., Birkel, H., & Hartmann, E. (2022). Industry 4.0 technologies as enablers of collaboration in circular supply chains: A systematic literature review. *International Journal of Production Research*, *60*(23), 6967–6995. DOI: 10.1080/00207543.2021.1999521

Haleem, A., Javaid, M., Singh, R. P., & Suman, R. (2022). Medical 4.0 technologies for healthcare: Features, capabilities, and applications. *Internet of Things and Cyber-Physical Systems*, *2*, 12–30. DOI: 10.1016/j.iotcps.2022.04.001

Jacob, C., Bourke, S., & Heuss, S. (2022). From Testers to Cocreators—the Value of and Approaches to Successful Patient Engagement in the Development of eHealth Solutions: Qualitative Expert Interview Study. *JMIR Human Factors*, *9*(4), e41481. DOI: 10.2196/41481 PMID: 36102548

Jalil, S., Rafi, S., LaToza, T. D., Moran, K., & Lam, W. (2023). Chatgpt and software testing education: Promises & perils. In *2023 IEEE International Conference on Software Testing, Verification and Validation Workshops (ICSTW)* (pp. 4130-4137). IEEE. DOI: 10.1109/ICSTW58534.2023.00078

Javaid, M., Haleem, A., & Singh, R. P. (2023). ChatGPT for healthcare services: An emerging stage for an innovative perspective. BenchCouncil Transactions on Benchmarks. *Standards and Evaluations*, *3*(1), 100105.

Junaid, M., Zhang, Q., Cao, M., & Luqman, A. (2023). Nexus between technology enabled supply chain dynamic capabilities, integration, resilience, and sustainable performance: An empirical examination of healthcare organizations. *Technological Forecasting and Social Change*, *196*, 122828. DOI: 10.1016/j.techfore.2023.122828

Kant, N., & Anjali, K. (2021). Blockchain Technology: A Strategic Resource. In Blockchain for Healthcare Systems (pp. 1-15). CRC Press. 13

Kaplan, R. M., & Hays, R. D. (2022). Health-related quality of life measurement in public health. *Annual Review of Public Health*, *43*(1), 355–373. DOI: 10.1146/annurev-publhealth-052120-012811 PMID: 34882431

Kasneci, E., Seßler, K., Küchemann, S., Bannert, M., Dementieva, D., Fischer, F., Gasser, U., Groh, G., Günnemann, S., Hüllermeier, E., Krusche, S., Kutyniok, G., Michaeli, T., Nerdel, C., Pfeffer, J., Poquet, O., Sailer, M., Schmidt, A., Seidel, T., & Kasneci, G. (2023). ChatGPT for good? On opportunities and challenges of large language models for education. *Learning and Individual Differences*, *103*, 102274. DOI: 10.1016/j.lindif.2023.102274

Kendzerska, T., Zhu, D. T., Gershon, A. S., Edwards, J. D., Peixoto, C., Robillard, R., & Kendall, C. E. (2021). The effects of the health system response to the COVID-19 pandemic on chronic disease management: A narrative review. *Risk Management and Healthcare Policy*, *14*, 575–584. DOI: 10.2147/RMHP.S293471 PMID: 33623448

Kotcher, J., Maibach, E., Miller, J., Campbell, E., Alqodmani, L., Maiero, M., & Wyns, A. (2021). Views of health professionals on climate change and health: A multinational survey study. *The Lancet. Planetary Health*, *5*(5), e316–e323. DOI: 10.1016/S2542-5196(21)00053-X PMID: 33838130

Kouba, P., Kohout, P., Haddadi, F., Bushuiev, A., Samusevich, R., Sedlar, J., Damborsky, J., Pluskal, T., Sivic, J., & Mazurenko, S. (2023). Machine Learning-Guided Protein Engineering. *ACS Catalysis*, *13*(21), 13863–13895. DOI: 10.1021/acscatal.3c02743 PMID: 37942269

Kwok, A. O., & Treiblmaier, H. (2023). Blockchain technology as a driver of economic development in small economies: A dynamic capabilities framework. *Journal of Decision Systems*, •••, 1–26.

Leffa, D. T., Grevet, E. H., Bau, C. H. D., Schneider, M., Ferrazza, C. P., da Silva, R. F., Miranda, M. S., Picon, F., Teche, S. P., Sanches, P., Pereira, D., Rubia, K., Brunoni, A. R., Camprodon, J. A., Caumo, W., & Rohde, L. A. (2022). Transcranial direct current stimulation vs sham for the treatment of inattention in adults with attention-deficit/hyperactivity disorder: The TUNED randomized clinical trial. *JAMA Psychiatry*, *79*(9), 847–856. DOI: 10.1001/jamapsychiatry.2022.2055 PMID: 35921102

Masih, E. A. (2022). Feasibility of using QR code for registration & evaluation of training and its ability to increase response rate–The learners' perception. *Nurse Education Today*, *111*, 105305. DOI: 10.1016/j.nedt.2022.105305 PMID: 35220149

Mele, G., Capaldo, G., Secundo, G., & Corvello, V. (2023). Revisiting the idea of knowledge-based dynamic capabilities for digital transformation. *Journal of Knowledge Management*.

Mostafiz, M. I., Musteen, M., Saiyed, A., & Ahsan, M. (2022). COVID-19 and the global value chain: Immediate dynamics and long-term restructuring in the garment industry. *Journal of Business Research*, *139*, 1588–1603. DOI: 10.1016/j.jbusres.2021.10.078

Patil et al. (2022). "Utilization of Artificial Intelligence in Healthcare System, Pharmaceutical Industry & Education". International Journal of Advanced Research in Science, Communication and Technology.

Pereira, R., Bianchi, I. S., & Araújo, V. M. D. S. (2021). Multi-framework implementation of the problem management process. *Форсайт*, *15*(3, 3 (eng)), 94–104. DOI: 10.17323/2500-2597.2021.3.94.104

Pesqueira, A., & Sousa, M. J. (2022). *12 Social Analytics Influencing KOLs Profiling in the Dissemination of Innovations and Scientific Knowledge in the Life Sciences Industry*. Innovations and Social Media Analytics in a Digital Society.

Pesqueira, A., & Sousa, M. J. (2022). Life Sciences Industry Blockchain Value Management, Investments, and Finance Impact Assessment: Global Questionnaire Survey of 1524 Industry Professionals and Executives. In Incorporating AI Technology in the Service Sector (pp. 67-107). Apple Academic Press.

Pesqueira, A. M., Sousa, M., & Pereira, R. (2023). Individual dynamic capabilities influential factors in blockchain technology innovation from hospital settings.

Secinaro, , Calandra, D., Secinaro, A., Muthurangu, V., & Biancone, P. (2021). The role of artificial intelligence in healthcare: A structured literature review. *BMC Medical Informatics and Decision Making*, *21*(1), 125. DOI: 10.1186/s12911-021-01488-9 PMID: 33836752

Shiwlani, A., Khan, M., Sherani, A. M. K., & Qayyum, M. U. (2023). Synergies of AI and Smart Technology: Revolutionizing Cancer Medicine, Vaccine Development, and Patient Care. International Journal of Social. *Humanities and Life Sciences*, *1*(1), 10–18.

Spiel, K., Hornecker, E., Williams, R. M., & Good, J. (2022). ADHD and technology research–investigated by neurodivergent readers. In *Proceedings of the 2022 CHI Conference on Human Factors in Computing Systems* (pp. 1-21). DOI: 10.1145/3491102.3517592

Tariq, , Awan, M. J., Alshudukhi, J., Alam, T. M., Alhamazani, K. T., & Meraf, Z. (2022). Software Measurement by Using Artificial Intelligence. *Journal of Nanomaterials*, *2022*(1), 7283171. DOI: 10.1155/2022/7283171

Ullah, H., Manickam, S., Obaidat, M., Laghari, S. U. A., & Uddin, M. (2023). Exploring the Potential of Metaverse Technology in Healthcare: Applications, Challenges, and Future Directions. *IEEE Access : Practical Innovations, Open Solutions*, *11*, 69686–69707. DOI: 10.1109/ACCESS.2023.3286696

Vallentin, A., Thórisson, K. R., & Latapie, H. (2023). Addressing the Unsustainability of Deep Neural Networks with Next-Gen AI. In International Conference on Artificial General Intelligence (pp. 296-306). Cham: Springer Nature Switzerland. DOI: 10.1007/978-3-031-33469-6_30

Vlasta, M. (2023). Methodological framework for European regulation of (artificial) intelligence and its limits.

Wada, M., Noda, Y., Iwata, Y., Tsugawa, S., Yoshida, K., Tani, H., Hirano, Y., Koike, S., Sasabayashi, D., Katayama, H., Plitman, E., Ohi, K., Ueno, F., Caravaggio, F., Koizumi, T., Gerretsen, P., Suzuki, T., Uchida, H., Müller, D. J., & Nakajima, S. (2022). Dopaminergic dysfunction and excitatory/inhibitory imbalance in treatment-resistant schizophrenia and novel neuromodulatory treatment. *Molecular Psychiatry*, *27*(7), 2950–2967. DOI: 10.1038/s41380-022-01572-0 PMID: 35444257

Wamba, S. F., Queiroz, M. M., Jabbour, C. J. C., & Shi, C. V. (2023). Are both generative AI and ChatGPT game changers for 21st-Century operations and supply chain excellence? *International Journal of Production Economics*, *265*, 109015. DOI: 10.1016/j.ijpe.2023.109015

Wani, . (2022). Utilization of Artificial Intelligence in Disease Prevention: Diagnosis, Treatment, and Implications for the Healthcare Workforce. *Health Care*. PMID: 35455786

Yulianti, T., & Sulistyawati, A. (2021). Enhancing public speaking ability through focus group discussion. [Pendidikan Dan Pengajaran]. *JURNAL PAJAR*, *5*(2), 287–295.

Chapter 12
Patient-Centered Healthcare:
Trust and Transparency Through Technology

Wasswa Shafik
https://orcid.org/0000-0002-9320-3186
Dig Connectivity Research Laboratory (DCRLab), Kampala, Uganda & School of Digital Science, Universiti Brunei Darussalam, Gadong, Brunei

ABSTRACT

This chapter explores the critical intersection of technology, trust, and transparency in advancing patient-centered healthcare. With digital innovations such as electronic health records, artificial intelligence, wearable devices, and blockchain, healthcare providers can now enhance patient engagement, improve care accuracy, and increase access. However, while these technologies offer unprecedented potential for personalized and proactive healthcare, they also pose challenges related to privacy, data security, and the ethical use of information. Through examining how these technologies can both build and compromise patient trust, this study identifies key strategies for enhancing transparency in healthcare delivery, fostering trust through secure and accessible digital solutions, and ensuring that healthcare remains both effective and ethically responsible. Ultimately, this paper underscores the need for a balanced approach that integrates technology with a commitment to patient autonomy, privacy, and clear communication.

1. INTRODUCTION

Patient-centered healthcare aims to provide personalized, tailored care that acknowledges the uniqueness of individual needs and preferences while involving patients and caregivers as essential partners in the provision of care and support. It is based on core principles of respect, dignity, and the empowerment of people to lead their care and treatment to the best of their abilities (Shafik et al., 2025). At the center of care is the person, with an emphasis on attending to people's goals, setting care pathways that facilitate the achievement of these goals, focusing on the capacity and what people can do rather than limitations and deficits, and adopting a strengths-based, rather than a needs-based, approach (Q. Lu et al., 2024). Key to enabling the above is the adoption of a patient-centered approach based on trust-enhancing and transparency values, which engender the belief of being treated with fairness, equity, and involvement in proceedings and care planning. The importance of striving toward making patients more informed

DOI: 10.4018/979-8-3373-0593-6.ch012

and more trusted, as a result, has been highlighted as a key marker to ensure better health outcomes (Sumner et al., 2024). By giving patients the information they need to feel engaged in their care, we can help foster greater trust in the healthcare system and achieve positive outcomes. Furthermore, the vision for Trust proposes that more accessible information is required to enable more effective and efficient communication, leading to better-informed patients. Involving the patient in decision-making and information provision expedites the decision-making process, increasing clarity and transparency, which, in turn, has a much more positive impact on patient needs and leads to a more satisfactory outcome (Zhao & Yam, 2024).

Coined in the 60s, the term patient-centered care has been repurposed and built upon in recent years to finally encompass many of the vital principles that underpin the most successful and persuasive healthcare models worldwide. What constitutes patient-centered care may look different in a sea of diverse practices, but at its core is a shared definition that requires placing the patient in the driver's seat and orienting care around things such as their needs, values, and desired outcomes (Kammerer et al., 2024). Additionally, it sees the importance of tapping into patient psychology and what makes them tick, with good practitioners taking into account the complete array of clinical, human, and environmental variables that collectively influence health outcomes when designing treatment plans. In addition to these clear must-haves, the prevailing opinion suggests that effective patient-centered care ought to be steeped in compassion and empathy, leverage patient and family participation, and result in care that is of high quality and personalized (Sarker, 2024). This new paradigm in care also strives to create an environment where trust can be gradually built over time, and decisions can be made with a greater level of transparency (Shafik, 2025b). When given the straightforward opportunity to choose, many patients rank the doctor-patient relationship as one of the strongest determinants in their degree of satisfaction with the medical care they receive. Unsurprisingly, the medical literature echoes this sentiment and researchers have found that effective patient-provider relationships have a positive impact on not only patient satisfaction scores but, perhaps more importantly, achievement of positive health outcomes (Kvæl et al., 2024). The opportunity to ask questions and exchange ideas is often strongly associated with comforting care experiences, while feeling as though you have a stronger say in your treatment course can reduce fear and anxiety, positively influence health by promoting realistic expectations, and, in some instances, augment adherence to treatment plans (Shafik, 2025c). In short, patient-centered care, initiated by a solid relationship, is good for those who give it and for those on the receiving end. Clearly, embracing patient preferences and needs is vital, but nailing the terminology and design principles to do so isn't always easy (O'Donnell et al., 2024). Technology, however, can be an engaging and, most notably, continuous way to foster relationships between patients and clinicians, and that's exactly what we will explore as Figure 1 presents selected healthcare technologies and their possible applications.

Figure 1. Healthcare enabling technologies

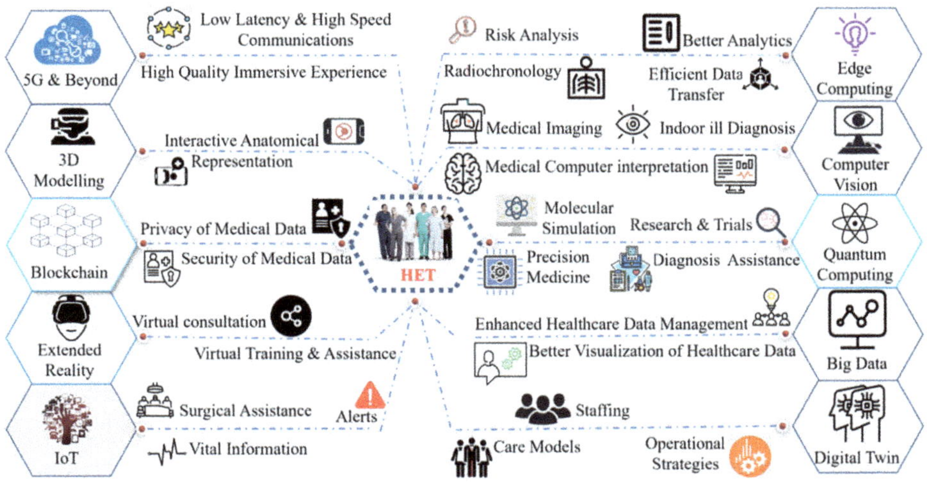

1.1. Definition and Principles

Patient-centered healthcare is a framework that places the patient at the center of the healthcare process, focusing on the personalization of care and treatment to meet unique and individual needs. This means tailoring solutions to the individual rather than the condition, focusing on how the illness impacts lives rather than life impacting the disease, actively collaborating with patients in care and treatment plans, and relying on patients to make decisions that align with their values and preferences (Agwiah & Boateng, 2024). Person- or patient-centered health is built on a set of philosophical principles that should guide interactions with patients:

1) Every person is unique.
2) Every person deserves to be respected and honored fully as a person.
3) Illness impacts individuals in different ways.
4) Every person lives in the context of their families, friends, and communities.
5) An essential aspect of care is the most effective engagement of each person in their journey toward healing and wellness, including the right to either accept or refuse proposed interventions.

There are three key mechanisms by which person- or patient-centered health benefits outcomes: collaboration, communication, and coping. Each of these is an element of the patient-centered approach. Considering these elements of patient-centered healthcare allows for a rather innovative approach to care, viewing healthcare as a unit rather than just including the activities of healthcare personnel in institutions. In working with patients on the nature of illness—rather than disease—care planning and tailoring diagnosis and treatments are identified as some of the practice innovations (Totzkay, 2024). Addressing elements of the patient-centered approach and holding them up to scrutiny is a path to conceptually understanding what it is or what it might be. Patient engagement is understood as a component of the patient-centered approach. However, an overriding philosophy of shared control and shared decision-making is inherent across the tenets developed by humanism (L. L. M. Lu et al., 2024). Two principles of patient participation are introduced:

1) Decision-making is shared, drawing a triangle of knowledge from the healthcare provider, the patient, and the evidence. Each person brings expertise.
2) Patients should be seen for who they are and not defined by the population set they might fall into.

At its core, patient-centered care is about engaging patients as part of their care and the treatment process. Likewise, engaged patients are more satisfied with their care, and satisfied patients are more likely to be engaged in their care (Shafik, 2024j). The initial steps in building patient engagement are rooted in trust and partnerships, thus using a tenet of patient-centered care to validate a component of patient engagement. Trust within the health system fosters better health outcomes and facilitates smoother engagement between parties (Williamson & Prybutok, 2024). All interactions can be considered confidential and respectful, with respect for talents and expertise and sharing of goals and responsibilities. All members within the triangle of knowledge share in the "ministry of care and the burden of loss" for the common purpose of the patient's best interest. Trust is multifaceted and is impacted by social and legal factors, as well as economic and personal attitudes, perceptions, and collaborative relationships (Barden et al., 2024). In short, patient-centered care is a framework that builds upon the underlying philosophy of human and patient-centric care. One core issue that underpins any of what follows is trust. Trust is a central tenet in any conversation about patient-centered care and engagement. Trust is impacted by openness, honesty, and true respect, building interrelationships that allow for some uncertainty and shared regard for roles in a collaborative relationship. Disclosing information with the aim of influencing thinking and feeling, even in a compassionate context, does not foster trust, such as aligning a philosophy and actions that demonstrate person-centered care (Kelsall-Knight & Stevens, 2024).

1.2. Importance of Trust and Transparency

Trust and transparency are key components of a patient-centered healthcare system. Patients' trust in their care providers promotes engagement, active participation in treatment decisions, and a greater likelihood that patients will follow their care providers' guidance. One common definition of trust in healthcare characterizes its three levels or dimensions: relational trust, based on mutual understanding, empathy, and regard; competence trust, predicated on parties' capability and expertise; and integrity trust, based on belief in the motivations and sincerity of one's care providers (Kovaleva et al., 2024). Healthcare institution integrity, competence, and fairness are often discussed in the context of trust and hospitals as well. Moreover, trust inoculates society against alienation, increases rational decision-making choices, and improves the legitimacy and compliance of political institutions. When it comes to transparency, one of its underlying theoretical goals is to restrain potential wrongdoing and misbehaviors, including efforts to harass doctors and aims to centralize institutional information overly (Valentin et al., 2024). In the healthcare context, transparency is often framed in terms of holding organizations that provide care to account: the release of information about quality and cost is thought to lead to increased oversight by patients, governments, and accrediting institutions for the good of all. When healthcare organizations are transparent, they reveal internal information about themselves to patients or other stakeholders with the expectation that others' decision-making and behavior will be changed by that information and motivated toward positive ends, from remaining as patients or families of patients to supplementing or substituting market-based mechanisms for finding information about facilities (Turk et al., 2024). Transparent healthcare institutions serve as trusted partners during decision-making encounters. Improved transparency, accountability, and trust in hospitals are also correlated with higher patient satisfaction scores and increased organizational innovation. Moreover, the electronic health information exchange slowed when security concerns mounted, and trust in regulations created barriers. The context also suggests that distrust of a care provider in the doctor-patient relationship may diminish the efficacy of treatment (Wang et al., 2024).

2. THE EVOLUTION OF TECHNOLOGY IN HEALTHCARE

Technological innovations in medicine can be traced back to prehistoric humans who used trepanation, a surgical process that involved drilling or scraping a hole in the bone of the skull to relieve pressure. Since then, they have had a profound impact on the delivery of care. In the 1910s, formal support groups advocating for hospital systems began to emerge worldwide. Twenty years later, in the 1930s and 1940s, insurance systems fundamentally changed the structures of health systems to operate based on insurance premiums (van Lummel et al., 2024). Technological advancements slowly began to integrate into healthcare settings, enabling greater access to care. For instance, a prototype of the ambulance telephone was introduced in 1946, connecting ambulances to doctors and hospitals by radio to coordinate the life support end route to the hospital. By the 1980s, an intricate telemedicine system was developed to bring astronauts into orbit together with physicians at mission control. Personal digital assistants were introduced in 1996, and in the 2000s, electronic health records became more widely adopted (Blanck et al., 2024). More recently, big data, artificial intelligence, and blockchain for recording transactions have become of increasing interest in relation to healthcare because they are applicable to numerous data, such as costs, demographics, and patient records. The ability of computers to recognize patterns, analyze huge amounts of data, interpret the data, and predict the results has major implications for healthcare. However, technological advancements alone do not address the root causes of ongoing low trust levels (Bense et al., 2024). Understanding recent trends in the use of data analytics, as well as changes in regulatory and use standards, is crucial for pinpointing how broader digital forces have the potential to foster transparency and trust in the patient context. The adoption of electronic health records increased roughly threefold between 2000 and 2015. The digitization of health information has not only helped organize clinical operations and gain significant improvements in operational efficiencies but has also made patient data more easily accessible to a wide range of stakeholders, including patients with secure portals (Sarker, 2024; Shafik, 2024h). Larger data sets and the development of sophisticated machine learning algorithms have further spurred connectivity with other disciplines such as epidemiology, bioinformatics, economics, and other life and social sciences.

2.1. Historical Context

In ancient times, healthcare was based on the knowledge and intuition of individual healers or caregivers. As the scientific method emerged, this tradition provided evidence-based knowledge of anatomy, physiology, pathology, and therapeutics. In the last 200 years, technological progress has brought revolutionary changes in healthcare practice. The division of the body into systems, the revolution of antiseptics, the invention of pharmaceuticals and vaccines, as well as the innovation of surgical techniques have saved millions of lives and have eradicated many infectious diseases from developed countries (Shafik, 2024i; Weber & Nøhr, 2024). For a long time, medical records were stored on paper, and progress was very slow, given that librarians bound them. In recent decades, however, healthcare services have completely transferred their paper-based records into advanced computing systems. This digital medical system has revolutionized the way healthcare is organized and delivered worldwide by streamlining administrative practices and improving patient care. Many technologies have played pivotal roles in these changes; one of the first technical inventions is the X-ray. X-rays transformed the quality of diagnostics compared to the visual and olfactory characteristics used for initial diagnosis (Shafik, 2024d; Umayal, 2024). Laboratory technology then boosted medicine by extending diagnostic disease characterization to the measurement of biological samples such as blood, urine, tissue, and cells. In other areas of practice, medical imaging systems and surgical applications progressed slowly from the likes of computed axial tomography to magnetic resonance imaging, fluoroscopy-guided surgery, robotics, and augmented reality. These technological changing trends have revolutionized clinical practices, improved diagnoses, and increased survival rates by reducing risks, errors, and treatment times. The integration of computers into healthcare practices faced numerous resistances and was met with several challenges, from initial design to current advanced applications (Sarker, 2024; Shafik, 2024c). However, practice is evolving, and vehicles of change posit that healthcare needs to change in terms of drawing the patient into the solution, as depicted in Figure 2.

Figure 2. Health innovation entities and stakeholders

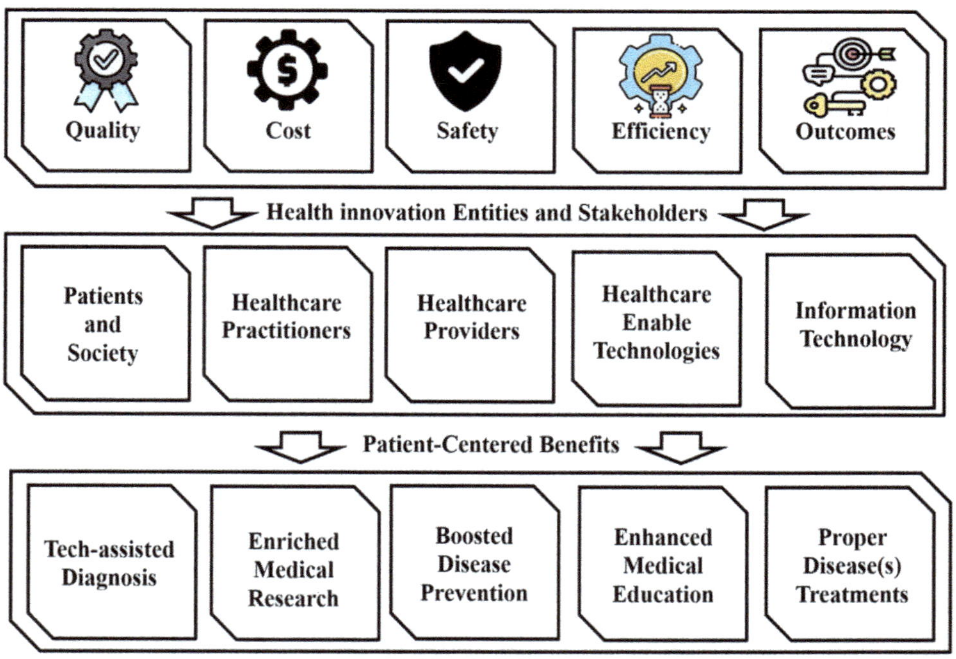

2.2. Current Technological Landscape

Electronic Health Records (EHRs), telemedicine, and mobile health applications are among the most prominent patient-centered health technology solutions at the moment. EHRs allow all necessary patient information to be stored in digital format, offering the opportunity to reduce paperwork, eliminate redundant information, and provide a convenient way for patients to share their health information with their various healthcare providers. Virtual care, or telemedicine, is another technology solution that puts patients first, giving them access to services they may have otherwise been unable to receive through in-person visits (Kammerer et al., 2024; Shafik, 2024f, 2024b). This includes virtual consultations with their healthcare providers, scheduled appointments for certain health services, and increased access to general practitioners via app-based virtual consultations. While the technologies above are designed to give patients more control over their healthcare offerings, various other tools and developments can be combined with these patient-centered technologies to deliver patient-centered care (Shafik, 2024g; Shafik & Kalinaki, 2024). The application of data analytics to these EHRs will provide insights into new diagnostic models and opportunities to personalize treatment plans. Meanwhile, innovative developments in artificial intelligence may help make these tools even more user-friendly, for example, by using voice to input data and interact with the technology (Marito & Widianto, 2024). This could improve health communications for those suffering from disability or literacy difficulties. It is important to note the significance of cybersecurity in relation to these technologies. Patient-centered care is not possible without trust, and cybersecurity is a conventional aspect of trust that has become even more widely discussed in the last year. However, while many tools are available to improve healthcare provision and personalized treatments, the lack of available resources is a considerable barrier to the development of many of these systems. There is also a chance that these systems are not reaching the right populations despite them being the ones who could benefit the most from personalized treatment plans (Määttä & Björkman, 2024; Shafik, 2023). In the United States, which has very high disparities in digital health engagement, African Americans express a strong desire for digital health policies, but only a small percentage of individuals own their health apps. This means that these technological tools are not able to address disparities directly but may exacerbate them. Finally, despite these many success stories, any final technological solution to improve the patient-centered health system will need to involve addressing the currently fragmented technologies available. In particular, this will be discussed in more detail in the next section with a focus on DRM (Shafik, 2024a; Umayal, 2024).

2.3. Patient Engagement Current Trends and Innovations

Engagement refers to the active inclusion of patients in matters related to their health and care. The healthcare landscape is being reshaped by trends that are driving and supporting novel and innovative ways to engage and include end users. Digital health tools can be useful for patient education and the dissemination of targeted and relevant health-related information. Modern-day telehealth platforms enable a more direct digital engagement with healthcare professionals, while apps on mobile phones can provide real-time emergency response buttons for chronic or high-need patients (Sarker, 2024). Additionally, there is ongoing research with a number of different patient populations evaluating the acceptability of using telemedicine systems to invite and engage participants in research studies, particularly those that are testing an intervention or new way of delivering health care. Furthermore, data science and technology are becoming increasingly significant in the effort to personalize care, to move from preventive care to preemptive care, and further to customize care to patients based on subphenotypes and genotypes in order to improve healthcare outcomes (Weber & Nøhr, 2024). In particular, the use of patient-generated real-world data and real-world evidence is increasingly being adopted in healthcare and health research settings with implications for ongoing monitoring or lifecycle safety checks of drugs, devices, or interventions in real-world settings. Artificial intelligence and machine learning have enormous potential to transform healthcare in the way it is delivered, making it more tailored to each patient. Furthermore, the widespread use of mobile phones alongside global internet connectivity infrastructure and the inclusion of new devices and tools to measure and collect patient-generated health data can be considered a catalyst for change and is already showing the potential to disrupt and change the landscape of healthcare (Tang et al., 2024). Table 1 highlights technologies advancing patient-centered care and their specific benefits, making it easier to understand the role of technology in healthcare.

Table 1. Key Technologies Supporting Patient-Centered Healthcare

Technology	Description	Impact on the Patients	User case in healthcare	Reference
Predictive Analytics	Using data to anticipate patient outcomes and needs	Proactive care, early intervention	Predictive models for readmission risks, disease outbreaks	(Umayal, 2024)
Augmented Reality (AR) and Virtual Reality (VR)	Interactive simulations for training and patient education	Pain management, rehabilitation, mental health support	VR for PTSD treatment, AR for patient anatomy education	(Sarker, 2024)
Robotic Process Automation (RPA)	Automating routine tasks in healthcare workflows	Reduced wait times, streamlined processes	RPA for scheduling, billing, record-keeping	(Megaro, 2023; Weber & Nøhr, 2024)
Natural Language Processing (NLP)	Technology that interprets patient-provider communications	Improved documentation, enhanced understanding	NLP for summarizing doctor-patient conversations	(Marito & Widianto, 2024)
Genomics and Personalized Medicine	Tailoring treatments based on genetic profiles	Targeted therapies, personalized medicine	Cancer genomics, pharmacogenomics	(Määttä & Björkman, 2024)
Blockchain for Health Data	Secures patient data using decentralized technology	Enhanced data privacy and security	Blockchain for EHRs, patient consent management	(Halas et al., 2024)
Remote Monitoring Systems	Monitoring of chronic conditions from a distance	Reduced hospital visits, early detection	Glucose monitors, heart rate monitors	(Kvæl et al., 2024)
Mobile Health Apps	Applications for health tracking, medication reminders	Enhanced engagement, convenient health management	MyChart, Medisafe app for medication reminders	(Tseng et al., 2024)
Patient Portals	Online platforms for accessing health records and communication with providers	Empowered decision-making, transparency	Access to test results, appointment scheduling	(Bense et al., 2024)
Wearable Devices	Devices tracking health metrics in real-time	Continuous health monitoring, proactive care	Fitbit, Apple Watch health monitoring	(Valentin et al., 2024)
Artificial Intelligence (AI)	Algorithms aiding diagnosis, treatment planning	Personalized care, predictive diagnostics	AI in imaging, chatbots for triage	(Totzkay, 2024)

continued on following page

Table 1. Continued

Technology	Description	Impact on the Patients	User case in healthcare	Reference
Telemedicine	Remote healthcare delivery through video, phone, and messaging	Convenience, accessibility, continuity of care	Video consultations, remote follow-ups	(Crompvoets et al., 2024)
Electronic Health Records (EHRs)	Digital records of patient health information	Improved care coordination, easy access	Epic, Cerner EHR systems	(Esmaeilzadeh, 2019)

3. BUILDING TRUST IN HEALTHCARE SYSTEMS

Understanding how to build trust among those who are utilizing healthcare services and, therefore, become patients is an active and expanding area of research. Developing trust is recognized as a fundamental tenet of healthcare, which should be 'safe, effective, patient-centered, timely, efficient, and equitable.' When trust is established between patients and those providing their care, those patients are more likely to adhere to recommendations made by clinicians, which in turn leads to better patient outcomes (Deshai & Rao, 2023). There are numerous reasons why trust may not be extended to professionals working within healthcare settings. The most significant of these is the ability to exert personal autonomy and share responsibility for decision-making. Strategies such as patient involvement in care decisions, improved information provision, and improved communication styles have all been suggested or empirically tested and, if successful, may be implemented to foster greater patient-provider relationships and, therefore, greater levels of trust and satisfaction. A wide variety of demographic, clinical, experiential, and situational factors impact how patients make decisions about whom to trust or not to trust (Okamura et al., 2024). The potential patient is a cognitive information processor and, as such, constructs inferences of trust based on not only how much or what kind of trust information is available but also the way in which it is presented. Furthermore, once trust has been established, it does not automatically secure future trustworthiness, especially if related actions are perceived as immoral, inequitable, or violating expectancies of fairness and accuracy. Therefore, in order to be effective, any initiatives directed at increasing trust in healthcare are likely to be multi-component (Williamson & Prybutok, 2024).

3.1. Challenges and Barriers

Healthcare environments commonly harbor obstacles to building and maintaining trust, making a trusting healthcare environment difficult to achieve. Sometimes, trust is hampered by communication difficulties or poor staff-patient relationships. The lack of empathy and concern regarding patients, particularly when the latter are perceived to be non-compliant, will also affect how trust is formed and maintained. In any case, dissatisfied patients reporting feeling devalued are significantly less likely to entrust their care to providers. Additionally, matters relating to the reputation or history of an organization, as well as structural issues such as access and bias, may also determine who places trust where (Okamura et al., 2024). Patients in populations often affected by historical biases and discrimination, for example, are less likely to put stock in the authenticity of the clinical encounter. Many racial and ethnic minorities and women enter the clinical setting already, wondering whether they are receiving second-rate care. In such cases, trust may be incrementally difficult to bestow. American Indian and Alaska Natives, one of the oldest minority groups and a group heavily reliant on Medicaid, are usually an understudied population with generally low levels of institutional trust in the federal government as well as government agencies (Deshai & Rao, 2023). Alaska Natives, on average, have lower levels of institutional trust compared to American Indians. Both sets of subpopulations have encountered systemic barriers to obtaining quality healthcare, and this has led to some of the lowest levels of trust across racial and ethnic minorities served by the system. These patients often do not trust practitioners or the quality of care because of the history of intergenerational trauma, historical abuses, or inappropriate treatment of their cultural heritage or customs. Often, patients are suspicious of health services because their healthcare institutions have chronically understaffed clinics, hospitals, or emergency rooms, which jeopardizes patient safety amidst the current technologies available, as illustrated in Figure 3 (Lau et al., 2019).

Figure 3. Patient-centered healthcare wearable devices

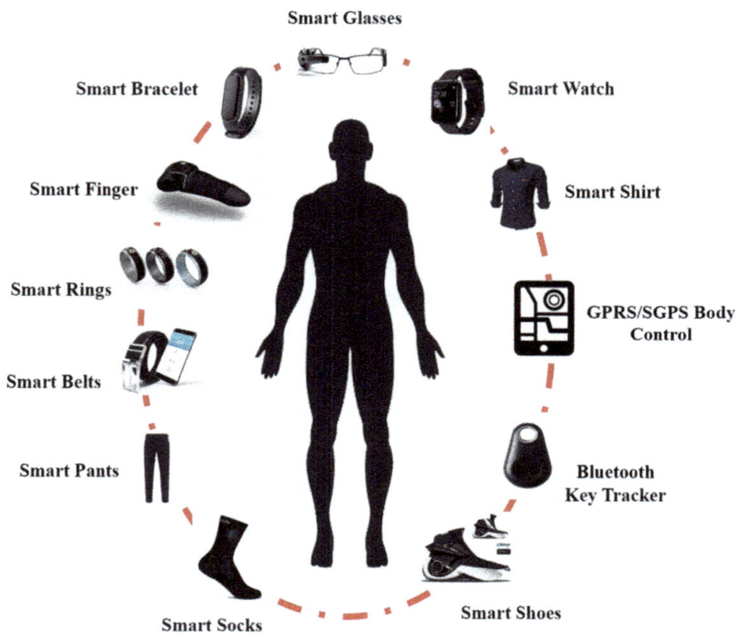

3.2. Benefits of Trustworthy Systems

Trust is associated with better health outcomes: trusted patients are more likely to follow clinical advice because they believe that their care provider has their best interests at heart. Conditions that foster trust develop open communication (Shafik, 2025e). Vast amounts of educational materials suggest that open communication helps patients feel comfortable expressing their concerns, which many acknowledge as a marker of patient-centered care, and increases the likelihood that providers and patients will forge a mutually agreeable treatment plan. Patients may be less likely to initiate legal claims for malpractice when they trust their providers (Khalsa et al., 2021). Commitment to improved patient education and access to healthcare resources is potentially associated with improved patient compliance with treatment plans and, therefore, better health outcomes. Patients who trust their providers will be more likely to engage in and maintain health-seeking behavior over time and also to bring a heightened level of loyalty to their healthcare 'brand' that includes the system as well as the personal individual clinicians. Furthermore, engaged patients are more likely to enroll in clinical trials, improving the knowledge base of both individual health conditions and health care overall (Dullabh et al., 2022). Transparency is correlated with patient trust in the healthcare system, which is of great importance when trying to engage and satisfy patients. Patients are also highly receptive to new technological forms of communication with their providers as long as there is a reasonable expectation of superior service. Therefore, if providing more information to the patient results in increased patient compliance and satisfaction, then there may be an associated increase in positive health outcomes (Shafik, 2024e). Because transparent systems can also be more trustworthy systems, the discussion of transparency provides a tool that we can use to evaluate and help build a model to describe how IT can help build trustworthy relationships between patients and the health care system and, thus, at the same time, improve health outcomes more generally (Esmaeilzadeh, 2019).

4. TRANSPARENCY IN HEALTHCARE

Patient-centered care has intrinsic merits when patient needs are at the forefront; however, healthcare providers claim that involving patients more is time-consuming and slows down productivity. Nevertheless, they believe that it is important and are committed to increased patient involvement. There is a tendency for greater openness in healthcare systems as providers and payers publish more and improved indicators of quality, outcomes, and performance to enable comparisons and raise profiles. This is now an international phenomenon, as all parts of the National Health Service are contractually obligated to supply information on their practices and standards of service (Deshai & Rao, 2023). Many developing countries have entered into reform processes to improve and extend health services. There is evidence that citizens are concerned about poor-quality healthcare and that they mistrust both healthcare providers and the health system. For these reforms to be successful, the new healthcare organizations have to be accountable and trustworthy (Singh et al., 2024). Transparency is fundamental because it strengthens the links between patients and providers, communities and health systems, and authorities and citizens, supports good governance, helps foster better communication, supports good record-keeping, encourages shared information, helps build stronger health information systems, improves health systems and the quality of healthcare fosters trust and mitigates suspicion benefits both patients and the health system facilitates good management and effective delivery (Khan et al., 2020; Shuker et al., 2018).

4.1. Importance and Benefits

Definition and importance advocates for a patient-centered healthcare system consistently promote transparency, a common term that has several definitions, specifically medical, legal, and ethical. In a comprehensive sense, transparency occurs when information is easily accessible, and patients and consumers can review and evaluate quality. Health services researchers often describe transparency as a characteristic of quality that promotes substantial improvements in care delivery. More specifically, patient advocates suggest that transparency builds trust between healthcare providers and patients. Major healthcare transformation proponents also endorse transparency as a crucial component of safe, efficient, and patient-centered care (Duffett, 2017; O'Riordan & Morin, 2023). This literature shows that transparency has several potential benefits. Patients who have complete information tend to be more confident in their care and show better health outcomes. Better-informed patients are also able to make complex healthcare decisions and control chronic conditions more consistently. In turn, health systems and providers can translate the volume of communication between patient and provider and the content of communication by system and provider into important measures of patient-centered care and pay-for-performance. In addition, patient reports and data quality ensure that a health system is meeting the goals of patient-centered care (like emphasis on patient decision-making and using health literacy standards) (Company Albir et al., 2024). Via transparency and tools such as process mapping, the stakeholders in healthcare delivery systems can view patient flow, patient-provider interaction, and care stages that can impact clinical outcomes. By providing data to the public and other healthcare organizations, delivery systems and providers can demonstrate a high degree of accountability to their local and national communities. For healthcare organizations, the benefits are numerous. They extend from patient care, financial, and legal risks that institutions and providers face to more directly gaining patient market share and growing their business (Weber & Nøhr, 2024). Building a system of transparency and open communication, including cost transparency, is an overt way of demonstrating an organization's philosophy, objectives, and commitment to patient-centered care. More importantly, this report suggests that healthcare providers and decision-makers are less likely to fully support patient-centered care where the case for quality is less definitive. In this case, those who finance, invest, license, and regulate these organizations may need to use arguments other than evidence of improved outcomes to persuade organizations to add transparency to their quality improvement activities (Okamura et al., 2024).

4.2. Barriers to Trust and Transparency

Many potential barriers in patient-centered doctor-patient relationships may impede trust and transparency. For instance, patients and doctors often speak different languages. Different health literacy or communication styles can interfere with clear and meaningful doctor-patient conversations. Cultural differences also play a role in choosing where a person seeks health care and determining if a person views a particular action as doctor shopping or hospital hopping. Further, different values, beliefs, and interpretations may lead to confusion, lack of communication, or misunderstandings (Umayal, 2024). Distrust may also occur because patients, who are often communicating with health care providers via email or weekend or overnight call lines, are simply looking for a quick and inexpensive fix to a difficult, expensive, and time-demanding health condition (Shafik, 2025a). Furthermore, especially in healthcare settings, privacy issues may prevent some patients from freely communicating with their doctors. The stigma of high-cost, difficult-to-treat conditions can also create communication barriers. This is further compounded by what some patients see as a lack of sympathy and empathy on the part of their healthcare provider, existing tools are available with several abilities, as illustrated in 4 (Q. Lu et al., 2024).

Figure 4. Abilities of patient-centered healthcare devices

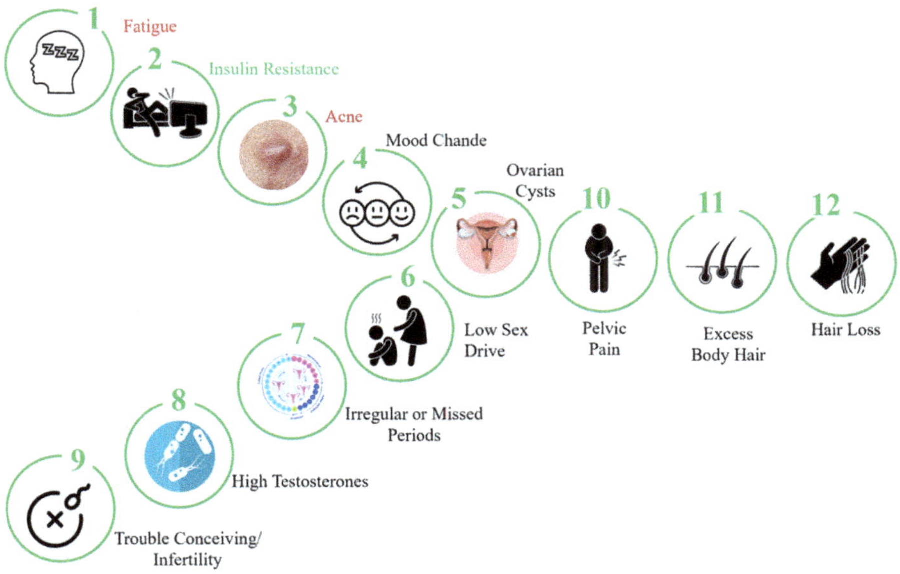

Doctors may invest significant time with patients to educate them on their health conditions, medications, options, side effects, costs, and disease progression. Patients, however, no matter the degree of this information and patient education, may not believe it or may not understand what the doctor is trying to communicate. This lack of communication is further compounded by the internet, which is fraught with many potential, if unwitting, cyberbullies or unvetted health information providers who provide misinformation about medications and diseases and who cannot truly appreciate how much time physicians spend with patients (Sumner et al., 2024; Zhao & Yam, 2024). In addition, unfortunately, many patients who are as educated as their healthcare provider in biomedical sciences may not trust their healthcare provider and may switch healthcare providers often. In general, barriers to trust may significantly affect patient engagement and satisfaction. It has been found that a lack of patient trust in primary care providers is a significant predictor of decreased adherence to one's primary care providers. This barrier is also true of lack of trust in alternative care providers; trust or lack of trust in all types of care providers affects whether a person will employ the care provider's suggested intervention. The extent of the potential harm by ethnicity, gender, age, and social status is a little-known area of clinical experience that needs studying (Sarker, 2024). Long-term follow-up studies could help paint a larger picture effect. For example, many people initially activate doctors as information brokers either after their access to medical data is impaired or when they are feeling relatively worse than they had in the past, compared with the point of diagnosis. By understanding what the potential barriers to trust are, we can learn to fix them or to build transparent rapport in subtle and intangible ways. The question then arises: what are the barriers to patient trust or understanding, and how can health information and informatics professionals help foster transparent doctor-patient partnerships in the era of individual patient care (Kvæl et al., 2024; O'Donnell et al., 2024)?

4.3. Challenges in Achieving Transparency

The most critical limitation lies in the technological infrastructure. Although there have been tremendous technological advancements in various fields, the infrastructure of healthcare IT systems is outdated. Consequently, older information systems are not designed to present or interpret the stream of patient-generated data in real-time (Shafik, 2025d). Technological barriers prevent the exchange of insightful data between patients and healthcare systems, reducing patients' participation and engagement in their health. Healthcare systems must comply with patient privacy constraints and government regulations. Due to the complexity of information and the possibility of misunderstandings, healthcare organizations fear the negative impacts of the misinterpretations of the shared data, and therefore, data-sharing protocols are not well established (Totzkay, 2024). Incentives for sharing data are not strong. From the patient's perspective, the information flow is one way, so it may not be important for patients to exchange their data. Technology infrastructure: Healthcare organizations should replace obsolete technologies and incorporate consumer products and cloud computing used in real-time data collection, analysis, and visualization. These technologies are vital to engage patients in their health. Workforce training: Healthcare organizations should train their healthcare staff on patient communication and tools to help patients better understand how to prevent complications. Policy: Healthcare organizations manage a vast amount of data, and therefore, policies must be established to guarantee access to this data (Williamson & Prybutok, 2024). Communication strategies: Hospitals must establish, conduct, and disseminate processes, expectations, and recommendations for patient care, as well as patient incentives to improve care, emphasizing the authenticity of the data's accuracy, relevance, and value in improving care and benefits. Table 2 provides an overview of trust factors in patient-centered healthcare, helping to clarify how technology can support or hinder patient trust and suggesting ways to strengthen it.

Table 2. Factors Influencing Patient Trust in Technology-Driven Healthcare Systems

Factor	Description	Impact on Trust	Strategies for Improvement	Reference
Regulatory Compliance	Adherence to legal and ethical standards for technology use in healthcare	Reassures patients of safety	Maintain transparency about certifications and standards	(Q. Lu et al., 2024)
Timeliness of Care	How quickly healthcare services are provided	Affects trust in technology as a supportive	Streamline tech support, real-time assistance	(Sumner et al., 2024)
Cultural Sensitivity	Ensuring technology is respectful of cultural values	Builds trust, improves adherence	Incorporate culturally appropriate content, language options	(Zhao & Yam, 2024)
Responsiveness to Patient Feedback	Actively responding to patient concerns and suggestions	Increases trust through responsiveness	Implement patient feedback loops, real-time support	(Kammerer et al., 2024)
Digital Literacy	Patient ability to understand and use healthcare technologies	Affects engagement and trust	Provide training resources, tech support	(Sarker, 2024)
Provide training resources and tech support.	Allowing patients control over their health information	Increased sense of empowerment	Enable opt-in choices, consent for data sharing	(Kvæl et al., 2024)

continued on following page

Table 2. Continued

Factor	Description	Impact on Trust	Strategies for Improvement	Reference
Interoperability of Systems	The ability for different healthcare technologies to work together seamlessly	Enhances care coordination	Implement standards like HL7, FHIR	(O'Donnell et al., 2024)
Reliability and Accuracy of Technology	Accuracy in technology-driven diagnostics and tools	Consistent performance builds confidence	Regular software updates, quality control checks	(Agwiah & Boateng, 2024)
Provider-Patient Communication	Open and respectful interactions between patients and healthcare providers	Builds a supportive relationship	Empathy training for providers, active listening	(Totzkay, 2024)
Accessibility	Ensuring equitable access to digital health solutions	Inclusive access enhances trust	Offer language support, digital literacy resources	(L. L. M. Lu et al., 2024)
Ease of Use	User-friendly design in digital health tools	Simple interfaces improve patient engagement	Develop intuitive apps and portals	(Williamson & Prybutok, 2024)
Transparency of Information	Clear communication on procedures and data usage	Transparency fosters confidence	Provide regular patient updates, use simple language	(Barden et al., 2024)
Data Privacy and Security	Protecting patient information from breaches	High security increases trust	Implement strong encryption, HIPAA compliance	(Kelsall-Knight & Stevens, 2024)

5. THE INTERSECTION OF TECHNOLOGY, TRUST, AND TRANSPARENCY

The ethical implications of integrating technology into health systems have ignited a spirited debate among healthcare professionals, computer scientists, patients, and other stakeholders. On the one hand, technology has the potential to foster trust and transparency in the healthcare system. For instance, by identifying ways in which patients can be protected, institutional practices made more transparent, and medical records more controllable by the patients themselves, trust in healthcare systems can be restored (Kovaleva et al., 2024). On the other hand, health technology comes with new ethical issues and potential risks associated with its rapid uptake, amplified by concerns about transparency and data security in light of recent security breaches and the illicit collection and use of data by several tech companies. This, in turn, has resulted in an increasing lack of trust in new regimes of data collection and surveillance, further informed by the increasing power of tech companies in Denmark, among other countries (Turk et al., 2024; Valentin et al., 2024).

5.1. Privacy and Patient Data Security

Privacy itself is another ethical concern associated with consumers' use of new technology, such as wearables that monitor body conditions. This is particularly an issue in AI, given that large amounts of data are needed to train an AI system. Such data can be hacked for a variety of malicious reasons, and plans made based on personal data collected to cause harm. As a result, ethical issues related to transferring or sharing personal information among different companies are increasingly evident. Using emerging technologies raises fundamental legal questions as well (Wang et al., 2024). Increasingly, these technologies are governed by a complex array of laws, regulations, and other legal instruments that protect patients and consumers. Where questions emerge, the courts are called on to decide on relevant legal ambiguities, often adjudicating between ethical and moral considerations to render holistic decisions (Bense et al., 2024; Blanck et al., 2024). Ensuring an organization or institution is in legal compliance is critical to patient trust. One major challenge to security in healthcare is the role of the trustworthiness of inputs into AI systems, the intent of those using the systems, and the ability of the company to safeguard that information. Technology's use—the strategy driving the interaction between trust, transparency, and technology—is thus vital to securing patient-centered healthcare systems, as well as building up concomitant trust. Balancing transparency and trust, however, with humane and responsible technology implementation is vital (Tseng et al., 2024).

5.2. Ethical Considerations

The inclusion of advanced technologies in healthcare has a wide range of ethical implications. Accordingly, it is important to prioritize the protection of patient privacy and autonomy in decisions about implementing technology and regulating data collection and use within the sector. This also has implications for the business models of technology companies. Initiatives and practices should prioritize the patient's right to share or not to share their data. Providers must be honest in openly discussing informed consent and the potential consequences of data sharing (Devlin et al., 2024). Another major ethical risk of using increasingly advanced algorithms to provide patient-centered healthcare is the potential for systematic bias against certain groups. Modern machine learning and artificial intelligence are dependent on data, which is collected in societies characterized by socioeconomic injustices. As a result, automated systems can inadvertently reinforce unfair social and racial practices that already govern health outcomes. The ethics of training healthcare providers in the context of these discussions are equally important (Crompvoets et al., 2024). Health training and education will be needed to ensure that professionals can approach patients and algorithms with an informed view of their biases and handle conflicts with the plan of care. A good way to approach these ethical concerns would be to prioritize the systematic integration of societal values and ethics into healthcare and technology. We believe that healthcare organizations should prioritize this as a way to gain patient trust and improve the patient-provider relationship. Technology for patients and providers should be designed considering the four pillars of medical ethics (Berk et al., 2024). Prioritizing these practices assures that patients who choose to integrate technology into their healthcare will receive patient-centered, personal, and ethical care. Ethical considerations should play a major role in decisions regarding the design and implementation of tools used for the protection of patient information. Correcting these practices can deepen trust and provide more evidence for the current gaps in the literature, regardless of the existing disabilities of the patients, as illustrated in Figure 5. The healthcare industry as a whole should prioritize an ethical culture, and ethics can be used as a selling point for our system to help build trust and engagement (Berk et al., 2024).

Figure 5. Sampled patient disabilities

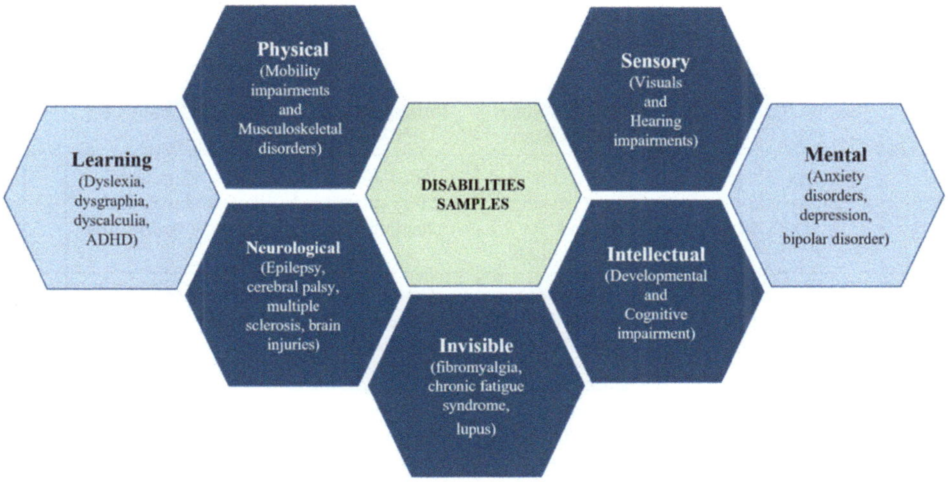

5.3. Legal Frameworks and Regulations

Legal frameworks and regulations. Regulations and laws (local, national, and international) strongly influence the use of technology in healthcare and research. In healthcare, the key reasons for using technology are to solve problems, provide better service, enhance communication, and share information. Emerging legal standards are implicitly shaping healthcare services to be more patient-focused. Historically, systems were often people-focused based on informal relationships between health professionals and patients (Khorram-Manesh et al., 2024). An increasingly data-driven, collaborative, and interdisciplinary relationship between healthcare providers and patients is likely to result in a more patient-focused system that is informed by patient preferences and values, as well as scientific knowledge and technologies for personalized medicine. Legal and regulatory requirements offer a useful point of reference in terms of 'best practice' for good governance. Perhaps the most important and recognized data protection law in the United States is the Health Insurance Portability and Accountability Act of 1996 (Halas et al., 2024; Hascher et al., 2024). This legislation addresses the administrative side of healthcare and the technical side, guaranteeing patients' right to access their records and requiring healthcare providers to keep data safe. Because of the detailed current impact this law has on healthcare, it drives transparency and accountability, which are policies currently being developed more broadly in healthcare through the Constitution and health regulatory authorities. Moreover, in rare cases in which there are legal requirements, individuals found to be out of compliance with such legislation and unable to demonstrate due diligence can face stiff penalties and, in severe cases, be imprisoned. Sanctions can be noted on state healthcare license applications or renewals; individuals found liable for breaches can also be subject to civil penalties such as monetary fines by government authorities (Määttä & Björkman, 2024). Perhaps the most important legal aspect of ensuring technical compliance with laws and regulations is avoiding possible legal liability for those who have developed and implemented technology and data privacy forms of law that govern the planned project or use of the software in question. In contrast to the global nature of laws, ethics vary globally (Tang et al., 2024). Table 3 demonstrates how the complexities and opportunities in using technology to foster trust and transparency in healthcare can be attained.

Table. **3.** *The Intersection of Technology, Trust, and Transparency in Healthcare*

Technology	How It Builds Trust	How It Enhances Transparency	Impact on the Patient	Potential Challenges	Reference
Biometric Authentication	Ensures secure and unique access to health data	Transparent, clear verification methods for patient records	Increased security prevents unauthorized access	Privacy issues, potential technical failures in verification	(Dullabh et al., 2022)
Cloud Storage for Health Records	Enables easy and secure storage of health records	Patients can access their records from anywhere	Convenient access, especially for chronic conditions	Security concerns, potential unauthorized access	(Esmaeilzadeh, 2019)
Machine Learning for Disease Detection	Offers early detection based on large data sets	Transparency in health risks and potential treatments	Early intervention, personalized disease management	High dependency on data quality, risk of false positives/ negatives	(Khan et al., 2020)
Chatbots and Virtual Assistants	Provides 24/7 support and quick answers to common health questions	Enhances transparency by providing consistent information	Immediate support reduced patient anxiety	Limited scope, risk of incorrect or incomplete responses	(Shuker et al., 2018)
Interoperability Standards (e.g., FHIR)	Ensures seamless data exchange between providers	Patients can access comprehensive health information	Improved care coordination, fewer information gaps	Compatibility issues, potential data privacy risks	(Duffett, 2017)
Digital Consent Forms	Allows patients control over data sharing and access	Clear documentation of patient consent	Empowers patients to make informed choices	The complexity of understanding terms, the potential misuse of consent data	(O'Riordan & Morin, 2023)
Augmented and Virtual Reality (AR/VR)	Provides transparent simulations for patient education	Patients can visualize treatments or medical conditions	Enhances patient understanding, manages expectations	High cost, accessibility limitations	(Company Albir et al., 2024)
Data Encryption	Ensures confidentiality of patient information	Transparency in how data is securely handled	Peace of mind, protection against unauthorized access	Potential slowdowns, complexity in data-sharing across systems	(Weber & Nøhr, 2024)
Genomics and Personalized Medicine	Tailors treatments to individual genetic profiles	A clear rationale for personalized treatments	Precision medicine for better outcomes	Privacy concerns need for informed consent	(Okamura et al., 2024)
Mobile Health Apps	Offers reliable information and resources	Easy access to personal data and health information	Convenience helps in tracking health goals	Inconsistent quality, potential for misinformation	(Tang et al., 2024)
Predictive Analytics	Builds trust through proactive care based on accurate predictions	Transparent explanations for predictive outcomes	Early detection, preventive care	Risks of misinterpretation, potential for data misuse	(Määttä & Björkman, 2024)

continued on following page

Table. Continued

Technology	How It Builds Trust	How It Enhances Transparency	Impact on the Patient	Potential Challenges	Reference
Patient Portals	Facilitates direct communication and access to personal health data	Transparent access to test results, medication, and records	Better engagement in healthcare management	Complexity for less tech-savvy patients, potential security risks	(Hascher et al., 2024)
Wearable Devices	Continuous monitoring promotes proactive health management	Patients can view personal health metrics in real-time	Increased engagement in personal health, early risk alerts	Data privacy, potential inaccuracies in consumer-grade devices	(Halas et al., 2024)
Telemedicine	Enables easy access to providers, fostering patient-provider trust	Patients can see and hear their providers virtually	Convenience accessibility for remote patients	Digital divide, security concerns in video consultations	(Khorram-Manesh et al., 2024)
Artificial Intelligence (AI)	Offers reliable, data-driven diagnostics and recommendations	Transparent algorithms can provide explanations for decisions	Improved diagnostic accuracy, personalized treatment plans	Algorithmic bias, lack of transparency in complex models	(Crompvoets et al., 2024)
Blockchain	Securely stores patient data with tamper-proof records	Ensures data integrity, traceable access history	Higher confidence in data accuracy and security	Limited adoption, complex implementation	(Devlin et al., 2024)
Electronic Health Records (EHRs)	Centralizes patient data, allowing consistent record-keeping	Patients have access to their medical history and updates	Empowered decision-making, streamlined care coordination	Privacy risks, potential data breaches	(Blanck et al., 2024)

6. CASE STUDIES AND BEST PRACTICES

Each section in this chapter offers a review of multiple studies, which shown in the healthcare environment have largely demonstrated the potential of HIT inclusion in patient care, trust building, and efficiency. A few of these studies reveal a different story, where the lack of use of successful technologies or unsuccessful implementation has brought insufficient results or even setbacks in patient trust. Regardless of the level of success, all outcomes can be viewed as instructive and essential for learning about how to conduct future activities in the healthcare context (Valentin et al., 2024). Furthermore, our findings reinforce the need for healthcare organizations to think critically about their HIT and health technology approaches, how they can be improved, how patient input can direct improvements and trust-building strategies, and the importance of constantly analyzing the role of such technologies in patient-centered endeavors. The case studies in this report attempt to showcase the wide range of organizations implementing technologies to build trust and transparency with patients in the healthcare system from a variety of sectors in a variety of countries and circumstances. Three out of the four case studies presented here represent models of successful trust-building technology integration in patient-centered care (Barden et al., 2024). These case studies explain the technology implemented, how it was used, its goals, and the ultimate outcomes. Lessons learned from the case studies are found in the narratives, as are the potential future experiments or expansions that the organizations may be considering as next steps. The fourth case study represents an instructive narrative of the setbacks associated with HIT. With one case revealing less-than-desirable results, this document delivers a hopeful mixture of both successful case studies as well as the complications and setbacks that must also be taken into account as HIT becomes further incorporated into healthcare systems worldwide (L. L. M. Lu et al., 2024).

6.1. Successful Implementation

In Great Britain, a relatively small practice develops online curricula for patients not comfortable using smart technology. A virtual visit program improves outcomes for patients with Parkinson's disease. Taiwan implemented the use of a digital self-care record to reduce poverty in the land. A unique online transparency initiative introduces patient-friendly data. An idea was proposed to post all patient and employee satisfaction data and then a bit about the practice. There was a pledge to keep things up to date and add other information and stories about their journey (Barden et al., 2024). "Patient and employee data and dashboard is public." A member of the College of Health Electronics is creating some patient videos. Redesigning care with patients: A Parkinson's disease research study implemented a virtual shared medical appointment with success. The institution's Parkinson's clinic was redesigned; patient types were served by the clinic better. Then, a virtual specialty review appointment was designed that mirrored aspects of earlier shared medical appointments. All components of the video visit were tested prior to implementation. Future: Implement the new EHR at the institution. Transfer the model to another clinic where it might work well. Known to transfer to clinic types (Kammerer et al., 2024; Zhao & Yam, 2024). The tool uses clinic schedules, pharmacy records, an alternate location for scheduling, the new device, and the new clinic notes. The future is unknown.

6.2. Lessons Learned

What have we learned from the case studies presented in the previous section? One clear message is that the technology needs to fit into the pre-existing healthcare delivery system in order to foster trust and transparency in care. Despite this, the adoption of new technology often requires changes to protocols, regulations, ethics, and workflows that are complicated and slow. Engaging stakeholders in the process of both technology "buy-in" and implementation at each stage, from development to scaling up, is an important and ongoing activity for staff in a patient-centered healthcare setting. The engagement of both medical and technical staff is key to ensuring the technology will meet their day-to-day needs and is more likely to be used (Barden et al., 2024). This includes not only training but also access to a help desk or IT specialist that providers, as well as patients, can seek for advice when they have technical difficulties. Results from monitoring and evaluation can help identify where change is needed and help test new processes and systems. Programs need built-in learning among all staff - including patients and support persons - that uses lessons from past implementation at the hospital and previous experiences with digital platforms. As the programs can become better and better by continuously learning, it is crucial to continue monitoring and evaluation work beyond implementation and during any period of sustainability. Case studies also showed that time is required for the integration of technology into care to be effective (Blanck et al., 2024; van Lummel et al., 2024). Continued training, tweaking, and involvement of key staff involves a regular time resource at the onset of implementation, and some staff members will be dedicating some of their time to the system on an ongoing basis. Consultants identified particular roles, such as a data analyst to evaluate program performance and a training officer to monitor and supervise data quality, as ones that need to be sustained. The use of a variety of media to support patients' use of the technology and free socialization opportunities increases the likelihood of a better patient uptake of the technology (Bense et al., 2024). Providing patients with home equipment, an internet connection, a personal account with a log-in, and technical support as necessary will also increase their access to a digital program.

7. FUTURE DIRECTIONS AND EMERGING TECHNOLOGIES

The nexus of technology and care has the promise of further fostering trust through transparency and positive clinical engagement of patients and providers. The third era of healthcare has already witnessed impressive technological advances in telemedicine, AI, and ML to develop predictive and personalized algorithms, radionics, body sensors, wearables, health and wellness mobile apps, and the Internet of Medical Things. These trends allow futuristic speculation about how they might further enhance our ability to deliver care with transparency and patient-centeredness (Devlin et al., 2024). Furthering the discussions about transparency and engagement among patients and providers using new and emerging technologies might spur new research, help to point to where these technologies could indeed potentially be used to benefit patient engagement and outcomes, and lead to ethical and legal considerations to ensure health systems align with patient-centered concepts proactively. Enthusiastic innovation in healthcare that enhances trust, transparency, safety, and relationships could drive a new era of patient-centered care. All stakeholders in the healthcare system crave a more responsive approach to the individual and believe that a vast range of new options, including research focusing on qualitative and sociological studies, provide further depth and insight into our understanding of the role of contemporary and emerging technologies in enhancing trust and transparency in healthcare, will be highly valuable to publish and could support the newly desired age of patient-centered care (Halas et al., 2024; Khorram-Manesh et al., 2024).

7.1. Potential Impact on Trust and Transparency

Health data systems need to ensure that patient information is handled with such care; a blatant disregard for information, a privacy breach, or data theft regarding the arrival of care at other undisclosed locations only breeds mistrust in caregivers and hinders care-seeking. Emerging technologies offer considerable potential to enhance trust and transparency. Blockchain, as a technology, is known to include health data because of the immutability of files released in a block on the shared ledger, helping to address privacy concerns and improve data security (van Lummel et al., 2024). AI can increase consumer involvement in care and inspire more transparent discussions if designed and successfully implemented for reasons such as trigger decisions and decision aids. Mobile apps are seen as a popular way to gather, manage, and access health data among young electronic patients who are busy. Individuals are experts in sharing personal and health information on a variety of apps, from authenticating children's vaccines on health assessment forms to managing chronic health plans. Plain language will always better hone a patient's application. Security links to convenience; only features that significantly boost the product and facilitate daily operation, such as registration and virtual queues, must be prioritized on the user-focused platform (Turk et al., 2024). Each of these proposed interventions has "shadow" risks, such as the unintentional disclosure of details, authentication of relevant data, or the capture of biased details syndrome. Similarly, many interventions may support the protection of privacy, but the congestion or prioritization of certain patient data could also lead to wider data problems. More research and design are needed to ensure that trust is strengthened and that the technological solutions designed to promote it accomplish their goals while not being exploited otherwise. A nuanced, comprehensive, and evidence-based debate about the promise and pitfalls of these emerging technologies is called for in the push to ensure better patient-centered health data systems (Kovaleva et al., 2024; Valentin et al., 2024).

7.2. Impact on Healthcare Delivery

These come in two main ways, entailing Access to Care and process excellence.

7.2.1. Access to Care

These technologies are viewed as having transformative potential. Reduced in-person visits and the use of telehealth technologies, which include virtual consults and online appointment registration, are seen as increasing healthcare delivery efficiencies. Telehealth has the potential to streamline communication between healthcare providers and reduce appointment scheduling times due to a reduction in the number of people accessing in-person care (Barden et al., 2024). These scenarios collectively illustrate how these emerging technologies are seen as streamlining healthcare delivery processes, increasing cost efficiencies in care delivery, and, most importantly, enhancing the overall convenience of often stressful experiences for patients. AI is believed to have a more powerful effect on greatly increasing healthcare delivery efficiencies and access to care for the population as a whole than any other emerging technology. AI will likely be one of the first areas to reduce wait times, propelling people to the access stage more rapidly (L. L. M. Lu et al., 2024).

7.2.2. Process Excellence

These technologies were seen as transforming the healthcare industry by changing delivery mechanisms and including novel channels for administering care. Technological changes such as online appointment registration were making it easier for patients to access care, and the information provided by process changes would become a valuable asset for further improvements. This goes beyond simple task automation aimed at enhancing convenience for both patients and staff. Such changes are facilitating the restructuring of roles and processes within healthcare (Agwiah & Boateng, 2024). The important element of these changes is the potential to create a new type of relationship between the patient and the technical system, which, in many ways, has elements of the types of relationships healthcare professionals have with patients. They extend beyond the current web-based technologies that recreate service delivery methods and enable more routing and administrative tasks such as choosing a provider, booking appointments, ordering renewals, checking test results, and making service-related inquiries. Development work to date focuses on consultant physician-patient interaction within hospitals and advances a vision of hospital services redesigned around patient pathways (L. L. M. Lu et al., 2024).

7.2. Opportunities for Further Research

A variety of promising research that has yet to be conducted would offer further insights into how technology fosters trust, transparency, and patient-centered approaches to care. Such a study is essential as technology plays an even larger role in healthcare. Such analyses must explore whether technology is effective in creating relationships, fostering trust, and supporting external visibility. Importantly, these analyses should consider how different technologies can be implemented to maximize individual patients' trust and transparency needs. Insight should be provided as to whether and how these solutions foster patients' understanding of and willingness to broadcast important personal healthcare information (Kovaleva et al., 2024). Longitudinal research that includes patient outcomes and impacts over time is also needed. This study will serve as a foundation for novel and established approaches. Work that examines patient acceptance, willingness to disclose information, and understanding of their digital footprint, among other factors, is essential. This research will have a direct impact on the development of technology to help patients comprehend how information about them is being used. It is also essential to emphasize the necessity of multidisciplinary collaboration in patient-oriented work. The creation and development of an authentic research community necessitates the integration of existing technologies, the conduct of fieldwork in actual clinic settings, and the discussion of outcomes that are both obtainable and beneficial. The transition to active academia or clinic must be well considered (Turk et al., 2024; Wang et al., 2024). We hope that this research will be used to advance a future that offers patient-centered treatment that is transparent and builds trust. As shown by this topic, this is critical. We are continuing our exploration of how to build upon it.

8. CONCLUSION

The case studies identified many of the common barriers to introducing new technologies, such as user resistance, the need for ongoing training, lack of resources, and cost concerns. Some case studies also highlighted the importance of preparing staff before a telemedicine service is implemented. Many of the case studies emphasized that planning and strategy development are instrumental in addressing these complexities. It is important to outline and share processes with patients and the community, as well as identify champions and endorsements from a broad range of professional stakeholders and consumers. This also helps in institutionalizing any changes. The role of governance, as well as clearly identified and supported staff roles, specific funding, and data collection, were also some features identified as important enablers in technology used by the case studies. Importantly, the findings from the individual case studies reveal that effective implementation of technology at each of the local sites properly took into account patient care and patient-centeredness. Incorporate risk management discussions into professional development activities so that staff and management teams are equipped to manage any increases in complaints and governance risks. While planning is crucial, it is also important to consistently and regularly find ways to contribute to a work culture that is based on trust, transparency, and empowerment. This will prepare both consumers and staff for the new telemedicine service and assist healthcare professionals in understanding how technologies such as telemedicine can complement existing care. Ongoing monitoring, evaluation, and modification of the implementation of new telemedicine services is essential to rectify any issues before they have a demonstrable impact on patient care. The suggestion includes implementing ongoing focus groups and interviews and an evaluation tool that is easily accessible to consumers and staff, as a proportion of patients will not be diverse in how they engage or use technology. Continuing to evaluate and obtain feedback from patients and staff on how the telemedicine service is functioning can also shed light on how to address current and potential issues in patient-centered care. Technology allows for scalable, less expensive, and more dynamic ways to support patients when they are ready to engage in their health. By providing reliable patients with the knowledge and information, they need to be able to take the next step and make a real difference.

REFERENCES

Agwiah, V. A., & Boateng, K.-H. T. (2024). Family Centered Care: The Perspective of Nurses in the Neonatal Intensive Care Unit of Tamale Teaching Hospital, Ghana: A Qualitative Exploration. *Asian Journal of Pediatric Research*, *14*(3), 27–36. Advance online publication. DOI: 10.9734/ajpr/2024/v14i3331

Albir, M. J. C., Andrés, J. L. P., & Solsona, M. D. E. (2024). [Translated article] Good humanisation practices in the healthcare of patients with rare diseases in Pharmacy Services. *Farmacia Hospitalaria*, *48*(1), T3–T8.

Barden, A., Kalman, J., Gierlinger, S., Baker, D., Giammarinaro, N., & Rousseau, N. (2024). From Monologue to Dialogue: The Pursuit of Relationship Centered Communication Across a Large, Integrated Healthcare System. *Journal of Patient Experience*, *11*, 23743735241226507. Advance online publication. DOI: 10.1177/23743735241226507 PMID: 38234981

Bense, J. E., Guilonard, N., Zwaginga, F., Stiggelbout, A. M., Louwerens, M., Mekelenkamp, H., Lankester, A. C., Pieterse, A. H., & de Pagter, A. P. J. (2024). The value of using patient-reported outcomes for health screening during long-term follow-up after paediatric stem cell transplantation for nonmalignant diseases. *Health Expectations*, *27*(1), e13902. Advance online publication. DOI: 10.1111/hex.13902 PMID: 38102818

Berk, A. L., Pickett, A., Kusters, I. S., & Gregory, M. E. (2024). Healthcare Experiences of Black Patients During and After Pregnancy: A Needs Assessment for Provider Training to Improve Quality of Care. *Journal of Racial and Ethnic Health Disparities*, *11*(2), 992–1004. Advance online publication. DOI: 10.1007/s40615-023-01579-5 PMID: 37010801

Blanck, E., Pirhonen Nørmark, L., Fors, A., Ekman, I., Ali, L., Swedberg, K., & Gyllensten, H. (2024). Self-efficacy and healthcare costs in patients with chronic heart failure or chronic obstructive pulmonary disease. *ESC Heart Failure*, *11*(1), 219–228. Advance online publication. DOI: 10.1002/ehf2.14574 PMID: 37940106

Crompvoets, P. I., Nieboer, A. P., van Rossum, E. F. C., & Cramm, J. M. (2024). Perceived weight stigma in healthcare settings among adults living with obesity: A cross-sectional investigation of the relationship with patient characteristics and person-centred care. *Health Expectations*, *27*(1), e13954. Advance online publication. DOI: 10.1111/hex.13954 PMID: 39102661

Deshai, N., & Rao, B. B. (2023). Transparency in healthcare and e-commerce: Detecting online fake reviews using a dense neural network model with relevance mapping. *Soft Computing*, *27*(14), 9861–9875. Advance online publication. DOI: 10.1007/s00500-023-08437-w

Devlin, M. K., McIntyre, N. J., Ramer, M. D., Kwon, Y. H., Nicholson, J. M., Mrkobrada, M., Kronick, J., Calvin, J. E., & Spicer, E. (2024). Applying the lessons of design thinking: A unique programme of care for acutely unwell, community-dwelling COVID-19 patients. *BMJ Open Quality*, *13*(1), e002500. Advance online publication. DOI: 10.1136/bmjoq-2023-002500 PMID: 38413092

Duffett, L. (2017). Patient engagement: What partnering with patient in research is all about. In *Thrombosis Research* (Vol. 150). DOI: 10.1016/j.thromres.2016.10.029

Dullabh, P., Sandberg, S. F., Heaney-Huls, K., Hovey, L. S., Lobach, D. F., Boxwala, A., Desai, P. J., Berliner, E., Dymek, C., Harrison, M. I., Swiger, J., & Sittig, D. F. (2022). Challenges and opportunities for advancing patient-centered clinical decision support: Findings from a horizon scan. *Journal of the American Medical Informatics Association : JAMIA*, *29*(7), 1233–1243. Advance online publication. DOI: 10.1093/jamia/ocac059 PMID: 35534996

Esmaeilzadeh, P. (2019). An Empirical Evaluation of Factors Influencing Patients' Reactions to the Implementation of Health Information Exchanges (HIEs). *International Journal of Human-Computer Interaction*, *35*(13), 1135–1146. Advance online publication. DOI: 10.1080/10447318.2018.1511181

Halas, G., Baldwin, A., Mackay, K., Cardenas, E., LaBine, L., Cherrett, P., Abraham, L., Fogarty, V., Singer, A., Katz, A., & Kirby, S. (2024). Patients' and caregivers' experiences of virtual care in a primary care setting during the COVID-19 pandemic: A patient-oriented research study. *Digital Health*, *10*, 20552076241232949. Advance online publication. DOI: 10.1177/20552076241232949 PMID: 38410792

Hascher, K., Jaiswal, J., LoSchiavo, C., Ezell, J., Duffalo, D., Greene, R. E., Cox, A., Burton, W. M., Griffin, M., John, T., Grin, B., & Halkitis, P. N. (2024). Lack of Informed and Affirming Healthcare for Sexual Minority Men: A Call for Patient-Centered Care. *Journal of General Internal Medicine*, *39*(11), 2023–2032. Advance online publication. DOI: 10.1007/s11606-024-08635-8 PMID: 38308157

Kammerer, E., Fawcett-Arsenault, J., Iliscupidez, L., & Ali, S. (2024). Healthcare Professionals' Perspectives on Improving Family-Centred Pain Care in a Tertiary Pediatric Centre. *Canadian Journal of Nursing Research*, *56*(2), 171–177. Advance online publication. DOI: 10.1177/08445621241228063 PMID: 38258330

Kelsall-Knight, L., & Stevens, R. (2024). Exploring the implementation of person-centred care in nursing practice. *Nursing Standard (Royal College of Nursing (Great Britain) : 1987)*, *39*(1). DOI: 10.7748/ns.2023.e12190

Khalsa, U., Pooni, R., Sandborg, C., Balboni, I., Wayman, K., & Lee, T. (2021). Supporting patient-centered care in the pediatric rheumatology setting: Patient, family and provider experiences with ournotes. *Arthritis and Rheumatology, 73*(SUPPL 9).

Khan, A. U., Shahid, A., Tariq, F., Ghaffar, A., Jamal, A., Abbas, S., & Javaid, N. (2020). Enhanced Decentralized Management of Patient-Driven Interoperability Based on Blockchain. In *Lecture Notes in Networks and Systems* (Vol. 97). DOI: 10.1007/978-3-030-33506-9_74

Khorram-Manesh, A., Gray, L., Goniewicz, K., Cocco, A., Ranse, J., Phattharapornjaroen, P., Achour, N., Sørensen, J., Peyravi, M., Hertelendy, A. J., Kupietz, K., Bergholtz, J., & Carlström, E. (2024). Care in emergencies and disasters: Can it be person-centered? *Patient Education and Counseling*, *118*, 108046. Advance online publication. DOI: 10.1016/j.pec.2023.108046 PMID: 37924742

Kovaleva, M. A., Nikolaeva, A. R., Uzdenova, B. R., Rafikova, N. F., Trostina, V. V., Marzieva, A. M., & Dorofeev, Y. N. (2024). Arterial blood pressure and its cerebral implications: A comprehensive examination of patient-centered approaches in clinical settings. *Revista Latinoamericana de Hipertensiòn*, *19*(1). Advance online publication. DOI: 10.5281/zenodo.10645465

Kvæl, L. A. H., Bergland, A., & Eldh, A. C. (2024). Preference-based patient participation in intermediate care: Translation, validation and piloting of the 4Ps in Norway. *Health Expectations*, *27*(1), e13899. Advance online publication. DOI: 10.1111/hex.13899 PMID: 37934200

Lau, F., Bartle-Clar, J. A., Bliss, G., Boricky, E. M., Courtney, K. L., Kuo, A., Kushniruk, A., Monkman, H., & Roudsari, A. (2019). *Improving Usability, Safety and Patient Outcomes with Health Information Technology. From Research to Practice*. IOS Press.

Lu, L. L. M., Henn, P., O'Tuathaigh, C., & Smith, S. (2024). Patient–healthcare provider communication and age-related hearing loss: A qualitative study of patients' perspectives. *Irish Journal of Medical Science*, *193*(1), 277–284. Advance online publication. DOI: 10.1007/s11845-023-03432-4 PMID: 37386348

Lu, Q., Link, E., Baumann, E., & Schulz, P. J. (2024). Linking patient-centered communication with cancer information avoidance: The mediating roles of patient trust and literacy. *Patient Education and Counseling*, *123*, 108230. Advance online publication. DOI: 10.1016/j.pec.2024.108230 PMID: 38484597

Määttä, S., & Björkman, I. (2024). We are not even allowed to call them patients anymore: Conceptions about person-centred care. *Health Expectations*, *27*(1), e13887. Advance online publication. DOI: 10.1111/hex.13887 PMID: 37854003

Marito, D. R., & Widianto, S. (2024). Link of Infection Prevention Climate to Patient-Centered Care: Role of Workplace Safety and Risk Mitigation. *Risk Management and Healthcare Policy*, *17*, 329–340. Advance online publication. DOI: 10.2147/RMHP.S439907 PMID: 38352960

Megaro, A. (2023). Transparency in AI systems for value co-creation in healthcare. In *Big Data and Decision-Making*. Applications and Uses in the Public and Private Sector., DOI: 10.1108/978-1-80382-551-920231007

O'Donnell, A., Gonyea, J., Wensley, T., & Nizza, M. (2024). High-quality patient-centered palliative care: Interprofessional team members' perceptions of social workers' roles and contribution. *Journal of Interprofessional Care*, *38*(1), 1–9. Advance online publication. DOI: 10.1080/13561820.2023.2238783 PMID: 37525994

O'Riordan, A., & Morin, A. (2023). Pandemic Patient Engagement Success: Maintaining Family Presence Through Partnership. *International Journal of Integrated Care*, *23*(S1), 703. Advance online publication. DOI: 10.5334/ijic.ICIC23270

Okamura, M., Fujimori, M., Otsuki, A., Saito, J., Yaguchi-Saito, A., Kuchiba, A., Uchitomi, Y., & Shimazu, T. (2024). Patients' perceptions of patient-centered communication with healthcare providers and associated factors in Japan – The INFORM Study 2020. *Patient Education and Counseling*, *122*, 108170. Advance online publication. DOI: 10.1016/j.pec.2024.108170 PMID: 38308974

Sarker, M. (2024). Reinventing Wellness: How Machine Learning Transforms Healthcare. *Journal of Artificial Intelligence General Science (JAIGS) ISSN:3006-4023, 3*(1). DOI: 10.60087/jaigs.v3i1.73

Shafik, W. (2023). Wearable Medical Electronics in Artificial Intelligence of Medical Things. In *Handbook of Security and Privacy of AI-Enabled Healthcare Systems and Internet of Medical Things*. https://doi.org/DOI: 10.1201/9781003370321-2

Shafik, W. (2024a). Artificial Intelligence-Enabled Internet of Medical Things (AIoMT) in Modern Healthcare Practices. In *Clinical Practice and Unmet Challenges in AI-Enhanced Healthcare Systems* (pp. 42–69). IGI Global. DOI: 10.4018/979-8-3693-2703-6.ch003

Shafik, W. (2024b). Artificial Intelligence-Enabled Internet of Medical Things for Enhanced Healthcare Systems. In *Smart Healthcare Systems* (pp. 119–134). CRC Press., DOI: 10.1201/9781032698519-9

Shafik, W. (2024c). Connected healthcare—the impact of Internet of Things on medical services. In *Artificial Intelligence and Internet of Things based Augmented Trends for Data Driven Systems* (pp. 181–217). CRC Press., DOI: 10.1201/9781003497318-10

Shafik, W. (2024d). Digital healthcare systems in a federated learning perspective. In *Federated Learning for Digital Healthcare Systems* (pp. 1–35). Elsevier., DOI: 10.1016/B978-0-443-13897-3.00001-1

Shafik, W. (2024e). IoT-Enabled Secure and Intelligent Smart Healthcare. In *Secure and Intelligent IoT-Enabled Smart Cities* (pp. 308–333). IGI Global., DOI: 10.4018/979-8-3693-2373-1.ch015

Shafik, W. (2024f). Smart Health Revolution: Exploring Artificial Intelligence of Internet of Medical Things. In *Healthcare Industry Assessment: Analyzing Risks, Security, and Reliability* (pp. 201–229). Springer. DOI: 10.1007/978-3-031-65434-3_9

Shafik, W. (2024g). The Future of Healthcare: AIoMT—Redefining Healthcare with Advanced Artificial Intelligence and Machine Learning Techniques. In *Artificial Intelligence and Machine Learning in Drug Design and Development* (pp. 605–634). Wiley., DOI: 10.1002/9781394234196.ch19

Shafik, W. (2024h). The Future of Healthcare: Data-Driven Trends and Innovation. In *Advancing Healthcare through Data-driven Innovations* (pp. 166–185). CRC Press. DOI: 10.1201/9781003475392-11

Shafik, W. (2025a). Artificial Intelligence Assisted Internet of Medical Things (AIoMTs) in Sustainable Healthcare Ecosystem. *Wellness Management Powered by AI Technologies*, 75–101.

Shafik, W. (2025b). Human-Artificial Intelligence Collaborations in Polycystic Ovary Syndrome (PCOS) Clinical Trials and Research. In *AI-Based Nutritional Intervention in Polycystic Ovary Syndrome (PCOS)* (pp. 307–330). Springer Nature Singapore. DOI: 10.1007/978-981-96-2120-0_13

Shafik, W. (2025c). Introduction to Machine Learning and Its Applications to Neuroscience. In *Machine Learning for Neurodegenerative Disorders* (pp. 1–32). CRC Press., DOI: 10.1201/9781032661025-1

Shafik, W. (2025d). Revolutionizing Skin Cancer Diagnosis With Artificial Intelligence: Insights Into Machine Learning Techniques. In *Impact of Digital Solutions for Improved Healthcare Delivery* (pp. 167–194). IGI Global.

Shafik, W. (2025e). Smart biomedical devices for smart healthcare. In *Machine Learning Models and Architectures for Biomedical Signal Processing* (pp. 421–448). Elsevier. DOI: 10.1016/B978-0-443-22158-3.00017-X

Shafik, W., & Kalinaki, K. (2024). Societal and Ethical Implications of Technology-Enhanced Agriculture and Healthcare: An African Context. *2024 IST-Africa Conference (IST-Africa)*, 1–11. DOI: 10.23919/IST-Africa63983.2024.10569306

Shafik, W., Singh, R., & Kumar, V. (2025). Artificial Intelligence Transparency and Explainability in Sustainable Healthcare. In *Transforming Healthcare Sector Through Artificial Intelligence and Environmental Sustainability* (pp. 165–191). Springer.

Shuker, C., Hamblin, R., Stolarek, I., & Simpson, A. (2018). Transparency in Healthcare 2017: Working with Consumers and Clinicians to Co-design a Transparent Future. *International Journal of Integrated Care, 18*(s1), 34. Advance online publication. DOI: 10.5334/ijic.s1034

Singh, R., Shafik, W., Crowther, D., & Kumar, V. (Eds.). (2024). *Transforming Healthcare Sector Through Artificial Intelligence and Environmental Sustainability* (1st ed., Vol. 1). Springer Nature Singapore., DOI: 10.1007/978-981-97-9555-0

Sumner, J., Bundele, A., Lim, H. W., Phan, P., Motani, M., & Mukhopadhyay, A. (2024). Developing an Artificial Intelligence-Driven Nudge Intervention to Improve Medication Adherence: A Human-Centred Design Approach. *Journal of Medical Systems*, *48*(1), 3. Advance online publication. DOI: 10.1007/s10916-023-02024-0 PMID: 38063940

Tang, C., Liu, Z., Hu, Q., Jiang, Z., Zheng, M., Xiong, C., Wang, S., Yao, S., Zhao, Y., Wan, X., Liu, G., Sun, Q., Wang, Z. L., & Li, L. (2024). Unconstrained Piezoelectric Vascular Electronics for Wireless Monitoring of Hemodynamics and Cardiovascular Health. *Small*, *20*(3), 2304752. Advance online publication. DOI: 10.1002/smll.202304752 PMID: 37691019

Totzkay, D. (2024). The potential influence of patient-centered communication, online provider communication, and social determinants of health on cancer screening. *Patient Education and Counseling*, *123*, 108238. Advance online publication. DOI: 10.1016/j.pec.2024.108238 PMID: 38452686

Tseng, T. Y., Mitchell, M. M., Chander, G., Latkin, C., Kennedy, C., & Knowlton, A. R. (2024). Patient-centered Engagement as a Mediator in the Associations of Healthcare Discrimination, Pain Care Denial, and Later Substance Use Among a Sample of Predominately African Americans Living with HIV. *AIDS and Behavior*, *28*(2), 429–438. Advance online publication. DOI: 10.1007/s10461-023-04235-5 PMID: 38060111

Turk, F., Sweetman, J., Chew-Graham, C. A., Gabbay, M., Shepherd, J., & van der Feltz-Cornelis, C. (2024). Accessing care for Long Covid from the perspectives of patients and healthcare practitioners: A qualitative study. *Health Expectations*, *27*(2), e14008. Advance online publication. DOI: 10.1111/hex.14008 PMID: 38481384

Umayal, K. (2024). Strategic Integration of Digital Health Technologies for Enhanced Patient-Centered Care in Modern Healthcare Management. *Shanlax International Journal of Management, 11*(iS1-Jan). DOI: 10.34293/management.v11iiS1-Jan.7142

Valentin, J. B., Mainz, J., Johnsen, S. P., Kristensen, K., & Kristensen, S. (2024). Rasch analysis of a patient-reported outcome measure for self-perceived health among psychiatric patients in Denmark. *BMJ Open Quality*, *13*(1), e002519. Advance online publication. DOI: 10.1136/bmjoq-2023-002519 PMID: 38350672 van Lummel, E. V. T. J., Ietswaard, L., Rigter, M., Tjan, D. H. T., van Delden, J. J. M., & Milota, M. (2024). Finding the balance between person-centred and treatment-centred discussions in advance care planning—A qualitative analysis of conversations within the MUTUAL (Multidisciplinary Timely Undertaken Advance Care Planning conversations) intervention using a narrative analysis. *Age and Ageing*, *53*(3), afae020. Advance online publication. DOI: 10.1093/ageing/afae020 PMID: 38452194

Wang, H., Pathak, M., Takami, T., Wiener, R. C., Shen, C., & Sambamoorthi, U. (2024). Ethnic Disparities in Patient-Centered Communication with Healthcare Providers: A Comparison of Non-Hispanic Asians and Non-Hispanic Whites. *Journal of Racial and Ethnic Health Disparities*. Advance online publication. DOI: 10.1007/s40615-023-01898-7 PMID: 38228862

Weber, D., & Nøhr, C. (2024). National Trial Overview: Towards Accessible and Patient-Centered Healthcare. *Studies in Health Technology and Informatics*, *310*. Advance online publication. DOI: 10.3233/SHTI231175 PMID: 38270025

Williamson, S. M., & Prybutok, V. (2024). Balancing Privacy and Progress: A Review of Privacy Challenges, Systemic Oversight, and Patient Perceptions in AI-Driven Healthcare. In *Applied Sciences (Switzerland)* (Vol. 14, Issue 2). DOI: 10.3390/app14020675

Zhao, C. X., & Yam, M. (2024). Role of patient specific 3D printed models in patient confidence, understanding and satisfaction of care in Singapore. *Journal of Orthopaedics*, *52*, 28–32. Advance online publication. DOI: 10.1016/j.jor.2024.02.010 PMID: 38404701

Chapter 13
Privacy-Preserving Machine Learning Models for Medical Data Ensuring Security in Smart Healthcare Systems

Hira Akhtar Butt
https://orcid.org/0009-0008-7793-1184
University of Central Punjab, Lahore, Pakistan

Zunaira Rashid
University of Management and Technology, Pakistan

Abdul Ahad
https://orcid.org/0000-0002-3914-2503
Northwestern Polytechnical University, Xian, China

Azeem Yousaf
University of Central Punjab, Sialkot, Pakistan

Ishal Imran
https://orcid.org/0009-0003-5356-2402
University of Management and Technology, Pakistan

ABSTRACT

Machine Learning (ML) is being adopted in the healthcare industry across diagnostics, treatment options, and analysis of patient information. The management of data increases risks to the patient's private information. This chapter explores the theoretical frameworks and consequences of privacy-enhancing ML methods, namely, differential privacy, Federated Learning (FL), and homomorphic encryption, to apply medical data for meaningful analysis while maintaining the non-disclosure of patient information. Differential privacy adds noise control to minimize identifying data corresponding to an individual. FL allows the training of models while avoiding data centralization, and homomorphic encryption will enable computations on top of encrypted data to guarantee data safety during processing. We also explain how blockchain could improve these privacy-preserving approaches; it can provide safe data sharing,

DOI: 10.4018/979-8-3373-0593-6.ch013

models, and audit and accountability of model management.

1. INTRODUCTION

Machine learning (ML) is the technology that has contributed so much to the healthcare sector today through accurate diagnosis, prescription, and patient outcome prediction. In healthcare, systems incorporating Medicine ML are rapidly becoming inevitable, ranging from the prediction of diseases to cancer detection and even the diagnosis of diabetic retinopathy (Moqurrab et al., 2022). Still, using ML in healthcare has one disadvantage—the problem of privacy, as patients' data is sensitive and protected by law. Most of these errors are unavoidable, but the challenge is significant because the use of artificial intelligence and other forms of machine learning for delivering healthcare services is now imminent, and the importance of data privacy cannot be overemphasized here (Ali et al., 2022).

The healthcare industry processes large volumes of sensitive information, such as patients' medical records, diagnoses, treatment histories, genetics, and identifiers (Wang et al., 2023). Such complex information adheres to specific rules concerning data protection, like the Health Insurance Portability and Accountability Act (HIPAA) in the USA or the General Data Protection Regulation (GDPR) in the European Union (EU) (Yigzaw et al., 2022). Even though these regulations seek to protect patient identity, the enhanced incorporation of massive datasets in ML models used in health care increases the vulnerability of privacy violations, data misuse, and patient rights infringement (Ahad et al., 2025). Despite the anonymization of medical data, there are ethical, legal, and social consequences when an unauthorized third party accesses the data or re-identified (Sweeney, 2002). Furthermore, centralized data repositories, which are the typical setting for most ML applications, threaten healthcare systems' security with potential data leaks that would compromise the personally identifiable information of numerous individuals (Yigzaw et al., 2022). Thus, the demand for pp-methods in ML is relatively high.

There has been a proposed privacy-preserving technique like Differential Privacy (DP), Federated Learning (FL), and Homomorphic Encryption (HE), which minimize the above risks while making sure that patients' data is also protected from being accessed by unauthorized individuals while developing the best ML models (Ahad et al., 2021). There are fundamentally revolutionary privacy-preserving methods; for example, differential privacy entails adding some noise to resultant datasets, ensuring that specific individuals cannot be discerned in data even when complex algorithms that target details in medical records are employed (Kifer & Machanavajjhala, 2011). This approach also allows the ML models to get their probabilities and analysis right while maintaining the privacy of the individual citizen (Ali et al., 2023).

Federated Learning is another approach that breaks potential data disclosure. That is why FL is different from centralized ML models: data are processed locally on devices while model updates are sent to the central server. Thus, a component that ensures that the patient data are not shared among the central servers, or third parties is guaranteed by this decentralized approach (McMahan et al., 2017). An example is federated learning, where in predictive healthcare analytics, several healthcare organizations contribute to the training of models but the data not show any patient's information (Ali et al., 2023).

This means encrypted data can be used in a computation without taking the data's encodings, thus making computations secure. This implies that any medical data can be processed in encrypted form, guaranteeing the data's independence and patient honesty during the computation process. Thus, homomorphic encryption is functional in settings that require healthcare providers to jointly cryptanalyze datasets, yet they should not get raw data from each other (Gentry, 2009).

Besides the approaches presented above, which guarantee the privacy-preserving of ML, blockchain has ample potential to increase the safety and openness of healthcare data (Butt, Ahad, Wasim, Madeira, et al., 2023). Through this form of distributed database, access to and utilization of medical data is considerably made transparent and accountable since data access records are imprinted within the blockchain ledger. This technology can be applied in developing controlled patient consent to gain access to patient data and coordinate access for research (Hölbl et al., 2018).

Figure 1. **Architecture of Privacy-Preserving Machine Learning Techniques in Healthcare. In this figure, each privacy-preserving technique including Differential Privacy (DP), Homomorphic Encryption (HE) and Federated Learning (FL) is illustrated within secure healthcare as interaction relationship**

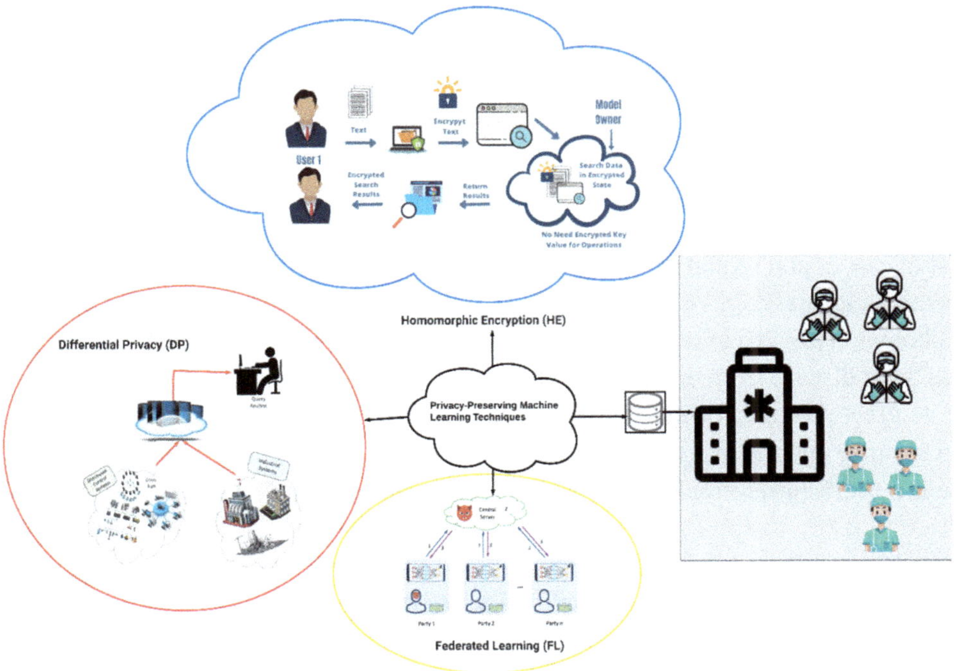

The ***Fig 1*** presents complex architecture suitable for applying privacy-preserving ML methods in healthcare settings. User interfaces with the secure system where the data is encrypted before being submitted to the data processing system in order to ensure it does not compromises the user's privacy. The architecture involves a cloud-based model owner that can point at data and search it by encrypting and decrypting the data thus adds to security by avoiding exposure of keys during operation. Central to this architecture are three primary privacy-preserving strategies: Differential Privacy (DP) which guarantees general data security while using the analyses of the aggregated database; Homomorphic Encryption (HE) through which computations are performed on the encrypted data without requiring decryption; And Federated Learning (FL), whereby several parties such as hospitals train a machine learning model on their data and exchange only updates of the model while keeping data private. Altogether these techniques help to maintain the support of a healthcare facility where patient data are privet while at the same time data for analysis and training different model are well availed. In general, this architecture strives to support data protection and security in healthcare applications which, in turn, will increase the trust of users within such applications as well as utilize machine learning to improve health results (Lin, 2024).

Since healthcare systems continuously turn to ML for sophisticated methods of detection and analysis of diseases, potential moral, legal, and privacy concerns regarding patient data should be discussed. This chapter will describe these techniques and elucidate how they can secure patients' information while promoting the development of machine learning in healthcare.

The Use Of Machine Learning In Developing Healthcare Systems

Machine Learning (ML) has adopted the healthcare sector as one of the most promising areas for implementing accurate diagnosis of diseases and more personalized treatments. Machine learning is a branch of AI, which is the ability of a computer to learn from data without being programmed to do so. Some of the principal areas where ML in healthcare are as follows: medical images (like finding out an abnormality in radiology images, MRI), the prognosis of diseases, customizing treatment procedures, and also generating patterns from large-scale patient databases (Esteva et al., 2019)

Another substantial improvement has occurred in recent years when deeper learning, one of the subtypes of ML, started to create tools for diagnostics that are equal to human expert ones and often even surpass them in some fields. For example, Convolutional Neural Networks (CNN) have accurately diagnosed skin cancer and retinal diseases from images (Litjens et al., 2017). In addition, ML is finding more applications in prescriptive analytics, for instance, in predicting patient clinical deterioration in an ICU (Rajkomar et al., 2018) or identifying patients with potential risk factors for diseases including diabetes and heart disease from data extracted from electronic health records EHRs (Choi et al., 2016).

Despite its great promise for increasing health outcomes using ML, it has several issues with data privacy and security and the question of the right and wrong use of personal health information. These issues remain a thorn in developing practical, scalable, and impactful ML applications in healthcare settings.

Importance of Data Privacy in Medical Applications

Medical data is vulnerable or sensitive since much of it is personal and usually attracts a privacy constraint. It describes some facets of patient characteristics that can be unique identifiers, diagnosis, treatment plan, genealogy, and any other private or confidential data as per HIPAA in the United States or GDPR in Europe. Loss of this kind of data could severely impact individuals, including fraud, such as identity theft, employment discrimination, and other harm to the person's well-being (Sweeney, 2002).

However, data privacy is particularly an acute problem in the case of ML. In most cases, ML algorithms depend on large datasets to build robust models. However, using these datasets poses the danger of exposing patient's sensitive information if adequately managed (Kifer & Machanavajjhala, 2011). Also, there are dangers about the possibility of re-identification of any available medical data in anonymized form. This concern is even more warranted in healthcare organizations, as the data processed is personal and relevant to organizational decision-making. Ironically, it is apparent that as ML technology becomes more integrated into the healthcare system, it is equally important to address the issues with data availability while at the same time protecting the patient's privacy.

The increase in ML technologies has highlighted privacy concerns; most healthcare ML applications are developed to obtain data from various sources and store them in a centralized database. Despite this strategy to amass more powerful models, there are advantages to centralizing AI models and their training data, which embrace data breaches and misuse risks asserted by Raji et al. (2020). They also show a critical gap in PPML that would preserve patient privacy while enhancing healthcare models.

Figure 2. **Measures of Security in Machine Learning Applied to Healthcare**

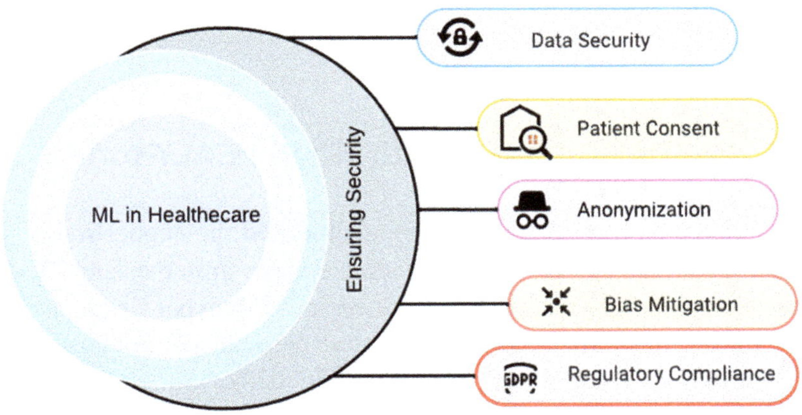

In ***Fig 2*** the elements from this diagram pertain to me and therefore ensures a secure implementation of ML in the health care sectors. At the core we have "ML in Healthcare", highlighting the essence of Machine Learning and how it can make a difference in the lives of patients. Surrounding it are crucial components that contribute to ensuring security: Data Security aims at preventing other unauthorized people or programs from accessing the information; Patient Consent ensures that the patient permits his or her data to be used; Anonymization involves the deletion of the actual identity of users with an aim of protecting their identity; Biases Mitigation to deter bias within an ML model that will in turn lead to unfair treatment; lastly, Regulatory Compliance, which guarantees ML adheres to legal requirements like GDPR to meet ethical practices All these combine into a coherent system that the protects the patient information in the best way possible while maximizing the usefulness of the machine learning technologies in the healthcare field.

Machine learning in health care is advancing, and with it, brings significant privacy challenges.' True to its promise, ML models can give better diagnosis and treatment, but they demand access to big datasets that contain patient's sensitive information. The key task here is to find the right level of ML with protection of personal health data against unauthorized access, breaches, abuse.

Purpose of the Chapter

This chapter aims to discuss and assess privacy preservation techniques in the context of using ML in innovative healthcare systems. With ML technologies getting embedded in today's health systems, ensuring data protection has been seen as a hot issue. This chapter introduces the essential PPML methods, including Differential Privacy (DP), Federated Learning (FL), Homomorphic Encryption (HE), and the use of blockchain as the privacy-enhancement frameworks that would ensure the privacy and protection of medical data. In this line of thought, this chapter will persuade the reader that building contextually advanced ML methods and systems that do not invade patients' privacy is possible by reviewing these methods based on their theoretical background, actual application, and regulatory/ethical concern. Lastly, it outlines a way forward for building safe, thoughtful, and responsible healthcare solutions with AI as the foundation.

2. CHALLENGES IN PRIVACY AND SECURITY IN HEALTHCARE

There are notable benefits, particularly in patients, midfield the application of technology in the delivery of health care, but then again, many challenges emerge from the same. The first is the rising rate of cyber attacks on healthcare systems. For instance, in 2024, cyber Criminals targeted Ascension Health Alliance and Cedars-Sinai Medical Center and stole the details of millions of patients, disruptive operations, and weak protection methods (Rundle, Dec. 27, 2024).

Furthermore, the recent surge of health applications and fitness trackers means that much personal health data is collected. HIPAA is not as applicable as people believe; it regulates only certain entities. However, this law does not protect much consumer health information; myriad state privacy laws govern it. Such a situation leads to handling the issue of data protection as a fragmented process where separate regulators regulate this or that aspect of protection (Jodka, 2024).

However, healthcare practitioners' daily usage of smartphones and other mobile devices poses other unique security risks. Furthermore, a survey of resident physicians in Germany established that although smartphones are essential tools of medicine practice, they present an acute security threat, such as unlawful accessibility of patient records and other emerging possible breaches due to inherent insecurity in smartphones (Kraushaar & Bohnet-Joschko, 2022).

Data sensitivity and patient privacy concerns

Medical data sensitivity is a consequence of the private and confidential character of the information received, including diagnoses, characterization of treatment, genetic information, and identifiable data that, in case of leakage, can cause a negative impact in the hands of other individuals. In the healthcare sector, there are high risks associated with the leakage of sensitive information, including credit card fraud, stigmatization, and discrimination, which squarely translate to social and psychological consequences in affected persons' lives (Rumbold & Pierscionek, 2017). The risks of these problems are compounded by the growing use of Electronic Health Records (EHRs) and AI involving advanced health systems because they extend data collection and analysis to millions of individuals (Fernández-Alemán et al., 2013) We have identified that EHR systems are most exposed to cyber threats as they operate as centralized databases storing a large volume of highly confidential data.

Figure 3. **Privacy Concerns Relating to Artificial Neural Networks in Medicine**

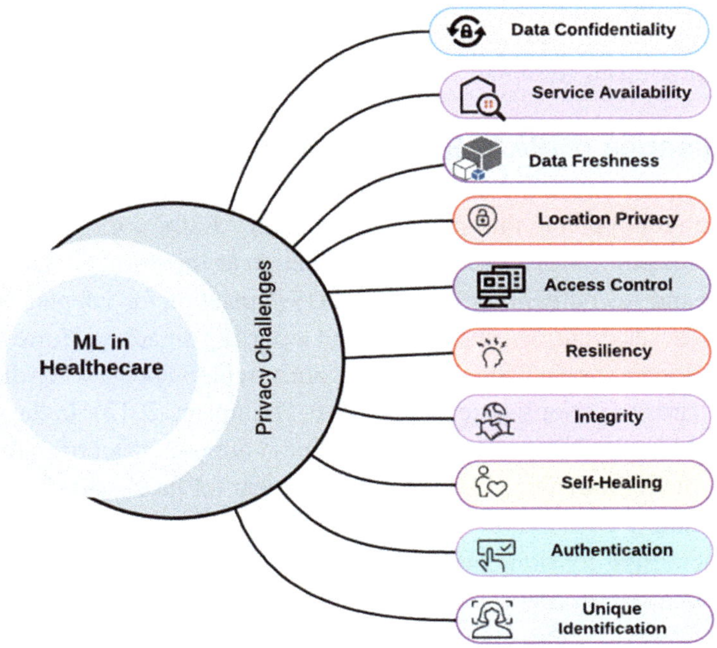

The diagram in ***Fig 3*** Presents key privacy risks that emerge with the integration of machine learning (ML) in healthcare. The middle of the diagram is dedicated to the term "ML in Healthcare," which states the main role of the concept in defining the changes in patient's treatment. Around this key notion, several issues need to be discussed to understand how to apply ML technologies efficiently and safely. Some challenges include Data Confidentiality, which concerns protecting sensitive patient information; Service Availability, which concerns the availability of health care services; and Data Freshness, which concerns using fresh data in data analysis. Further, the diagram also describes Location Privacy regarding patient location data privacy and Access Control regarding data access permission. Other challenges of Dependability are Resiliency – where a system should be able to handle failure; Integrity – where a system should remain honest and accurate; Self-Healing – where a system should be able to diagnose and correct all failures; Authentication – where a system should only allow authorized entities to access data; and finally, Unique Identification is important because it calls for the identification of a person with the least invasion of privacy. In combination, they all highlight the contingencies and challenges when adopting machine learning as a part of clinical decision-making and maintaining patients' privacy and security of generated data.

Further, common de-identification and anonymization techniques used in preserving the patient's information have been revealed to possess some shortcomings (Narayanan & Shmatikov, 2008). Showed how real people can be found in anonymized datasets withdrawn from online databases re-correlated with another public dataset, thus questioning the efficiency of current PPML methods. Furthermore, the patient's consent is often inadequate or not obtained in data sharing and research situations, constituting ethical violations. For example, (Gaye et al., 2014) Reported findings from a cross-sectional survey revealed that a number of the participants were not clear on how their data was used in secondary research; therefore, there is a need to establish clear guidelines on data management. Such issues only highlight the need for healthcare organizations to employ better privacy practices for keeping their patients' trust and staying ethical, both of which require incorporating stronger cryptographical practices and distributed data processing systems.

Regulatory challenges (HIPAA, GDPR, etc) and compliance

It emphasizes the requirements that mark the regulatory framework of healthcare data to protect privacy and promote the ethical use of sensitive information as the primary challenge. HIPAA – Health Insurance Portability and Accountability Act – is the US legislation for safeguarding health information with the standards for access controls, encryption, and reporting breaches. However, these requirements are often complex, and operative challenges for healthcare providers appear when they attempt to introduce unified security standards to various systems (Rinehart-Thompson, 2013). In the same way, the General Data Protection Regulation (GDPR) in the European Union imposes strict rules for data protection, such as a right to erasure, the right to data portability, and consent for processing.

A work by (Chaudhuri, 2018) Shows the problem of aligning GDPR with current practices in the healthcare sector, increasing tensions between access to information for medical needs and privacy concerns. Data transfer across borders takes the process up a notch because organizations face numerous situations where the GDPR is either interpreted or implemented differently by different member states (Hoofnagle et al., 2019). However, sanctions for failure to observe these laws are stiff; under GDPR, a company can be fined up to €20 million or 4% of global turnover, making the risks both financial and reputational (*General Data Protection Regulation.*, 2016).

The issues of HIPAA and GDPR are not uniform across the globe. As a result, it is exceedingly difficult to achieve compliance if there are joint operations between different healthcare systems of other countries. According to (McGraw, 2013) Piecemeal regulations work against MM technologies like AI since organizations dealing with such innovations are bound to face legal challenges. These regulatory hurdles underscore the necessity of healthcare entities to commit resources to enhanced compliance initiatives beyond limited privacy programs, decisive managerial or employee training, and superficial integration of privacy mechanisms to resolve corresponding issues under global demands.

Ethical considerations in the use of medical data

Ethical implementation of medical data balances research's possible benefits with patients privacy rights. The first of healthcare's four fundamental moral principles is respect for autonomy, meaning a patient's data cannot be used without consent. That said, honoring meaningful consent has remained elusive in practice, especially when data collection is massive. In cases of secondary data use (Ploug, 2020) most patients are not informed about how their data is shared or reused because consent forms are lengthy and unclear. Also, the principle of beneficence requires the custodians of health information to utilize such data to promote the highest good for patients. However, the ethical issue arises because the same data can be used for advertising purposes, such as forming advertisers' interests in opposition to the patients (Grady, 2015). Another significant ethical implication is the ability to misuse data, which is based on the fact that anonymized data sets are usually identifiable through more complex analysis (El Emam et al., 2011).

When decisions are made to limit the amount of data from certain cultures or populations, prejudices of equity and justice are at stake, thus possibly increasing health inequality. Justice is also an ethical principle requiring all population groups to benefit equally from medical research and technological innovations (Prainsack & Buyx, 2017). Lastly, other ethical issues emerge when applying artificial intelligence, including algorithmic bias and accountability.

As rightly pointed out by (Mittelstadt et al., 2016) Where AI systems make critical healthcare staking decisions, there must be ways to enable accountability to capture the risks of opaque and unfair decision-making or harm. Such ethical concerns warrant comprehensive regulatory and policy mechanisms that protect the appropriate use and sharing of medical data in respectful, beneficial, and justified ways to build trust between patients and healthcare givers (Butt, Ahad, Wasim, Shayea, et al., 2023).

3. PRIVACY-PRESERVING MACHINE LEARNING (PPML) TECHNIQUES

PPML solutions are intended to solve two problems simultaneously: utilizing big datasets to promote the development of AI-based healthcare solutions while protecting patient data privacy. The most popular solutions include differential privacy, federated learning, and homomorphic encryption, which differ in data protection and anonymity.

DP is a technique that synthesizes datasets and protects the inputs of individual records while retaining some utility for analysts. This approach guarantees that in the dataset generated, no single individual's information can be identified even when the attacker has some secondary information. According to (Dwork & Roth, 2014) DP is defined as a mathematical of privacy, which can be realized by injecting noise into the query outputs or during model training. For instance, in the healthcare domain, DP has been seamlessly incorporated into genomic research so that statistics can be computed on otherwise irreversibly identifying genetic data (Abadi et al., 2016).

Another unique method is FL, which enables a model's training in distributed devices or organizations without sharing the original data to a crucial point. In FL, the data remains local, and only the model updating procedure is conducted on the central server, which does not cause any violation of data protection regulations such as GDPR. One application is in the context of predictive healthcare analytics; similar to Google's GDELT, hospitals jointly train models for early disease diagnostics while keeping patients' data private (McMahan et al., 2017). Research by (Sheller et al., 2020) explains that FL has been applied, for instance, in enhancing MRI diagnostic scans without patient identification data being transferred to headquarters.

Homomorphic encryption (HE) provides a mathematical computation that can be done by cryptographic means on an encrypted data item without decrypting it. This helps ensure that the data stays protected through the processing chain. HE is more valuable when multiple healthcare providers require dataset analysis but cannot share raw data due to data sensitivity. For instance, (Gentry, 2009) The idea of fully homomorphic encryption as the means of securely evaluating functions was proposed, while subsequent developments ensured that fully homomorphic encryption is computationally viable in specific medical settings. For instance, (Akgün et al., 2015) Used HE to study the genomic data for disease risks and avenues without involving the original sequences.

In addition to these fundamental approaches, blockchain has appeared as a complementary method to improve privacy levels in ML. With the help of blockchain, information is transparent and cannot be easily altered. Utilizing smart contracts guarantees the introduction of a highly effective approach to security access to sensitive healthcare data. From (Liang et al., 2017) Blockchain has to be deployed with FL to capture the model migration process and ensure security in institutional collaboration.

These privacy-preserving techniques can manage specific privacy concerns from the data, making them suitable for addressing various umbrella facets of privacy when combined. They can significantly boost the credibility of AI in the healthcare domain. Nevertheless, issues like computational costs, complexity of scalability, and users' acceptance are still open questions.

Differential Privacy (DP)

Data privacy, specifically Differential Privacy (DP), is a mathematical theory conceived primarily to prevent the leakage of persons' information when analyzing data. By definition, a mechanism satisfies DP if an observer cannot tell whether a particular individual's information is in the data set, even with background information (Dwork & Roth, 2014). The idea is simple: the basic idea in noise addition is to introduce randomness into the computation, which can never give an extrapolated detailed profile of any individual. Such property enables exchanging/aggregating data or using it inside an organization without compromising privacy; this makes DP especially useful in healthcare, where data is especially sensitive.

The simplest mode of DP is adding noise into the answer or a reasonable computation done to the data. This noise is proportional to the sensitivity of the function that is to be computed, which can, in many cases, use distributions such as Laplace or Gaussian. The privacy parameter reduces the amount of noise. This parameter is often represented by ϵ, which measures the privacy leakage and is defined based on the minimum amount of randomness of the difference between the actual and modified joint distribution (Abadi et al., 2016). A lower ϵ is stronger privacy because of additional noise, but it sacrifices some data authenticity. For example, in the case of healthcare, DP can be used to prevent identity disclosure issues where statistical computation on a given data set, like the prevalence of a particular disease or patients' outcome several months after admittance to a hospital, cannot reveal individual attributes of the patients even if an observer who has some extra information on the patients tries to perform an inversion attack.

Figure 4. **Application of Differential Privacy (DP) in Data Analysis**

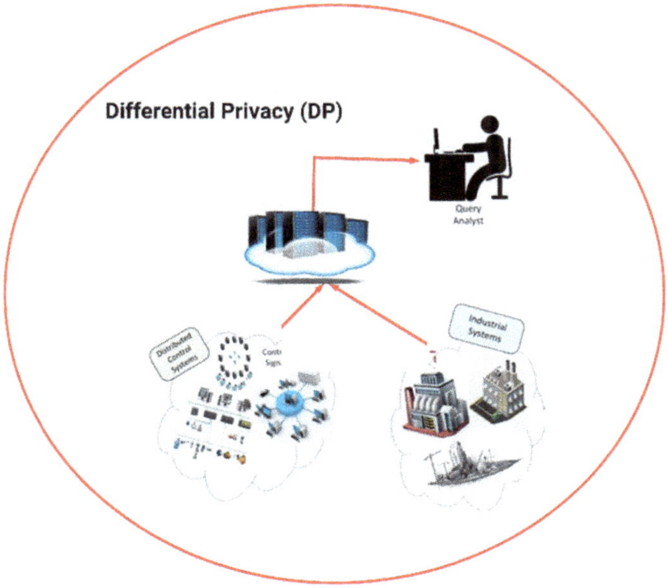

The diagram of DP in ***Fig 4*** It gives an idea of how DP prevents individual privacy during data analysis. In its simplest form, DP allows a query analyst to retrieve and examine data residing in a secure cloud database while preserving citizens' privacy. This flow chart shows where the data moves through the system and where the analyst interacts with a cloud-based storage and retrieval system. This cloud dedicates relevant data for use in Industrial Systems and Distributed Control Systems, among others. That is where transparency shines, and these systems rely on DP's safe and privacy-preserving function to deliver insights while avoiding identifying unique individuals. While adding noise to the result, Differential Privacy guarantees that the absence or presence of anyone's information does not greatly impact the result, thereby strengthening the protection of personal and sensitive data within data analysis in various industries.

Differential privacy has been implemented and evaluated in several healthcare-related use cases to safeguard identifiable patient data. One of the most specific fields to which DP was applied is genomic research, as personal genetic data is among the most recognizable. (Johnson, Pollard, Shen, Lehman, Feng, Ghassemi, Moody, Szolovits, Anthony Celi, et al., 2016) Illustrated how DP could be applied to safely disclose summary statistics, preserve patient privacy, and conduct extensive analysis simultaneously. Another example is using DP within the Electronic Health Record (EHR) systems framework (Erlingsson et al., 2014). I have done a study and introduced a tool called RAPPOR to gather and analyze the aggregate frequencies of sensitive medical behaviors without leaking individual information. Moreover, DP has been embedded into federated learning paradigms for health care, enabling the federated learning and training of predictors across different institutions while respecting patients' privacy (McMahan et al., 2017). Hopefully, these examples illustrate DP's capacity to respond to concerns about the burgeoning application of big data in health care.

Table 1. Summary of Key Research on Differential Privacy (DP) in healthcare

Ref.	Year	Objectives	Performance	Major Limitations
(Dwork & Roth, 2014)	2014	To provide a mathematical framework ensuring individual data privacy in statistical analysis.	It describes the theoretical groundwork of DP and illustrates the possibility of private data analysis.	The density of noise may impact the accuracy of the data collected; privacy and functionality of the databases are incompatible.
(Abadi et al., 2016)	2016	DP can be used in machine learning frameworks to protect personal data.	Enhances the ability to add noise to real-world applications of ML that address data analysis privacy.	The variant for the privacy parameter ϵ is not straightforward; often takes time to attain the privacy levels desired.
(Johnson et al., 2016)	2016	In order to deploy DP to reveal summary statistics while retaining patients' anonymity in genomic data.	Explains how to keep privacy in genomic research while disclosing and maintaining security for sensitive information.	It should be noted that the applicability of public versus private might differ depending on the data type; genomic data is especially privacy sensitive.
(Erlingsson et al., 2014)	2014	To introduce a tool for collecting sensitive medical behavior data without compromising individual privacy.	It facilitates the easy and efficient obtainment of data grouped while maintaining the anonymity of respondents' responses.	However, depending on the context and distribution of the information, averages can persistently anonymize information that secretly sanitizes personal identity.
(McMahan et al., 2017)	2017	To allow federated learning while promoting privacy for patients in different healthcare settings.	It supports multiple training strategies simultaneously and provides patient confidentiality with other datasets.	Issues of model complexity in the training process and data management; possibility of variability of the model's performance from institution to institution.

The following ***Table 1*** provides a summary of the key findings on the state of DP research relevant to healthcare. Every entry also points out the reference, year, title, aims and objectives, performance indicators, and key limitations of each research finding.

Federated Learning (FL)

When the training data is sensitive, Federated Learning (FL) is a distributed method to train a machine learning model where the actual data is never collected centrally: it is kept locally on the devices, while the updates of the model parameters are accumulated at a central server (McMahan et al., 2017). With the help of this paradigm, it is possible to solve significant problems such as privacy and security since data that envisages valuable information, such as patients' records in healthcare, are not transferred or accumulated. Some of the benefits that FL offers over conventional aged, centralized learning are. The method is more suitable than FL in areas such as healthcare, where data privacy is paramount. First, it eliminates the possibility of data leakage since data will be stored where it originated. Second, it adheres much better to compliance with standards such as GDPR and HIPAA, which imply very restrictive policies regarding data sharing and storage. Finally, FL also supports institutions to work together on meaningful and effective generalized models without leaking data information (Butt, Ahad, Wasim, Madeira, et al., 2023).

In FL, model training takes place iteratively in the participating nodes – devices or organizations that own the local data set. Every node retrains the model using its local data and only sends the update (for instance, gradients or weights) to the server. The server then takes these updates, often through mechanisms such as Federated averaging, and combines them to produce a global model that can learn from all participants (McMahan et al., 2017). This continues until convergence in a process known as the iterative process or until the model has stabilized. To strengthen privacy even more, FL can be combined with techniques like Differential Privacy, in which noise is added to the model updates, and Secure Aggregation, which ensures that the said updates are encrypted during transfer (Kairouz et al., 2021). The damages arising from centralized training can indeed be effectively minimized by FL, thus making the concept very effective (Butt, Ahad, Wasim, Shayea, et al., 2023).

Figure 5. **FL Architecture**

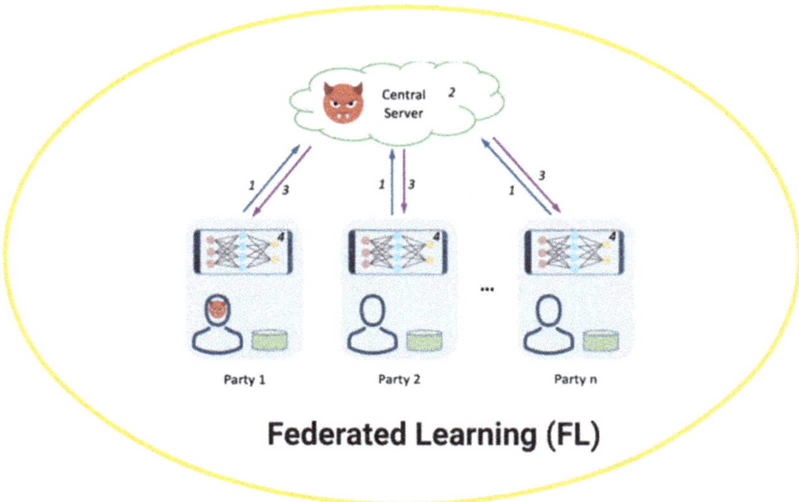

Fig 5 shows the architecture of Federated Learning (FL), the decentralized approach to AI/ML, where several parties train a model while the data remains centrally with the parties. In this setup, Party 1, Party 2, and Party n denote different data holders performing local model training on their own data set. These training processes are parallel, and each party updates its model parameters from the data it possesses. The central server coordinates the interaction between the parties, which combines the model updates without receiving the raw data, thus protecting privacy. Schematic arrows depict the delivery of model parameters between the involved parties and the central server. This framework will enable organizations to harness the benefits of machine learning without exposing sensitive data to the public domain, hence improving privacy and security in shared intelligent environments.

FL has been deployed in healthcare following its proven convenience, especially in projects involving multiple institutions but limited data sharing. Its primary use is in computer-aided diagnosis, specifically in medical imaging. (Butt, Ahad, Wasim, Madeira, et al., 2023) used FL to develop a Deep-Learning (DL) model to segment brain tumors from MRI scans from several hospitals (Butt, Ahad, Wasim, Shayea, et al., 2023). The patient data is stored at the local level of each institution through decentralized data storage. The study successfully achieved high model accuracy, which is near to central data storage, while maintaining patient confidentiality. Likewise, FL has been applied in the prediction of EHR data. (Stripelis et al., 2024) Showed how FL can be used to build models for estimating CV risk factors while preserving data locally in multiple hospitals instead of sharing the information with other parties (Sheller et al., 2020).

FL also applies to the use of wearables in the health sector. For example, (Brisimi et al., 2018) Used FL to train models concerning the health status of individual clients based on data collected by wearable gadgets. This approach made it possible to create concrete individual predictions like blood glucose level prediction and keep users' raw data secure on the user's device (Shome et al.). All these examples serve to demonstrate how FL has the potential to revolutionize private healthcare data analysis by allowing enhanced learning, collaboration, and stepped advancement in the field of personalized medicine (Panayides et al., 2020).

Table 2. Summary of Key Research on Federated Learning (FL) in Healthcare

Ref.	Year	Objectives	Performance	Major Limitations
(McMahan et al., 2017)	2017	To allow for training of the ML models from the locally stored data In order to avoid the centralization of the data.	Effective model training is illustrated along with data privacy conscious approaches; solves privacy problem related to sensitive data usage.	Challenges in coordinating the sections to produce updates; effective communication of the protocols are important.
(Butt et al., 2023)	2023	To examine how FL can be used in the context of the healthcare system, to follow the legal requirements and increase the safety of data.	Effectively deploys and progresses deep learning algorithms bimodal reflectivity for medical imaging as well as patient anonymity.	Deficiencies in switches relate the model convergence difficulties with the heterogeneity of data distribution between the institutions.
(Stripelis et al., 2024)	2024	The framework, FL, can be used to estimate cardiovascular risk factors without compromise to patient data.	Does it in a way that allows for the accurate estimation of CV risk factors but without prejudice to the patients' data protection rights.	Some draw back on imprecise model in the case where local datasets are small or unbalanced.
(Brisimi et al., 2018)	2018	To process health statistics derived from these wearables and provide user safety for their raw data in their devices.	Does allow for customized forecasts, for example the level of glucose in blood, while preserving anonymity.	In wearables, dependency on devices and variation in wearables' use can potentially impact data credibility and consequently device models.
(Kairouz et al., 2021)	2021	To enhance the privacy of FL, a method that involves utilizing between Differential Privacy and Secure Aggregation.	Doubles up as a way to increase the privacy of Models during update and aggregation operations.	At a higher level of security, certain evaluation trade-offs, current and future model complexity.

Table 2 table gives a summary of the important studies done on Federated Learning (FL), especially in the healthcare domain. The meta-data for each entry consist of references, year of publication, title, aims and objectives, key performance indicators, and proximal, distal, and relative research limitations attributable to the studies.

Homomorphic Encryption (HE)

Homomorphic Encryption is an approach that involves encrypting plaintext information using a cryptographic algorithm to ciphertext where mathematical operations are performed. For example, if two values, x and y., are encrypted as E(x) and E(y), operations such as addition or multiplication can be performed directly. E(y), addition, or multiplication can be directly made on the ciphertexts. $(E(x) + E($

y)) to produce E(x+y). This encrypted result can be decrypted to give the correct plaintext result faster than taking a casualty x+y. Fully Homomorphic Encryption follows this concept of complete obfuscation by safely allowing further computations, such as polynomial functions in computations (Gentry, 2009).

In healthcare, this mechanism guarantees that the patient data is encrypted every time it is stored, transmitted, and processed. For example, it is possible to have a cloud server perform data analytics on encrypted health records, but such a server does not get a chance to deal with the raw data. This has a unique application in projects where many organizations are involved and must exchange data to analyze them to provide value to many clients but should not disclose any patient details (Lu et al., 2015).

Figure 6. **Homomorphic Encryption (HE) for Secure Data Processing**

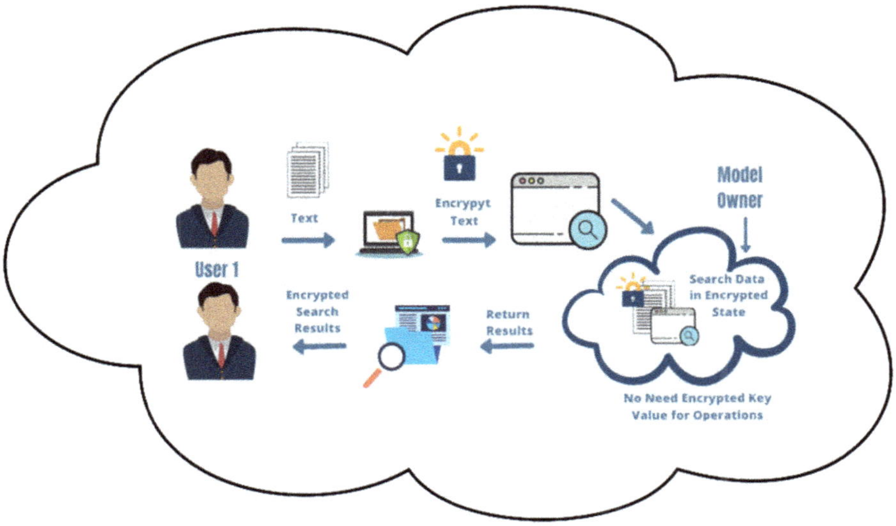

The following ***Fig 6*** look at explaining the HE general idea and Analyse it using the selected diagram in cloud computing environment when it comes to secure data processing. The process starts with the user feeding the system with sensitive text data that is encrypted before being sent. This encryption make sure that the data does not fall into the wrong hands as it transits to the cloud. The Model Owner in cloud also has the capacity to search and perform operation on the data when it is in encrypted form without exposing any key. Finally, after further processing, the encrypted search results are passed back to the user for further protection of the original data through the entire result processing process. This architecture reinforces the strength of Homomorphic Encryption since meaningful computation can be performed on encrypted data and still not reduce privacy making its application powerful in secure data management and analysis throughout several applications.

Homomorphic Encryption is mainly used in healthcare applications, particularly in sensitive areas. One area is in genomic data analysis, where, for instance, the increase in the number of genes identified as causing a specific disease complicates the differential diagnostics. The genomic data is unique regarding privacy, mainly since the data contains identifiers and is linked to individuals. Researching's HE facilitates computation on encrypted genomic sequences and helps researchers find genetic markers of diseases while preserving the actual sequences of genomes of individual patients (Akgün et al., 2015).

HE is also used in prediction, in which patients' records are encrypted and used to train predictive AI systems for diseases. For instance, in oncology, encrypted tumor-related data can be used to evaluate patterns and assess potential improvements to cancer treatment policy without compromising the identifiable information of the patients. (Naehrig). Another example is in telemedicine, where HE guarantees the privacy of consultations and diagnoses conducted on servers outside the health system (Yue et al., 2016).

Moreover, HE is used in drug discovery and clinical trial data analysis. Biopharmaceutical firms can conduct coordinated research on common databases by safely simultaneously evaluating patients' reactions to certain medications while extending customer privacy. This application is most suitable in the case of rare diseases, as data from different centers need to be amalgamated for valid inference (Chirra, 2023).

Long considered pure privacy, Homomorphic Encryption has drawbacks, such as a high computational cost and scalability concerns. Current solutions of FHE are computationally expensive, making them inaccessible to real-time healthcare systems. However, the current research findings focus on improving points and developing more effective algorithms and hardware acceleration to enable the broad application of HE in the health sector.

Table 3. Summary of Key Research on Homomorphic Encryption (HE) in Healthcare

Ref.	Year	Objectives	Performance	Major Limitations
(Gentry, 2009)	2009	To propose a cryptographic scheme that would enable arithmetic on plain messages and ciphertexts without converting these to plaintext.	Laid down the first of the so-called Fully Homomorphic Encryption (FHE) techniques for secure evaluation.	Substantial computation cost; it cannot be employed in real-time processes due to high complexity.
(Lu et al., 2015)	2015	To apply HE in healthcare analytics, how can patient data be protected from being checked during the process of analysis.	Showcased the capacity to analyze encrypted health records' data without compromising raw data.	Not very easy to practice due to computational complexity; the use in large data set might be problematic.
(Akgün et al., 2015)	2015	To allow for calculations of encrypted genomic sequences to be used in identification of disease markers.	Allowed the consideration of a large number of patients' data in genomic analysis without compromising their identification data.	Size and density of the genomic data and possibility of encountering a large number of algorithm calls; resource-intensive.
(Yue et al., 2016)	2016	Telemedicine consultations, examination or diagnosis which are maintained on external servers must be protected on a privacy basis.	Increased patient privacy of communication in cases of telemedicine intervention.	Reliance on computation; cannot be used in real-time times The algorithms require a strong computational power to operate smoothly.
(Chirra, 2023)	2023	For secure analysis of clinical trial data when one or many organizations are dealing with the data of the patients.	It was possible to carry out group research on patient response to medications while at the same time preserving patient's confidentiality.	Due to the high dimensionality, it is computationally expensive, and is sometimes less scalable; new methods have to be continuously sought for its implementation.

This ***Table 3*** gives a brief on important research done on Homomorphic Encryption (HE), and the various uses in health care. Every entry has the number of references, year of publication, title, objectives of the study, key performance outcomes and relevant concerns or limitations that are related to each of the studies embraced.

4. BLOCKCHAIN AND DATA PRIVACY

Blockchain is a decentralized digital-based record-keeping method offering secure, transparent, and tamper-free services. In the chain, every block has a series of secured transactions that cannot be changed by anyone unless transformed by the network participants (S. Nakamoto, 2008). This decentralized structure removes the dependence on a central body, increasing reliability and other people's trust. Traditional blockchain work is based on consensus algorithms like the proof of work or proof of stake to approve the authenticity of the transactions and ensure that the system is not compromised. Blockchain was initially developed to be used only for cryptocurrencies, but today, it has found its use in multiple sectors, such as healthcare, because of its potential to maintain the integrity of the data and its ability to keep it private (Zhang et al., 2018).

It seeks to examine how Blockchain enhances data privacy and security in diverse ways. First, it uses a cryptographic hash to preserve data from getting modified by unauthorized people. Also, due to decentralization in the case of blockchain, no concentrated points may be compromised, as is the case of many database hacks (Zhang et al., 2018). Moreover, blockchain comprises permissioned networks whereby only predetermined people with access authorizations can view or submit transactions. In healthcare, the same feature facilitates access to specific patient details that are available only to authorized individuals. Smart contracts also complement the patient's privacy since they automate the decision-making process, including procedures like patient consent before their data can be shared, depending on specific conditions predefined. (Hu et al., 2018).

Blockchain allows for the safe sharing of data in the healthcare sector through the creation of safer ground, away from third-party interferences (Khan et al., 2021). For example, blockchain in electronic health records enables multiple physicians to share a patient record for research or collaboration treatment with a record of permanent transactions log indicating who accessed the data and why (Hölbl et al., 2018). In model management, blockchain can contain the machine learning models and their changes and be traced at any point in the model's life cycle. This is particularly important in FL frameworks where, through blockchain, the mathematic contribution of different participants receives accurate tracking and auditing (Liang et al., 2017).

Another capability that supports accountability is present in blockchain, which is auditability. For instance, each transaction is stamped and assigned to the specific user who made it, thus offering an incredibly detailed action trail. Concerning this audit trail, where data is breached or misused, the culprit or the irresponsible person can be easily identified, upholding credibility among the stakeholders and discouraging the irresponsible lot (Singh et al., 2024).

The idea of Blockchain can be regarded as highly beneficial for auditing in the sphere of healthcare as well as for compliance with ethical standards. Due to the incorruptibility of the technique, the usage data can be monitored transparently while preserving compliance with legal requirements, including HIPAA or GDPR. For instance, blockchain can apply regulations in compliance procedures since the smart contract can alert authorities on violations or control user access (Ichikawa et al., 2017). Furthermore, it is impossible to change records of consent, access, or data sharing through blockchain solutions, which means blockchain brings credible evidence to escalate ethical issues.

Blockchain can also apply to ethical data sharing in research. For instance, it can offer consent solutions that enable patients to give or withdraw their data access as necessary, all within a record of their transactions (Fareed et al., 2019). Such a level of control is compatible with values of autonomy and accountability, so the data is being utilized properly and frantically.

Concept of Blockchain Technology

Blockchain is a distributed digital ledger technology with digital records of transactions executed in an organization. In this chain, each block has a pointer to the previous block; it contains the address of the computer managing the block and the time the transactions occurred while the recorded information is stored in the transaction databases. The fact that it is based on distributed database and shared between users means that there is no way for a single authority to change the data and make it not transparent to others (Satoshi Nakamoto, 2008). In consensus models such as PoW or PoS, blockchain guarantees that only lawful transactions are incorporated into the chain. This technology, initially used for cryptocurrencies like Bitcoin, has now become a game changer in areas of work excluding finance and especially in the field of health care where security and accuracy of data are paramount(Nakamoto & Bitcoin, 2008).

How blockchain enhances data privacy and security

Blockchain contributes to strengthening data protection and privacy and fastens data cryptographic processing due to decentralization. Data hashing creates the ability to make a message, once recorded in a blockchain block, almost immutable to further modifications. This makes it secure and protects it; it cannot be tampered with, guaranteeing total integrity. Blockchain is every point distributed and does not have single access points to it, making it resistant to the hacking that is prevalent in most centrally controlled systems (Zhang et al., 2018).

Also, privacy is upheld since blockchain provides only permissioned blockchains, which provide access to only authenticated individuals. These permissioned networks enable specific organizations to have the power to decide who can access the data to view or add transactions or even validate the transactions. Furthermore, the smart contracts incorporated into the blockchain can solve problems of patient consent for data exchange, compliance with personal data protection, including GDPR and HIPAA, and security (Hölbl et al., 2018).

Figure 7. **Block-chain based Data Sharing Architecture for Healthcare**

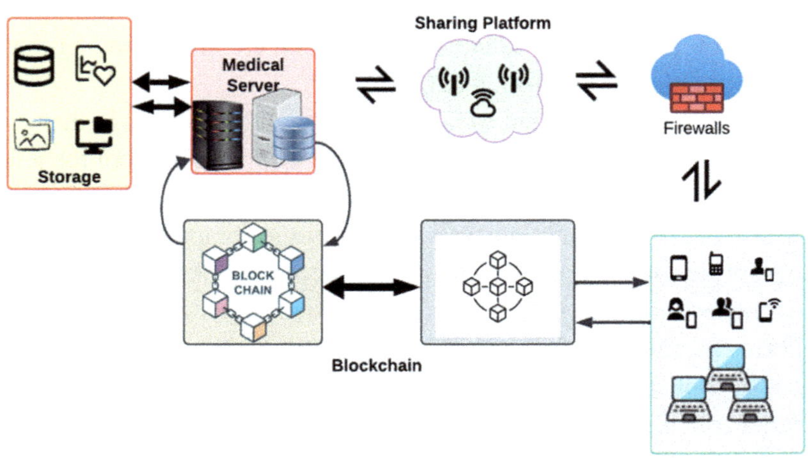

In *Fig 7* the diagram depicts a complex architecture for secure exchange of data in healthcare context introduced blockchain to improve privacy and data security. The central part of the software solution is a blockchain, which is to become a distributed database for managing medical information. It starts with Storage wherein confidential medical data are stored, while a Medical Server is used in dealing and processing of this information. It means that data passes between the storage and the medical server to enable easy access to the data to the owner without compromising its integrity. A Sharing Platform connects different users as well as stakeholders while leveraging the usage of Firewalls to prevent hacking incidents. The application of the blockchain environment means that any data provided to be used by the end-users of the devices, be it a mobile, tablet or a computer, is indeed accurate and cannot be tampered with in any way. This architecture is a good example of modern trends in creating secure data storage in healthcare, where the combination of blockchain and privacy-preserving methods is used to build trust for sharing medical data.

Safe Data Sharing, Model Management, and Accountability in Smart Healthcare Using Blockchain

In the medical profession, blockchain has enabled secure data sharing as the platform is transparent and incredibly resistant to alterations. For example, hospitals can transmit patient records to researchers while protecting the patients' data, as blockchain can also record data access and sharing (Hu et al., 2023). This sharing approach allows ease of working together among healthcare givers without compromising the patient's data (Vishwa, 2021).

In model management, especially in applications such as FL in ML, blockchain captures the contribution and evolution of models across organizations. The model's progression between iterations must be recorded on the blockchain to create a verifiable path of the model, thus avoiding modification by outside actors (Zhang et al., 2021). Blockchain also encourages accountability by providing data models and transaction history for review. This is particularly beneficial in flagging bias or error in learning algorithms utilized in clinical decisions (Pawar et al., 2021).

The usefulness of Blockchain in Controlling and Guaranteeing Ethical Standards Compliance for Auditing

Auditing compliance with ethical standards in the health sector would not be possible without blockchain. Collectively, these facts mean that each DA or DS event is recorded on the blockchain, leaving no room for violating laws such as GDPR and HIPAA. (Ichikawa et al., 2017). This trail is beneficial when solving controversy or looking into cyber-crime problems such as hacking.

Moreover, by enabling smart contracts, blockchain developed a way to use automation in regulation. 'These contracts can set conditions, for instance, whereby patient data can only be shared with the patient's consent or when there is a report of a data breach incident to the authorities. Granting, withdrawing, or varying their consent on data usage involves dynamic consent mechanisms that are more under autonomy and accountability ethics (Fareed et al., 2019)The blockchain provides confidence to patients, researchers, and healthcare consumers by making the processes transparent and ethical. It keeps the patient in charge of their data while allowing the health systems to meet moral and legal requirements.

5. CASE STUDIES AND APPLICATIONS

Case Study 1: A Federated Learning System for Brain Tumor Segmentation

The use case of FL to accelerate research in medical imaging using de-identified patient images across multiple institutions is a recent and pioneering work. (Sheller et al., 2020) Applied FL to fine-tune deep learning models for brain Tumor segmentation on MRI datasets drawn from different hospitals. This approach was GDPR compliant since patient data was never sent to other centers; only model parameters were shared between centers while the performance was like centralized training. This approach promoted cooperation between hospitals while at the same time not violating patient confidentiality in a way that demonstrated FL benefits in various forms of sensitive applications in healthcare institutions.

Case Study 2: Differential Privacy in Genomic Data Sharing

DP has been used in genomic studies where data sharing could be conducted securely. To address these concerns, (Johnson, Pollard, Shen, Lehman, Feng, Ghassemi, Moody, Szolovits, Celi, et al., 2016) Proposed a DP framework that produced plummeted genomic summaries by adding calibrated noise to avoid individual genetic data information leakage. This was particularly so for consented collections like the International Genome Sample Resource, whose data sharing across institutions was previously restricted by privacy issues.

Case Study 3: Blockchain for the Exchange of Secure Health Information

Blockchain implementation for secure health data exchange has been successfully implemented in Estonia's healthcare system. The Estonian government uses blockchain technology to preserve electronic health records (EHRs), and here, all the activities related to the patient's data are recorded and cannot be changed (Hölbl et al., 2018). This system improved patient trust, revolutionized the information exchange between healthcare providers and researchers worldwide, and presented a standard model for privacy-preserving EHR management.

Application 1: Homomorphic Encryption in Telemedicine

The other application of HE concerns telemedicine, in which HE has made it possible to perform computations that do not reveal the patient's information. The authors (Tang et al., 2016) provided an example of applying HE for processing encrypted medical images in cloud web servers. This made it possible to keep patient data safe while being processed, a key challenge of telemedicine since it uses third-party platforms to execute prescriptions. The study pointed out how HE could enable remote care to be safe and sustainable at the same time (Akgün et al., 2015).

Application 2: Privacy-Preserving Machine Learning for Diabetes Prediction

Many models for diagnosing diabetes and other chronic diseases involve collecting large volumes of patient information, which raises privacy concerns. (Brisimi et al., 2018) Used FL to create the model employing EHR data from numerous HCOs. It helped keep data local and still have precisely accurate models, which was the goal of the approach defended. This application shows that privacy-preserving technologies are helpful for the development of more accurate predictions in the sphere of medicine (Wang et al., 2017).

Application 3: Blockchain for Drug Traceability and Clinical Trials

Blockchain technology has increased the transparency and accountability of drug tracking and clinical trials. In Pfizer's pilot project, blockchain was used to monitor pharmaceutical products' supply chain and guarantee that all processes and stages were recorded safely (Blossey et al., 2019). In the same way, the integrity of trial data was preserved through the constant use of blockchain to avoid alteration of clinical trial processes; all processes were conducted standard, ethical, and regulatory. As will be shown in this application, blockchain can cover various aspects of privacy and accountability in the healthcare field (Gurtu & Johny, 2019).

Some Existing Current Healthcare Systems Implementing Privacy-Preserving ML Models

Diabetic Retinopathy Diagnosis Using Federated Learning with Google

Google has applied FL to train the machine learning models for diagnosing diabetic retinopathy using images from different hospitals without aggregation of patients' data (Lim et al., 2020). The failure to transfer raw data but rather encrypted model updates managed to respect patients' anonymity and enhance diagnostic outcomes (Feng et al., 2020).

DP-Driven Genomic Study Involving the NIH

The NIH is using DP to help with broader genomics research while maintaining individual genetic information privacy. The NIH All of Us program employs DP methods of messaging aggregate health information to the researchers while considering the impact of using sensitive data (Ram et al., 2020).

Homomorphic Encryption in Predictive Analytical Model

Based in Canada, the AI in Medicine platform applies homomorphic encryption to analyze patients' encrypted data and make chronic disease management predictions. By processing data at the highest security level, the platform complies with Canadian data protection laws and develops AI-supported healthcare technologies (Chen et al., 2012).

Case Studies Illustrating the Success and Challenges of Implementing Differential Privacy, FL, and Homomorphic Encryption

Differential Privacy in Census Data (Success and Challenge)

Differential privacy has been applied by the U.S. Census Bureau in 2020 to produce estimates of the total population, preserving the privacy of specific persons (Rinehart-Thompson, 2013). Concerning the success, anonymity helped; issues stem from a tension between less precise data for minorities in small populations, an issue integral to healthcare.

The Role of FL in Multi-Hospital Collaboration (Successful Sample)

FL was implemented in a project by NVIDIA and the King's College London to train AI models for brain tumor segmentation (Jodka, 2024). The model enhanced the accuracy of diagnostic tests without compromising patients' information privacy. However, some limitations were encountered, they covered issues with heterogeneity when dealing with data distributions and computational complexities inherent in decentralized training.

This is much more challenging in the real world since homomorphic encryption differs in Genome-Wide Association Studies. (European Commission, 2016) Employed HE for GWA studies to enable them to determine genetic markers associated with traits of interest without using raw genetic data. Indeed, privacy was maintained, but computational burden and scalability were also issues that hindered real-time analyses of massive data.

Real-World Applications of Blockchain in Healthcare Privacy

Estonia's National Blockchain for EHRs

Estonia Reveals National Blockchain for EHR The establishment of Estonia National Blockchain for EHR will ensure that patients have complete, real-time ownership of their records and that their data is kept entirely secret where necessary.

Estonia has adopted a blockchain-powered solution for storing patients' electronic health records or EHRs. The system guarantees that the entire audit trail is achieved, and the patients are always aware of who has accessed their files and for what reasons. With this system, (Hölbl et al., 2018) observe that the level of trust, as well as the level of data transparency in health care, has been enhanced (Kruse et al., 2017).

Pfizer's GTT: Blockchain for Drug Traceability

The I blockchain utilized by Pfizer correctly and securely records every process, from production to the distribution process. This approach is equally effective at reducing the chances of counterfeit drugs and enhancing accountability in drug safety (Blossey et al., 2019).

Dynamic Consent Management via Blockchain

Patients can grant consent to share genomic data in real time through a blockchain platform created by Nebula Genomics. This platform engages smart contracts to ensure that the consent conditions are adhered to in a way that realizes the highest levels of autonomy while ensuring that the data privacy laws of a country are met (Al Omar et al., 2017).

6. REGULATION, ETHICS, AND POLICY CONSIDERATIONS

Legal Requirements Related to the Application of Medical Data

Healthcare industry laws such as the Health Insurance Portability and Accountability Act (Hippa) in the United States or the General Data Protection Regulation (GDPTR) in the European Union provide guidelines on how medical data is collected, stored, and used to enhance its security to the patient. HIPAA provides standards for protecting the privacy and security of patient's health information for a wide range of organizations, including healthcare providers, health plans, and other entities; this includes controlling who has access to the information or can encrypt this data and how and when individuals must notify others of a breach. HIPAA allows the use of electronic personal health information only by entities that meet the authorization criteria, thereby eliminating misuse of patients' information for unjustified health care purposes (McGraw, 2013).

Likewise, GDPR is a comprehensive legal regime designed to protect personal data within the EU, based on the principles of transparency, accountability, and control of individuals. It requires consent before collecting personal data and encourages such data controllers to allow the data subjects the right to be forgotten (Hoofnagle et al., 2019) In addition, GDPR applies to third-party processors, which means that the privacy requirements will continue until the data is processed and disposed of. These frameworks call attention to the need to protect patients' personally identifiable health information while promoting the development of new and improved healthcare solutions.

Privacy issues of using PP methods

DP, FL and HE are privacy-preserving technologies associated with numerous ethical concerns. Identified techniques can be considered ethical since they respect autonomy, beneficence, and justice: people's data would not be disclosed, however, contributing to improving clinical practice. For instance, FL allows model training by sharing information and training without compromising the patient's data. (Kairouz et al., 2021).

However, ethical concerns are raised whenever these methods affect data utility or get some form of bias. For example, the anonymization process used in DP may cause specific characteristics of datasets to be concealed, which may lower the efficiency of the diagnostic AI models. Second, privacy-protecting measures might hurt vulnerable groups by preventing the use of data, thereby perpetuating health inequalities (Prainsack & Buyx, 2017). To overcome these challenges, it is mandatory to consider the methods and ensure equity and fair treatment for the benefit of all populations without prejudice.

Balancing Innovation in AI with Patient Confidentiality and Safety

This work shows how it is possible to develop methods and tools for using artificial intelligence in medical practice without violating the rights and confidentiality of patients. AI may radically change healthcare delivery through evidence-based individual treatment, risk profiling, and early diagnoses. However, the effectiveness and applicability of these approaches mainly depend on significant volumes of personal patient data, and this causes privacy and data misuse. (Mittelstadt et al., 2016).

The described privacy-preserving AI techniques offer a way to meet these conflicting objectives. For instance, blockchain can be applied when conducting data transactions where there is a need to improve contract transparency. However, the utility and accuracy of the data still need to be maintained, and an auditable report on the construction of the AI model needs to be generated. Differential privacy can be used to protect the identity of patients in the training data set to support the development of AI technology without incriminating the patients (Dwork & Roth, 2014). Most remarkably, healthcare providers should ensure that human patients put their confidence in such software solutions, recognizing that healthcare facilities are using safe, legal, and reliable artificial intelligence technologies.

Legal and Ethical Concerns with the Emergent Approaches to Enhance Privacy Protection

The use and application of privacy-preserving solutions in the area of healthcare present the individual with many challenges that are legal and ethical. Finally, from a legal perspective, organizations must use the Data Protection Acts and Regulations like the HIPAA or GDPR, which considers data protection. At the same time, cross-border, the use of FL, for example, entails compliance with GDPR provisions on data transfer, which sets demanding conditions for cross-border data exchange (Charles & Natarajan, 2024).

However, its application requires an ethical standard that ensures all parties understand the techniques applied equally. The patient should know how their data is processed and how their privacy is to be protected. Blockchain-based dynamic consent structures can promote patients' control over their data, increase trust, and ensure ethical compliance (Hoofnagle et al., 2019).

However, these methods also have limitations and biases that healthcare providers must consider. For example, it is essential to ensure that privacy-preserving AI models are trained on diverse datasets to prevent bias in providing healthcare to people. (Fareed et al., 2019)To that end, incorporating the spotlighted legal and ethical concerns, privacy-preserving technologies can be safely adopted and utilized in structural healthcare systems to advance innovation while remaining faithful to patients' trust. (Rajkomar et al., 2019).

7. FUTURE DIRECTIONS IN PRIVACY-PRESERVING MACHINE LEARNING (ML) FOR HEALTHCARE

Trends in Machine Learning Models Toward Privacy Preservation

Privacy-preserving ML is a fast-growing field due to the need for secure and more sensitive data processing in healthcare. A new tendency is the progression of synergistic privacy protection architectures utilizing different methodologies like DP, FL, and HE. These integrated methods can help address the adverse characteristics of individual techniques' attempts to scale up the privacy-preserving framework, which these different approaches seek to solve (Kairouz et al., 2021). For example, recent FL frameworks integrate DP into the system to introduce noise in model updates, reducing privacy considerations during cooperative training (Butt et al., 2024).

The fourth trend is the increasing use of privacy-enhancing technologies that can be used by devices located on the edge, including smartphones or smart medically equipped wearables. These devices can functionally and securely compute localized analytics via SMPC and encrypted machine learning and perform real-time data analysis without transferring valuable data to the central server (Zhao et al., 2018). In the same sense, privacy structures in using blockchain are trending since they can enable safe and verifiable data exchanges across healthcare-related companies (Chattopadhyay, 2024).

Opportunities for Future Research on the Implementation of ML in Healthcare Privacy

Despite significant advancements, privacy-preserving ML in healthcare presents several opportunities for future research:

- Algorithms such as HE and DP are generally computationally intensive and thus can hardly be adopted in large-scale healthcare solutions. Possible directions for future studies include lightweight implementations of these methods and research on advanced hardware accelerators for improving the efficiency of these techniques (Anzt et al., 2020).
- While inclusive privacy-preserving techniques could help proactively conceal certain features in the dataset or hamper the variety of data, those same methods can increase biases inherent in various healthcare datasets. Further studies are required to develop strategies to protect personal data and be equally advantageous for minority groups interested in improved healthcare solutions (Mehrabi et al., 2021).
- The application of privacy-preserving ML to personalized medicine is still a research problem. Future research is expected to incorporate means such as FL and HE into the personalized treatment plan to ensure the safe analysis of genetic, behavioral, and environmental data (Yang et al., 2019).
- Other promising areas include developing further sophisticated patient-oriented systems full of possibilities that patients can dynamically invoke regarding their data usage. Blockchain and smart contracts could make the consent process more dynamic and real-time, thus empowering patients while supporting more ethical partnerships for research purposes (Fareed et al., 2019).

AI and Data Privacy: Helping to Shape Smart Healthcare Systems

It will be seen that AI and data privacy will hold important mandates for changing the landscape of innovative healthcare systems. Analytic tools, which include prediction analysis, prescription treatments, and diagnosis, require high-quality data sets. Privacy-preserving ML ensures that such advancements can be integrated into the domain without undermining patient-particular information, thereby improving confidence and utilization of the innovation in healthcare centers (Mittelstadt et al., 2016).

Therefore, advanced healthcare smart systems will incorporate privacy-preserving AI to promote secure and efficient healthcare. For instance, privacy-preserving AI can directly assist facilities in Intensive Care Units (ICUs) in drawing decisions on prompt patient care involving comprehensively encrypted data sets to predict patient health decline (Brisimi et al., 2018) In addition, the opportunities to implement blockchain applications in healthcare will improve the compatibility of data sharing between establishments such as hospitals, insurance companies, and patients.

Ahead of us is the interaction between AI, privacy-preserving ML, quantum computing, and 5G connectivity to redefine competent healthcare. More advanced cryptographic techniques with quantum bits may strengthen data protection; fifth-generation communication technology will allow the sharing of AI-compatible data with high speed and protection. Such innovations, when coupled with strong privacy considerations, will help develop healthcare intelligent systems that are also moral.

8. CONCLUSION

Privacy-preserving ML techniques are increasingly essential in the current relevance of health systems, which utilize patient data that is often deemed sensitive. Patients' anonymity has become one of the biggest challenges in these sectors as the healthcare business advances further into data-driven technologies. Approaches like DP, FL, and HE offer the security platforms needed to manage these issues while enabling the use of the data. These methods, in turn, are supported by blockchain technology in increasing transparency, accountability, and security in data sharing and model management.

These techniques solve privacy concerns about unauthorized data access, breaches, and re-identification risks. They also allow for secure and decentralized data processing to comply with HIPAA and GDPR regulations and practice ethical patient treatments. Moreover, these methods reduce trust concerns about the use of patients' data for research and AI development, thus inviting more patients and institutions to contribute to data sharing.

Privacy-preserving ML could revolutionize the use of healthcare and other industries in a specific setting since it will utilize less data about individuals. Thus, due to the commitment made through integrating innovation with patient anonymity, the specified methods create the foundation of ethical and security adoption of AI in healthcare. The overarching idea is to enable research and practice professionals to leverage AI and related technologies in clinical diagnostics and treatment planning as well as data analytics with a level of privacy protection adequate to address the increasing concerns associated with data privacy and security. While these techniques develop and become more effective, the problems of more intelligent, more secure, and more ethically sound health systems are outlined.

Hence, privacy-preserving ML methods are not only solutions to present problems but also foundations for the future intelligent, secure healthcare system fully trusted by patients, doctors, healthcare providers, and policymakers. With such approaches, continued research, development, and implementation of these techniques will guarantee that AI and ML development and integration fulfill basic tenets of privacy, ethical medical practice, and safe patient treatment.

REFERENCES

Abadi, M., Chu, A., Goodfellow, I., McMahan, H. B., Mironov, I., Talwar, K., & Zhang, L. (2016). Deep learning with differential privacy. *Proceedings of the 2016 ACM SIGSAC conference on computer and communications security*

Ahad, A., Jiangbin, Z., Mughees, A., Puspitasari, I., & Tayyab, M. (2025). Secure Horizons: Integrating Blockchain With AI for Enhanced Smart Healthcare Systems. In AI Techniques for Securing Medical and Business Practices (pp. 357-390). IGI Global. doi:DOI: 10.1145/2976749.2978318

Ahad, A., Tahir, M., Sheikh, M. A. S., Mughees, A., & Ahmed, K. I. (2021). Optimal route selection in 5G-based smart health-care network: a reinforcement learning approach. 2021 26th IEEE Asia-Pacific Conference on Communications (APCC)

Akgün, M., Bayrak, A. O., Ozer, B., & Sağıroğlu, M. Ş. (2015). Privacy preserving processing of genomic data: A survey. *Journal of Biomedical Informatics*, *56*, 103–111.

Al Omar, A., Rahman, M. S., Basu, A., & Kiyomoto, S. (2017). Medibchain: A blockchain based privacy preserving platform for healthcare data. Security, Privacy, and Anonymity in Computation, Communication, and Storage: SpaCCS 2017 International Workshops, Guangzhou, China, December 12-15, 2017, Proceedings 10

Ali, M., Naeem, F., Tariq, M., & Kaddoum, G. (2022). Federated learning for privacy preservation in smart healthcare systems: A comprehensive survey. *IEEE Journal of Biomedical and Health Informatics*, *27*(2), 778–789.

Ali, Z., Ahad, A., Madeira, F., & Shayea, I. (2023). Enhancing Transparency and Trustworthiness of Healthcare IoT Data with AWS: A Proposed Model. EAI International Conference on IoT Technologies for HealthCare

Anzt, H., Cojean, T., Yen-Chen, C., Dongarra, J., Flegar, G., Nayak, P., Tomov, S., Tsai, Y. M., & Wang, W. (2020). Load-balancing sparse matrix vector product kernels on gpus. [TOPC]. *ACM Transactions on Parallel Computing*, *7*(1), 1–26.

Blossey, G., Eisenhardt, J., & Hahn, G. (2019). Blockchain technology in supply chain management: An application perspective.

Brisimi, T. S., Chen, R., Mela, T., Olshevsky, A., Paschalidis, I. C., & Shi, W. (2018). Federated learning of predictive models from federated electronic health records. *International Journal of Medical Informatics*, *112*, 59–67. DOI: 10.1016/j.ijmedinf.2018.01.007 PMID: 29500022

Butt, H. A., Ahad, A., Wasim, M., Madeira, F., & Chamran, M. K. (2023). 5G and IoT for Intelligent Healthcare: AI and Machine Learning Approaches—A Review. *International Conference on Smart Objects and Technologies for Social Good*

Butt, H. A., Ahad, A., Wasim, M., Shayea, I., Coelho, P. J., Pires, I. M., & Garcia, N. M. (2023). Federated machine learning in 5G smart healthcare: A security perspective review. *Procedia Computer Science*, *224*, 580–586. DOI: 10.1016/j.procs.2023.09.084

Butt, H. A., Harthy, K. S. A., Shah, M. A., Hussain, M., Amin, R., & Rehman, M. U. (2024). Enhanced DDoS Detection Using Advanced Machine Learning and Ensemble Techniques in Software Defined Networking. *Computers, Materials & Continua*, *81*(2), 3003–3031. DOI: 10.32604/cmc.2024.057185

Charles, S., & Natarajan, J. (2024). Identification of key gene modules and novel transcription factors in tetralogy of fallot using machine learning and network topological features. *Medinformatics*, *1*(1), 27–34. DOI: 10.47852/bonviewMEDIN32021554

Chattopadhyay, S. (2024). *Decoding medical diagnosis with machine learning classifiers*. Medinformatics. DOI: 10.47852/bonviewMEDIN42022583

Chaudhuri, A. (2018). *Internet of Things, for Things, and by Things*. Auerbach Publications. DOI: 10.1201/9781315200644

Chen, Y., Peng, B., Wang, X., & Tang, H. (2012). *Large-Scale Privacy-Preserving Mapping of Human Genomic Sequences on Hybrid Clouds*. NDSS.

Chirra, B. R. (2023). Enhancing Healthcare Data Security with Homomorphic Encryption: A Case Study on Electronic Health Records (EHR) Systems. *Revista de Inteligencia Artificial en Medicina*, *14*(1), 549–559.

Dwork, C., & Roth, A. (2014). The algorithmic foundations of differential privacy. *Foundations and Trends® in Theoretical Computer Science*, *9*(3–4), 211-407.

El Emam, K., Jonker, E., Arbuckle, L., & Malin, B. (2011). A systematic review of re-identification attacks on health data. *PLoS One*, *6*(12), e28071. DOI: 10.1371/journal.pone.0028071 PMID: 22164229

Erlingsson, Ú., Pihur, V., & Korolova, A. (2014). Rappor: Randomized aggregatable privacy-preserving ordinal response. *Proceedings of the 2014 ACM SIGSAC conference on computer and communications security*

Fareed, N., Walker, D., Sieck, C. J., Taylor, R., Scarborough, S., Huerta, T. R., & McAlearney, A. S. (2019). Inpatient portal clusters: Identifying user groups based on portal features. *Journal of the American Medical Informatics Association : JAMIA*, *26*(1), 28–36.

Feng, J., Rong, C., Sun, F., Guo, D., & Li, Y. (2020). PMF: A privacy-preserving human mobility prediction framework via federated learning. *Proceedings of the ACM on Interactive, Mobile, Wearable and Ubiquitous Technologies*, *4*(1), 1–21. DOI: 10.1145/3381006 PMID: 35846237

Fernández-Alemán, J. L., Señor, I. C., Lozoya, P. Á. O., & Toval, A. (2013). Security and privacy in electronic health records: A systematic literature review. *Journal of Biomedical Informatics*, *46*(3), 541–562. DOI: 10.1016/j.jbi.2012.12.003 PMID: 23305810

Gaye, A., Marcon, Y., Isaeva, J., LaFlamme, P., Turner, A., Jones, E. M., Minion, J., Boyd, A. W., Newby, C. J., Nuotio, M.-L., Wilson, R., Butters, O., Murtagh, B., Demir, I., Doiron, D., Giepmans, L., Wallace, S. E., Budin-Ljøsne, I., Oliver Schmidt, C., & Burton, P. R. (2014). DataSHIELD: Taking the analysis to the data, not the data to the analysis. *International Journal of Epidemiology*, *43*(6), 1929–1944. DOI: 10.1093/ije/dyu188 PMID: 25261970

General Data Protection Regulation. (2016). https://eur-lex.europa.eu/legal-content/EN/TXT/?uri=CELEX%3A32016R0679

Gentry, C. (2009). Fully homomorphic encryption using ideal lattices. Proceedings of the forty-first annual ACM symposium on Theory of computing, Grady, C. (2015). Enduring and emerging challenges of informed consent. *The New England Journal of Medicine*, *372*(9), 855–862. PMID: 19196665

Gurtu, A., & Johny, J. (2019). Potential of blockchain technology in supply chain management: A literature review. *International Journal of Physical Distribution & Logistics Management*, *49*(9), 881–900. DOI: 10.1108/IJPDLM-11-2018-0371

Hölbl, M., Kompara, M., Kamišalić, A., & Nemec Zlatolas, L. (2018). A systematic review of the use of blockchain in healthcare. *Symmetry*, *10*(10), 470. DOI: 10.3390/sym10100470

Hoofnagle, C. J., Van Der Sloot, B., & Borgesius, F. Z. (2019). The European Union general data protection regulation: What it is and what it means. *Information & Communications Technology Law*, *28*(1), 65–98. DOI: 10.1080/13600834.2019.1573501

Hu, M., Ren, Y., & Chen, C. (2023). Privacy-Preserving Medical Data-Sharing System with Symmetric Encryption Based on Blockchain. *Symmetry*, *15*(5), 1010. DOI: 10.3390/sym15051010

Hu, Y., Liyanage, M., Mansoor, A., Thilakarathna, K., Jourjon, G., & Seneviratne, A. (2018). Blockchain-based smart contracts-applications and challenges. *arXiv preprint arXiv:1810.04699.*

Ichikawa, D., Kashiyama, M., & Ueno, T. (2017). Tamper-resistant mobile health using blockchain technology. *JMIR mHealth and uHealth*, *5*(7), e7938. DOI: 10.2196/mhealth.7938 PMID: 28747296

Jodka, S. H. (2024). *HIPAA-free zone? Think again: the surprising state laws regulating collection of health and fitness data.* https://www.reuters.com/legal/litigation/hipaa-free-zone-think-again-surprising-state-laws-regulating-collection-health-2024-10-25/?utm_source=chatgpt.com

Johnson, A. E., Pollard, T. J., Shen, L., Lehman, L.-H., Feng, M., Ghassemi, M., Moody, B., Szolovits, P., Anthony Celi, L., & Mark, R. G. (2016). MIMIC-III, a freely accessible critical care database. *Scientific Data*, *3*(1), 1–9. DOI: 10.1038/sdata.2016.35 PMID: 27219127

Johnson, A. E., Pollard, T. J., Shen, L., Lehman, L.-H., Feng, M., Ghassemi, M., Moody, B., Szolovits, P., Celi, L. A., & Mark, R. G. (2016). Data descriptor: MIMIC-III, a freely accessible critical care database. *Scientific Data*, *3*(160035), 1–9.

Kairouz, P., McMahan, H. B., Avent, B., Bellet, A., Bennis, M., Bhagoji, A. N., Bonawitz, K., Charles, Z., Cormode, G., & Cummings, R. (2021). Advances and open problems in federated learning. *Foundations and trends® in machine learning, 14*(1–2), 1-210.

Khan, S. N., Loukil, F., Ghedira-Guegan, C., Benkhelifa, E., & Bani-Hani, A. (2021). Blockchain smart contracts: Applications, challenges, and future trends. *Peer-to-Peer Networking and Applications*, *14*(5), 2901–2925. DOI: 10.1007/s12083-021-01127-0 PMID: 33897937

Kifer, D., & Machanavajjhala, A. (2011). No free lunch in data privacy. *Proceedings of the 2011 ACM SIGMOD International Conference on Management of data*

Kraushaar, J., & Bohnet-Joschko, S. (2022). Smartphone use and security challenges in hospitals: A survey among resident physicians in Germany. *International Journal of Environmental Research and Public Health*, *19*(24), 16546.

Kruse, C. S., Smith, B., Vanderlinden, H., & Nealand, A. (2017). Security techniques for the electronic health records. *Journal of Medical Systems*, *41*(8), 1–9. DOI: 10.1007/s10916-017-0778-4 PMID: 28733949

Liang, X., Zhao, J., Shetty, S., Liu, J., & Li, D. (2017). Integrating blockchain for data sharing and collaboration in mobile healthcare applications. 2017 IEEE 28th annual international symposium on personal, indoor, and mobile radio communications (PIMRC), Lim, W. Y. B., Luong, N. C., Hoang, D. T., Jiao, Y., Liang, Y.-C., Yang, Q., Niyato, D., & Miao, C. (2020). Federated learning in mobile edge networks: A comprehensive survey. *IEEE Communications Surveys and Tutorials*, *22*(3), 2031–2063.

Lin, H. (2024). Artificial intelligence with great potential in medical informatics: A brief review. *Medinformatics*, *1*(1), 2–9. DOI: 10.47852/bonviewMEDIN42022204

Lu, W.-J., Yamada, Y., & Sakuma, J. (2015). Privacy-preserving genome-wide association studies on cloud environment using fully homomorphic encryption. *BMC Medical Informatics and Decision Making*.

McGraw, D. (2013). Building public trust in uses of Health Insurance Portability and Accountability Act de-identified data. *Journal of the American Medical Informatics Association : JAMIA*, *20*(1), 29–34.

McMahan, B., Moore, E., Ramage, D., Hampson, S., & Arcas, B. A. (2017). Communication-efficient learning of deep networks from decentralized data. Artificial intelligence and statistics,

Mehrabi, N., Morstatter, F., Saxena, N., Lerman, K., & Galstyan, A. (2021). A survey on bias and fairness in machine learning. *ACM Computing Surveys*, *54*(6), 1–35.

Mittelstadt, B. D., Allo, P., Taddeo, M., Wachter, S., & Floridi, L. (2016). The ethics of algorithms: Mapping the debate. *Big Data & Society*, *3*(2), 2053951716679679. DOI: 10.1177/2053951716679679

Moqurrab, S. A., Tariq, N., Anjum, A., Asheralieva, A., Malik, S. U., Malik, H., Pervaiz, H., & Gill, S. S. (2022). A deep learning-based privacy-preserving model for smart healthcare in Internet of medical things using fog computing. *Wireless Personal Communications*, *126*(3), 2379–2401. DOI: 10.1007/s11277-021-09323-0 PMID: 36059591

Naehrig, M. Improved Security for a Ring-Based Fully Homomorphic Encryption Scheme.

Nakamoto, S. (2008). *Bitcoin: A peer-to-peer electronic cash system*. Satoshi Nakamoto.

Nakamoto, S. (2008). *Bitcoin: A peer-to-peer electronic cash system.*https://bitcoin.org/bitcoin.pdf

Nakamoto, S., & Bitcoin, A. (2008). A peer-to-peer electronic cash system. *Bitcoin.–URL:https://bitcoin.org/bitcoin. pdf*, *4*(2), 15.

Narayanan, A., & Shmatikov, V. (2008). Robust de-anonymization of large sparse datasets. 2008 IEEE Symposium on Security and Privacy (sp 2008), Panayides, A. S., Amini, A., Filipovic, N. D., Sharma, A., Tsaftaris, S. A., Young, A., Foran, D., Do, N., Golemati, S., & Kurc, T. (2020). AI in medical imaging informatics: Current challenges and future directions. *IEEE Journal of Biomedical and Health Informatics*, *24*(7), 1837–1857.

Pawar, P., Edoh, T. O., Singh, M., & Parolia, N. (2021). Hitching medical iot devices to blockchain for personal health information management. *Blockchain Technology for IoT Applications*, 191-205.

Ploug, T. (2020). In Defence of informed consent for health record research-why arguments from 'easy rescue','no harm'and 'consent bias' fail. *BMC Medical Ethics*, *21*(1), 75. DOI: 10.1186/s12910-020-00519-w PMID: 32819343

Prainsack, B., & Buyx, A. (2017). *Solidarity in biomedicine and beyond* (Vol. 33). Cambridge University Press. DOI: 10.1017/9781139696593

Rajkomar, A., Dean, J., & Kohane, I. (2019). Machine learning in medicine. *The New England Journal of Medicine*, *380*(14), 1347–1358. DOI: 10.1056/NEJMra1814259 PMID: 30943338

Ram, H., Sahadevan, S., Gale, N., Caggiano, M. P., Yu, X., Ohno, C., & Heisler, M. G. (2020). An integrated analysis of cell-type specific gene expression reveals genes regulated by REVOLUTA and KANADI1 in the Arabidopsis shoot apical meristem. *PLOS Genetics*, *16*(4), e1008661. DOI: 10.1371/journal.pgen.1008661 PMID: 32294082

Rinehart-Thompson, L. A. (2013). *Health information management and compliance: Challenges in HIPAA implementat(2013).*https://pmc.ncbi.nlm.nih.gov/articles/PMC3797550/

Rumbold, J. M. M., & Pierscionek, B. (2017). The effect of the general data protection regulation on medical research. *Journal of Medical Internet Research*, *19*(2), e47. DOI: 10.2196/jmir.7108 PMID: 28235748

Rundle, J. (Dec. 27, 2024). *Healthcare Providers Face Stiffer Cyber Rules Even as They Cry for Help.* https://www.wsj.com/articles/healthcare-providers-face-stiffer-cyber-rules-even-as-they-cry-for-help -b466197a?utm_source=chatgpt.com

Sheller, M. J., Edwards, B., Reina, G. A., Martin, J., Pati, S., Kotrotsou, A., Milchenko, M., Xu, W., Marcus, D., Colen, R. R., & Bakas, S. (2020). Federated learning in medicine: Facilitating multi-institutional collaborations without sharing patient data. *Scientific Reports*, *10*(1), 12598. DOI: 10.1038/s41598-020-69250-1 PMID: 32724046

Shome, A., Amiri, S., & Belloum, A. S. Systematic Literature Review of Privacy-Preserving Deep Learning in Medical Image Analysis.

Singh, K., Krishna, C., & Kumar, D. (2024). Professional Ethics, Challenges and Opportunities for Blockchain Technology in Healthcare Sector: A Systematic Review. *Recent Advances in Computer Science and Communications (Formerly: Recent Patents on Computer Science), 17*(1), 72-86.

Stripelis, D., Gupta, U., Saleem, H., Dhinagar, N., Ghai, T., Anastasiou, C., Sánchez, R., Ver Steeg, G., Ravi, S., & Naveed, M. (2024). A federated learning architecture for secure and private neuroimaging analysis. *Patterns (New York, N.Y.)*, *5*(8), 101031. DOI: 10.1016/j.patter.2024.101031 PMID: 39233693

Sweeney, L. (2002). k-anonymity: A model for protecting privacy. *International Journal of Uncertainty, Fuzziness and Knowledge-based Systems*, *10*(05), 557–570. DOI: 10.1142/S0218488502001648

Tang, H., Jiang, X., Wang, X., Wang, S., Sofia, H., Fox, D., Lauter, K., Malin, B., Telenti, A., Xiong, L., & Ohno-Machado, L. (2016). Protecting genomic data analytics in the cloud: State of the art and opportunities. *BMC Medical Genomics*, *9*(1), 1–9. DOI: 10.1186/s12920-016-0224-3 PMID: 27733153

Vishwa, A. (2021). *MediBlock-A Privacy-aware Blockchain to store patients data and effective diagnosis methods*. University of Technology Sydney.

Wang, B., Song, W., Lou, W., & Hou, Y. T. (2017). Privacy-preserving pattern matching over encrypted genetic data in cloud computing. IEEE INFOCOM 2017-IEEE Conference on Computer Communications

Wang, W., Li, X., Qiu, X., Zhang, X., Brusic, V., & Zhao, J. (2023). A privacy preserving framework for federated learning in smart healthcare systems. *Information Processing & Management*, *60*(1), 103167. DOI: 10.1016/j.ipm.2022.103167

Yang, Q., Liu, Y., Chen, T., & Tong, Y. (2019). Federated machine learning: Concept and applications. [TIST]. *ACM Transactions on Intelligent Systems and Technology*, *10*(2), 1–19. DOI: 10.1145/3298981

Yigzaw, K. Y., Olabarriaga, S. D., Michalas, A., Marco-Ruiz, L., Hillen, C., Verginadis, Y., De Oliveira, M. T., Krefting, D., Penzel, T., & Bowden, J. (2022). Health data security and privacy: Challenges and solutions for the future. *Roadmap to Successful Digital Health Ecosystems*, 335-362.

Yue, X., Wang, H., Jin, D., Li, M., & Jiang, W. (2016). Healthcare data gateways: Found healthcare intelligence on blockchain with novel privacy risk control. *Journal of Medical Systems*, *40*(10), 1–8. DOI: 10.1007/s10916-016-0574-6 PMID: 27565509

Zhang, P., Schmidt, D. C., White, J., & Lenz, G. (2018). Blockchain technology use cases in healthcare. [). Elsevier.]. *Advances in Computers*, *111*, 1–41. DOI: 10.1016/bs.adcom.2018.03.006

Zhang, R., Xue, R., & Liu, L. (2021). Security and privacy for healthcare blockchains. *IEEE Transactions on Services Computing*, *15*(6), 3668–3686. DOI: 10.1109/TSC.2021.3085913

Zhao, J., Mortier, R., Crowcroft, J., & Wang, L. (2018). Privacy-preserving machine learning based data analytics on edge devices. Proceedings of the 2018 AAAI/ACM Conference on AI, Ethics, and Society DOI: 10.1145/3278721.3278778

Chapter 14
Redefining Healthcare Data Storage and Access With Decentralized Technologies

Abdul Razzaq
https://orcid.org/0000-0002-4465-6365
Northwestern Polytechnical University, China

Muhammad Numair
Beijing Normal University, China

Salman Ahmed
University of Suffolk, UK

Muhammad Usman Akhtar
https://orcid.org/0000-0002-5389-1156
Northwestern Polytechnical University, China

ABSTRACT

Advances in the healthcare sector need to secure efficient and decentralized systems to handle the large number of images and test reports. Traditional cloud-based healthcare systems pose crucial challenges, such as higher maintenance costs, significant storage demand, and, most importantly, privacy concerns. This chapter introduced the comprehensive patient-centric system for decentralized storage, secure medical data sharing, integrating blockchain technology and distributed file systems. The healthcare system leverages the IPFS and Ethereum blockchain to empowering scalable privacy protection of globally available storage of medical metadata. The framework enhances the accessibility and usability of incorporating a mobile offering for the patients, hospitals, and other stakeholders to interact with the decentralized system through the blockchain-integrated mobile application.This chapter provides an innovative approach to addressing the healthcare centralized data management limitations while ensuring patient privacy and data security.

DOI: 10.4018/979-8-3373-0593-6.ch014

1. INTRODUCTION

The widespread adoption of Information Technology (IT) in healthcare has significantly improved people's overall health worldwide by making services more effective. Patient information systems allow stakeholders to individually track the health conditions and therapies over time, offering insights into patient diagnosis and therapy. There is abundant evidence that the latest clinical system enhances the safety and privacy protection of the patient-centeredness of therapy (Casalino et al., 2003). However, the potential of personal health information is often underutilised due to fragmented information and data management challenges in healthcare systems. Health information systems are often split across hospitals, medical clinics, labs, and pharmacies. It's worth noting that the healthcare sector has historically lagged well behind other industries in information collection, processing, transport, and management, and this gap is particularly evident in data transmission and communication technology (DOC, 1999).

It plays an important part in today's medical business. At the beginning of the 1970s, different technologies were integrated into the healthcare sectors, such as the Hospital information system (HIS) and digital imaging modalities; the other technologies are important Magnetic Resonance Imaging (MRI), Computed Tomography (CT), and Picture archiving and communication systems (PACSs) these technologies are integrated into health sectors. Today, the global healthcare sector shares information through computer technologies. The internet has transformed into a significant repository of information and an economical means of communication. The rising significance of the internet and information technology has introduced new technological concerns, with cybersecurity attacks and unauthorized utilization of electronic data sharing being vital concerns for the healthcare sectors. This underscores the crucial role of healthcare professionals and IT specialists in managing and securing these technological integrations (Heart, Ben-Assuli, & Shabtai, 2017).

Cloud servers primarily distribute information through nodes to manage the vast volume of data. However, the issue with centralized systems is that a single person is typically authorized to handle a large volume of data, leading to a single point of failure and vulnerabilities. To mitigate this risk, third parties store the information on the cloud server (Zhu, Wu, Gai, & Choo, 2019) . In contrast, blockchain, a decentralized ledger technology, eliminates the need for third-party services. It provides trust, transparency, privacy, and security, making it an empowering solution for systems (Siyal et al., 2019). Blockchain is a decentralized storage of data in independently distributed ledger network nodes. However, a key challenge is that network nodes have a limited capacity to store large amounts of data (Dai, Zhang, Wang, & Jin, 2018, Razzaq et al., 2022). The unique features of blockchain, such as its decentralization and security, make it a promising solution for the increasing demand in the healthcare sector to store and process large imaging data in the future. This demand will surge for storing and processing sensitive image information (Liu et al., 2022; Cao et al., 2022).

As a result, the secure storage and uninterrupted transmission of medical images are critical concerns. The current methods for handling medical images and patient information in centralized storage are inadequate, leading to serious privacy, transparency, and security risks. Over the past few decades, any company developing medical image processing systems has encountered significant challenges, particularly the potential for healthcare record data breaches within large medical data centres (Seh et al., 2020).

Figure 1. Overview of the patient-centric system

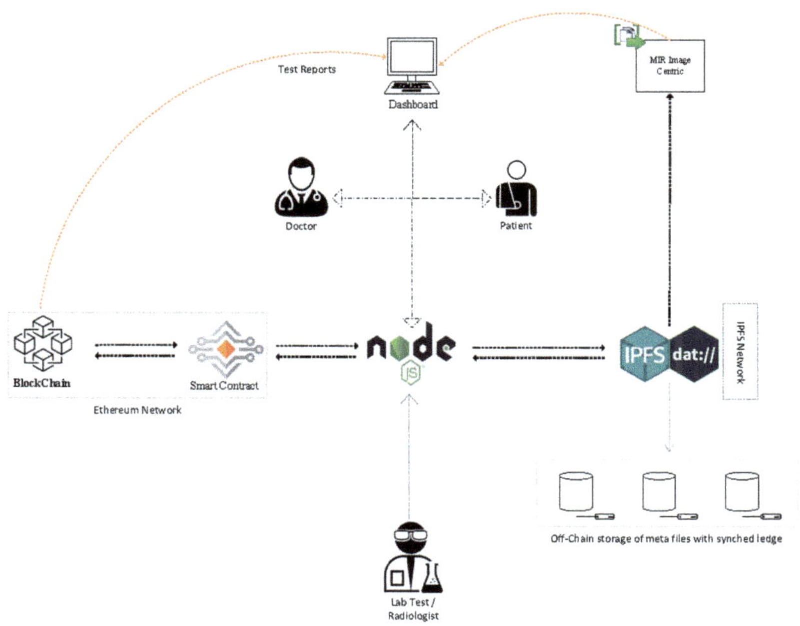

Consequently, a patient-centric system is necessary (see Figure 1), in which patients have total control over the medical images and can track them online without relying on a centralized system. The shift toward decentralized technology, such as blockchain technology (Mettler, 2016), is not just a significant trend but a beacon of hope for the future of healthcare. It has the potential to provide the framework for lowering the previously mentioned problematic challenges and driving widespread acceptance of a patient-centric system. Medical photos far exceed the volume of those accessible on a public blockchain (Halamka, Lippman, & Ekblaw, 2017), but this is a challenge we can overcome with the right technology and mindset.

The Inter-Planetary File System (IPFS) is a decentralized distributed platform that addresses the issue of centralized storage (Benet, 2014). IPFS was developed to facilitate hypermedia storage and sharing inside a distributed peer-to-peer (P2P) content-addressable file system. The decentralized off-chain storing capabilities of IPFS provides the distinct advantage of compatibility with several blockchain networks. IPFS provides distributed data access methods that are durable, intelligent, and efficient in online services. However, significant challenges remain in storing vital medical images utilizing these distributed storage technologies, including unauthorized access and concerns about patient image confidentiality. The urgency and seriousness of the issue are highlighted by the importance of lessening the chances of data hacking or breaches and significantly controlling the data transfer between healthcare, hospitals, medical organizations, and practitioners. A private, secure storage system in a healthcare system provides the vital features of its huge capacity, fewer expenses, and limitations associated with gathering medical images by eliminating the need for a centralized healthcare system (Shini, Thomas, & Chithraranjan, 2012).

2. BLOCKCHAIN ADOPTION IN HEALTHCARE

Blockchain technology has revolutionized the healthcare system's vital role in the privacy and security sectors. Several studies have recognized this technology's potential in the healthcare industry (Zheng et al., 2018). The existing healthcare sector and the traditional system might be vital standards to shift to blockchain technology (Yue, Wang, Jin, Li, & Jiang, 2016). Digital healthcare institutions must implement decentralized blockchain and information and communication technologies ICTs, paving the way for a modern digital healthcare ecosystem for the patients and the service providers (Chen, Xu, Shi, Zhao, & Zhao, 2018). The blockchain application in the healthcare system offers a vital service to may assist the patient's physicians and healthcare organization in several ways to assess the patient information, including the critical record, claims, and payments administration, medical IoT security management (Hathaliya, Tanwar, Tyagi, & Kumar, 2019). Bitcoin's incredible success in blockchain technology has become the promising technologies introduced to the decentralized system; mining nodes are essential for keeping a copy distributed in the ledger and performing functions, such as verifying and validating each transaction. The results established that tamper-proof ledger provide decentralized security, precise timestamping, and members' capacity to share (Nakamoto, 2008). Multiple sectors have used blockchain technology, including the healthcare and supply chain, the most famous sectors, and the logistics, document, and accounting sectors (Khan & Salah, 2018). Blockchain technology is used to resolve issues related to data sharing and key features of trust and privacy owing to its robust and decentralized framework, creating an exciting future for the healthcare industry (Salah et al., 2019). Table 1 presents a comparative analysis of blockchain-based storage and traditional healthcare data storage solutions, highlighting differences in security, data integrity, interoperability, scalability, cost efficiency, regulatory compliance, data access speed, centralization, and risk of data loss.

Table 1. Comparison of blockchain-based storage with traditional healthcare data storage solutions.

Feature	Blockchain-Based Storage	Cloud-Based Storage	Traditional On-Premises Storage
Security	High (decentralized, encrypted, tamper-proof)	Moderate (centralized encryption, risk of breaches)	Moderate (firewalls, access control, but vulnerable to internal threats)
Data Integrity	Ensured (immutable ledger, cryptographic hashing)	Moderate (data can be altered by administrators)	Moderate (risk of accidental loss or manipulation)
Interoperability	High (smart contracts, standardized access)	Moderate (dependent on API integrations)	Low (often siloed, difficult cross-system access)
Scalability	Moderate (depends on blockchain type and consensus mechanism)	High (cloud services scale dynamically)	Low (limited by physical infrastructure)
Cost Efficiency	Moderate to High (initial setup cost, lower maintenance)	High (subscription-based, lower initial investment)	Low (high setup and maintenance costs)
Regulatory Compliance	High (traceability, auditability, GDPR, HIPAA support)	Moderate (varies by provider, potential compliance gaps)	Moderate (requires extensive documentation and audits)
Data Access Speed	Moderate (depends on network congestion)	High (optimized for fast retrieval)	High (direct access to local storage)
Centralization	Decentralized (distributed ledger technology)	Centralized (controlled by service providers)	Centralized (managed by healthcare organizations)
Risk of Data Loss	Low (redundancy across nodes)	Moderate (data loss possible if provider fails)	High (risk of hardware failure, physical damage)

Centralized healthcare data management presents significant risks, including data breaches, unauthorized access, and inefficiencies in data sharing. According to a *2023 IBM Cost of a Data Breach Report*, the average cost of a healthcare data breach was **$10.93 million**, the highest among all industries. Additionally, in 2022 alone, the U.S. Department of Health and Human Services reported **707 healthcare data breaches**, exposing over **51.9 million records**. Blockchain technology offers a decentralized approach to healthcare data management, enhancing security, interoperability, and transparency. Future blockchain innovations include:

- **Decentralized Patient Records** – Patients will have full ownership of their medical records, allowing access through smart contracts without intermediaries.
- **Interoperability Across Healthcare Providers** – Blockchain-based frameworks will enable seamless and real-time data exchange between hospitals and research institutions.
- **Drug Supply Chain Transparency** – Blockchain will mitigate counterfeit drugs, ensuring the authenticity of pharmaceuticals through immutable ledger tracking.
- **Smart Contracts for Insurance and Billing** – Automated claims processing via blockchain will eliminate fraud and reduce administrative costs.

During the COVID-19 pandemic, several blockchain projects emerged to tackle healthcare challenges:

- **MiPasa** (IBM & WHO collaboration) – A blockchain-based platform for sharing verified COVID-19 infection data while maintaining privacy.
- **VaccineGuard** (Estonia's Guardtime) – Used blockchain to track vaccine distribution and prevent fraud.
- **VeChain's E-HCert** – A blockchain-based digital COVID-19 test record deployed in hospitals in Cyprus to ensure accurate verification of test results.

These real-world implementations validate blockchain's potential to revolutionize healthcare, making it more secure, transparent, and efficient.

A blockchain network mining node performs, verifies, and retains data inside the blocks. To execute a smart contract, a transaction is executed to the corresponding Ethereum address, and the contract, a key component of blockchain technology, is performed with the specified input for that transaction. The smart contract utilization of Ethereum, an open-source, decentralized platform, capabilities and facilitates the deployment of smart contracts (Bocek, Rodrigues, Strasser, & Stiller, 2017). In blockchain networks, transactions are compiled of interconnected blocks through a chain link to proceed with the block record. Blockchain is characteristic of immutability, an important security key attribute of decentralized networks that protects against unauthorized access and modifications. Any modification of any type of data restricts invalid transactions since the hash becomes immutable, and unauthorized access of values in the headers of succeeding blocks would alter due to the hash function's methodology. Consequently, an assailant could not alter the data without compromising the whole chain (Guntur, Dornadula, & Nimbagal, 2022).

Figure 2. Process of data recording to the blockchain ledger.

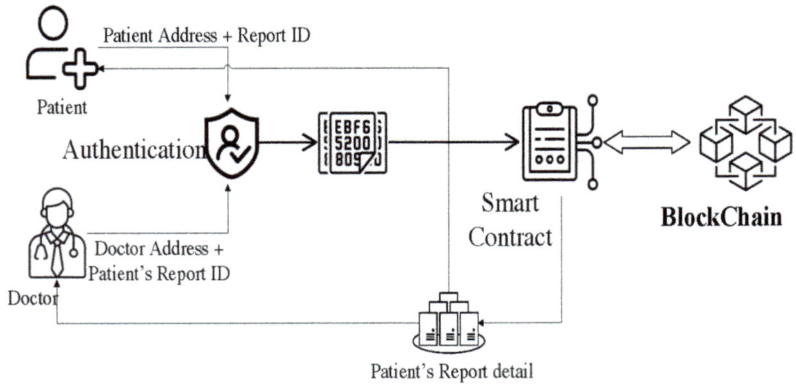

The proposed system illustrates that in healthcare, stakeholders, including doctors and patients, can access their test reports by retrieving them from the blockchain ledger. The process begins when the user can easily access a healthcare test report by entering their report number or choosing the second way to enter their identity, which is stored on the blockchain ledger (see Figure 2). The system clearly shows that only authorized users can access medical reports, and it implements robust security measures to ensure they are protected from unauthorized access, thereby instilling confidence in its reliability.

3. CHALLENGES IN HEALTHCARE DATA MANAGEMENT

The legacy system in the healthcare industry provides only internal resource exchange, resulting in inconsistency with healthcare external systems. Decentralized systems integration may result in enhanced and integrated healthcare, necessitating collaboration across healthcare organizations. Transferring medical data across various entities, including healthcare providers, doctors, and research institutions, is a critical difficulty. However, the progressive use of blockchain technology to tackle this problem, with its flexible, secure, decentralized data processing and governance methodology, offers a hopeful future for healthcare data integration. Blockchain technology advances healthcare in several ways, bringing hope for a more integrated and efficient healthcare system.

Blockchain technology has altered data management and storage techniques into a digital and immutable format. The beginning of digitalization and cloud storage has made transferring enormous amounts of data from traditional methods to electronic devices easier. In the medical industry, patient data is often digitized and stored in secure systems that can only be accessed by authorized personnel. The recording, storing, and accessing of medical data has been revolutionized by this technology, increasing efficiency and security. However, it's crucial to understand the potential drawbacks of digitization. Table 2 provides a comparative analysis of centralized vs. decentralized management of digital identity, which is the primary explanation for the difference between centralized and decentralized systems.

Table 2. Identity management systems (Centralized vs Decentralized).

Feature	Central Identity Management	Blockchain-based Distributed Identity Management
Governance	Central Governance	Decentral Governance
Identity Change	Change Management on Central Server	Change Management with Individual Consent
Key Management	Reset the password to recover the lost identity/key.	Digital assets are vanished if the key is lost.
Storage	Server is Central	Distributed Nodes.
Freedom	Risk of stolen Identities	Users to reclaim stolen/lost Identities.

Patient mobility is one of the vital issues. When patients transfer from one institute to another, their information may get scattered across many institutions, making accessing their medical records difficult. Patients can lose access to their electronic medical reports when they relocate, even though they are generated during patient visits and are stored in electronic medical records. This could result in an incomplete medical history, making it difficult for physicians to determine a patient's best action. The issue is exacerbated by the absence of interoperability across various healthcare systems. Responding to COVID-19 has been very challenging due to the centralization of the present healthcare data systems. Issues including data inconsistencies, delayed reporting, and privacy violations have hindered global response strategies. Blockchain technology solves these issues by decentralizing the sharing and storing of private health data. For instance, in Estonia, blockchain has been integrated into the healthcare system to ensure the security and accessibility of patient data. Challenges to blockchain integration with healthcare systems are guaranteeing compatibility with existing systems and sticking to laws like GDPR. A workable way to compromise privacy concerns and decentralization's benefit is to store personal data off-chain while keeping on-chain hashes.

Furthermore, the global healthcare system collects patient data from various sources worldwide (Akhtar et al., 2025). These sources are included in healthcare databases such as electronic health records, clinical trials and the medical literature. Knowledge graphs and patient information across the vapors data and matching them based on their collected information, including attribute name, age, gender, and other personal details, is a significant part of data collection (Akhtar et al., 2022). However, since these attributes may be expressed differently in different languages, advanced natural language processing (NLP) is crucial in standardizing formats, tokenizing text, and extracting relevant feature techniques. In clinical settings, NLP can support healthcare providers in making more informed decisions by providing a comprehensive view of the patient's medical history (Liu et al., 2024). Yet, NLP faces challenges regarding computational resources and scalability, which can lead to increased memory consumption and resource usage, particularly in low-resource healthcare systems (Mohammed et al., 2024). These challenges underline the need for further research and development in this area.

The global response to COVID-19 has brought to light significant challenges in healthcare data management, including privacy issues, interoperability obstacles, and scalability demands (Razzaq, Abdul, et al., 2022). However, there is a solution on the horizon. Blockchain technology is a game-changer with decentralized data interchange and reduced dependence on vulnerable centralized systems. It effectively addresses issues related to immutable functions. It ensures compliance with privacy regulations like the GDPR, particularly regarding sensitive data such as COVID-19 test results and vaccination records. These solutions, which integrate off-chain and on-chain storage hashes, are currently under investigation, offering a future where data security and regulatory compliance are in balance. (Zhu et al., 2020).

4. ROLE OF SECURE SMART CONTRACTS IN HEALTHCARE DATA

The smart contract is a computer program protocol executed automatically when the conditions or rules are met in their code. These rules and contracts are designed to run independently when certain rules and conditions have fulfilled the criteria. The contract creates trust and transparency between involved parties without needing the middleman or any third party. In the healthcare sector, smart contracts help hospitals and doctors share medical data securely while they keep patient privacy intact. Smart contracts provide full control to the users who can access their medical records by securing unauthorized individuals who can't view patient data. The healthcare system is more secure due to implementing these contracts. They automate patient data sharing, appointment scheduling, and billing processes, eliminating intermediaries such as insurance companies and billing systems. Smart contracts can handle the payments and approve the claims automatically by reducing the need for human intervention and reducing administrative costs. Smart contracts play a vital role in the health sector in saving payment records for every transaction; whoever is involved can track them and make sure they follow the rules. This particular role in healthcare was protecting data, ensuring its accuracy and transparency. Smart contracts can improve clinical trial research collaboration and automate sharing anonymized patient data, which helps the researcher secure and conduct efficient research.

The patient has to track their health care data, and the researcher can access relevant information quickly. Furthermore, the smart contract makes the healthcare product supply chain management more secure and transparent. For instance, the contracts may automate the complete information of drug origin and its journal from the maker to the ultimate customer to reduce the danger of fake medical data entering the supply chain. This ensures compliance with the law and encourages trust between patients and the medical staff. Smart contracts ensure that interactions are automated clearly and securely in healthcare, improving trust between these parties. The smart contract helps smooth health information sharing between patients, providers, and payers, ultimately improving patient-centered care. Recently, the main problem occurring in the health care systems is the inability to securely share patient data across different organizations, causing delays in treatment and disturbing the patient experience. Smart contracts and blockchain technology fully command who can access and use their healthcare record data. They enable the sharing of real-time critical information like test results, prescriptions, and medical history; they help healthcare providers make faster and more informed decisions. Smart contracts minimize errors and delays and automate secure data sharing. The significant benefits of smart contracts to automation of insurance claim processing claims and payment systems are that patients can track their full history based on the transaction procedure. The inefficient handling of claims leads to dispute payment delays and higher administrative costs; the smart contract simplifies, solves, and verifies claims based on clear criteria such as insurance coverage and patient eligibility. Once the conditions are successfully met, the payments automatically reduce human involvement and the chance of fraud. Smart contracts make communication easier between the patient's healthcare providers and insurance companies, leading to more transparent and accurate claims processing and improving the system's overall efficiency. The smart contract offers a more transparent and efficient procedure.

Smart contracts could improve secure, efficient healthcare data management to reduce the rising cost. The traditional healthcare system often relies on manual data processing, and privacy security features are the main problems leading to inefficiencies and higher costs. Smart contracts can automate tasks like reducing the processing of payments, verifying claims, and managing medical records easily, saving time and other resources. It reduces the overall healthcare cost, and doctors focus more on patient care and expertise in the pharmaceutical industry. Smart contracts track and verify the supply chain of medicines important for the patient's health, especially with the global issue of counterfeit drugs. Blockchain transparency features are utilised in the healthcare system for real-time tracking of medication that makes a secure and clear record of every transaction. This ensures the patients receive real treatments and helps prevent fake drugs from entering the market (Ahad, Abdul, et al., 2025, Ahad, Abdul, et al., 2021, Ahad, Abdul, et al., 2023). While the user can easily track the source of drugs where they come from sources, and it provides full authentication to trace the primary source of drugs, they can quickly fix the supply chain issues. The smart contract improves patient outcomes, reduces cost, and increases trust efficiency when the healthcare industry grows. The healthcare system integrates with the blockchain technology smart contract to automate the delivery of patient data sharing service and track the complete medical record through the smart contracts. However, to fully unlock the potential issues, competent contact must be addressed, such as regulatory compliance integration with the current healthcare system and acceptance by the healthcare organization. The research and development teams continue to focus on how smart contracts could play a vital role in creating the next generation of healthcare solutions, benefiting both patients and healthcare providers.

5. REGULATORY AND ETHICAL CHALLENGES IN BLOCKCHAIN HEALTHCARE IMPLEMENTATION

Blockchain technology presents a groundbreaking opportunity to increase data security and patient autonomy in medical systems. This innovation comes with significant privacy rules and regulations introduced properly to assure compliance with existing laws and maintain moral standards.

COMPLIANCE WITH REGULATIONS LIKE GDPR AND HIPAA

Despite its decentralized nature and immutability, Blockchain holds the potential to enhance healthcare data privacy significantly. However, the EU's General Data Protection Regulation (GDPR) and the US Health Insurance Portability and Accountability Act (HIPAA) may pose challenges. Still, blockchain-based electronic health record (EHR) systems can improve compatibility, privacy, and control of the healthcare system. When deployed in real-world scenarios, these systems can revolutionize how healthcare data is accessed and managed (Ettaloui et al., 2024).

The primary concern regarding blockchain immutability is the GDPR protection rule, which states that the 'right to be forgotten' when data is recorded on the blockchain ledger cannot be altered or deleted, which is against GDPR. The 'right to be forgotten' is a key principle of the GDPR that allows individuals to request the deletion or removal of personal data when there is no compelling reason for its continued processing. The research explained that blockchain technology's decentralized and immutable nature introduced unique challenges when adhering to privacy and security regulations such as the Health Insurance Portability and Accountability Act (HIPAA) and the General Data Protection Regulation (GDPR).

The blockchain off-chain concern provides the solution to store the data outside the blockchain ledger, where only the hashed references are stored on the blockchain ledger. This 'off-chain' concept refers to data not stored directly on the blockchain but instead referenced by the blockchain. According to the legal norms, this approach allows data to be changed or removed while maintaining the blockchain rights and integrity. Applying the HIPAA confidentiality rules in a permissioned blockchain where access is linked to automated participants can be implemented. The researcher explored that blockchain technology continues to grow in the healthcare sector, and the organization needs to understand how to ensure the security and privacy of patient health information on the blockchain while maintaining compliance with these regulations. The HIPAA mandates uncompromising the healthcare sector to ensure the confidentiality and integrity of the data. Blockchain technology's distributed ledger and transparency can improve data privacy, strong encryption, and access to the control mechanism, which is crucial to keeping the information secure.

Smart contracts in the healthcare sector automate administrative tasks and improve remote patient tracking. These 'smart contracts' are self-executing contracts with the terms of the agreement between the patient and the healthcare provider directly written into code. In the healthcare sector, the Internet of Things devices may appropriately handle data from the wearable device and connect it with blockchain technology. These contracts may alert the medical staff and prepare patient data for immediate action when anomalies are found. The smart contract manages health insurance claims where minor insurance payout hospitalizations brought on certain medical occurrences; by implementing predefined conditions, smart contracts ensure patients' and health care information, which are the more effective ways for the health care sectors.

ETHICAL CONSIDERATIONS

Blockchain technology provides vital ethical implications for the healthcare sector beyond adherence to the law. Utilizing blockchain technology must be guided by the following principles: prioritizing patient autonomy, privacy, and equality. Blockchain technology improves patient autonomy by allowing individuals to access their personal record information to control medical data. The patients' trust, privacy, and transparency are increased when they can decide who can access their data. However, this freedom elaborates that people must understand the implications of sharing data, necessitating comprehensive patient education programs to ensure informed decisions. Security and privacy are essential elements of medical ethics. Although blockchain technology might increase data security in the healthcare sector, privacy is a concern since people could be re-identified using anonymized healthcare data. Ethical deployment requires ongoing monitoring and providing strong identification techniques to prevent unauthorized violations. Blockchain technology is growing in the care sector; thus, it's more important to address the potential consequences and the moral issues surrounding its adoption. Equity in healthcare sector access and outcome is a global ethical need. The decentralized nature of blockchain has robust features to reduce healthcare sector disparities and enhance the storage and accessibility of medical images. However, variations in digital literacy and technology access might exacerbate the disadvantages. The global health disparities highlight administrative shortcomings, faulty IT systems, and unnecessary global issues.

Collaboration among different departments, including engineers, lawmakers, medical experts, and ethicists, is crucial for successfully utilizing blockchain technology in healthcare sectors. It's vital to give ethical issues like consent management, fair access to medical advancements, and preventing data monopolies early consideration. The development of blockchain-based systems prioritizing inclusivity should prevent the marginalization of disadvantaged populations. Blockchain technology supports global health goals by creating ethical standards and guidelines across countries. In the healthcare system, transparency, privacy, and security in managing sensitive patient information are priorities, and everyone involved should know how the data is properly governed. Blockchain with artificial intelligence also helps process data fairly, reducing bias in healthcare services. Patient education about digital tools and improving digital literacy is also important, as informed users are more likely to use blockchain systems responsibly. Lastly, strong evidence is needed to ensure new technologies follow core healthcare values and to address any ethical challenges that arise quickly.

This also calls to question the commercialization of data and the potential for abuse, particularly among those with lower incomes. The concern about the ethical guidelines is that patients' consent must always be completely voluntary and that they cannot be forced to provide information to benefit from it. Other questions are raised about the vital ethics of blockchain technology's environmental implications. Many blockchain systems use proof-of-work algorithms that utilize energy at a time when environmental sustainability is pivotal. To address this, energy-efficient protocols like hybrid consensus, which combines proof-of-work and proof-of-stake, or proof-stake, which assigns transaction validation based on the amount of cryptocurrency a person holds, must be preferred in blockchain-based healthcare systems.

The decentralized blockchain technology's utilization in the medical sector raises the accountability problem. If there are mistakes in security, privacy, and transparency problems or data misuse, it cannot easily figure out who is responsible in a system that is not centralized. This lack of a clear accountability structure can lead to ethical concerns. Therefore, it is important to establish an ethical network story integrated with other networks like the Internet of Things (IoT), artificial intelligence (AI), and machine learning; these should also be considered in the ethical framework (Razzaq, Abdul, et al., 2023). These technologies can bring benefits for the ethical difficulties to the medical field. In summary, blockchain brings changes for healthcare professionals who are paying attention to conflicts like firmness, privacy sustainability, and accountability.

A complete teamwork approach, including ethicists, regulators, healthcare professionals, and technology experts, is important to building a modern and ethically sound medical system. Government organizations and international bodies must work together to establish a global ethical standard and ensure privacy rules and regulations to reap the benefits of the blockchain sectors without compromising medical ethics and human rights.

GLOBAL VARIATIONS IN BLOCKCHAIN ADOPTION IN HEALTHCARE

However, blockchain has seen conservative but growing interest in healthcare applications in the US, where it is subject to HIPAA regulations. The goal has been to improve interoperability across diverse healthcare information systems while maintaining adherence to security and privacy laws.

As blockchain technology becomes more accepted in healthcare, the willingness of stakeholders to adopt new technologies, the state of healthcare infrastructure, and regional regulations will influence how it is applied. The different levels of development in technical infrastructure can slow the adoption of blockchain. Areas with reduced digitalized healthcare systems may face more challenges, particularly integrating systems and ensuring that data can be shared. On the other hand, more technologically advanced regions will have a stronger infrastructure and be more ready to use blockchain solutions due to their higher acceptance of digital health.

Furthermore, the privacy regulation and protection acts make more of an impact on the blockchain application how they made are blockchain applications (Razzaq, Abdul, et al., 2024). The European Union GDPR clearly defines the rules for the blockchain application to handle personal data and other documents information correctly. It is concerned about the blockchain ensuring that personal information is secure and managed openly and honestly. The balance strictly applied between the data minimization requirements of the GDPR and the inherently high levels of security and openness of blockchain technology is a challenge. To address these issues, hybrid blockchain systems are being explored to secure the data off-chain and only essential data, such as cryptographic hashes and on-chain. This ultimately guarantees compliance with the data privacy acts roles and regulations to maintain the benefits of blockchain immutable ledger. The main obstacle to blockchain adoption in the US healthcare sector is assuring compliance with the Insurance Portability and Accountability Act (HIPAA) to protect data sensitivity. The HIPAA's privacy security and transparency requirements are essential when transferring and storing medical data over decentralized networks. The transparency and variability of blockchain technology can make it challenging to comply with HIPAA's mandate that patients have the right to request the removal of their healthcare data on a blockchain platform. This dilemma now focuses on developing a solution that allows blockchain to comply with HIPAA regulations.

Another effective strategy to consider is permission blockchain models, which provide limited and regulated access to patient data. These private blockchains must be verified with the existing healthcare information system, which may necessitate updating or modifying the entire infrastructure. There is a pressing need to increase interest in exploring how blockchain can enhance the interoperability of healthcare systems despite the challenges posed by regulations. The existing healthcare system data transmission methods often suffer from incredible fragmentation delays and errors, which can lead to poor patient care.

Blockchain technology could solve these problems by empowering the secure and reliable sharing of patient data across different healthcare sectors and service providers. This autonomously improves the quality of care and reduces administrative costs, as patients, doctors, and insurance companies would have access to up-to-date and accurate information. Blockchain is potentially growing in different countries, especially in the medical sector, as more countries develop legal frameworks that empower and facilitate the protection of patient privacy and confidentiality. The success of blockchain technology in the healthcare sector will depend on how well it integrates with other advanced technologies like cloud computing, AI, and the IoT. For instance, blockchain can enhance the security and reliability of

AI models by ensuring the quality of the data used for training. It can also facilitate the secure and real-time sharing of health data collected by IoT devices, thereby improving decision-making in patient care.

Integrating with decentralized blockchain can improve the responsiveness and flexibility of the healthcare sector. For instance, using blockchain and AI together could empower more accurate predictive analytics by ensuring the data quality used to train AI models. In the same way, the real-time health data gathered by IoT devices can be securely shared across blockchain networks, providing reliable and unalterable data that will improve decision-making in patient care. Utilizing blockchain technology in the healthcare sector can have vital advantages, especially when it comes to lessening fraud and unauthorized access and promoting transparency. The multiple stakeholders can increase confidence in study results by utilizing blockchain technology to document every step of a clinical trial, from patient consent to the final report. This guarantees the data is verifiable and immutable. This could lead to better results in the pharmaceutical industry, where issues such as fraud and data manipulation have long persisted. It could also help eradicate counterfeit drugs and ensure that patients can receive safe and effective treatments by tracing the origin of pharmaceuticals throughout the supply chain. Other potential blockchain applications in healthcare include managing patient records, ensuring drug traceability, and facilitating secure and transparent billing processes.

6 EMERGING TRENDS IN DECENTRALIZED HEALTHCARE TECHNOLOGIES

The integration of wearable technology, the IoT, and AI in healthcare is undergoing a significant transformation, with blockchain technology playing a pivotal role. The global impact of COVID-19 has underscored the strides made in digital health. A notable blockchain application is the creation of Digital Health Passports (DHPs), which incorporate immunity and vaccination certificates (see Figure 3 and Figure 4). These passports facilitate the secure and permanent sharing of COVID-19 test and vaccination information, all stored on decentralized networks like IPFS. Smart contracts powered by Ethereum automate health data verification, leading to faster responses from medical authorities.

Figure 3. Overview of the solution based on some experimental studies of our research.

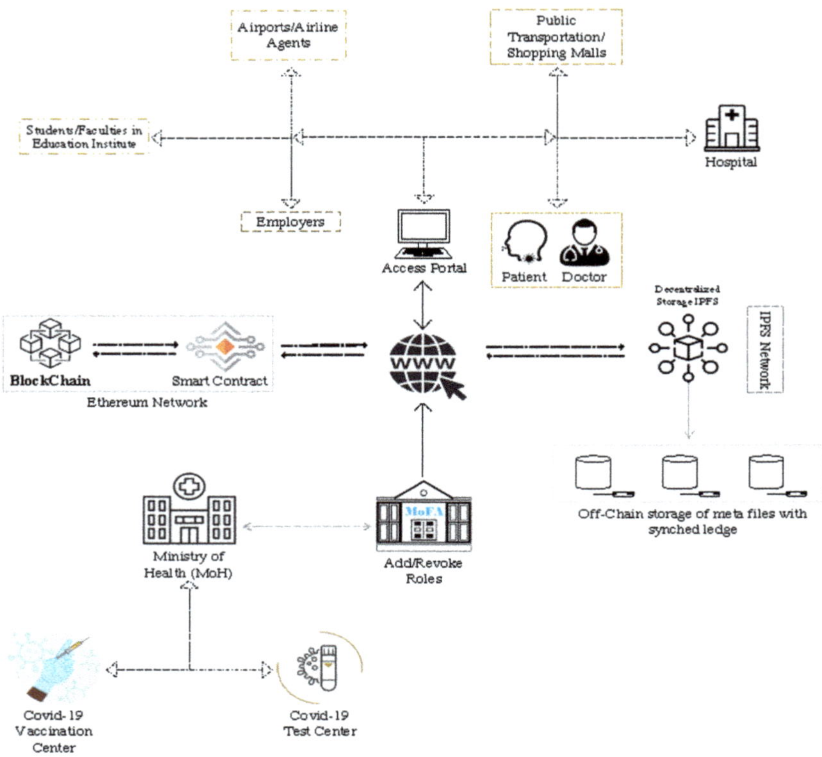

This collaborative effort addresses critical healthcare challenges like real-time data access, security, and privacy. Research indicates that the wearables, blockchain, and AI combination could significantly enhance chronic disease treatment as healthcare transitions from hospital-centric to patient-centric models. These changes place patients at the core of the healthcare system, enabling better monitoring and personalized care (Zheng et al., 2018; Yue, Wang, Jin, Li, & Jiang, 2016). Integrating the healthcare system with the decentralized blockchain and other technologies like the wearable Internet of Things is paramount. Wearable Internet of Things devices continuously gather vital signs, activity levels, and other health data securely stored on blockchain networks. The decentralized platform ensures data confidentiality and immutability, empowering healthcare professionals to make swift decisions. For instance, wearable health monitors can record real-time data like heart rate and glucose levels, facilitating early intervention during critical health events. The decentralized security features of blockchain protect confidential health information from unauthorized access (Azaria, Ekblaw, Vieira, & Lippman,2016; Esposito, De Santis, Tortora, Chang, & Choo, 2018).

Figure 4. Data sharing sequence process

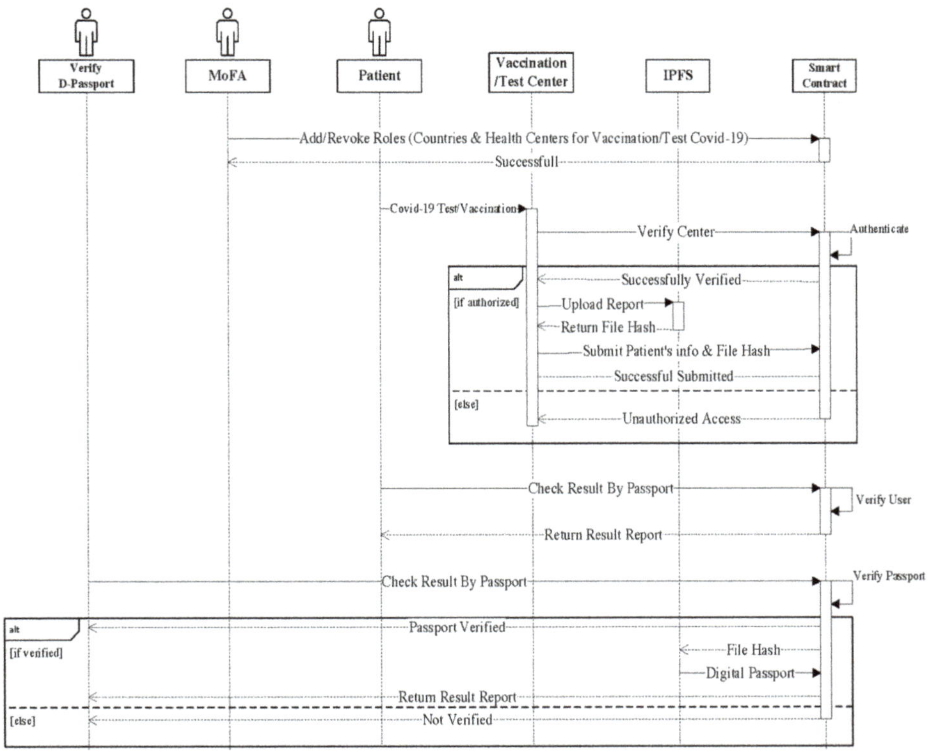

Platforms like HNMblock help track disease data in real-time without it being tampered with, which is important for responding quickly to outbreaks. Its features make sure that health data stays secure and useful. This is key for health programs, as these platforms help governments and health groups create better policies and understand disease trends. (Radanović & Likić, 2018). Additionally, wearable IoT devices with blockchain capabilities increase the quality and usability of electronic health records (EHRs) by providing healthcare organizations with secure, decentralized data exchange (Halamka, Lippman, & Ekblaw, 2017).

AI is critical to this convergence because AI-powered analytics can identify trends and address healthcare issues when applied to blockchain-stored health data. For instance, by analyzing IoT-generated data on blockchain networks, AI algorithms may detect when chronic diseases will begin, enabling proactive preventive therapies. This connection improves healthcare decision-making by automating diagnoses, optimizing resource allocation, and enabling predictive healthcare. Wearable technology, blockchain, and AI advance remote patient monitoring by giving continuous insights into patients' health issues without requiring frequent in-person consultations (Chen et al., 2018; Zhang et al., 2017). Blockchain makes it easier to trade data in predictive healthcare securely and collaboratively. Unified learning models and private blockchain protocols enable decentralized AI training without compromising data privacy. These models are especially relevant to personalized medicine, which uses extensive data from several sources to develop patient-specific treatment plans. Institutions may unify easily with these decentralized frameworks while protecting the patient's critical data (Esposito, De Santis, Tortora, Chang, & Choo, 2018) (Yue, Wang, Jin, Li, & Jiang, 2016).

Wearable IoT-enabled gadgets are revolutionizing healthcare delivery by collecting vast amounts of health data, such as heart rate, oxygen saturation, and sleep patterns. This data is securely stored on blockchain networks, ensuring it cannot be changed and making it easier to share with insurance companies or healthcare providers. More importantly, this method empowers patients by giving them more control over their health information, fostering a sense of independence and control. Moreover, wearable technology that uses blockchain meets regulatory standards like GDPR and HIPAA, which focus on data security and patient consent management. With blockchain-enabled apps, patients can control who can access their health data, promoting a patient-centered approach to care (Hathaliya, Tanwar, Tyagi, & Kumar, 2019; Kuo, Ohno-Machado, & Kim, 2017).

Blockchain and IoT technologies are not just transforming individualized patient care; they are revolutionizing public health administration. For example, IoT devices linked to blockchain networks may observe environmental factors like air quality and disease spread to provide policymakers with relevant data. This link increases the transparency of health data and facilitates prompt responses to public health emergencies (Akhtar et al., 2019). Moreover, pharmaceutical companies may use blockchain to trace medical records on the supply chain to guarantee the safety and authenticity of medicines and reduce the likelihood that fake products will reach the market. The potential of blockchain to revolutionize public health administration is an exciting prospect for the future (Azaria, Ekblaw, Vieira, & Lippman,2016; Esposito, De Santis, Tortora, Chang, & Choo, 2018).

Despite the benefits, applying decentralized technology to healthcare presents challenges. One issue is interoperability, where decentralized platforms may have difficulty working with older systems. Another is scalability, particularly when dealing with large amounts of IoT data. To address these problems, innovative solutions like smart contract-based dynamic verification services are being developed. These smart contracts utilize decentralized networks to verify data from IoT devices while ensuring its accuracy and integrity, a crucial role that blockchain plays in healthcare innovation. With its immutable and transparent nature, blockchain technology is instrumental in maintaining health data security and integrity in a decentralized system, reassuring data safety (Kuo, Ohno-Machado, & Kim, 2017).

Decentralized healthcare technologies are not just a concept but are used to treat chronic diseases. For instance, wearable IoT devices can continuously monitor patients with chronic conditions, while blockchain ensures the data is secure and easily accessible. AI-powered prediction prototype analyses this data to find potential health risks early, allowing healthcare providers to take preventive action. By combining blockchain, AI, and IoT, healthcare systems can enhance patient outcomes, lowering the chances of hospital readmissions (Zheng et al., 2018; Xu, Weber, & Staples, 2019). The healthcare sector has seen the rise of new business models due to the merging of wearable tech, blockchain, and IoT. Decentralized solutions enable safe and transparent collaboration between patients, insurers, pharmaceutical companies, and medical professionals. For example, blockchain can support automated insurance claims processing, ensuring transparency and reducing administrative costs. Likewise, wearable sensors combined with blockchain technology provide real-time alerts and notifications, enabling quick actions that could save lives. Advancements in decentralized healthcare technology are changing how data is managed, shared, and used in medicine. By integrating blockchain with wearables, AI, and IoT, there are enormous capabilities to outcome patient results, healthcare delivery, and data security. While challenges like interoperability and scalability remain, ongoing research and innovation are paving the way for a decentralized, patient-focused healthcare system that meets the needs of the modern medical sector (Azaria, Ekblaw, Vieira, & Lippman,2016; Xu, Weber, & Staples, 2019).

7 DECENTRALIZED DATA MANAGEMENT IN HEALTHCARE

One of the most difficult tasks in healthcare is maintaining sensitive patient data safely and properly. Traditional centralized systems often lack the security, scalability, and interoperability required for modern healthcare environments. Decentralized systems, particularly those based on blockchain technology, provide several advantages. The decentralized blockchain technology has transparent, secure, immutable methods of handling and storing medical data (Agbo, Mahmoud, & Eklund, 2019). The decentralized nature of blockchain technology reduces the vulnerabilities and unauthorized access related to the centralized repositories while ensuring the data accessibility and integrity by the blockchain network to store the data accessibility and integrity of medical information. Blockchain decentralized systems eliminate the single point of failure seen in the traditional healthcare system and improve protection against attacks and data breaches. Patients have greater control over the availability of their medical information because of blockchain's exact access control via smart contracts (Zhang, Walker, White, Schmidt, & Lenz, 2017). The decentralized healthcare record management promotes transparency and accountability, building trust between patients and healthcare personnel. The platform allows patients, doctors, and medical administration to easily trace complete transaction histories and find the origin and flow of information. Every transaction or data exchange recorded on an immutable blockchain ledger reduces the risk of fraud or data manipulation. It ensures that every access is monitored and validated to protect private medical data. The resilience of decentralized systems may be increased by distributing data across several nodes. This distribution ensures operations continue during hardware failures or attacks against specific nodes. In an emergency, this allows medical professionals to have constant access to vital patient data.

Finally, decentralization promotes interoperability by enabling secure data sharing across several healthcare organizations without relying on a single centralized authority. This encourages collaboration between laboratories, research institutions, and medical centres, improving treatment quality and accelerating medical advancement. The role of blockchain in this process is significant, as it ensures the security and integrity of shared data, fostering optimism about the future of healthcare.

Figure 5. An overview of the detailed solution.

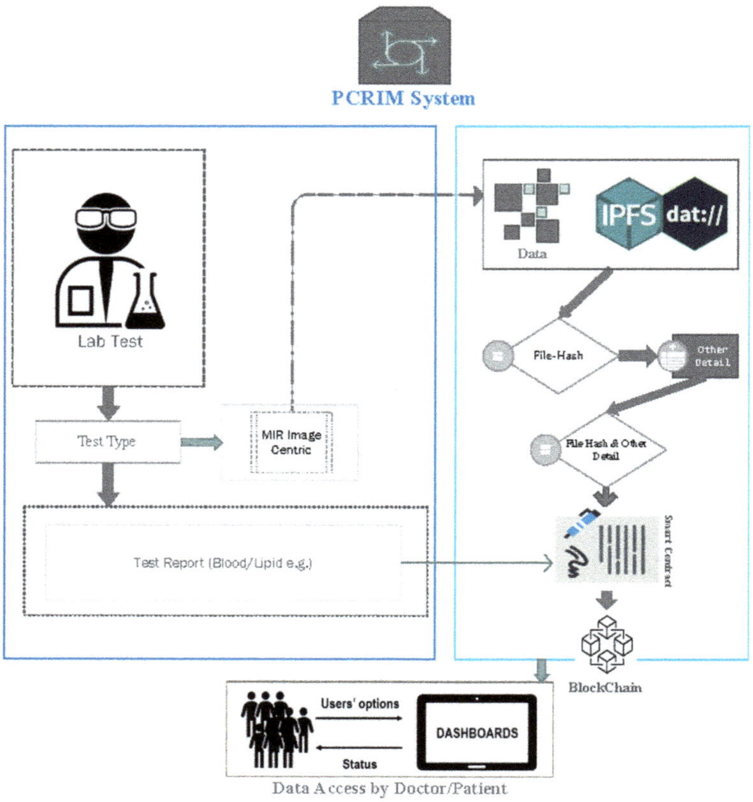

Figure 5 illustrates the data access by the patients and how they interact with the decentralized system to upload medical data on a decentralized application. The laboratory handles the first patient report, and the laboratory assistant takes the sample of the patient's blood test and runs the test for the required reports. Then, the laboratory assistant stores the record on the blockchain leader against the patient's ID and appointment ID. Another interaction with the system is the radiologist connects the medical image to other examinations and test purposes and then uploads the medical image to IPFS using the decentralized application DApp system and provides the rest of the required complete details against the patient's ID and the appointment ID which is stored on the blockchain ledger. This service completes the cycle by providing that the events continually repeat and automatically after a fixed time or are triggered by receiving medical image data from the server. The dashboard provides complete data to doctors and patients who can access the available data publicly. The platform is open access, allowing doctors, patients, and medical administrative staff to easily download and access data on the decentralized platform. The medical image and other resources can be accessed through the user-friendly web portal, where the user needs to enter their patient ID and other details, ensuring a comfortable and confident experience.

8. BENEFITS OF BLOCKCHAIN IN MEDICAL DATA STORAGE

Blockchain's decentralized nature provides a platform for storing and sharing data, facilitating interoperability across multiple healthcare systems. This is particularly crucial in medical imaging, where hospitals, laboratories, and research institutions must securely transmit and preserve large amounts of data. Blockchain significantly improves data integrity, streamlines processes, and reduces data redundancy in this industry. By eliminating data redundancy, blockchain technology enhances the efficiency of healthcare data management, making it a valuable tool for healthcare providers (Azaria, Ekblaw, Vieira, & Lippman,2016).

Research shows that integrating blockchain technology into existing healthcare systems enhances medical data transfers' efficacy while adhering to strict privacy and data security regulations. Decentralized storage systems and cryptographic techniques that ensure data security and integrity are used to achieve this (Esposito, De Santis, Tortora, Chang, & Choo, 2018). Blockchain technology introduced critical problems such as patient confidentiality and data ownership. However, it also ensures that patients have control over their medical data because decentralized systems limit access to only approved individuals or organizations. This not only empowers patients but also promotes transparency, fostering confidence between patients and healthcare providers and ensuring the integrity of the healthcare system.

The quality of medical data is enhanced by blockchain technology's capacity to create unchangeable records, especially in circumstances like insurance claims or legal disputes. In healthcare, the main advantage of medical imaging is storing it in blockchain-distributed storage features to enable the secure transfer of imaging data while lowering the risk of unauthorized access to image data breaches. During COVID-19, blockchain technology effectively secured the accessibility and integrity of vaccination records for several stakeholders. Blockchain technology plays a vital role in this matter; vaccination status verification is made possible with the help of a smart contract that is automatically executed transparently and reduces administrative burdens. Furthermore, the e-blockchain increases trust by providing an unchangeable audit trail of vaccination records, essential for public health campaigns and international travel. In COVID-19, the blockchain changed the shape of the distribution of vast amounts of generic data required to track the situation of patient information and store it on the IPFS Interplanetary file system (Azaria et al., 2016; Razzaq et al., 2023). Blockchain also significantly reduces administrative costs by automating data, removing redundancies, and guaranteeing real-time data access to all stakeholders. By simplifying processes and reducing operating costs, this enhancement increases the efficiency of healthcare services and offers promising financial benefits.

9 SMART CONTRACTS AND HEALTHCARE AUTOMATION

The smart contract is vital in the healthcare system's automating of procedures. The smart contract automatically executes the automated healthcare sector. The smart contract automates several procedures, such as patient permission, accessing information, processing insurance claims, and securely transmitting medical data, which are made simple by these self-executing contracts. The smart contract removes the middlemen and reduces the risk of mistakes and administrative expenses (Yue, Wang, Jin, Li, & Jiang, 2016). Smart contracts execute several factors, which are designed according to the setup of the roles or deny access to medical data in the context of patient consent. These contracts speed up medical work and professionalism while guaranteeing that the individuals have complete data ownership (Kuo,

Ohno-Machado, & Kim, 2017). Smart contracts automate the settlement of insurance claims by improving transparency and privacy (Tith et al., 2020). The immutable audit trail of smart contracts provides transparency in every transaction, securely documented and available for regulatory and compliance obligations. This is important in clinical research where openness and harsh commitment to professionals are necessary. Automating patient permission to use study data and sand mart contracts throughout the procedure may ensure that researchers adhere to ethical norms without requiring human intervention.

Smart contracts also play a significant role in improving pharmaceutical supply networks for traceability purposes. Automating verification procedures for the healthcare sector and professionals can reduce the risks associated with counterfeit or fraudulent medications and ensure that patients receive only genuine ones. These solutions improve operations and foster more confidence by eliminating the risk of errors or delays caused by human processes. This versatility of smart contracts, from automating healthcare procedures to enhancing pharmaceutical supply networks, underscores their potential to revolutionize various aspects of healthcare. A major advancement in healthcare automation, smart contracts boost productivity, strengthen data security, and give patients and providers more control.

Figure 6. Data sharing sequence process.

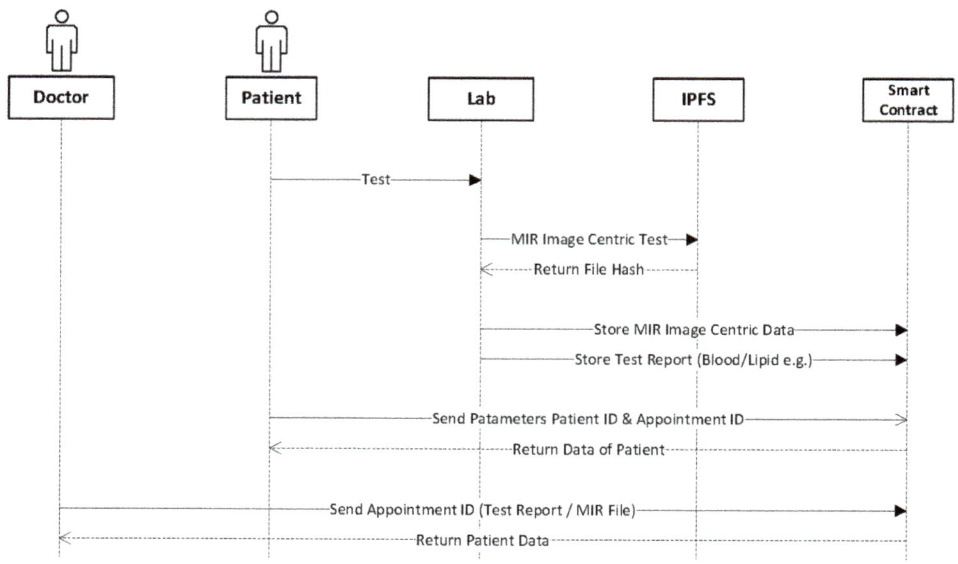

Figure 6 illustrates the network entities and their interaction. It shows the sequence of the different entities, such as the Doctor, patients' laboratory IPFS, and smart contract. These entities directly communicate with each other, like the doctor-patient entities, who access the data from the blockchain ledger and use the web portal. The laboratory entities are used to uphold the mediator data, such as the images on IPFS. After the upload, the file hash is returned to the parents and stored on the blocking ledger.

10. CHALLENGES AND FUTURE DIRECTIONS

Blockchain technology has several advantages, but there are drawbacks as well. The scalability of blockchain networks is a major worry since the system's processing and storage capacity would not be able to handle the increasing volume of medical data. Another issue is how blockchain solutions integrate with existing healthcare IT systems, which could use outdated technology (Radanović & Likić, 2018). To address these issues, ongoing research attempts to develop more scalable blockchain architectures and improve how blockchain is integrated with other technologies, such as cloud computing and artificial intelligence. These enhancements are intended to provide healthcare data management with an architecture that is more flexible and robust (Xu, Weber, & Staples, 2019).

The healthcare sector's features depend upon the smooth integration of blockchain technology with other advanced technologies such as machine intelligence and the Internet of Things. These technologies will provide the more robust creation of patient-centric, intelligent healthcare systems that can adapt to the changing needs of the healthcare sector. The healthcare sector is integrating blockchain and other technologies, such as healthcare scalability and interoperability issues, and is solving these issues. For instance, real-time patient data can be securely transmitted over blockchain networks via wearable health monitors and other Internet of Things devices, facilitating better monitoring and timely treatment of chronic disease. Using machine learning algorithms to examine the blockchain data and provide predictive insights that help clinicians detect early signs of diseases, such as different diseases, such as diabetes or cardiovascular problems, could lead to better preventive treatments.

Blockchain technology has the vast potential to support the global health sector, such as disease outbreak detection and immunization campaigns. Due to the features of blockchain immutability and transparency, it provides a secure platform for data sharing across the healthcare industry. Furthermore, by preventing the sale of forged medicines and ensuring the legality of medicines in supply chains, blockchain technology builds trust in healthcare in different sectors of institutions. However, legal and technical barriers to implementation still exist in the current healthcare sector. On the other hand, the healthcare industry is focused on developing compatible solutions to integrate blockchain with existing IT infrastructure, and governments need to make clear recommendations for blockchain compliance with data security regulations such as privacy protection rules such as HIPAA and GDPR. The combination of blockchain technology with IoT, AI, and other technologies has enabled a breakthrough in the healthcare sector, allowing for patient-centric, secure, and efficient systems that can adapt to new difficulties. Furthermore, despite the challenges, blockchain technology can potentially revolutionize healthcare systems as they are decentralized globally as it develops and is further researched. Technology developers, clinicians, and regulatory bodies must continue to cooperate to provide the solution and ensure that blockchain technology can meet the main demands of the healthcare industry in the future while maintaining security, privacy, and trust among all stakeholders.

The adoption of blockchain technology in the healthcare sector faces various obstacles, but there is a potential to advance healthcare systems globally as they develop and further research is conducted. Blockchain technology developers, clinicians, and regulatory bodies should continue to integrate these technologies and collaborate to ensure that blockchain solutions can meet the demands of the medical industry in the future while maintaining security, privacy, and trust among all stakeholders, including the patient-doctors and hospital administration. One of the most exciting aspects of using blockchain technology in healthcare is its potential to improve patient engagement significantly. Patients traditionally have limited control over their medical records because they are often distributed across the healthcare system, making accessing or managing all the related resources difficult. Blockchain technology offers a solution by giving patients ownership and control over their data, which they can share with healthcare providers as needed. This empowerment of patients can lead to a more collaborative care model, where patients can actively make healthcare decisions. The blockchain decentralized the system by giving patients control over their data and enabling true health monitoring through IoT devices. Blockchain can transform healthcare from a reactive to a proactive, preventative approach, offering a promising future for patient care.

Blockchain technology has a decentralized system to speed up medical billing and claims processing while enhancing patient communication. The main problems in the healthcare sector are delays, fraud, and billing errors, which decrease the healthcare sector's efficiency and privacy. These problems can be mitigated by utilizing blockchain technology to create a visible and immutable ledger, ensuring that every transaction is documented and validated from the blockchain ledger. Blockchain technology will save administrative costs by eliminating inconsistencies and streamlining reimbursement. Blockchain technology can easily reduce the risk of fraud by automating and securing invoicing processes using smart contracts, which guarantee that payments are only issued for services provided. The blockchain could have a significant impact on the pharmaceutical supply chain. Blockchain technology's ability to track and verify pharmaceuticals could greatly reduce the number of counterfeit drugs reaching the market. The global problem that threatens patient safety is drug fraud. The blockchain can make the pharmaceutical supply chain more trustworthy by offering a transparent, secure ledger that documents the entire path of a drug from producer to distributor to pharmacy. In addition to protecting patients, blockchain technology will guarantee the effectiveness and safety of the drugs they are given.

Blockchain technology can improve the privacy and security of medical research and its effectiveness. Problems including fraud, data tampering, and the lack of openness often plague a key component of medical research, clinical trials. When researchers utilize blockchain technology to document every step of a study, they can be sure that the data is immutable and is available to all authorized participants. It reduces the obstacles of forgery and unauthorized access in the healthcare sector. It can lead to the protection of clinical trial data from unauthorized access. Blockchain technology can trace the origin of trial data and the legitimacy of medical research by making it illegal to use false or fraudulent data. Blockchain technology in healthcare will only increase as it develops and can be integrated with other advanced technologies such as cloud computing, AI, and machine learning. When these technologies are combined, they will create more intelligent, flexible healthcare systems that can anticipate patient needs, provide immediate information, and improve the quality of care. Artificial intelligence leads data and machine learning systems, for instance, to examine patient data held on blockchain networks to predict potential health risks and provide personalized treatment approaches. Large amounts of medical data can be handled and stored through cloud computing while balancing the security of the blockchain's decentralized healthcare system structure.

11. CONCLUSIONS

This chapter introduced the transformation and potential utilization of blockchain technology in addressing the vital challenges in the healthcare sector for decentralized data management. The healthcare system needs to redefine the traditional to the decentralized system, such as the blockchain distributed storage solution, expand the centralized database's width to introduce the interplanetary file system and smart contracts and revise the healthcare privacy security and stability and interoperability in the healthcare sectors. This innovation empowers patients with greater control over their medical data and enhances privacy, transparency, and trust among the stakeholders. Furthermore, the transformation also needs the intention of blockchain technology with other emerging technologies like the IoT and AI, introducing novel opportunities for real-time data sharing, predictive analysis, and personalized care. This chapter also discusses the implications of blockchain technology facing the scalability regulator and ethical challenges. Addressing these challenges and barriers is a collaborative effort that requires the involvement of policymakers and technology in the healthcare profession. As this research advancement in this field advances, blockchain technology has the potential to refine the healthcare system, shifting from reactive to proactive patient-centralized models that propose data security, privacy, and collaboration.

REFERENCES

Agbo, C. C., Mahmoud, Q. H., & Eklund, J. M. (2019, April). Blockchain technology in healthcare: A systematic review. [). MDPI.]. *Health Care*, *7*(2), 56. PMID: 30987333

Ahad, A., Jiangbin, Z., Mughees, A., Puspitasari, I., & Tayyab, M. (2025). Secure Horizons: Integrating Blockchain With AI for Enhanced Smart Healthcare Systems. In AI Techniques for Securing Medical and Business Practices (pp. 357-390). IGI Global.

Ahad, A., Tahir, M., Sheikh, M. A. S., Mughees, A., & Ahmed, K. I. (2021, October). Optimal route selection in 5g-based smart health-care network: a reinforcement learning approach. In 2021 26th IEEE Asia-Pacific Conference on Communications (APCC) (pp. 248-253). IEEE.

Akhtar, M. U., & Khalil, M. I. K. Link Prediction Techniques in Complex Networks.

Akhtar, M. U., Liu, J., Xie, Z., Cui, X., Liu, X., & Huang, B. (2025). Multilingual entity alignment by abductive knowledge reasoning on multiple knowledge graphs. *Engineering Applications of Artificial Intelligence*, *139*, 109660. DOI: 10.1016/j.engappai.2024.109660

Akhtar, M. U., Liu, J., Xie, Z., Liu, X., Ahmed, S., & Huang, B. (2022). Entity alignment based on relational semantics augmentation for multilingual knowledge graphs. *Knowledge-Based Systems*, *252*, 109494. DOI: 10.1016/j.knosys.2022.109494

Ali, Z., Ahad, A., Madeira, F., & Shayea, I. (2023, October). Enhancing Transparency and Trustworthiness of Healthcare IoT Data with AWS: A Proposed Model. In EAI International Conference on IoT Technologies for HealthCare (pp. 44-56). Cham: Springer Nature Switzerland.

Azaria, A., Ekblaw, A., Vieira, T., & Lippman, A. (2016, August). Medrec: Using blockchain for medical data access and permission management. In *2016 2nd international conference on open and big data (OBD)* (pp. 25-30). IEEE.

Benet, J. (2014). IPFS—Content Addressed, Versioned, P2P File System(DRAFT 3). Available online: https://arxiv.org/abs/1407.3 561 (accessed on 21 March 2020).

Bocek, T., Rodrigues, B. B., Strasser, T., & Stiller, B. (2017, May). Blockchains everywhere-a use-case of blockchains in the pharma supply-chain. In 2017 IFIP/IEEE symposium on integrated network and service management (IM) (pp. 772-777). IEEE.

Cao, Z., Wang, Y., Zheng, W., Yin, L., Tang, Y., Miao, W., Liu, S., & Yang, B. (2022). The algorithm of stereo vision and shape from shading based on endoscope imaging. *Biomedical Signal Processing and Control*, *76*, 103658. DOI: 10.1016/j.bspc.2022.103658

Casalino, L., Gillies, R. R., Shortell, S. M., Schmittdiel, J. A., Bodenheimer, T., Robinson, J. C., Rundall, T., Oswald, N., Schauffler, H., & Wang, M. C. (2003). External incentives, information technology, and organized processes to improve health care quality for patients with chronic diseases. *Journal of the American Medical Association*, *289*(4), 434–441. DOI: 10.1001/jama.289.4.434 PMID: 12533122

Chen, W., Xu, Z., Shi, S., Zhao, Y., & Zhao, J. (2018, December). A survey of blockchain applications in different domains. In *Proceedings of the 2018 International Conference on Blockchain Technology and Application* (pp. 17-21).

Dai, M., Zhang, S., Wang, H., & Jin, S. (2018). A low storage room requirement framework for distributed ledger in blockchain. *IEEE Access : Practical Innovations, Open Solutions*, *6*, 22970–22975. DOI: 10.1109/ACCESS.2018.2814624

DOC (U.S. Department of Commerce). (1999). *The Emerging Digital Economy II: Appendices.* U.S. Department of Commerce.

Esposito, C., De Santis, A., Tortora, G., Chang, H., & Choo, K. K. R. (2018). Blockchain: A panacea for healthcare cloud-based data security and privacy? *IEEE Cloud Computing*, *5*(1), 31–37. DOI: 10.1109/MCC.2018.011791712

Ettaloui, N., Arezki, S., & Gadi, T. (2024). An Overview of Blockchain-Based Electronic Health Record and Compliance with GDPR and HIPAA. In Farhaoui, Y., Hussain, A., Saba, T., Taherdoost, H., & Verma, A. (Eds.), *Artificial Intelligence, Data Science and Applications. ICAISE 2023. Lecture Notes in Networks and Systems* (Vol. 838). Springer., DOI: 10.1007/978-3-031-48573-2_58

Guntur, L. N., Dornadula, G., & Nimbagal, R. N. (2022). Blockchain Technology: A Breakthrough in the Healthcare Sector. In Idrees, S. M., & Nowostawski, M. (Eds.), *Transformations Through Blockchain Technology* (pp. 137–160). Springer. DOI: 10.1007/978-3-030-93344-9_6

Halamka, J. D., Lippman, A., & Ekblaw, A. (2017). The Potential for Blockchain to Transform Electronic Health Records. *Harvard Business Review*, *3*, 2–5. Retrieved March 20, 2020, from https://hbr.org/2017/03/the-potential-for-blockchain-to-transform-electronic-health-records

Hathaliya, J. J., Tanwar, S., Tyagi, S., & Kumar, N. (2019). Securing electronics healthcare records in Healthcare 4.0: A biometric-based approach. *Computers & Electrical Engineering*, *76*, 398–410. DOI: 10.1016/j.compeleceng.2019.04.017

Heart, T., Ben-Assuli, O., & Shabtai, I. (2017). A Review of PHR, EMR and EHR Integration: A More Personalized Healthcare and Public Health Policy. *Health Policy and Technology*, *6*(1), 20–25. DOI: 10.1016/j.hlpt.2016.08.002

Khan, M., & Salah, K. (2018, May). IoT security: Review, blockchain solutions, and open challenges. *Future Generation Computer Systems*, *82*, 395–411. DOI: 10.1016/j.future.2017.11.022

Kuo, T. T., Kim, H. E., & Ohno-Machado, L. (2017). Blockchain distributed ledger technologies for biomedical and health care applications. *Journal of the American Medical Informatics Association : JAMIA*, *24*(6), 1211–1220. DOI: 10.1093/jamia/ocx068 PMID: 29016974

Liu, Y., Liu, Z., Zhang, Q., Su, J., Cai, Z., & Li, X. (2024). Blockchain and trusted reputation assessment-based incentive mechanism for healthcare services. *Future Generation Computer Systems*, *154*, 59–71. DOI: 10.1016/j.future.2023.12.023

Liu, Y., Tian, J., Hu, R., Yang, B., Liu, S., Yin, L., & Zheng, W. (2022). Improved Feature Point Pair Purification Algorithm Based on SIFT During Endoscope Image Stitching. *Frontiers in Neurorobotics*, *16*, 840594. DOI: 10.3389/fnbot.2022.840594 PMID: 35242022

Mettler, M. (2016, September). Blockchain technology in healthcare: The revolution starts here. In 2016 IEEE 18th international conference on e-health networking, applications and services (Healthcom) (pp. 1-3). IEEE.

Mohammed, M. A., Lakhan, A., Zebari, D. A., Abd Ghani, M. K., Marhoon, H. A., Abdulkareem, K. H., & Martinek, R. (2024). Securing healthcare data in industrial cyber-physical systems using combining deep learning and blockchain technology. *Engineering Applications of Artificial Intelligence*, *129*, 107612. DOI: 10.1016/j.engappai.2023.107612

Nakamoto, S. (2008). *Bitcoin: A peer-to-peer electronic cash system*. Whitepaper.

Radanović, I., & Likić, R. (2018). Opportunities for use of blockchain technology in medicine. *Applied Health Economics and Health Policy*, *16*(5), 583–590. DOI: 10.1007/s40258-018-0412-8 PMID: 30022440

Razzaq, A., Ahmad, A., Malik, A. W., Fahmideh, M., & Ramadan, R. A. (2023). Software engineering for internet of underwater things to analyze oceanic data. *Internet of Things : Engineering Cyber Physical Human Systems*, *24*, 100893. DOI: 10.1016/j.iot.2023.100893

Razzaq, A., Mohsan, S. A. H., Ghayyur, S. A. K., Al-Kahtani, N., Alkahtani, H. K., & Mostafa, S. M. (2022, December). Blockchain in healthcare: a decentralized platform for digital health passport of COVID-19 based on vaccination and immunity certificates. In Healthcare (Vol. 10, No. 12, p. 2453). MDPI.

Razzaq, A., Mohsan, S. A. H., Ghayyur, S. A. K., Alsharif, M. H., Alkahtani, H. K., Karim, F. K., & Mostafa, S. M. (2022). Blockchain-Enabled Decentralized Secure Big Data of Remote Sensing. *Electronics (Basel)*, *11*(19), 3164. DOI: 10.3390/electronics11193164

Razzaq, A., Zhang, T., Numair, M., Alreshidi, A., Jing, C., Aljaloud, A., & Qurat Ul Ain, M. (2024). Transforming academic assessment: The metaverse-backed Web 3 secure exam system. *Computer Applications in Engineering Education*, *32*(6), e22797.

Salah, K., Rehman, M. H. U., Nizamuddin, N., & Al-Fuqaha, A. (2019). Blockchain for AI: Review and Open Research Challenges. *IEEE Access : Practical Innovations, Open Solutions*, *7*, 10127–10149. DOI: 10.1109/ACCESS.2018.2890507

Seh, A. H., Zarour, M., Alenezi, M., Sarkar, A. K., Agrawal, A., & Khan, A. R. (2020). Healthcare Data Breaches: Insights and Implications. *Health Care*, *8*, 133. PMID: 32414183

Shini, S. G., Thomas, T., & Chithraranjan, K. (2012). Cloud Based Medical Image Exchange-Security Challenges. *Procedia Engineering*, *38*, 3454–3461. DOI: 10.1016/j.proeng.2012.06.399

Siyal, A. A., Aisha, Z. J., Muhammad, Z., Kainat, A., Aiman, K., & Georgia, S. (2019). Applications of blockchain technology in medicine and healthcare: Challenges and future perspectives. *Cryptography*, *3*(1), 3. DOI: 10.3390/cryptography3010003

Tith, D., Lee, J. S., Suzuki, H., Wijesundara, W. M. A. B., Taira, N., Obi, T., & Ohyama, N. (2020). Patient consent management by a purpose-based consent model for electronic health record based on blockchain technology. *Healthcare Informatics Research, 26*(4), 265–273. DOI: 10.4258/hir.2020.26.4.265 PMID: 33190460

Xu, X., Weber, I., & Staples, M. (2019). *Architecture for blockchain applications*. Springer. DOI: 10.1007/978-3-030-03035-3

Yue, X., Wang, H., Jin, D., Li, M., & Jiang, W. (2016). Healthcare data gateways: Found healthcare intelligence on blockchain with novel privacy risk control. *Journal of Medical Systems, 40*(10), 218. DOI: 10.1007/s10916-016-0574-6 PMID: 27565509

Zhang, P., Walker, M. A., White, J., Schmidt, D. C., & Lenz, G. (2017, October). Metrics for assessing blockchain-based healthcare decentralized apps. In *2017 IEEE 19th international conference on e-health networking, applications and services (Healthcom)* (pp. 1-4). IEEE. DOI: 10.1109/HealthCom.2017.8210842

Zheng, Z., Xie, S., Dai, H., Chen, X., & Wang, H. (2018). Blockchain challenges and opportunities: A survey. *International Journal of Web and Grid Services, 14*(4), 352. DOI: 10.1504/IJWGS.2018.095647

Zhu, L., Wu, Y., Gai, K., & Choo, K. K. R. (2019). Controllable and trustworthy blockchain-based cloud data management. *Future Generation Computer Systems, 91*, 527–535. DOI: 10.1016/j.future.2018.09.019

Zhu, L., Wu, Y., Gai, K., & Choo, K. K. R. (2020). Controllable and trustworthy blockchain-based cloud data management. *Future Generation Computer Systems*.

Chapter 15
The Convergence of Blockchain and Artificial Intelligence:
Transforming Healthcare

Ananya Pandey
https://orcid.org/0000-0002-2419-6314
Christ University, Bangalore, India

Jipson Joseph
https://orcid.org/0009-0005-1795-5051
Christ University, Bangalore, India

ABSTRACT

Blockchain and Artificial Intelligence (AI) together are revolutionizing healthcare by improving safety, privacy, and electronic health records' security. Adoption of private blockchain enhances accessibility and efficiency while demonstrating the industry's dedication to data protection. In addition to addressing important sector issues, this convergence offers improved illness detection, response, and overall healthcare efficacy. Additional research into cutting-edge AI features combined with blockchain promises to improve results and influence the way healthcare is delivered globally in the future while ensuring data security, privacy, and innovation. In light of the aforementioned, this chapter looks at how blockchain technology and AI can be combined to solve current issues with healthcare data security and privacy. It offers insights into best practices and strategies for utilizing blockchain and AI's revolutionary potential in healthcare by examining various recent studies and developing trends.

INTRODUCTION

According to the World Health Organization (WHO), "health innovation" enhances healthcare's efficacy, affordability, sustainability, quality, and safety. "New or improved" health policies, procedures, systems, goods and technology, services, and delivery methods that lead to better healthcare are all included in this description (WHO, 2016; McSherry & Douglas, 2016). Other considerations include advancements in patient happiness, education, research, and care access. To put it simply, the ultimate purpose of health innovation is to maximize the performance of the health system in order to better

DOI: 10.4018/979-8-3373-0593-6.ch015

fulfill the needs and wants of both public and private healthcare systems. In order to improve treatment, diagnosis, education, outreach, prevention, research quality and delivery, and access to healthcare, innovations in the field should, in theory, result in scalable solutions and improvements in health policies, systems, products, technologies, services, and delivery methods. Poor-quality treatment is responsible for between 5.7 and 8.4 million deaths yearly in low- and middle-income countries (LMICs), and 107 million years of life are lived with a handicap, mostly among those with untreated diabetes and mental illness (National Academies of Sciences, Engineering, and Medicine, 2018). The first step in raising the standard of healthcare worldwide is to earn the capacity to describe and measure the burden of poor treatment. Innovation is invention plus spread and adoption (Kelly & Young, 2017). It could be a brand-new concept, item, service, or care plan in the healthcare industry that outperforms the status quo. Two essential characteristics of successful innovations are their usability and desirability. Slow acceptance and dissemination are not unique to the healthcare industry. To reach 40% consumer acceptance, it took the telephone 64 years, electricity 45 years, computers 23 years, mobile phones 16 years, radios 12 years, and the internet 13 years (De Gusta, 2012). However, compared to healthcare, other industries have advanced in better, quicker, and more intelligent innovation. Successful businesses figure out what their customers want and use that information to develop. They pinpoint the main problems, collaborate with clients, other interested parties, and specialists to resolve them, create an adoption and diffusion plan, and implement it. These companies have created and offered their staff an innovative culture.

Healthcare data security aims to safeguard the information, networks, and computers used by healthcare organizations and providers. Regulations under the Health Insurance Portability and Accountability Act (HIPAA) are one of the main forces behind healthcare data security. These guidelines offer broad guidance on how to handle private medical information. Many patients now have access to sophisticated, individualized healthcare thanks to recent developments in healthcare delivery, which has enhanced their wellbeing. The next stage in healthcare is the smooth integration of these cutting-edge technologies, including blockchain, artificial intelligence (AI), and wearable sensor devices with Internet of Things (IoT) support. In light of the above perspective, this chapter explores how AI and blockchain are converging to transform the healthcare sector. It further identifies the potential benefits, challenges and future directions related to advancing technology in healthcare.

BLOCKCHAIN TECHNOLOGY IN HEALTHCARE

An innovative database technique called blockchain technology makes it possible for transparent information sharing within a company network. Data, which is kept in a blockchain database, in the form of blocks and are connected in a chain. There are certain principles of this technology such as decentralization, integrity, cryptography, security, privacy and inclusiveness (Angraal et al., 2017). Since blockchain is a peer-to-peer (P2P) network, no single user or participant controls a transaction; instead, power is shared among all network members. This implies that no single stakeholder can hack, alter, or shut down the chain of blocks. Because of its distributed (decentralized) nature, the blockchain network is immune to fraud and hacking (Sarode et al., 2021). Further, every member of the blockchain-powered network has the freedom to decide; in this case, user intuition serves as the only guide and confidence in the system is not compelled. The tight integrity is evident in the ways of this complete P2P network's operation and the rewards to each user for their efforts. This fundamental idea underpins the design of blockchain, which offers users a high degree of confidentiality and authenticity (Laroiya et al., 2020).

It makes use of cryptography's power to guarantee data integrity and closely knit security. Although the blockchain transaction system is quite harsh on careless users, it is advantageous and lucrative for legitimate users. This indicates that everyone who acts like a good user and receives the proper rewards is treated fairly by the blockchain system (Guo & Yu, 2022). However, one will be punished if they use it for malicious purposes. Since blockchain is a distributed network, there isn't a single point of failure, and no one individual can act carelessly and harm the network as a whole. Any damage resulting from a password compromise will only affect that particular individual (Budhi, 2022). The network transaction is extremely safe with blockchain PKI (Public Key Infrastructure) encryption unless one is foolish enough to divulge the private key, for which there is currently no technology. For the most part, one can rely on blockchain technology to make sure the transactions are executed securely (Kfoury & Khoury, 2018).

Everyone can independently participate in the global economy without facing prejudice thanks to the blockchain's inclusive approach. Due to the complete elimination of the requirement for a bank account, Bitcoin enables everyone, including the wealthiest and poorest, to invest and participate in this global economy. Without the involvement of a third party or the payment of a negligible transaction charge, individuals are free to choose to transact with anybody they like and prefer. The participation of everyone in this global economy, which will be just, safe, and equitable for everyone, will be the primary contribution of the blockchain to the world (Lichtfous et al., 2018).

Ensuring data privacy has become crucial in today's digital environment as organizations and customers conduct business online for a variety of reasons including shopping, payment transfers, and information verification. A great approach to carry out any agreement between two parties is through the Blockchain's Smart Contract, which essentially permits transactions to proceed only if specific predetermined benchmarks have been met and approved by both sides.

Patient Data Management

Patient data management is among the most successful uses of blockchain technology in the healthcare industry. Blockchain encryption technologies make it possible to store data securely, whether it is bank account information, social security numbers, or medical records of patients (Liu et al., 2020). By keeping away unauthorized people from accessing the data, distributed ledger technology guarantees the safe transfer of patient medical records. Additionally, blockchain guarantees data immutability. This ensures that patient data is accurate and authentic across time as once it is recorded, it cannot be changed without network consensus. Furthermore, while preserving data accuracy, blockchain enables the smooth exchange of patient records between various healthcare providers (Kasyapa & Vanmathi, 2024).

Clinical Trial Records

When studying a novel disease or conducting clinical trials of new medications, researchers frequently have to gather a large amount of data. The trial data's integrity is protected from manipulation and tampering by the immutability feature. Additionally, blockchain facilitates the recording of all clinical trial modifications and the tracking of the specifics of those modifications (Nugent et al., 2016). In addition, blockchain's consensus process makes sure that several people must agree before any modifications are made to clinical study records. This encourages dependability and trust by validating each change and designating it as genuine (Maslove et al., 2018).

Supply Chain Management

The healthcare system faces a serious issue with fake medications, which are not only common but also potentially harmful. Toxic substances used in counterfeit medications may have an adverse impact on a patient's health. After they expire, the illegal medications are occasionally repackaged with false labeling, which can have serious negative health effects (Ziavrou et al., 2022). The National Crime Prevention Council estimates that over 10% of medications in the world's supply chain are fake. Up to 70% of the drugs in the supply chain in several nations are counterfeit. Applying blockchain in healthcare can overcome these challenges and help optimize supply chain management (Mackey et la., 2015). Every step of the drug supply chain may be tracked by blockchain-based systems, which facilitates the detection and elimination of counterfeit medications. Furthermore, blockchain technology in healthcare can aid in monitoring drug life cycle.

Telemedicine

People who live in remote places may find it easier to get high-quality treatment through telemedicine. But because it depends on patients and healthcare professionals exchanging private health information, it is susceptible to cyberattacks. This danger can be eliminated by using blockchain technology in healthcare since it offers a more secure and decentralized platform for data sharing. Additionally, blockchain offers a safe framework for simple wearable IoT device integration, which facilitates remote patient progress monitoring (Paul et al., 2023).

Interoperability

For better diagnosis, treatments, and general care, patients occasionally need to see several doctors and require thorough medical history information. One of the biggest challenges, though, is keeping track of a patient's whole medical history and sharing it with other medical professionals (Balogh et al., 2015). Blockchain in healthcare solves important issues including inconsistent data formats, data privacy, and security, among others, to enable interoperable health data transmission. Multiple users can access the same dataset thanks to blockchain's decentralized nature. This improves data availability by removing the requirement for a central authority to store data and lowering the possibility of a single point of failure (Punia et al., 2024).

Limitations of Blockchain in Healthcare

Blockchain is a relatively new technology that has not yet reached its full potential. Since blockchain is a relatively new technology, the healthcare industry faces numerous obstacles.

Lack of Technical Knowledge

It is not anticipated that every user will possess costly software and hardware. The newest technologies are also unfamiliar to many users. For instance, a large number of elderly men and women do not use computers or laptops. Mining cryptocurrencies requires GPUs, which not all laptops have (Bracci et al., 2022). This is a significant blockchain challenge. The newest technologies should be known to the users.

The media should take effective measures to vigorously promote these new technologies. Businesses ought to make an effort to lower the cost of the technology as well (Sadhya & Sadhya, 2018).

Paperless Method Adoption

Paper records are preferred by many physicians and consumers. The medical records are better kept in a file system. Not all pharmacies are completely paperless. Prescriptions are used by the majority of pharmacies to maintain track of their inventory (Balasubramanian et al., 2021). Additionally, patients retain the paperwork for their convenience. It is therefore difficult to transition to a blockchain network that is entirely paperless. Small blockchains should be used by doctors to become accustomed to the newest technology. They ought to attempt to use as few documents as possible. They can use paper for documentation pertaining to surgery, such as X-ray plates. However, since blockchains are easy to store, the health sector should use them for prescriptions and other file information (Elvas et al., 2023).

Involvement of Government

Majority of the hospitals are in the public sector owned by the State. Therefore, the government is involved in putting rules into effect. Some governments are determined to embrace the newest technological advancements. But no central authority or other parties are there to make choices. Therefore, blockchain cannot be applied in Government controlled Hospitals since it is a highly decentralized, distributed ledger (Andrew et al., 2023). Blockchain typically makes the decisions. The governments should take the lead in implementing the blockchain technology in the hospitals. Blockchain offers a special blend of distributivity and security, in order for the government to keep data for use in research and other endeavors (Kshetri, 2023).

Cost Reduction

Blockchain technology is still quite expensive. Users need expensive hardware and software for mining. To mine cryptocurrencies, expensive GPUs are required. Every block needs electricity in order to mine. However, miners do not receive adequate incentives. As a result, this technology is quite expensive (McGhin et al., 2019). Blockchain businesses should concentrate on cutting costs because technology is developing daily. In order to encourage more miners to participate in the blockchain, the corporations should also raise the reward (Habib et al., 2022).

Central Healthcare

The majority of healthcare systems are dispersed. Numerous hospitals are spread over several locations. Thus, keeping a blockchain up to date is an extremely demanding undertaking. Maintaining all of the medical records together in order to implement blockchain technology would be hard without a streamlined method (Hölbl et al., 2018). For example, a patient goes to hospital "A" in one place. The next time, he might go to Hospital "A" itself, but in a different place. Two distinct places are represented by two blockchains. It will therefore be difficult to retrieve the prior medical records. Hospitals should use blockchain in specific areas so they can identify issues and address them appropriately. The networks ought to be dispersed, and every hospital ought to keep a sizable blockchain to store data so that they can have access to medical records if required (Tagde et al., 2021).

ARTIFICIAL INTELLIGENCE IN HEALTHCARE

AI is a scientific discipline that focuses on building computers and machines that can reason, learn, and behave in ways that would typically need human intelligence or that involve data whose scale exceeds what humans can evaluate. The vast area of AI includes computer science, data analytics and statistics, hardware and software engineering, linguistics, neurology, and even philosophy and psychology (Xu et al., 2021). Through the completion of tasks that are normally completed by humans, but in a fraction of the time and cost, AI makes life easier for patients, physicians, and hospital managers. AI in healthcare can be used to power surgery-assisting robots, discover novel connections between genetic codes, automate administrative work, customize treatment alternatives, and much more (Bajwa et al., 2021). The application of machine learning, natural language processing, deep learning, and other AI technologies to improve patient and healthcare provider experiences is referred to as AI in healthcare. Health practitioners can better manage their resources and tackle different facets of healthcare more pro-actively thanks to AI's data-processing and prediction skills. Health administrators can find electronic health data more quickly, physicians can diagnose patients more quickly and accurately, and patients can receive more individualized and timely care because of these technologies (Ehrenstein et al., 2019).

Medical Diagnosis

Approximately 400,000 hospitalized patients experience avoidable harm each year, and 100,000 of them pass away. Given this, one of AI's most intriguing medical uses is the potential to enhance the diagnostic procedure (Nassimbwa Kabanda, n.d.). Large caseloads and incomplete medical histories can result in fatal human errors. AI is immune to those factors and can identify and anticipate illnesses more quickly than the majority of medical practitioners. Medical diagnostics is the process of assessing illnesses or conditions by looking at test findings, medical history, and symptoms. Finding the root cause of a medical issue and accurately diagnosing it in order to treat it effectively are the objectives of medical diagnostics (Choudhury & Asun, 2020). This may entail a number of diagnostic tests, including blood tests, biopsy procedures, and imaging tests (such as MRIs, CT scans, and X-rays). These tests' outcomes assist medical professionals in deciding on the best course of action for their patients. Apart from aiding in the diagnosis of medical diseases, medical diagnostics can also be utilized to track the course of a condition, evaluate the efficacy of treatment, and identify possible health issues before they worsen (Pinto-Coelho, 2023). By increasing the diagnostic process's speed, efficiency, and prediction accuracy, the recent AI revolution has the potential to completely transform the medical diagnostics industry. AI algorithms can evaluate medical pictures, such as X-rays, MRIs, ultrasounds, CT scans, and DXAs, and help medical professionals diagnose illnesses more rapidly and precisely (Gore, 2020). Medical 2D/3D imaging, bio-signals (such as ECG, EEG, EMG, and EHR), vital indicators (such as blood pressure, body temperature, pulse rate, and respiration rate), demographic data, medical history, and laboratory test results are just a few of the vast volumes of patient data that AI can assess. This could aid in decision-making and yield precise forecast outcomes. This can assist medical professionals in making better decisions on patient care (Al-Antari, 2023).

Drug Discovery

The medication development industry is hampered by research that requires thousands of human hours and rapidly rising development expenses. Only 10% of the pharmaceuticals that go through clinical trials are successfully brought to market, and the average cost of doing so is estimated to be $1.3 billion (Wong et al., 2014). AI is accelerating this process by assisting in the design of medications, anticipating potential negative effects, and selecting the best candidates for clinical trials as a result of technological advancements. Predicting the toxicity and effectiveness of possible therapeutic molecules is one of the main uses of AI in medicinal chemistry. Traditional drug development methods frequently depend on time-consuming and labor-intensive experimentation to evaluate a compound's possible effects on the human body (Vora et al., 2023). In addition to being a time-consuming and expensive procedure, the outcomes are frequently unpredictable and highly variable. These restrictions can be solved by AI methods like machine learning. By analyzing vast amounts of data, machine learning algorithms are able to spot patterns and trends that human researchers might miss. This can make it possible to propose novel bioactive chemicals with little adverse effects considerably more quickly than with classical protocols (Blanco-Gonzalez et al., 2023).

Patient Experience

AI can help with digital communications by providing patients with personalized health advice, schedule reminders, and recommended next steps. AI's capacity to support medical diagnosis also enhances the pace and precision of patient visits, resulting in quicker and more individualized treatment (Maleki Varnosfaderani & Forouzanfar, 2024). Additionally, hospitals, clinics, and doctors are able to treat more patients everyday by effectively offering smooth patient experience. AI is transforming healthcare by making it more individualized, efficient, and accessible. Virtual health assistants, AI-assisted scheduling, and remote monitoring allow patients to receive care that is customized to meet their individual needs, cutting down on waiting times and raising patient satisfaction levels (Bajwa et al., 2021). Both patients and healthcare professionals may find lengthy waiting times and ineffective appointment scheduling to be annoying. AI-assisted patient scheduling minimizes waiting times and improves patient flow in hospitals by using algorithms to evaluate patient data and identify the best times for appointments. In addition to improving the patient experience, this helps hospitals make better use of their resources, which increases their ability to satisfy patient requirements and provide higher-quality care (Ferriera et al., 2023).

Virtual Health Assistants

For patients, navigating the healthcare system can be difficult and intimidating. Virtual health assistants are online resources that offer individualized assistance, answering questions and helping patients along their medical path. Virtual health assistants encourage a more proactive approach to healthcare management by providing patients with real-time support and information, enabling them to take charge of their health and well-being (Samala & Rawas, 2024). Virtual health assistants can help patients find proper care and access health information. Although they are still in their infancy, virtual assistants in healthcare are predicted to become widely used by 2029 (Bohr & Memarzadeh, 2020). The medical virtual assistant industry is anticipated to generate revenue at a compound annual growth rate of 26.29% between 2019 and 2029, according to a report titled Global Virtual Assistants in Healthcare industry

– Analysis and Forecast, 2019-25 (PRNewswire, 2024). The interactive and user-friendly interface of medical virtual assistants makes it easier to hold a conversation with patients and ask them questions one at a time. However, virtual assistants can make sure that only confirmed individuals make appointments at their facility by implementing an OTP verification mechanism. According to 78% of doctors, using a medical virtual assistant to make appointments can be very beneficial. However, if one wants to easily track planned appointments and follow-ups, they can integrate a virtual assistant with a CRM system (Davis et al., 2020).

Data Management

There are occasions when the jungle of trillions of data points can obscure extremely important information. Additionally, the creation of novel medications, preventative medicine, and accurate diagnosis are slowed down when crucial data points cannot be connected (OECD, 2018). AI dismantles data silos and connects information that used to take years to process in minutes due to its capacity to handle enormous volumes of data. In addition to improving daily operations and patient experiences, this can cut down on the time and expense of healthcare administrative procedures (Bajwa et al., 2021). Healthcare data management has always been a difficult and complicated undertaking. The sheer amount, diversity, and speed of data created in the healthcare industry are frequently too much for traditional approaches to handle. Accurately recording, storing, and retrieving patient records, medical histories, treatment plans, and billing information places a significant load on healthcare practitioners (Yogesh & Karthikeyan, 2012).

The volume of data is one of the main obstacles. The volume of data produced by healthcare operations is massive and still increasing at an exponential rate. This data is available in a number of formats, including unstructured data (such as medical photographs and doctor's notes) and structured data (such as coded entries and numerical values) (Mathew & Pillai, 2015). This variability is frequently too much for traditional data management systems to handle efficiently. The accuracy of the data is another major obstacle. Errors in manual data input and processing can have major repercussions for patient care and billing (Li et al., 2022). The overall quality of care can be compromised by inaccurate data, which can lead to misdiagnosis, inappropriate treatments, and financial disparities. Another area where conventional approaches are inadequate is data integration. The usage of numerous databases and systems by healthcare providers makes it challenging to compile data into a single, cohesive view. Decision-making is delayed and full insights are lacking as a result of this fragmentation, which makes it difficult to access and analyze data efficiently (Tatineni, 2022).

Robotic Surgery

From open heart surgery to minimally invasive treatments, hospitals use AI and robots to assist. While seated at a computer console, surgeons can operate the mechanical arms of a robot that provides them with a magnified, three-dimensional picture of the operative site. The entire procedure is then guided by the surgeon and other team members who collaborate closely with the robot. Robot-assisted operations have reduced pain, shortened recuperation times, and decreased surgical-related complications (Moglia et al., 2021). Using robotics in surgery offers a number of intraoperative advantages, including enhanced dexterity, ergonomics, and a realistic magnified three-dimensional vision. Reduced rates of blood loss and transfusions, shorter inpatient stays, and fewer complications are all examples of established perioperative outcomes (Diana & Marescaux, 2015). With over 12 million procedures carried out by 60,000 doctors worldwide on the da Vinci system alone, robotic surgery is progressively replacing traditional laparoscopic surgery as the preferred minimally invasive method for routine operations (Sheetz et al., 2020). Robotics is a fundamental technology in digital surgery that is ready to be integrated with AI to improve or potentially completely transform intraoperative surgical practice (Ashrafiana, 2024).

Limitations of AI in healthcare

For the clinical and technical validation of AI models, clinicians need high-quality datasets. However, gathering patient data and photos to test AI algorithms becomes difficult because medical data is fragmented across multiple EHRs and IT platforms. Another challenge is that interoperability issues may prevent medical data from one institution from being interoperable with other systems (Diaz et al., 2021). The healthcare industry has to focus on methods for standardizing medical data in order to expand the quantity of data available for testing AI systems. It is not always possible to apply the metrics used to evaluate an AI model's performance in healthcare contexts. The AI chasm is the difference between the technical accuracy of AI tests and the clinical efficacy shown in the actual world (Mirin, 2021). Developers and physicians should work together to look at how AI algorithms improve patient care in order to close this gap. They can accomplish this by employing decision curve analysis to evaluate the correctness of AI models. By comparing the datasets and calculating the likelihood that an AI model will succeed in the real world, this approach allows them to assess the clinical utility of a prediction model. Peer-reviewed studies, prospective research, and established approaches on AI in healthcare are insufficient (Khosravi et al., 2024). Most of the research has been done after the fact and has been based on past patient medical records. Prospective research is necessary for doctors to examine the present patients over time in order to fully appreciate the benefits of AI diagnosis in practical situations. Additionally, physicians should use telehealth visits, remote monitoring technology (sensors and trackers), and physical examinations to keep an eye on their patients' health in order to conduct trustworthy prospective research (Ko et al., 2023).

CONVERGENCE OF BLOCKCHAIN AND AI IN HEALTHCARE

A paradigm shift in healthcare is being brought about by the combination of blockchain technology and AI, which addresses important issues with protecting electronic health records (EHRs) and data privacy, and enabling safe data transfer (Bathula et al., 2024). AI makes use of a wide range of suggested algorithms, decision-making skills, and vast amounts of data for enabling healthcare providers to view patient medical records on the blockchain. The revolutionary technologies of blockchain and AI are developing at a rate never seen before. Every technology advances our understanding of data organization and system optimization (Jabarulla & Lee, 2021). Their combined effect increases productivity, security, transparency, and trust, opening up new options. Integration becomes essential to achieving the full potential of both professions as they rapidly gain widespread acceptance. Nevertheless, integrating these cutting-edge technologies necessitates managing technological challenges (Khogali & Mekid, 2023).

To increase interoperability, trust, and responsible management across extended product life cycles, standards must significantly change.

AI-blockchain market is expected to grow at a 60% CAGR to $27 billion by 2027 (Hussain & Al-Turjman, 2021). Demand is dependent on blockchain application cases for AI that call for real-time analytics and distributed trust. The numerous and diverse applications of blockchain technology for AI show how these two fields can complement one another. Blockchain integration offers a safe basis for everything from supply chain optimization to improving data privacy in AI applications (Khanh & Khang, 2021). In the era of digital transformation, privacy is a top priority for Power of Data and AI. Blockchain technology improves data privacy in AI applications by offering decentralized storage options. Blockchain disperses data among numerous nodes, greatly lowering the danger of unwanted access, in contrast to traditional databases that are susceptible to breaches (Andrew et al., 2023). Furthermore, once data is recorded, it cannot be changed or removed without network participants' consent due to blockchain's immutability. By enabling businesses to keep an accurate audit trail of data access and alterations, this feature improves accountability and traceability (Punia et al., 2024). By providing decentralized identity solutions, blockchain also gives consumers more control over their personal information. Users' privacy choices are respected because they have the ability to decide what information they want to share and with whom. Organizations may secure sensitive data while enabling AI algorithms to examine it safely by integrating blockchain technology with cutting-edge encryption methods (Gurtu & Johnny, 2019).

By combining the two technical ecosystems, the shortcomings of blockchain and AI can be effectively overcome. AI algorithms use data or information to learn, understand, and draw conclusions (Salah et al., 2019). Machine learning algorithms work better when data is obtained from a data repository or a reliable, secure, trustworthy, and reputable platform. Blockchain serves as a distributed ledger that all mining nodes can use to store and trade data in a way that is agreed upon, verified, and cryptographically safe (Kayikci & Khoshgoftaar, 2024). Data on the blockchain is unchangeable and is stored with a high degree of robustness and integrity. The outcomes may be reliable and unquestionable when smart contracts are used to perform analytics and make decisions utilizing machine-learning algorithms (Junaid et al., 2022). With the combination of blockchain and AI, a secure, unchangeable, decentralized system can be created for the sensitive data that AI-driven methods need to gather, store, and utilize. Medical, personal, banking and financial, trade, and legal data are just a few of the industries that benefit from this method's core data and information security advancements. Adding AI skills to the health sector can be advantageous, even though blockchain can guarantee safety and integrity (Tagde et al., 2021).

AI is currently mostly used to identify abnormalities in CT and X-ray images, a task that it can complete at least as well as humans and guarantee a more individualized level of treatment (Turransky & Amini, 2022). Experts predict that significant innovations will surface in the future because of the potential for significant advantages in reducing medical costs and improving the standard of medical care (Junaid et al., 2022). In order to improve the more efficient use of patient data, diagnosis accuracy, and the provision of better recommendations based on evidence-based research findings, Google, Microsoft, Apple, Amazon, and numerous startups are actively investigating AI for medical applications. These applications follow developments in robotic surgery and smartphone apps that provide digital advice (Bajwa et al., 2021). By 2026, the US healthcare system may save $150 billion annually because of critical clinical health AI applications. The difficulties of interoperability and protection in healthcare must be addressed by AI, which is beginning to gain traction (Bevere & Faccilongo, 2024). The combination of complex algorithms, large data sets, and effective machinery has produced a contemporary method for integrating technologies in healthcare.

FUTURE OF BLOCKCHAIN AND AI IN HEALTHCARE

A blockchain network can be used in healthcare industry to exchange and store patient data. In the healthcare sector, blockchain applications can precisely detect grave errors, even those that are harmful. Blockchain is essential for managing clinical trial fraud for improved patient outcomes (Haleem et al., 2021). Blockchain gives people authority over their medical records, enabling them to limit access and improve transparency. In around five to ten years, blockchain and AI will be used to enhance healthcare, leading to more secure data, personal access to this data, and significant operational efficiencies (Haleem et al., 2021). Blockchain technology's common feature would assist in providing decentralized, untampered ledger patient data administration. This would increase institutional trust and allay worries about security lapses or illegal access. Smart contracts could allow patients to own all of their medical records and give providers access only when necessary (Andrew et al., 2023). Since researchers might access bigger amounts of anonymized datasets while still protecting patient privacy, this type of safe data exchange could accelerate the advancement of research. AI is becoming more and more useful in evaluating large data sets and finding trends (Arora et al., 2024). AI will therefore be the driving force behind precision medicine in the future, enabling early diagnosis and effective treatment planning. For example, the machine learning algorithms would then create predictive models for a variety of ailments, such as diabetes or cancer, and use them for early intervention by utilizing the distinctive characteristics of the data stored on blockchain networks (Johnson et al., 2021). *Firstly*, these AI applications would improve diagnostic imaging; *second*ly, they would decrease repetitive chores; and *thirdly*, they would aid in clinical decision-making, which would reduce diagnostic errors. Also, it can use blockchain-enabled AI-powered tools to provide instantaneous, real-time images of patients' health state based on various metrics gathered via a wearable, saving time and enabling individualized care (Uppal et al., 2023).

The technology's combination facilitates the simplification of medication development and eases drug trials. With the aid of blockchain technology, all trial phases are transparently recorded, and AI will quickly analyze trial data to find beneficial chemicals and forecast patient reactions. This would significantly reduce the amount of time and money needed to introduce new medications to the market (Tagde et al., 2021). Additionally, blockchain's traceability capabilities can combat counterfeit medications, guaranteeing pharmaceutical legitimacy throughout the supply chain. Besides, this could help with other synergies like invoicing and claims administration. While transparent billing handles fraud, AI can improve revenue cycle management by identifying inefficiencies and automating administrative procedures (Haq & Esuka, 2018). Lower expenses for payers and providers follow, which contribute to lower patient costs. To fully utilize blockchain and AI in healthcare, interoperability, ethical, and regulatory challenges must be resolved. Both stakeholder support and platform standardization will be necessary. Additionally, stringent regulations will be needed to oversee the ethical application of blockchain and AI, particularly when handling private patient information (Soori et al., 2024). Together, blockchain technology and AI will revolutionize the healthcare industry by effectively developing a system that is both patient-centered and extremely safe. This combination between the promising pathways could be greatly modified, offering the healthcare sector major advances, especially when considering the possible breakthroughs, the business may achieve in terms of tailored medication, operational efficiency, and innovation (Bathula et al., 2024). These technologies' development, integration, and advancement are probably going to provide widespread relief from some, if not all, of the problems facing contemporary healthcare, opening doors for a decade that will fundamentally alter the landscape (Junaid et al., 2022).

CONCLUSION

The dynamic merging of two innovative technologies—blockchain and AI—is poised to bring about a significant revolution in the healthcare sector. AI, which uses data analytics, machine learning, and natural language processing to transform healthcare procedures, diagnoses, and patient care, is the perfect match for blockchain, which is praised for its unparalleled security, data integrity, and decentralized structure.

Blockchain technology is built to solve important problems in the administration of healthcare data. It ensures data integrity, privacy, and accessibility by providing a safe, unchangeable ledger for sharing and storing private patient data. Additionally, it gives patients fine-grained control over their medical records, guaranteeing informed consent and promoting communication between researchers, payers, and healthcare providers. There is no denying of the revolutionary potential of blockchain technology in the healthcare industry. Healthcare firms may improve patient care, expedite data sharing, safeguard sensitive medical data, and streamline operations by utilizing blockchain technology. It can potentially help patients and healthcare professionals save a lot of time and money. However, AI's ability to evaluate enormous amounts of medical data lays the groundwork for improved clinical decision-making, personalized medicine, and predictive analytics. In healthcare systems, AI-driven algorithms have been crucial in spotting illness trends, forecasting patient outcomes, and optimizing resource allocation. But there are also various drawbacks to the combination of blockchain technology and AI in healthcare. Concerns include scalability, interoperability, ethical issues, and regulatory compliance. Facilitating the use of these technologies through cooperative research and creative solutions can lead to improvements in patient outcomes, healthcare ecosystem efficiency, and healthcare quality.

REFERENCES

Al-Antari, M. A. (2023). Artificial intelligence for medical diagnostics—Existing and future al technology. *Diagnostics (Basel)*, *13*(4), 688. DOI: 10.3390/diagnostics13040688 PMID: 36832175

Andrew, J., Isravel, D. P., Sagayam, K. M., Bhushan, B., Sei, Y., & Eunice, J. (2023). Blockchain for healthcare systems: Architecture, security challenges, trends and future directions. *Journal of Network and Computer Applications*, *215*, 103633. DOI: 10.1016/j.jnca.2023.103633

Angraal, S., Krumholz, H. M., & Schulz, W. L. (2017). Blockchain technology: Applications in health care. *Circulation: Cardiovascular Quality and Outcomes*, *10*(9), e003800. DOI: 10.1161/CIRCOUTCOMES.117.003800 PMID: 28912202

Arora, A., Wagner, S. K., Carpenter, R., Jena, R., & Keane, P. A. (2024). The urgent need to accelerate synthetic data privacy frameworks for medical research. *The Lancet. Digital Health*. PMID: 39603900

Ashrafian, H. (2024). Artificial intelligence in surgery: The future is now. *European Surgical Research*, *65*, 22–39.

Bajwa, J., Munir, U., Nori, A., & Williams, B. (2021). Artificial intelligence in healthcare: Transforming the practice of medicine. *Future Healthcare Journal*, *8*(2), e188–e194. DOI: 10.7861/fhj.2021-0095 PMID: 34286183

Balasubramanian, S., Shukla, V., Sethi, J. S., Islam, N., & Saloum, R. (2021). A readiness assessment framework for Blockchain adoption: A healthcare case study. *Technological Forecasting and Social Change*, *165*, 120536. DOI: 10.1016/j.techfore.2020.120536

Balogh, E., Miller, B., & Ball, J. (2015). The diagnostic process. improving diagnosis in health care national academies of sciences, engineering, and medicine.

Bathula, A., Gupta, S. K., Merugu, S., Saba, L., Khanna, N. N., Laird, J. R., Sanagala, S. S., Singh, R., Garg, D., Fouda, M. M., & Suri, J. S. (2024). Blockchain, artificial intelligence, and healthcare: The tripod of future—a narrative review. *Artificial Intelligence Review*, *57*(9), 238. DOI: 10.1007/s10462-024-10873-5

Bevere, D., & Faccilongo, N. (2024). Shaping the Future of Healthcare: Integrating Ecology and Digital Innovation. *Sustainability (Basel)*, *16*(9), 3835. DOI: 10.3390/su16093835

Blanco-Gonzalez, A., Cabezon, A., Seco-Gonzalez, A., Conde-Torres, D., Antelo-Riveiro, P., Pineiro, A., & Garcia-Fandino, R. (2023). The role of AI in drug discovery: Challenges, opportunities, and strategies. *Pharmaceuticals (Basel, Switzerland)*, *16*(6), 891. DOI: 10.3390/ph16060891 PMID: 37375838

Bohr, A., & Memarzadeh, K. (2020). The rise of artificial intelligence in healthcare applications. In *Artificial Intelligence in healthcare* (pp. 25–60). Academic Press. DOI: 10.1016/B978-0-12-818438-7.00002-2

Bracci, E., Tallaki, M., Ievoli, R., & Diplotti, S. (2022). Knowledge, diffusion and interest in blockchain technology in SMEs. *Journal of Knowledge Management*, *26*(5), 1386–1407. DOI: 10.1108/JKM-02-2021-0099

Budhi, V. (2022). *Advantages and disadvantages of Blockchain technology*. Forbes Technology Council.

Choudhury, A., & Asan, O. (2020). Role of artificial intelligence in patient safety outcomes: Systematic literature review. *JMIR Medical Informatics*, *8*(7), e18599. DOI: 10.2196/18599 PMID: 32706688

Davis, C. R., Murphy, K. J., Curtis, R. G., & Maher, C. A. (2020). A process evaluation examining the performance, adherence, and acceptability of a physical activity and diet artificial intelligence virtual health assistant. *International Journal of Environmental Research and Public Health*, *17*(23), 9137. DOI: 10.3390/ijerph17239137 PMID: 33297456

DeGusta, M. (2012). *Are smartphones spreading faster than any technology in human history?* Massachusetts Institute of Technology Review.

Diana, M., & Marescaux, J. (2015). Robotic surgery. *British Journal of Surgery*, *102*(2), e15–e28. DOI: 10.1002/bjs.9711 PMID: 25627128

Diaz, O., Kushibar, K., Osuala, R., Linardos, A., Garrucho, L., Igual, L., Radeva, P., Prior, F., Gkontra, P., & Lekadir, K. (2021). Data preparation for artificial intelligence in medical imaging: A comprehensive guide to open-access platforms and tools. *Physica Medica*, *83*, 25–37. DOI: 10.1016/j.ejmp.2021.02.007 PMID: 33684723

Ehrenstein, V., Kharrazi, H., Lehmann, H., & Taylor, C. O. (2019). Obtaining data from electronic health records. In *Tools and technologies for registry interoperability, registries for evaluating patient outcomes: A user's guide, 3rd edition, Addendum 2 [Internet]*. Agency for Healthcare Research and Quality (US).

Elvas, L. B., Serrão, C., & Ferreira, J. C. (2023, January). Sharing health information using a blockchain. [). MDPI.]. *Health Care*, *11*(2), 170. PMID: 36673538

Ferreira, D. C., Vieira, I., Pedro, M. I., Caldas, P., & Varela, M. (2023, February). Patient satisfaction with healthcare services and the techniques used for its assessment: A systematic literature review and a bibliometric analysis. [). MDPI.]. *Health Care*, *11*(5), 639. PMID: 36900644

Gore, J. C. (2020). Artificial intelligence in medical imaging. *Magnetic Resonance Imaging*, *68*, A1–A4. DOI: 10.1016/j.mri.2019.12.006 PMID: 31857130

Guo, H., & Yu, X. (2022). A survey on blockchain technology and its security. *Blockchain: research and applications, 3*(2), 100067.

Gurtu, A., & Johny, J. (2019). Potential of blockchain technology in supply chain management: A literature review. *International Journal of Physical Distribution & Logistics Management*, *49*(9), 881–900. DOI: 10.1108/IJPDLM-11-2018-0371

Habib, G., Sharma, S., Ibrahim, S., Ahmad, I., Qureshi, S., & Ishfaq, M. (2022). Blockchain technology: Benefits, challenges, applications, and integration of blockchain technology with cloud computing. *Future Internet*, *14*(11), 341. DOI: 10.3390/fi14110341

Haleem, A., Javaid, M., Singh, R. P., Suman, R., & Rab, S. (2021). Blockchain technology applications in healthcare: An overview. *International Journal of Intelligent Networks*, *2*, 130–139. DOI: 10.1016/j.ijin.2021.09.005

Haq, I., & Esuka, O. M. (2018). Blockchain technology in the pharmaceutical industry to prevent counterfeit drugs. *International Journal of Computer Applications*, *180*(25), 8–12. DOI: 10.5120/ijca2018916579

Hölbl, M., Kompara, M., Kamišalić, A., & Nemec Zlatolas, L. (2018). A systematic review of the use of blockchain in healthcare. *Symmetry*, *10*(10), 470. DOI: 10.3390/sym10100470

Hussain, A. A., & Al-Turjman, F. (2021). Artificial intelligence and blockchain: A review. *Transactions on Emerging Telecommunications Technologies*, *32*(9), e4268. DOI: 10.1002/ett.4268

Jabarulla, M. Y., & Lee, H. N. (2021, August). A blockchain and artificial intelligence-based, patient-centric healthcare system for combating the COVID-19 pandemic: Opportunities and applications. []. Mdpi.]. *Health Care*, *9*(8), 1019. PMID: 34442156

Johnson, K. B., Wei, W. Q., Weeraratne, D., Frisse, M. E., Misulis, K., Rhee, K., Zhao, J., & Snowdon, J. L. (2021). Precision medicine, AI, and the future of personalized health care. *Clinical and Translational Science*, *14*(1), 86–93. DOI: 10.1111/cts.12884 PMID: 32961010

Junaid, S. B., Imam, A. A., Balogun, A. O., De Silva, L. C., Surakat, Y. A., Kumar, G., & Mahamad, S. (2022, October). Recent advancements in emerging technologies for healthcare management systems: A survey. []. MDPI.]. *Health Care*, *10*(10), 1940. PMID: 36292387

Kasyapa, M. S., & Vanmathi, C. (2024). Blockchain integration in healthcare: A comprehensive investigation of use cases, performance issues, and mitigation strategies. *Frontiers in Digital Health*, *6*, 1359858. DOI: 10.3389/fdgth.2024.1359858 PMID: 38736708

Kayikci, S., & Khoshgoftaar, T. M. (2024). Blockchain meets machine learning: A survey. *Journal of Big Data*, *11*(1), 9. DOI: 10.1186/s40537-023-00852-y

Kelly, C. J., & Young, A. J. (2017). Promoting innovation in healthcare. *Future Healthcare Journal*, *4*(2), 121–125. DOI: 10.7861/futurehosp.4-2-121 PMID: 31098448

Kfoury, E., & Khoury, D. (2018, July). Distributed public key infrastructure and PSK exchange based on blockchain technology. In *2018 IEEE International Conference on Internet of Things (iThings) and IEEE Green Computing and Communications (GreenCom) and IEEE Cyber, Physical and Social Computing (CPSCom) and IEEE Smart Data (SmartData)* (pp. 1116-1120). IEEE. DOI: 10.1109/Cybermatics_2018.2018.00203

Khanh, H. H., & Khang, A. (2021). The role of artificial intelligence in blockchain applications. In *Reinventing Manufacturing and Business Processes through Artificial Intelligence* (pp. 19–38). CRC Press. DOI: 10.1201/9781003145011-2

Khogali, H. O., & Mekid, S. (2023). The blended future of automation and AI: Examining some long-term societal and ethical impact features. *Technology in Society*, *73*, 102232. DOI: 10.1016/j.techsoc.2023.102232

Khosravi, M., Zare, Z., Mojtabaeian, S. M., & Izadi, R. (2024). Artificial intelligence and decision-making in healthcare: A thematic analysis of a systematic review of reviews. *Health Services Research and Managerial Epidemiology*, *11*, 23333928241234863. DOI: 10.1177/23333928241234863 PMID: 38449840

Ko, H. Y. K., Tripathi, N. K., Mozumder, C., Muengtaweepongsa, S., & Pal, I. (2023). Real-Time Remote Patient Monitoring and Alarming System for Non Communicable Lifestyle Diseases. *International Journal of Telemedicine and Applications*, *2023*(1), 9965226. PMID: 38020047

Kshetri, N. (2023). Blockchain's role in enhancing quality and safety and promoting sustainability in the food and beverage industry. *Sustainability (Basel)*, *15*(23), 16223. DOI: 10.3390/su152316223

Laroiya, C., Saxena, D., & Komalavalli, C. (2020). Applications of blockchain technology. In *Handbook of research on blockchain technology* (pp. 213–243). Academic press. DOI: 10.1016/B978-0-12-819816-2.00009-5

Li, C., Chen, Y., & Shang, Y. (2022). A review of industrial big data for decision making in intelligent manufacturing. *Engineering Science and Technology, an International Journal*, *29*, 101021. DOI: 10.1016/j.jestch.2021.06.001

Lichtfous, M., Yadav, V., & Fratino, V. (2018). Can blockchain accelerate financial inclusion globally. *Deloitte Inside Magazine*, *19*(02), 1–8.

Liu, H., Crespo, R. G., & Martínez, O. S. (2020, July). Enhancing privacy and data security across healthcare applications using blockchain and distributed ledger concepts. [). MDPI.]. *Health Care*, *8*(3), 243. PMID: 32751325

Mackey, T. K., Liang, B. A., York, P., & Kubic, T. (2015). Counterfeit drug penetration into global legitimate medicine supply chains: A global assessment. *The American Journal of Tropical Medicine and Hygiene*, *92*(6_Suppl, Suppl 6), 59–67. DOI: 10.4269/ajtmh.14-0389 PMID: 25897059

Maleki Varnosfaderani, S., & Forouzanfar, M. (2024). The role of AI in hospitals and clinics: Transforming healthcare in the 21st century. *Bioengineering (Basel, Switzerland)*, *11*(4), 337. DOI: 10.3390/bioengineering11040337 PMID: 38671759

Maslove, D. M., Klein, J., Brohman, K., & Martin, P. (2018). Using blockchain technology to manage clinical trials data: A proof-of-concept study. *JMIR Medical Informatics*, *6*(4), e11949. DOI: 10.2196/11949 PMID: 30578196

Mathew, P. S., & Pillai, A. S. (2015, March). Big Data solutions in Healthcare: Problems and perspectives. In *2015 International conference on innovations in information, embedded and communication systems (ICIIECS)* (pp. 1-6). IEEE. DOI: 10.1109/ICIIECS.2015.7193211

McGhin, T., Choo, K. K. R., Liu, C. Z., & He, D. (2019). Blockchain in healthcare applications: Research challenges and opportunities. *Journal of Network and Computer Applications*, *135*, 62–75. DOI: 10.1016/j.jnca.2019.02.027

McSherry, R. O. B., & Douglas, M. (2011). Innovation in nursing practice: A means to tackling the global challenges facing nurses, midwives and nurse leaders and managers in the future. *Journal of Nursing Management*, *19*(2), 165–169. DOI: 10.1111/j.1365-2834.2011.01241.x PMID: 21375618

Mirin, K. (2021). Implementation of AI in Healthcare: Challenges and Potential.

Moglia, A., Georgiou, K., Georgiou, E., Satava, R. M., & Cuschieri, A. (2021). A systematic review on artificial intelligence in robot-assisted surgery. *International Journal of Surgery*, *95*, 106151. DOI: 10.1016/j.ijsu.2021.106151 PMID: 34695601

Nassimbwa Kabanda, D. (n.d.). The Impact of AI on Reducing Medical Errors. *SSRN*.

National Academies of Sciences, Engineering, and Medicine. (2018). The Current State of Global Health Care Quality. In *Crossing the Global Quality Chasm: Improving Health Care Worldwide*. National Academies Press (US).

Nugent, T., Upton, D., & Cimpoesu, M. (2016). Improving data transparency in clinical trials using blockchain smart contracts. *F1000 Research*, *5*, 5. DOI: 10.12688/f1000research.9756.1 PMID: 28357041

OECD. (2018). Innovation and Access to Medicines. *OECD*. https://www.oecd.org/content/dam/oecd/en/publications/reports/2018/11/pharmaceutical-innovation-and-access-to-medicines_g1g98d77/9789264307391-en.pdf

Paul, M., Maglaras, L., Ferrag, M. A., & Almomani, I. (2023). Digitization of the healthcare sector: A study on privacy and security concerns. *ICT Express*, *9*(4), 571–588. DOI: 10.1016/j.icte.2023.02.007

Pinto-Coelho, L. (2023). How artificial intelligence is shaping medical imaging technology: A survey of innovations and applications. *Bioengineering (Basel, Switzerland)*, *10*(12), 1435. DOI: 10.3390/bioengineering10121435 PMID: 38136026

PRNewswire. (2024, June). Medical Virtual Assistant Market. https://www.prnewswire.com/news-releases/medical-virtual-assistant-market-size-to-grow-usd-2668-4-million-by-2029-at-a-cagr-of-27-9--valuates-reports-302168403.html

Punia, A., Gulia, P., Gill, N. S., Ibeke, E., Iwendi, C., & Shukla, P. K. (2024). A systematic review on blockchain-based access control systems in cloud environments. *Journal of Cloud Computing (Heidelberg, Germany)*, *13*(1), 146. DOI: 10.1186/s13677-024-00697-7

Sadhya, V., & Sadhya, H. (2018). Barriers to adoption of blockchain technology.

Salah, K., Rehman, M. H. U., Nizamuddin, N., & Al-Fuqaha, A. (2019). Blockchain for AI: Review and open research challenges. *IEEE Access : Practical Innovations, Open Solutions*, *7*, 10127–10149. DOI: 10.1109/ACCESS.2018.2890507

Samala, A. D., & Rawas, S. (2024). Generative AI as Virtual Healthcare Assistant for Enhancing Patient Care Quality. *International Journal of Online & Biomedical Engineering*, *20*(5), 174–187. DOI: 10.3991/ijoe.v20i05.45937

Sarode, R. P., Poudel, M., Shrestha, S., & Bhalla, S. (2021). Blockchain for committing peer-to-peer transactions using distributed ledger technologies. *International Journal on Computer Science and Engineering*, *24*(3), 215–227.

Sheetz, K. H., Claflin, J., & Dimick, J. B. (2020). Trends in the adoption of robotic surgery for common surgical procedures. *JAMA Network Open*, *3*(1), e1918911–e1918911. DOI: 10.1001/jamanetworkopen.2019.18911 PMID: 31922557

Tagde, P., Tagde, S., Bhattacharya, T., Tagde, P., Chopra, H., Akter, R., Kaushik, D., & Rahman, M. H. (2021). Blockchain and artificial intelligence technology in e-Health. *Environmental Science and Pollution Research International*, *28*(38), 52810–52831. DOI: 10.1007/s11356-021-16223-0 PMID: 34476701

Tatineni, S. (2022). INTEGRATING AI, BLOCKCHAIN AND CLOUD TECHNOLOGIES FOR DATA MANAGEMENT IN HEALTHCARE. [JCET]. *Journal of Computer Engineering and Technology*, *5*(01).

Turransky, A., & Amini, M. H. (2022). Artificial intelligence and cybersecurity: tale of healthcare applications. *Cyberphysical smart cities infrastructures: Optimal operation and intelligent decision making*, 1-11.

Uppal, S., Kansekar, B., Mini, S., & Tosh, D. (2023). HealthDote: A blockchain-based model for continuous health monitoring using an interplanetary file system. *Healthcare Analytics*, *3*, 100175. DOI: 10.1016/j.health.2023.100175

Vora, L. K., Gholap, A. D., Jetha, K., Thakur, R. R. S., Solanki, H. K., & Chavda, V. P. (2023). Artificial intelligence in pharmaceutical technology and drug delivery design. *Pharmaceutics*, *15*(7), 1916. DOI: 10.3390/pharmaceutics15071916 PMID: 37514102

Wong, H. H., Jessup, A., Sertkaya, A., Birkenbach, A., Berlind, A., & Eyraud, J. (2014). Examination of clinical trial costs and barriers for drug development final. *Office of the Assistant Secretary for Planning and Evaluation, US Department of Health & Human Services*, 1-92.

World Health Organization (WHO). (2016). Innovation. http://www.who.int/ topics/innovation/en/

Xu, Y., Liu, X., Cao, X., Huang, C., Liu, E., Qian, S., Liu, X., Wu, Y., Dong, F., Qiu, C.-W., Qiu, J., Hua, K., Su, W., Wu, J., Xu, H., Han, Y., Fu, C., Yin, Z., Liu, M., & Zhang, J. (2021). Artificial intelligence: A powerful paradigm for scientific research. *Innovation (Cambridge (Mass.))*, *2*(4), 100179. DOI: 10.1016/j.xinn.2021.100179 PMID: 34877560

Yogesh, M. J., & Karthikeyan, J. (2022). Health informatics: engaging modern healthcare units: a brief overview. *Frontiers in Public Health*, *10*, 854688. DOI: 10.3389/fpubh.2022.854688 PMID: 35570921

Ziavrou, K. S., Noguera, S., & Boumba, V. A. (2022). Trends in counterfeit drugs and pharmaceuticals before and during COVID-19 pandemic. *Forensic Science International*, *338*, 111382. DOI: 10.1016/j.forsciint.2022.111382 PMID: 35882074

Compilation of References

Abadi, M., Chu, A., Goodfellow, I., McMahan, H. B., Mironov, I., Talwar, K., & Zhang, L. (2016). Deep learning with differential privacy. *Proceedings of the 2016 ACM SIGSAC conference on computer and communications security*

Abbas, A., Alroobaea, R., Krichen, M., Rubaiee, S., Vimal, S., & Almansour, F. M. (2024). Blockchain-assisted secured data management framework for health information analysis based on Internet of Medical Things. *Personal and Ubiquitous Computing*, *28*(1), 59–72. DOI: 10.1007/s00779-021-01583-8

Abbas, H., Hussain, M., Zahid, S., & Ahmed, R. H. (2023). Enhancing Food Security: A Blockchain-Enabled Traceability Framework to Mitigate Stockpiling of Food Commodities. *2023 International Conference on IT and Industrial Technologies (ICIT)*, 1–7. DOI: 10.1109/ICIT59216.2023.10335828

Abou-Nassar, E. M., Iliyasu, A. M., El-Kafrawy, P. M., Song, O.-Y., Bashir, A. K., & Abd El-Latif, A. A. (2020). DITrust chain: Towards blockchain-based trust models for sustainable healthcare IoT systems. *IEEE Access : Practical Innovations, Open Solutions*, *8*, 111223–111238. DOI: 10.1109/ACCESS.2020.2999468

Adarsh, S., Joseph, S. G., John, F., Lekshmi, M., & Asharaf, S. (2021). A Transparent and Traceable Coverage Analysis Model for Vaccine Supply-Chain Using Blockchain Technology. *IT Professional*, *23*(4), 28–35. DOI: 10.1109/MITP.2021.3094194

Adeniyi, A., Arowoogun, J., Chidi, R., Okolo, C., & Babawarun, O. (2024). *The impact of electronic health records on patient care and outcomes: A comprehensive review*. World Journal of Advanced Research and Reviews.

Adere, E. M. (2022). Blockchain in healthcare and IoT: A systematic literature review. *Journal od. Array (New York, N.Y.)*, *14*(9), 100–139. DOI: 10.1016/j.array.2022.100139

Adil, M., Khan, M. K., Kumar, N., Attique, M., Farouk, A., Guizani, M., & Jin, Z. (2024). Healthcare internet of things: Security threats, challenges and future research directions. *IEEE Internet of Things Journal*, *11*(11), 19046–19069. DOI: 10.1109/JIOT.2024.3360289

Adrian Gheorghe, F. S. A. P., & Unal Tatar, O. F. K. (2021). Blockchain for a Resilient, Efficient, and Effective Supply Chain: Evidence from Cases. In: Acquisition Research Program.

AG. A. G., Su, H. K., & Kuo, W. K. (2022, May). Blockchain-based Healthcare System for Elderly Care. In 2022 IEEE 4th Eurasia Conference on Biomedical Engineering, Healthcare and Sustainability (ECBIOS) (pp. 144-147). IEEE.

Agarwal, A., Joshi, R., Arora, H., & Kaushik, R. (2023, February). Privacy and security of healthcare data in cloud based on the blockchain technology. In *2023 7th International Conference on Computing Methodologies and Communication (ICCMC)* (pp. 87-92). IEEE. DOI: 10.1109/ICCMC56507.2023.10083822

Agarwal, U., Rishiwal, V., Tanwar, S., Chaudhary, R., Sharma, G., Bokoro, P. N., & Sharma, R. (2022). Blockchain technology for secure supply chain management: A comprehensive review. *IEEE Access : Practical Innovations, Open Solutions*, *10*, 85493–85517. DOI: 10.1109/ACCESS.2022.3194319

Agbo, C. C., Mahmoud, Q. H., & Eklund, J. M. (2019). Blockchain technology in healthcare: A systematic review. In Healthcare (Switzerland) (Vol. 7, Issue 2). MDPI. DOI: 10.3390/healthcare7020056

Agbo, C. C., Mahmoud, Q. H., & Eklund, J. M. (2019, April). Blockchain technology in healthcare: A systematic review. []). MDPI.]. *Health Care*, *7*(2), 56. PMID: 30987333

Agrawal, K., Aggarwal, M., Tanwar, S., Sharma, G., Bokoro, P., & Sharma, R. (2022). An Extensive Blockchain Based Applications Survey: Tools, Frameworks, Opportunities, Challenges and Solutions. *IEEE Access : Practical Innovations, Open Solutions*, *10*, 116858–116906. DOI: 10.1109/ACCESS.2022.3219160

Agwiah, V. A., & Boateng, K.-H. T. (2024). Family Centered Care: The Perspective of Nurses in the Neonatal Intensive Care Unit of Tamale Teaching Hospital, Ghana: A Qualitative Exploration. *Asian Journal of Pediatric Research*, *14*(3), 27–36. Advance online publication. DOI: 10.9734/ajpr/2024/v14i3331

Ahad, A., Jiangbin, Z., Mughees, A., Puspitasari, I., & Tayyab, M. (2025). Secure Horizons: Integrating Blockchain With AI for Enhanced Smart Healthcare Systems. In *AI Techniques for Securing Medical and Business Practices* (pp. 357-390). IGI Global.

Ahad, A., Jiangbin, Z., Mughees, A., Puspitasari, I., & Tayyab, M. (2025). Secure Horizons: Integrating Blockchain With AI for Enhanced Smart Healthcare Systems. In AI Techniques for Securing Medical and Business Practices (pp. 357–390). IGI Global.

Ahad, A., Jiangbin, Z., Mughees, A., Puspitasari, I., & Tayyab, M. (2025). Secure Horizons: Integrating Blockchain With AI for Enhanced Smart Healthcare Systems. In AI Techniques for Securing Medical and Business Practices (pp. 357-390). IGI Global. doi:DOI: 10.1145/2976749.2978318

Ahad, A., Tahir, M., Sheikh, M. A. S., Mughees, A., & Ahmed, K. I. (2021). Optimal route selection in 5G-based smart health-care network: a reinforcement learning approach. 2021 26th IEEE Asia-Pacific Conference on Communications (APCC)

Ahad, A., Tahir, M., Sheikh, M. A. S., Mughees, A., & Ahmed, K. I. (2021). Optimal route selection in 5G-based smart health-care network: A reinforcement learning approach. 2021 26th IEEE Asia-Pacific Conference on Communications (APCC)

Ahad, A., Tahir, M., Sheikh, M. A. S., Mughees, A., & Ahmed, K. I. (2021). Optimal route selection in 5G-based smart health-care network: a reinforcement learning approach. *2021 26th IEEE Asia-Pacific Conference on Communications (APCC)*, 248–253.

Ahad, A., Tahir, M., Sheikh, M. A. S., Mughees, A., & Ahmed, K. I. (2021, October). Optimal route selection in 5g-based smart health-care network: a reinforcement learning approach. In 2021 26th IEEE Asia-Pacific Conference on Communications (APCC) (pp. 248-253). IEEE.

Ahad, A., Tahir, M., Sheikh, M. A. S., Mughees, A., & Ahmed, K. I. (2021, October). Optimal route selection in 5G-based smart health-care network: a reinforcement learning approach. In *2021 26th IEEE Asia-Pacific Conference on Communications (APCC)* (pp. 248-253). IEEE.

Ahad, A., Tahir, M., Sheikh, M. A. S., Mughees, A., & Ahmed, K. I. (2021, October). Optimal route selection in 5G-based smart healthcare network: A reinforcement learning approach. In *2021 26th IEEE Asia-Pacific Conference on Communications (APCC)* (pp. 248–253). IEEE. https://doi.org/DOI: 10.1109/APCC49754.2021.9609815

Ahad, A., Jiangbin, Z., Mughees, A., Puspitasari, I., & Tayyab, M. (2025). Secure horizons: Integrating blockchain with AI for enhanced smart healthcare systems. In *AI techniques for securing medical and business practices* (pp. 357–390). IGI Global.

Ahmad, A. Y. B., Verma, N., Sarhan, N., Awwad, E. M., Arora, A., & Nyangaresi, V. O. (2024). An IoT and Blockchain-Based Secure and Transparent Supply Chain Management Framework in Smart Cities Using Optimal Queue Model. *IEEE Access : Practical Innovations, Open Solutions*, *12*, 51752–51771. DOI: 10.1109/ACCESS.2024.3376605

Ahmad, M., Jabeen, M., Qasim, M., & Hasnain, M. (2024). Integrating Modern Technology in Education: Enhancing Learning, Engagement, and Accessibility in the Digital Age. *International Research Journal of Management and Social Sciences*, *5*(2), 267–271.

Ahmed, A., Aamir, A., Raza, T., & Khan, M. H. D. (2021). Blockchain Based RFID Prototype For Medicine Traceability along the Healthcare Supply Chain. *2021 7th International Conference on Aerospace Science and Engineering, ICASE 2021*. DOI: 10.1109/ICASE54940.2021.9904249

Ahmed, M., Reno, S., Ferdous, M., & Shama, R. M. (2022). Detection of Counterfeit Medicine Using a Private and Permissioned Blockchain. *2022 2nd Asian Conference on Innovation in Technology, ASIANCON 2022*. DOI: 10.1109/ASIANCON55314.2022.9909424

Ahmed, I., Ahmad, A., & Jeon, G. (2020). An IoT-based deep learning framework for early assessment of COVID-19. *IEEE Internet of Things Journal*, *8*(21), 15855–15862. DOI: 10.1109/JIOT.2020.3034074 PMID: 35782174

Ahmed, I., Turki, M., Baklouti, M., Dammak, B., & Alshahrani, A. (2024). Towards an Optimized Blockchain-Based Secure Medical Prescription-Management System. *Future Internet*, *16*(7), 243. DOI: 10.3390/fi16070243

Ahmed, R. H., Hussain, M., & Zahid, S. (2023). Transforming Blood Donation Processes with Blockchain and IoT Integration: A augmented Approach to Secure and Efficient Healthcare Practices. *2023 International Conference on IT and Industrial Technologies (ICIT)*, 1–8. DOI: 10.1109/ICIT59216.2023.10335787

Ahram, T., Sargolzaei, A., Sargolzaei, S., Daniels, J., & Amaba, B. (2017). *Blockchain technology innovations*. Paper presented at the 2017 IEEE Technology & Engineering Management Conference (TEMSCON). DOI: 10.1109/TEMSCON.2017.7998367

Akbar, M. A., Leiva, V., Rafi, S., Qadri, S. F., Mahmood, S., & Alsanad, A. (2022). Towards roadmap to implement blockchain in healthcare systems based on a maturity model. *Journal of Software (Malden, MA), 34*(12), 1–15. DOI: 10.1002/smr.2500

Akgün, M., Bayrak, A. O., Ozer, B., & Sağıroğlu, M. Ş. (2015). Privacy preserving processing of genomic data: A survey. *Journal of Biomedical Informatics, 56*, 103–111.

Akhtar, M. U., & Khalil, M. I. K. Link Prediction Techniques in Complex Networks.

Akhtar, M. U., Liu, J., Xie, Z., Cui, X., Liu, X., & Huang, B. (2025). Multilingual entity alignment by abductive knowledge reasoning on multiple knowledge graphs. *Engineering Applications of Artificial Intelligence, 139*, 109660. DOI: 10.1016/j.engappai.2024.109660

Akhtar, M. U., Liu, J., Xie, Z., Liu, X., Ahmed, S., & Huang, B. (2022). Entity alignment based on relational semantics augmentation for multilingual knowledge graphs. *Knowledge-Based Systems, 252*, 109494. DOI: 10.1016/j.knosys.2022.109494

Akram, W., Joshi, R., Haider, T., Sharma, P., Jain, V., Garud, N., & Narwaria, N. S. (2024). Blockchain technology: A potential tool for the management of pharma supply chain. *Research in Social & Administrative Pharmacy, 20*(6), 156–164. DOI: 10.1016/j.sapharm.2024.02.014 PMID: 38423927

Akshaya, R. S., Shetty, S. K., & Patil, A. P. (2022, November). Preserving and Sharing Of Medical Data Using Blockchain Technology. In *2022 IEEE North Karnataka Subsection Flagship International Conference (NKCon)* (pp. 1-5). IEEE.

Al Alkeem, E., Yeun, C. Y., & Zemerly, M. J. (2015). Security and privacy framework for ubiquitous healthcare IoT devices. 2015 10th international conference for internet technology and secured transactions (ICITST)

Al Omar, A., Rahman, M. S., Basu, A., & Kiyomoto, S. (2017). Medibchain: A blockchain based privacy preserving platform for healthcare data. Security, Privacy, and Anonymity in Computation, Communication, and Storage: SpaCCS 2017 International Workshops, Guangzhou, China, December 12-15, 2017, Proceedings 10

Al Shahrani, A. M., Rizwan, A., Sánchez-Chero, M., Rosas-Prado, C. E., Salazar, E. B., & Awad, N. A. (2022). An internet of things (IoT)-based optimization to enhance security in healthcare applications. *Mathematical Problems in Engineering, 2022*(1), 6802967.

Alaa, H., Habaebi, M. H., Rafiqul, I., Hasbullah, N. F., & Zabidi, S. A. (2022). Systematic Review on AI-Blockchain Based E-Healthcare Records Management Systems. *IEEE Access : Practical Innovations, Open Solutions, 10*(10), 1–33. DOI: 10.1109/ACCESS.2022.3201878

Alabdulatif, A., Khalil, I., & Rahman, M. S. (2022). Security of Blockchain and AI-Empowered Smart Healthcare Application-Based Analysis. *Applied Sciences (Basel, Switzerland), 21*(11), 1–32. DOI: 10.3390/app122111039 PMID: 36330151

Alagar, V., Alsaig, A., Ormandjiva, O., & Wan, K. (2018). Context-based security and privacy for healthcare IoT. 2018 IEEE International Conference on Smart Internet of Things (SmartIoT)

Alam, N., Hasan Tanvir, M. R., Shanto, S. A., Israt, F., Rahman, A., & Momotaj, S. (2021). Blockchain based counterfeit medicine authentication system. *ISCAIE 2021 - IEEE 11th Symposium on Computer Applications and Industrial Electronics*, 214–217. DOI: 10.1109/ISCAIE51753.2021.9431789

Al-Antari, M. A. (2023). Artificial intelligence for medical diagnostics—Existing and future aI technology. *Diagnostics (Basel)*, *13*(4), 688. DOI: 10.3390/diagnostics13040688 PMID: 36832175

Alassaf, N., & Gutub, A. (2019). Simulating light-weight-cryptography implementation for IoT healthcare data security applications. [IJEHMC]. *International Journal of E-Health and Medical Communications*, *10*(4), 1–15.

Alawida, M., Mejri, S., Mehmood, A., Chikhaoui, B., & Isaac Abiodun, O. (2023). A Comprehensive Study of ChatGPT: Advancements, Limitations, and Ethical Considerations in Natural Language Processing and Cybersecurity. *Information (Basel)*, *14*(8), 462. DOI: 10.3390/info14080462

Albir, M. J. C., Andrés, J. L. P., & Solsona, M. D. E. (2024). [Translated article] Good humanisation practices in the healthcare of patients with rare diseases in Pharmacy Services. *Farmacia Hospitalaria*, *48*(1), T3–T8.

Alexaki, S., Alexandris, G., Katos, V., & Petroulakis, N. E. (2018, September). Blockchain-based electronic patient records for regulated circular healthcare jurisdictions. In *2018 IEEE 23rd International Workshop on Computer Aided Modeling and Design of Communication Links and Networks (CAMAD)* (pp. 1-6). IEEE. DOI: 10.1109/CAMAD.2018.8514954

Alhadhrami, Z., Alghfeli, S., Alghfeli, M., Abedlla, J. A., & Shuaib, K. (2017, November). Introducing blockchains for healthcare. In *2017 international conference on electrical and computing technologies and applications (ICECTA)* (pp. 1-4). IEEE. DOI: 10.1109/ICECTA.2017.8252043

Alhat, P. (2024). *Blockchain Technology*. INTERANTIONAL JOURNAL OF SCIENTIFIC RESEARCH IN ENGINEERING AND MANAGEMENT., DOI: 10.55041/IJSREM30694

Ali, F., Aloqaily, M., Alfandi, O., & Ozkasap, O. (2020). Cyberphysical Blockchain-Enabled Peer-to-Peer Energy Trading. *arXiv*, arXiv: 2001.00746.

Ali, Z., Ahad, A., Madeira, F., & Shayea, I. (2023). Enhancing Transparency and Trustworthiness of Healthcare IoT Data with AWS: A Proposed Model. EAI International Conference on IoT Technologies for HealthCare

Ali, Z., Ahad, A., Madeira, F., & Shayea, I. (2023, October). Enhancing Transparency and Trustworthiness of Healthcare IoT Data with AWS: A Proposed Model. In EAI International Conference on IoT Technologies for HealthCare (pp. 44-56). Cham: Springer Nature Switzerland.

Ali, Z., Ahad, A., Madeira, F., & Shayea, I. (2023, October). Enhancing Transparency and Trustworthiness of Healthcare IoT Data with AWS: A Proposed Model. In *EAI International Conference on IoT Technologies for HealthCare* (pp. 44-56). Cham: Springer Nature Switzerland. DOI: 10.1007/978-3-031-71911-0_4

Ali, A., Almaiah, M. A., Hajjej, F., Pasha, M. F., Fang, O. H., Khan, R., Teo, J., & Zakarya, M. (2022). An industrial IoT-based blockchain-enabled secure searchable encryption approach for healthcare systems using neural network. *Sensors (Basel)*, *22*(2), 572. DOI: 10.3390/s22020572 PMID: 35062530

Ali, , Ali, H., Saeed, A., Ahmed Khan, A., Tin, T. T., Assam, M., Ghadi, Y. Y., & Mohamed, H. G. (2023, September). Blockchain-Powered Healthcare Systems: Enhancing Scalability and Security with Hybrid Deep Learning. *Sensors (Basel)*, *23*(18), 7740. DOI: 10.3390/s23187740 PMID: 37765797

Ali, M., Naeem, F., Tariq, M., & Kaddoum, G. (2022). Federated learning for privacy preservation in smart healthcare systems: A comprehensive survey. *IEEE Journal of Biomedical and Health Informatics*, *27*(2), 778–789.

Ali, Z., Ahad, A., Madeira, F., & Shayea, I. (2023). Enhancing Transparency and Trustworthiness of Healthcare IoT Data with AWS: A Proposed Model. *EAI International Conference on IoT Technologies for HealthCare*, 44–56.

Almalawi, A., Khan, A. I., Alsolami, F., Abushark, Y. B., & Alfakeeh, A. S. (2023). Managing security of healthcare data for a modern healthcare system. [PubMed]. *Sensors (Basel)*, *23*(7), 3612.

Al-Marridi, A. Z., Mohamed, A., & Erbad, A. (2024). Optimized blockchain-based healthcare framework empowered by mixed multi-agent reinforcement learning. *Journal of Network and Computer Applications*, *224*, 103834. DOI: 10.1016/j.jnca.2024.103834

Alromaihi, S., Elmedany, W., & Balakrishna, C. (2018). Cyber security challenges of deploying IoT in smart cities for healthcare applications. 2018 6th International Conference on Future Internet of Things and Cloud Workshops (FiCloudW)

Alshazly, H., Linse, C., Barth, E., & Martinetz, T. (2021). Explainable COVID-19 detection using chest CT scans and deep learning. *Sensors (Basel)*, *21*(1), 455. DOI: 10.3390/s21020455 PMID: 33440674

Al-Sumaidaee, G., Alkhudary, R., Zilic, Z., & Swidan, A. (2023). Performance analysis of a private blockchain network built on Hyperledger Fabric for healthcare. *Information Processing & Management*, *60*(2), 103160. DOI: 10.1016/j.ipm.2022.103160

Alyami, A., Rahman, S., & Yadlapalli, A. (2023). The Effect of Blockchain Technology on Hospital Supply Chain Performance. Paper presented at the Proceedings of the International Conference on Industrial Engineering and Operations Management.

Alzahrani, A. G. M., Alenezi, A., Mershed, A., Atlam, H., & Wills, G. (2020). A framework for data sharing between healthcare providers using blockchain.

Amini, M., & Jahanbakhsh Javid, N. (2023). A multi-perspective framework established on diffusion of innovation (DOI) theory and technology, organization and environment (TOE) framework toward supply chain management system based on cloud computing technology for small and medium enterprises. Organization and Environment (TOE) Framework Toward Supply Chain Management System Based on Cloud Computing Technology for Small and Medium Enterprises (January 2023). *International Journal of Information Technology and Innovation Adoption*, *11*, 1217–1234.

Andrew, I. (2023). Blockchain for healthcare systems: Architecture, security challenges, trends and future directions. *Journal of Network and Computer Applications*, *215*(6), 103633. DOI: 10.1016/j.jnca.2023.103633

Angelov, P., & Almeida Soares, E. (2020). SARS-CoV-2 CT-scan dataset: A large dataset of real patients CT scans for SARS-CoV-2 identification. *MedRxiv*, 2020.04.24.20078584. https://doi.org/DOI: 10.1101/2020.04.24.20078584

Angraal, S., Krumholz, H. M., & Schulz, W. L. (2017). Blockchain technology: Applications in health care. *Circulation: Cardiovascular Quality and Outcomes*, *10*(9), e003800. DOI: 10.1161/CIRCOUTCOMES.117.003800 PMID: 28912202

Anoop, V. S., & Asharaf, S. (2022). Integrating artificial intelligence and blockchain for enabling a trusted ecosystem for healthcare sector. In *Intelligent Healthcare: Infrastructure, Algorithms and Management* (pp. 281–295). Springer Nature Singapore. DOI: 10.1007/978-981-16-8150-9_13

Anzt, H., Cojean, T., Yen-Chen, C., Dongarra, J., Flegar, G., Nayak, P., Tomov, S., Tsai, Y. M., & Wang, W. (2020). Load-balancing sparse matrix vector product kernels on gpus. [TOPC]. *ACM Transactions on Parallel Computing*, *7*(1), 1–26.

Arbabi, M. S., Lal, C., Veeraragavan, N. R., Marijan, D., Nygård, J. F., & Vitenberg, R. (2022). A survey on blockchain for healthcare: Challenges, benefits, and future directions. *IEEE Communications Surveys and Tutorials*, *25*(1), 386–424. DOI: 10.1109/COMST.2022.3224644

Armand, T. P. T., Carole, K. S., Bhattacharjee, S., Mozumder, M. A. I., Amaechi, A. O., & Kim, H. C. 2024, February. The benefits of integrating AI, IoT, and Blockchain in healthcare supply chain management: A multi-dimensional analysis with case study. In *2024 26th International Conference on Advanced Communications Technology (ICACT)* (pp. 300-304). IEEE.

Arora, A., Wagner, S. K., Carpenter, R., Jena, R., & Keane, P. A. (2024). The urgent need to accelerate synthetic data privacy frameworks for medical research. *The Lancet. Digital Health.* PMID: 39603900

Arora, G., Dhariwal, N., & Marken, G. (2024). IoT Security Challenges in Healthcare: Navigating Risks, Strategies, and Innovations for a Safer Connected Health Ecosystem. *2024 International Conference on Emerging Innovations and Advanced Computing (INNOCOMP)*

Ashfaq, F., Ahad, A., Hussain, M., & Madeira, F. (2023). Transforming Diabetes Care: A Review of IoT-Based Mobile Health Systems. EAI International Conference on IoT Technologies for HealthCare

Ashfaq, F., Ahad, A., Hussain, M., & Madeira, F. (2023, October). Transforming Diabetes Care: A Review of IoT-Based Mobile Health Systems. In *EAI International Conference on IoT Technologies for HealthCare* (pp. 14-32). Cham: Springer Nature Switzerland. DOI: 10.1007/978-3-031-71911-0_2

Ashrafian, H. (2024). Artificial intelligence in surgery: The future is now. *European Surgical Research*, *65*, 22–39.

Attaran, M. (2020). Blockchain technology in healthcare: Challenges and opportunities. *International Journal of Healthcare Management*, (11), 1–15. DOI: 10.1080/20479700.2020.1843887

Avellino, I., Bailly, G., Canlorbe, G., Belgihti, J., Morel, G., & Vitrani, M. A. (2019, May). Impacts of telemanipulation in robotic assisted surgery. In *Proceedings of the 2019 CHI conference on human factors in computing systems* (pp. 1-15). DOI: 10.1145/3290605.3300813

Awotunde, J. B., Jimoh, R. G., Folorunso, S. O., Adeniyi, E. A., Abiodun, K. M., & Banjo, O. O. (2021). Privacy and security concerns in IoT-based healthcare systems. In *The fusion of internet of things, artificial intelligence, and cloud computing in health care* (pp. 105–134). Springer.

Azaria, A., Ekblaw, A., Vieira, T., & Lippman, A. (2016, August). Medrec: Using blockchain for medical data access and permission management. In 2016 2nd international conference on open and big data (OBD) (pp. 25-30). IEEE.

Baheti, P., Sikka, M., Arya, K. V., & Rajesh, R. (2020, February). Federated Learning on Distributed Medical Records for Detection of Lung Nodules. In *VISIGRAPP* (Vol. 4, pp. 445–451). VISAPP. DOI: 10.5220/0009144704450451

Bajwa, J., Munir, U., Nori, A., & Williams, B. (2021). Artificial intelligence in healthcare: Transforming the practice of medicine. *Future Healthcare Journal, 8*(2), e188–e194. DOI: 10.7861/fhj.2021-0095 PMID: 34286183

Bala, I., Pindoo, I., Mijwil, M. M., Abotaleb, M., & Yundong, W. (2024). Ensuring security and privacy in Healthcare Systems: A Review Exploring challenges, solutions, Future trends, and the practical applications of Artificial Intelligence. *Jordan Medical Journal, 58*(3).

Balan, A. (2024). Revolutionizing Medical Data Management with Secure Self-Sovereign Applications for Patient Empowerment. *2024 E-Health and Bioengineering Conference (EHB)*, 1–4.

Balasubramanian, S., Shukla, V., Sethi, J. S., Islam, N., & Saloum, R. (2021). A readiness assessment framework for Blockchain adoption: A healthcare case study. *Technological Forecasting and Social Change, 165*, 120536. DOI: 10.1016/j.techfore.2020.120536

Ball, P. (2021). What the COVID-19 pandemic reveals about science, policy and society. *Interface Focus, 11*(6), 20210022. DOI: 10.1098/rsfs.2021.0022 PMID: 34956594

Balogh, E., Miller, B., & Ball, J. (2015). The diagnostic process. improving diagnosis in health care national academies of sciences, engineering, and medicine.

Banoth, R., & Dave, M. (2022). A Survey on Decentralized Application based On Blockchain Platform. *2022 International Conference on Sustainable Computing and Data Communication Systems (ICSCDS)*, 1171-1174. DOI: 10.1109/ICSCDS53736.2022.9760861

Barden, A., Kalman, J., Gierlinger, S., Baker, D., Giammarinaro, N., & Rousseau, N. (2024). From Monologue to Dialogue: The Pursuit of Relationship Centered Communication Across a Large, Integrated Healthcare System. *Journal of Patient Experience, 11*, 23743735241226507. Advance online publication. DOI: 10.1177/23743735241226507 PMID: 38234981

Basu, A., Mullick, S. S., Das, S., & Das, S. (2022). Do pre-processing and class imbalance matter to the deep image classifiers for COVID-19 detection? An explainable analysis. *IEEE Transactions on Artificial Intelligence*, •••, 1–15. DOI: 10.1109/TAI.2022.3149971

Bathula, A., Gupta, S. K., Merugu, S., Saba, L., Khanna, N. N., Laird, J. R., Sanagala, S. S., Singh, R., Garg, D., Fouda, M. M., & Suri, J. S. (2024). Blockchain, artificial intelligence, and healthcare: The tripod of future—a narrative review. *Artificial Intelligence Review*, *57*(9), 238. DOI: 10.1007/s10462-024-10873-5

Benet, J. (2014). IPFS—Content Addressed, Versioned, P2P File System(DRAFT 3). Available online: https://arxiv.org/abs/1407.3 561 (accessed on 21 March 2020).

Bense, J. E., Guilonard, N., Zwaginga, F., Stiggelbout, A. M., Louwerens, M., Mekelenkamp, H., Lankester, A. C., Pieterse, A. H., & de Pagter, A. P. J. (2024). The value of using patient-reported outcomes for health screening during long-term follow-up after paediatric stem cell transplantation for nonmalignant diseases. *Health Expectations*, *27*(1), e13902. Advance online publication. DOI: 10.1111/hex.13902 PMID: 38102818

Bentov, I., Lee, C., Mizrahi, A., & Rosenfeld, M. (2014). Proof of activity: Extending bitcoin's proof of work via proof of stake [extended abstract] y. *Performance Evaluation Review*, *42*(3), 34–37. DOI: 10.1145/2695533.2695545

Berk, A. L., Pickett, A., Kusters, I. S., & Gregory, M. E. (2024). Healthcare Experiences of Black Patients During and After Pregnancy: A Needs Assessment for Provider Training to Improve Quality of Care. *Journal of Racial and Ethnic Health Disparities*, *11*(2), 992–1004. Advance online publication. DOI: 10.1007/s40615-023-01579-5 PMID: 37010801

Besher, K. M., Subah, Z., & Ali, M. Z. (2020). IoT sensor initiated healthcare data security. *IEEE Sensors Journal*, *21*(10), 11977–11982. DOI: 10.1109/JSEN.2020.3013634

Bevere, D., & Faccilongo, N. (2024). Shaping the Future of Healthcare: Integrating Ecology and Digital Innovation. *Sustainability (Basel)*, *16*(9), 3835. DOI: 10.3390/su16093835

Bhattamisra, , Banerjee, P., Gupta, P., Mayuren, J., Patra, S., & Candasamy, M. (2023). Artificial Intelligence in Pharmaceutical and Healthcare Research. *Big Data and Cognitive Computing*, *7*(1), 10. DOI: 10.3390/bdcc7010010

Bhutta, M., Khwaja, A., Nadeem, A., Ahmad, H., Khan, M., Hanif, M., Song, H., Alshamari, M., & Cao, Y. (2021). A Survey on Blockchain Technology: Evolution, Architecture and Security. *IEEE Access : Practical Innovations, Open Solutions*, *9*, 61048–61073. DOI: 10.1109/ACCESS.2021.3072849

Bidve, V., Kakakde, K., Sarasu, P., Kediya, S., Tamkhade, P., & Nair, S. (2023). Patient Data Management Using Blockchain Technology. *Indonesian Journal of Electrical Engineering and Computer Science*, *32*(3), 1746–1754. DOI: 10.11591/ijeecs.v32.i3.pp1746-1754

Blanck, E., Pirhonen Nørmark, L., Fors, A., Ekman, I., Ali, L., Swedberg, K., & Gyllensten, H. (2024). Self-efficacy and healthcare costs in patients with chronic heart failure or chronic obstructive pulmonary disease. *ESC Heart Failure*, *11*(1), 219–228. Advance online publication. DOI: 10.1002/ehf2.14574 PMID: 37940106

Blanco-Gonzalez, A., Cabezon, A., Seco-Gonzalez, A., Conde-Torres, D., Antelo-Riveiro, P., Pineiro, A., & Garcia-Fandino, R. (2023). The role of AI in drug discovery: Challenges, opportunities, and strategies. *Pharmaceuticals (Basel, Switzerland)*, *16*(6), 891. DOI: 10.3390/ph16060891 PMID: 37375838

Blossey, G., Eisenhardt, J., & Hahn, G. (2019). Blockchain technology in supply chain management: An application perspective.

Bocek, T., Rodrigues, B. B., Strasser, T., & Stiller, B. (2017, May). Blockchains everywhere-a use-case of blockchains in the pharma supply-chain. In 2017 IFIP/IEEE symposium on integrated network and service management (IM) (pp. 772-777). IEEE.

Bohr, A., & Memarzadeh, K. (2020). The rise of artificial intelligence in healthcare applications. In *Artificial Intelligence in healthcare* (pp. 25–60). Academic Press. DOI: 10.1016/B978-0-12-818438-7.00002-2

Bommareddy, S., Khan, J. A., & Anand, R. (2022). A review on healthcare data privacy and security. *Networking Technologies in Smart Healthcare*, 165-187.

Bottou, L. (2010). Large-scale machine learning with stochastic gradient descent. In *Proceedings of-COMPSTAT'2010: 19th International Conference on Computational StatisticsParis France,August 22-27, 2010Keynote, Invited and Contributed Papers* (pp. 177-186). Physica-Verlag HD. DOI: 10.1007/978-3-7908-2604-3_16

Bouguerra, A., Hughes, M., Cakir, M. S., & Tatoglu, E. (2022). Linking entrepreneurial orientation to environmental collaboration: A stakeholder theory and evidence from multinational companies in an emerging market. *British Journal of Management*.

Bracci, E., Tallaki, M., Ievoli, R., & Diplotti, S. (2022). Knowledge, diffusion and interest in blockchain technology in SMEs. *Journal of Knowledge Management*, *26*(5), 1386–1407. DOI: 10.1108/JKM-02-2021-0099

Breaux, R., Shroff, D. M., Cash, A. R., Swanson, C. S., Carlton, C., Bertollo, J. R., & Dahiya, A. V. (2023). Telehealth delivery of the RELAX intervention for families of adolescents diagnosed with ADHD: Preliminary treatment outcomes and evidence of acceptability and feasibility. *Evidence-Based Practice in Child and Adolescent Mental Health*, *8*(1), 24–38. DOI: 10.1080/23794925.2021.1970053

Brisimi, T. S., Chen, R., Mela, T., Olshevsky, A., Paschalidis, I. C., & Shi, W. (2018). Federated learning of predictive models from federated electronic health records. *International Journal of Medical Informatics*, *112*, 59–67. DOI: 10.1016/j.ijmedinf.2018.01.007 PMID: 29500022

Bristow, A. S., Buys, K. C., & Mays, L. C. (2023). OLD CLASS: An Innovative Approach to the Chronic Disease History of Present Illness. *The Journal for Nurse Practitioners*, *19*(5), 104545. DOI: 10.1016/j.nurpra.2023.104545

Budhi, V. (2022). *Advantages and disadvantages of Blockchain technology*. Forbes Technology Council.

Buterin, V. (2014). A next-generation smart contract and decentralized application platform. *white paper, 3*(37), 2-1.

Butt, H. A., Ahad, A., Wasim, M., Madeira, F., & Chamran, M. K. (2023, October). 5G and IoT for Intelligent Healthcare: AI and Machine Learning Approaches—A Review. In *International Conference on Smart Objects and Technologies for Social Good* (pp. 107-123). Cham: Springer Nature Switzerland. DOI: 10.1007/978-3-031-52524-7_8

Butt, H. A., Ahad, A., Wasim, M., Madeira, F., & Chamran, M. K. (2023). 5G and IoT for Intelligent Healthcare: AI and Machine Learning Approaches—A Review. *International Conference on Smart Objects and Technologies for Social Good*

Butt, H. A., Ahad, A., Wasim, M., Shayea, I., Coelho, P. J., Pires, I. M., & Garcia, N. M. (2023). Federated machine learning in 5G smart healthcare: A security perspective review. *Procedia Computer Science*, *224*, 580–586. DOI: 10.1016/j.procs.2023.09.084

Butt, H. A., Harthy, K. S. A., Shah, M. A., Hussain, M., Amin, R., & Rehman, M. U. (2024). Enhanced DDoS Detection Using Advanced Machine Learning and Ensemble Techniques in Software Defined Networking. *Computers, Materials & Continua*, *81*(2), 3003–3031. DOI: 10.32604/cmc.2024.057185

Cao, B., Wang, Z., Zhang, L., Feng, D., Peng, M., Zhang, L., & Han, Z. (2021). Blockchain Systems, Technologies, and Applications: A Methodology Perspective. *IEEE Communications Surveys and Tutorials*, *25*(1), 353–385. DOI: 10.1109/COMST.2022.3204702

Cao, Z., Wang, Y., Zheng, W., Yin, L., Tang, Y., Miao, W., Liu, S., & Yang, B. (2022). The algorithm of stereo vision and shape from shading based on endoscope imaging. *Biomedical Signal Processing and Control*, *76*, 103658. DOI: 10.1016/j.bspc.2022.103658

Casalino, L., Gillies, R. R., Shortell, S. M., Schmittdiel, J. A., Bodenheimer, T., Robinson, J. C., Rundall, T., Oswald, N., Schauffler, H., & Wang, M. C. (2003). External incentives, information technology, and organized processes to improve health care quality for patients with chronic diseases. *Journal of the American Medical Association*, *289*(4), 434–441. DOI: 10.1001/jama.289.4.434 PMID: 12533122

Casino, F., Dasaklis, T. K., & Patsakis, C. (2019). A systematic literature review of blockchain-based applications: Current status, classification and open issues. *Telematics and Informatics*, *36*, 55–81. DOI: 10.1016/j.tele.2018.11.006

Centobelli, P., Cerchione, R., Del Vecchio, P., Oropallo, E., & Secundo, G. (2022). Blockchain technology for bridging trust, traceability and transparency in circular supply chain. *Information & Management*, *59*(7), 103508. DOI: 10.1016/j.im.2021.103508

Chacko, A., & Hayajneh, T. (2018). Security and privacy issues with IoT in healthcare. *EAI Endorsed Transactions on Pervasive Health and Technology*, *4*(14), e2. DOI: 10.4108/eai.13-7-2018.155079

Chan, M., Estève, D., Fourniols, J.-Y., Escriba, C., & Campo, E. (2012). Smart wearable systems: Current status and future challenges. *Artificial Intelligence in Medicine*, *56*(3), 137–156. DOI: 10.1016/j.artmed.2012.09.003 PMID: 23122689

Charles, S., & Natarajan, J. (2024). Identification of key gene modules and novel transcription factors in tetralogy of fallot using machine learning and network topological features. *Medinformatics*, *1*(1), 27–34. DOI: 10.47852/bonviewMEDIN32021554

Charles, W., Van Der Waal, M., Flach, J., Bisschop, A., Van Der Waal, R., Es-Sbai, H., & McLeod, C. (2023). Blockchain-Based Dynamic Consent and its Applications for Patient-Centric Research and Health Information Sharing: Protocol for an Integrative Review. *JMIR Research Protocols*, *13*, e50339. Advance online publication. DOI: 10.2196/50339 PMID: 38315514

Chattopadhyay, A. K., Nag, A., Ghosh, D., & Chanda, K. (2019). A secure framework for IoT-based healthcare system. Proceedings of International Ethical Hacking Conference 2018: eHaCON 2018, Kolkata, India, Chattopadhyay, S. (2024). Decoding medical diagnosis with machine learning classifiers. *Medinformatics*. DOI: 10.1007/978-981-13-1544-2_31

Chattopadhyay, S. (2024). *Decoding medical diagnosis with machine learning classifiers*. Medinformatics. DOI: 10.47852/bonviewMEDIN42022583

Chattu, V. K. (2021). A Review of Artificial Intelligence, Big Data, and Blockchain Technology Applications in Medicine and Global Health. *Big Data and Cognitive Computing*, *5*(3), 41. DOI: 10.3390/bdcc5030041

Chaudhuri, A. (2018). *Internet of Things, for Things, and by Things*. Auerbach Publications. DOI: 10.1201/9781315200644

Chen, L., Lee, W. K., Chang, C. C., Choo, K. K. R., & Zhang, N. (2019). Blockchain based searchable encryption for electronic health record sharing. *Future Generation Computer Systems*, *95*, 420–429. DOI: 10.1016/j.future.2019.01.018

Chen, S.-G., Chen, J.-Y., Yang, Y.-P., Chien, C.-S., Wang, M.-L., & Lin, L.-T. (2020). Use of radiographic features in COVID-19 diagnosis: Challenges and perspectives. *Journal of the Chinese Medical Association*, *83*(7), 644–647. DOI: 10.1097/JCMA.0000000000000336 PMID: 32349032

Chen, W., Xu, Z., Shi, S., Zhao, Y., & Zhao, J. (2018, December). A survey of blockchain applications in different domains. In *Proceedings of the 2018 International Conference on Blockchain Technology and Application* (pp. 17-21).

Chen, Y., Ding, S., Xu, Z., Zheng, H., & Yang, S. (2019). Blockchain-based medical records secure storage and medical service framework. *Journal of Medical Systems*, *43*(1), 1–9. DOI: 10.1007/s10916-018-1121-4 PMID: 30467604

Chen, Y., Peng, B., Wang, X., & Tang, H. (2012). *Large-Scale Privacy-Preserving Mapping of Human Genomic Sequences on Hybrid Clouds*. NDSS.

Chen, Y., Yang, X., Chen, B., Miao, C., & Yu, H. (2017, November). PdAssist: Objective and quantified symptom assessment of Parkinson's disease via smartphone. In *2017 IEEE International Conference on Bioinformatics and Biomedicine (BIBM)* (pp. 939-945). IEEE. DOI: 10.1109/BIBM.2017.8217783

Chen, Z., Xu, W., Wang, B., & Yu, H. (2021). A blockchain-based preserving and sharing system for medical data privacy. *Future Generation Computer Systems*, *124*, 338–350. DOI: 10.1016/j.future.2021.05.023

Cheung, H. H., & Choi, S. H. (2011). Implementation issues in RFID-based anti-counterfeiting systems. *Computers in Industry*, *62*(7), 708–718. DOI: 10.1016/j.compind.2011.04.001

Chiacchio, F., D'Urso, D., Oliveri, L. M., Spitaleri, A., Spampinato, C., & Giordano, D. (2022). A non-fungible token solution for the track and trace of pharmaceutical supply chain. *Applied Sciences (Basel, Switzerland)*, *12*(8), 4019. DOI: 10.3390/app12084019

Chirra, B. R. (2023). Enhancing Healthcare Data Security with Homomorphic Encryption: A Case Study on Electronic Health Records (EHR) Systems. *Revista de Inteligencia Artificial en Medicina*, *14*(1), 549–559.

Choi, J., Choi, C., Kim, S., & Ko, H. (2019). Medical information protection frameworks for smart healthcare based on IoT. *Proceedings of the 9th International Conference on Web Intelligence, Mining and Semantics*

Choudhury, A., & Asan, O. (2020). Role of artificial intelligence in patient safety outcomes: Systematic literature review. *JMIR Medical Informatics*, *8*(7), e18599. DOI: 10.2196/18599 PMID: 32706688

Chowdhury, M. E., Rahman, T., Khandakar, A., Mazhar, R., Kadir, M. A., Mahbub, Z. B., Islam, K. R., Khan, M. S., Iqbal, A., Emadi, N. A., Reaz, M. B. I., & Islam, M. T. (2020). Can AI help in screening viral and COVID-19 pneumonia? *IEEE Access : Practical Innovations, Open Solutions*, *8*, 132665–132676. DOI: 10.1109/ACCESS.2020.3010287

Cifuentes-Faura, J. (2022). European Union policies and their role in combating climate change over the years. *Air Quality, Atmosphere & Health*, *15*(8), 1–8. DOI: 10.1007/s11869-022-01156-5 PMID: 35035604

Ciotti, M., Ciccozzi, M., Terrinoni, A., Jiang, W.-C., Wang, C.-B., & Bernardini, S. (2020). The COVID-19 pandemic. *Critical Reviews in Clinical Laboratory Sciences*, *57*(6), 365–388. DOI: 10.1080/10408363.2020.1783198 PMID: 32645276

Coronavirus. (2020). 13,968 cases and 223 deaths. Retrieved from https://www.worldometers.info/coronavirus/country/ethiopia

Creswell, J. W., & Clark, V. L. P. (2017). *Designing and conducting mixed methods research.* Sage publications.

Creswell, J. W., & Creswell, J. D. (2017). *Research design: Qualitative, quantitative, and mixed methods approaches.* Sage publications.

Crompvoets, P. I., Nieboer, A. P., van Rossum, E. F. C., & Cramm, J. M. (2024). Perceived weight stigma in healthcare settings among adults living with obesity: A cross-sectional investigation of the relationship with patient characteristics and person-centred care. *Health Expectations*, *27*(1), e13954. Advance online publication. DOI: 10.1111/hex.13954 PMID: 39102661

Culp, W. (2020). Coronavirus disease 2019. *Practice*, *14*(6), e01218. PMID: 32784318

Dagher, G., Mohler, J., Milojkovic, M., & Marella, P. (2018). Ancile: Privacy-Preserving Framework for Access Control and Interoperability of Electronic Health Records Using Blockchain Technology. *Sustainable Cities and Society*, *39*, 283–297. DOI: 10.1016/j.scs.2018.02.014

Dai, M., Zhang, S., Wang, H., & Jin, S. (2018). A low storage room requirement framework for distributed ledger in blockchain. *IEEE Access : Practical Innovations, Open Solutions*, *6*, 22970–22975. DOI: 10.1109/ACCESS.2018.2814624

Daraojimba, A., Enahoro, Q., Ogugua, J., Anyanwu, E., Akomolafe, O., & Odilibe, I. (2023). *The impact of electronic health records on healthcare delivery and patient outcomes: A review.* World Journal of Advanced Research and Reviews., DOI: 10.30574/wjarr.2024.21.2.0478

Davis, C. R., Murphy, K. J., Curtis, R. G., & Maher, C. A. (2020). A process evaluation examining the performance, adherence, and acceptability of a physical activity and diet artificial intelligence virtual health assistant. *International Journal of Environmental Research and Public Health, 17*(23), 9137. DOI: 10.3390/ijerph17239137 PMID: 33297456

Dayan, I., Roth, H. R., Zhong, A., Harouni, A., Gentili, A., Abidin, A. Z., Liu, A., Costa, A. B., Wood, B. J., Tsai, C.-S., Wang, C.-H., Hsu, C.-N., Lee, C. K., Ruan, P., Xu, D., Wu, D., Huang, E., Kitamura, F. C., Lacey, G., & Li, Q. (2021). Federated learning for predicting clinical outcomes in patients with COVID-19. *Nature Medicine, 27*(10), 1735–1743. DOI: 10.1038/s41591-021-01506-3 PMID: 34526699

Debnath, B., Shakur, M. S., Bari, A. M., Saha, J., Porna, W. A., Mishu, M. J., Islam, A. R. M. T., & Rahman, M. A. (2023). Assessing the critical success factors for implementing industry 4.0 in the pharmaceutical industry: Implications for supply chain sustainability in emerging economies. *PLoS One, 18*(6), e0287149. DOI: 10.1371/journal.pone.0287149 PMID: 37319165

DeGusta, M. (2012). *Are smartphones spreading faster than any technology in human history?* Massachusetts Institute of Technology Review.

Deng, X., & Ouyang, Y. (2022). Cross-Border Supply Chain System Constructed by Complex Computer Blockchain for International Cooperation. *Computational Intelligence and Neuroscience, 2022*, 1–10. Advance online publication. DOI: 10.1155/2022/6221211 PMID: 35449736

Deshai, N., & Rao, B. B. (2023). Transparency in healthcare and e-commerce: Detecting online fake reviews using a dense neural network model with relevance mapping. *Soft Computing, 27*(14), 9861–9875. Advance online publication. DOI: 10.1007/s00500-023-08437-w

Deshmukh, V., Pathak, S., & Bhattacharya, P. (2025). Bl-Boost: A blockchain-based XG-Boost EHR scheme in Healthcare 5.0 ecosystems. *International Journal of Computing, 17*(1), 1–15.

Devlin, M. K., McIntyre, N. J., Ramer, M. D., Kwon, Y. H., Nicholson, J. M., Mrkobrada, M., Kronick, J., Calvin, J. E., & Spicer, E. (2024). Applying the lessons of design thinking: A unique programme of care for acutely unwell, community-dwelling COVID-19 patients. *BMJ Open Quality, 13*(1), e002500. Advance online publication. DOI: 10.1136/bmjoq-2023-002500 PMID: 38413092

Dhingra, S., Raut, R., Kumar, M., & Naik, B. K. R. (2024). Factors impacting Indian healthcare supply chain performance and influence in the public and private sector: The mediating role of blockchain technology adoption. *Benchmarking*. Advance online publication. DOI: 10.1108/BIJ-10-2023-0687

Diana, M., & Marescaux, J. (2015). Robotic surgery. *British Journal of Surgery, 102*(2), e15–e28. DOI: 10.1002/bjs.9711 PMID: 25627128

Dian, F. J., Vahidnia, R., & Rahmati, A. (2020). Wearables and the Internet of Things (IoT), applications, opportunities, and challenges: A Survey. *IEEE Access : Practical Innovations, Open Solutions, 8*, 69200–69211.

Díaz, J. S. P., & García, Á. L. (2023). Study of the performance and scalability of federated learning for medical imaging with intermittent clients. *Neurocomputing, 518*, 142–154. DOI: 10.1016/j.neucom.2022.11.011

Diaz, O., Kushibar, K., Osuala, R., Linardos, A., Garrucho, L., Igual, L., Radeva, P., Prior, F., Gkontra, P., & Lekadir, K. (2021). Data preparation for artificial intelligence in medical imaging: A comprehensive guide to open-access platforms and tools. *Physica Medica*, *83*, 25–37. DOI: 10.1016/j.ejmp.2021.02.007 PMID: 33684723

Dillard-Wright, J., & Shields-Haas, V. (2021). Nursing with the people: Reimagining futures for nursing. *Advances in Nursing Science*, *44*(3), 195–209. DOI: 10.1097/ANS.0000000000000361 PMID: 33624989

Dimitrov, D. V. (2019). Blockchain applications for healthcare data management. *Healthcare Informatics Research*, *25*(1), 51–56. DOI: 10.4258/hir.2019.25.1.51 PMID: 30788182

DOC (U.S. Department of Commerce). (1999). *The Emerging Digital Economy II: Appendices*. U.S. Department of Commerce.

Dong, S., Abbas, K., Li, M., & Kamruzzaman, J. (2023). Blockchain technology and application: An overview. *PeerJ. Computer Science*, *9*, e1705. Advance online publication. DOI: 10.7717/peerj-cs.1705 PMID: 38077532

Duan, S., Chamran, M. K., & Alobaedy, M. M. (2024). Enhancing Blockchain Interoperability Through Cross-Chain Outsourcing and Communication. *2024 IEEE 6th Symposium on Computers & Informatics (ISCI)* (pp. 276-281). Kuala Lumpur: IEEE. doi:DOI: 10.1109/ISCI62787

Dubovitskaya, A., Xu, Z., Ryu, S., Schumacher, M., & Wang, F. (2018, April). Secure and trustable electronic medical records sharing using blockchain. *AMIA ... Annual Symposium Proceedings - AMIA Symposium. AMIA Symposium*, *2017*, 650. PMID: 29854130

Duffett, L. (2017). Patient engagement: What partnering with patient in research is all about. In *Thrombosis Research* (Vol. 150). DOI: 10.1016/j.thromres.2016.10.029

Dullabh, P., Sandberg, S. F., Heaney-Huls, K., Hovey, L. S., Lobach, D. F., Boxwala, A., Desai, P. J., Berliner, E., Dymek, C., Harrison, M. I., Swiger, J., & Sittig, D. F. (2022). Challenges and opportunities for advancing patient-centered clinical decision support: Findings from a horizon scan. *Journal of the American Medical Informatics Association : JAMIA*, *29*(7), 1233–1243. Advance online publication. DOI: 10.1093/jamia/ocac059 PMID: 35534996

Durrani, M. Y., Yasmin, S., & Rho, S. (2022). An Internet of Medical Things-based liver tumor detection system using semantic segmentation. *Journal of Internet Technology*, *23*(1), 163–175.

Dwork, C., & Roth, A. (2014). The algorithmic foundations of differential privacy. *Foundations and Trends® in Theoretical Computer Science, 9*(3–4), 211-407.

Eager, B., & Brunton, R. (2023). Prompting higher education towards AI-augmented teaching and learning practice. Journal of University Teaching & Learning Practice, 20(5), 02.

Ebrahimi, S., & Bridgelall, R. (2021). A fuzzy Delphi analytic hierarchy model to rank factors influencing public transit mode choice: A case study. *Research in Transportation Business & Management*, *39*, 100496. DOI: 10.1016/j.rtbm.2020.100496

Ehrenstein, V., Kharrazi, H., Lehmann, H., & Taylor, C. O. (2019). Obtaining data from electronic health records. In *Tools and technologies for registry interoperability, registries for evaluating patient outcomes: A user's guide, 3rd edition, Addendum 2 [Internet]*. Agency for Healthcare Research and Quality (US).

Ekblaw, A., Azaria, A., Halamka, J. D., & Lippman, A. (2016, August). A Case Study for Blockchain in Healthcare:"MedRec" prototype for electronic health records and medical research data. In *Proceedings of IEEE open & big data conference* (Vol. 13, p. 13).

Ekramifard, A., Amintoosi, H., Seno, A. H., Dehghantanha, A., & Parizi, R. M. (2020). A systematic literature review of integration of blockchain and artificial intelligence. *Blockchain cybersecurity, trust and privacy*, pp.147-160.

El Emam, K., Jonker, E., Arbuckle, L., & Malin, B. (2011). A systematic review of re-identification attacks on health data. *PLoS One*, *6*(12), e28071. DOI: 10.1371/journal.pone.0028071 PMID: 22164229

Elayan, H., Aloqaily, M., & Guizani, M. (2021). Sustainability of healthcare data analysis IoT-based systems using deep federated learning. *IEEE Internet of Things Journal*, *9*(10), 7338–7346. DOI: 10.1109/JIOT.2021.3103635

ElBaih, M. (2023). The Role of Privacy Regulations in AI Development (A Discussion of the Ways in Which Privacy Regulations Can Shape the Development of AI). Available at *SSRN* 4589207. DOI: 10.2139/ssrn.4589207

Elhoseny, M., Ramírez-González, G., Abu-Elnasr, O. M., Shawkat, S. A., Arunkumar, N., & Farouk, A. (2018). Secure medical data transmission model for IoT-based healthcare systems. *IEEE Access : Practical Innovations, Open Solutions*, *6*, 20596–20608. DOI: 10.1109/ACCESS.2018.2817615

Elvas, L. B., Serrão, C., & Ferreira, J. C. (2023, January). Sharing health information using a blockchain. [). MDPI.]. *Health Care*, *11*(2), 170. PMID: 36673538

Engelhardt, M. A. (2017). Hitching healthcare to the chain: An introduction to blockchain technology in the healthcare sector. *Technology Innovation Management Review*, *7*(10), 22–34. DOI: 10.22215/timreview/1111

Erlingsson, Ú., Pihur, V., & Korolova, A. (2014). Rappor: Randomized aggregatable privacy-preserving ordinal response. *Proceedings of the 2014 ACM SIGSAC conference on computer and communications security*

Esmaeilzadeh, P. (2019). An Empirical Evaluation of Factors Influencing Patients' Reactions to the Implementation of Health Information Exchanges (HIEs). *International Journal of Human-Computer Interaction*, *35*(13), 1135–1146. Advance online publication. DOI: 10.1080/10447318.2018.1511181

Esposito, C., De Santis, A., Tortora, G., Chang, H., & Choo, K. K. R. (2018). Blockchain: A panacea for healthcare cloud-based data security and privacy? *IEEE Cloud Computing*, *5*(1), 31–37. DOI: 10.1109/MCC.2018.011791712

Esteva, A., Chou, K., Yeung, S., Naik, N., Madani, A., Mottaghi, A., Liu, Y., Topol, E., Dean, J., & Socher, R. (2021). Deep learning-enabled medical computer vision. *NPJ Digital Medicine*, *4*(1), 1–9. DOI: 10.1038/s41746-020-00376-2 PMID: 33420381

Esteva, A., Robicquet, A., Ramsundar, B., Kuleshov, V., DePristo, M., Chou, K., Cui, C., Corrado, G., Thrun, S., & Dean, J. (2019). A guide to deep learning in healthcare. *Nature Medicine*, *25*(1), 24–29. DOI: 10.1038/s41591-018-0316-z PMID: 30617335

Ettaloui, N., Arezki, S., & Gadi, T. (2024). An Overview of Blockchain-Based Electronic Health Record and Compliance with GDPR and HIPAA. In Farhaoui, Y., Hussain, A., Saba, T., Taherdoost, H., & Verma, A. (Eds.), *Artificial Intelligence, Data Science and Applications. ICAISE 2023. Lecture Notes in Networks and Systems* (Vol. 838). Springer., DOI: 10.1007/978-3-031-48573-2_58

European Commission. (2016). *The General Data Protection Regulation.* https://ec.europa.eu/justice/dataprotection/reform/files/regulation_oj_en.pdf

Faneela, , Khan, M. A., Alsuhibany, S. A., El Shafai, W., Rehman, M. U., & Ahmad, J. (2023). An immutable framework for smart healthcare using blockchain technology. *Computer Systems Science and Engineering*, *46*(1), 165–179. DOI: 10.32604/csse.2023.035066

Farahani, B., Firouzi, F., Chang, V., Badaroglu, M., Constant, N., & Mankodiya, K. (2018). Towards fog-driven IoT eHealth: Promises and challenges of IoT in medicine and healthcare. *Future Generation Computer Systems*, *78*, 659–676. DOI: 10.1016/j.future.2017.04.036

Fareed, N., Walker, D., Sieck, C. J., Taylor, R., Scarborough, S., Huerta, T. R., & McAlearney, A. S. (2019). Inpatient portal clusters: Identifying user groups based on portal features. *Journal of the American Medical Informatics Association : JAMIA*, *26*(1), 28–36.

Fatoum, H., Hanna, S., Halamka, J. D., Sicker, D. C., Spangenberg, P., & Hashmi, S. K. (2021). Blockchain integration with digital technology and the future of health care ecosystems: Systematic review. *Journal of Medical Internet Research*, *23*(11), e19846. DOI: 10.2196/19846 PMID: 34726603

Feki, I., Ammar, S., Kessentini, Y., & Muhammad, K. (2021). Federated learning for COVID-19 screening from Chest X-ray images. *Applied Soft Computing*, *106*, 107330. DOI: 10.1016/j.asoc.2021.107330 PMID: 33776607

Feng, J., Rong, C., Sun, F., Guo, D., & Li, Y. (2020). PMF: A privacy-preserving human mobility prediction framework via federated learning. *Proceedings of the ACM on Interactive, Mobile, Wearable and Ubiquitous Technologies*, *4*(1), 1–21. DOI: 10.1145/3381006 PMID: 35846237

Fernández-Alemán, J. L., Señor, I. C., Lozoya, P. Á. O., & Toval, A. (2013). Security and privacy in electronic health records: A systematic literature review. *Journal of Biomedical Informatics*, *46*(3), 541–562. DOI: 10.1016/j.jbi.2012.12.003 PMID: 23305810

Ferreira, D. C., Vieira, I., Pedro, M. I., Caldas, P., & Varela, M. (2023, February). Patient satisfaction with healthcare services and the techniques used for its assessment: A systematic literature review and a bibliometric analysis. [). MDPI.]. *Health Care*, *11*(5), 639. PMID: 36900644

Firouzi, F., Jiang, S., Chakrabarty, K., Farahani, B., Daneshmand, M., Song, J., & Mankodiya, K. (2022). Fusion of IoT, AI, edge–fog–cloud, and blockchain: Challenges, solutions, and a case study in healthcare and medicine. *IEEE Internet of Things Journal*, *10*(5), 3686–3705. DOI: 10.1109/JIOT.2022.3191881

Frid-Adar, M., Diamant, I., Klang, E., Amitai, M., Goldberger, J., & Greenspan, H. (2018). GAN-based synthetic medical image augmentation for increased CNN performance in liver lesion classification. *Neurocomputing*, *321*, 321–331. DOI: 10.1016/j.neucom.2018.09.013

Gakire, M. (2024). *The Use of Blockchain in Securing Patient Data*. Research Output Journal of Public Health and Medicine., DOI: 10.59298/ROJPHM/2024/324750

Gandhi, D. A., & Ghosal, M. (2018). Intelligent healthcare using IoT: An extensive survey. In *2018 Second International Conference on Inventive Communication and Computational Technologies (ICICCT)* (pp. 800–802).

Ganesan, R., Devi, T., Kumar, S. R., & Gayathri, N. (2022). Securing Healthcare Information Using Blockchain Technology: A Deep Insight. In *Blockchain Security in Cloud Computing* (pp. 253-263): Springer. DOI: 10.1007/978-3-030-70501-5_12

Gaye, A., Marcon, Y., Isaeva, J., LaFlamme, P., Turner, A., Jones, E. M., Minion, J., Boyd, A. W., Newby, C. J., Nuotio, M.-L., Wilson, R., Butters, O., Murtagh, B., Demir, I., Doiron, D., Giepmans, L., Wallace, S. E., Budin-Ljøsne, I., Oliver Schmidt, C., & Burton, P. R. (2014). DataSHIELD: Taking the analysis to the data, not the data to the analysis. *International Journal of Epidemiology*, *43*(6), 1929–1944. DOI: 10.1093/ije/dyu188 PMID: 25261970

Gebhardt, M., Kopyto, M., Birkel, H., & Hartmann, E. (2022). Industry 4.0 technologies as enablers of collaboration in circular supply chains: A systematic literature review. *International Journal of Production Research*, *60*(23), 6967–6995. DOI: 10.1080/00207543.2021.1999521

General Data Protection Regulation. (2016). https://eur-lex.europa.eu/legal-content/EN/TXT/?uri=CELEX%3A32016R0679

Gentry, C. (2009). Fully homomorphic encryption using ideal lattices. Proceedings of the forty-first annual ACM symposium on Theory of computing, Grady, C. (2015). Enduring and emerging challenges of informed consent. *The New England Journal of Medicine*, *372*(9), 855–862. PMID: 19196665

George, E., Idemudia, C., & Ige, A. (2024). *Blockchain technology in financial services: enhancing security, transparency, and efficiency in transactions and services*. Open Access Research Journal of Multidisciplinary Studies., DOI: 10.53022/oarjms.2024.8.1.0042

Ghadge, A., Bourlakis, M., Kamble, S., & Seuring, S. (2023). Blockchain implementation in pharmaceutical supply chains: A review and conceptual framework. *International Journal of Production Research*, *61*(19), 6633–6651. DOI: 10.1080/00207543.2022.2125595

Ghadi, Y. Y., Mazhar, T., Shahzad, T., Amir khan, M., Abd-Alrazaq, A., Ahmed, A., & Hamam, H. (2024). Muhammad Amir khan, Alaa Abd-Alrazaq, Arfan Ahmed, and Habib Hamam. "The role of blockchain to secure internet of medical things.". *Scientific Reports*, *14*(1), 18422. DOI: 10.1038/s41598-024-68529-x PMID: 39117650

Goddard, M. (2017). The EU General Data Protection Regulation (GDPR): European regulation that has a global impact. *International Journal of Market Research*, *59*(6), 703–705. DOI: 10.2501/IJMR-2017-050

Gopalan, S. S., Raza, A., & Almobaideen, W. (2021). IoT security in healthcare using AI: A survey. 2020 International Conference on Communications, Signal Processing, and their Applications (ICCSPA), Ho, E. S. (2022). Data security challenges in deep neural network for healthcare IoT systems. *Security and Privacy Preserving for IoT and 5G Networks: Techniques, Challenges, and New Directions*, 19-37.

Gore, J. C. (2020). Artificial intelligence in medical imaging. *Magnetic Resonance Imaging*, *68*, A1–A4. DOI: 10.1016/j.mri.2019.12.006 PMID: 31857130

Govindan, K., Nasr, A. K., Saeed Heidary, M., Nosrati-Abarghooee, S., & Mina, H. (2023). Prioritizing adoption barriers of platforms based on blockchain technology from balanced scorecard perspectives in healthcare industry: A structural approach. *International Journal of Production Research*, *61*(11), 3512–3526. DOI: 10.1080/00207543.2021.2013560

Guermazi, R., Chaabane, I., & Hammami, M. (2018). AECID: Asymmetric entropy for classifying imbalanced data. *Information Sciences*, *467*, 373–397. DOI: 10.1016/j.ins.2018.07.076

Guntur, L. N., Dornadula, G., & Nimbagal, R. N. (2022). Blockchain Technology: A Breakthrough in the Healthcare Sector. In Idrees, S. M., & Nowostawski, M. (Eds.), *Transformations Through Blockchain Technology* (pp. 137–160). Springer. DOI: 10.1007/978-3-030-93344-9_6

Guo, H., & Yu, X. (2022). A survey on blockchain technology and its security. *Blockchain: research and applications, 3*(2), 100067.

Guo, Y., Gao, Y., & Shen, D. (2015). Deformable MR prostate segmentation via deep feature learning and sparse patch matching. *IEEE Transactions on Medical Imaging*, *35*(5), 1077–1089. PMID: 26685226

Guo, Z., Li, X., Huang, H., Guo, N., & Li, Q. (2019). Deep learning-based image segmentation on multimodal medical imaging. *IEEE Transactions on Radiation and Plasma Medical Sciences*, *3*(2), 162–169. DOI: 10.1109/TRPMS.2018.2890359 PMID: 34722958

Gupta, S., Bali, A., & Singh, A. (n.d.). *Fake Product Detection System Using Blockchain Fake Product Detection Using Blockchain View project Fake Product Detection System Using Blockchain*. Retrieved from https://www.researchgate.net/publication/366064456

Gupta, A., Misra, S., Pathak, N., & Das, D. (2023). Fedcare: Federated learning for resource-constrained healthcare devices in iomt system. *IEEE Transactions on Computational Social Systems*, *10*(4), 1587–1596. DOI: 10.1109/TCSS.2022.3232192

Gurtu, A., & Johny, J. (2019). Potential of blockchain technology in supply chain management: A literature review. *International Journal of Physical Distribution & Logistics Management*, *49*(9), 881–900. DOI: 10.1108/IJPDLM-11-2018-0371

Gwassi, O. A. H., Uçan, O. N., & Navarro, E. A. (2024). Cyber-XAI-Block: An end-to-end cyber threat detection & fl-based risk assessment framework for iot enabled smart organization using xai and blockchain technologies. *Multimedia Tools and Applications*, •••, 1–42. DOI: 10.1007/s11042-024-20059-4

Habib, G., Sharma, S., Ibrahim, S., Ahmad, I., Qureshi, S., & Ishfaq, M. (2022). Blockchain technology: Benefits, challenges, applications, and integration of blockchain technology with cloud computing. *Future Internet*, *14*(11), 341. DOI: 10.3390/fi14110341

Haider, K. Z., Malik, K. R., Khalid, S., Nawaz, T., & Jabbar, S. (2019). Deepgender: Real-time gender classification using deep learning for smartphones. *Journal of Real-Time Image Processing*, *16*(1), 15–29. DOI: 10.1007/s11554-017-0714-3

Halamka, J. D., Lippman, A., & Ekblaw, A. (2017). The Potential for Blockchain to Transform Electronic Health Records. *Harvard Business Review*, *3*, 2–5. Retrieved March 20, 2020, from https://hbr.org/2017/03/the-potential-for-blockchain-to-transform-electronic-health-records

Halas, G., Baldwin, A., Mackay, K., Cardenas, E., LaBine, L., Cherrett, P., Abraham, L., Fogarty, V., Singer, A., Katz, A., & Kirby, S. (2024). Patients' and caregivers' experiences of virtual care in a primary care setting during the COVID-19 pandemic: A patient-oriented research study. *Digital Health*, *10*, 20552076241232949. Advance online publication. DOI: 10.1177/20552076241232949 PMID: 38410792

Haleem, A., Javaid, M., Singh, R. P., & Suman, R. (2022). Medical 4.0 technologies for healthcare: Features, capabilities, and applications. *Internet of Things and Cyber-Physical Systems*, *2*, 12–30. DOI: 10.1016/j.iotcps.2022.04.001

Haleem, A., Javaid, M., Singh, R. P., Suman, R., & Rab, S. (2021). Blockchain technology applications in healthcare: An overview. *International Journal of Intelligent Networks*, *2*, 130–139. DOI: 10.1016/j.ijin.2021.09.005

Haq, I., & Esuka, O. M. (2018). Blockchain technology in the pharmaceutical industry to prevent counterfeit drugs. *International Journal of Computer Applications*, *180*(25), 8–12. DOI: 10.5120/ijca2018916579

Hasan, K., Chowdhury, M. J. M., Biswas, K., Ahmed, K., Islam, M. S., & Usman, M. (2022). A blockchain-based secure data-sharing framework for Software Defined Wireless Body Area Networks. *Computer Networks*, *211*, 109004. DOI: 10.1016/j.comnet.2022.109004

Hascher, K., Jaiswal, J., LoSchiavo, C., Ezell, J., Duffalo, D., Greene, R. E., Cox, A., Burton, W. M., Griffin, M., John, T., Grin, B., & Halkitis, P. N. (2024). Lack of Informed and Affirming Healthcare for Sexual Minority Men: A Call for Patient-Centered Care. *Journal of General Internal Medicine*, *39*(11), 2023–2032. Advance online publication. DOI: 10.1007/s11606-024-08635-8 PMID: 38308157

Hathaliya, J. J., Tanwar, S., Tyagi, S., & Kumar, N. (2019). Securing electronics healthcare records in Healthcare 4.0: A biometric-based approach. *Computers & Electrical Engineering*, *76*, 398–410. DOI: 10.1016/j.compeleceng.2019.04.017

Havaeji, H., Dao, T.-M., & Wong, T. (2023). Supervised learning by evolutionary computation tuning: An application to blockchain-based pharmaceutical supply chain cost model. *Mathematics*, *11*(9), 2021. DOI: 10.3390/math11092021

Heart, T., Ben-Assuli, O., & Shabtai, I. (2017). A Review of PHR, EMR and EHR Integration: A More Personalized Healthcare and Public Health Policy. *Health Policy and Technology*, *6*(1), 20–25. DOI: 10.1016/j.hlpt.2016.08.002

Hemdan, E. E.-D., Shouman, M. A., & Karar, M. E. (2020). COVIDx-Net: A framework of deep learning classifiers to diagnose COVID-19 in X-ray images. *arXiv preprint*, arXiv:2003.11055.

Hennebelle, A., Ismail, L., Materwala, H., Al Kaabi, J., Ranjan, P., & Janardhanan, R. (2024). Secure and privacy-preserving automated machine learning operations into end-to-end integrated IoT-edge-artificial intelligence-blockchain monitoring system for diabetes mellitus prediction. *Computational and Structural Biotechnology Journal*, *23*, 212–233. DOI: 10.1016/j.csbj.2023.11.038 PMID: 38169966

Hölbl, M., Kompara, M., Kamišalić, A., & Nemec Zlatolas, L. (2018). A systematic review of the use of blockchain in healthcare. *Symmetry*, *10*(10), 470. DOI: 10.3390/sym10100470

Hoofnagle, C. J., Van Der Sloot, B., & Borgesius, F. Z. (2019). The European Union general data protection regulation: What it is and what it means. *Information & Communications Technology Law*, *28*(1), 65–98. DOI: 10.1080/13600834.2019.1573501

Hossain, M. J., Wadud, M. A. H., & Alamin, M. (2021). HDM-Chain: A Secure Blockchain-based Healthcare Data Management framework to ensure Privacy and Security in the Health Unit. *2021 5th International Conference on Electrical Engineering and Information and Communication Technology, ICEEICT 2021*. DOI: 10.1109/ICEEICT53905.2021.9667820

Hossain, M. S., & Muhammad, G. (2020). Deep learning based pathology detection for smart connected healthcare. *IEEE Network*, *34*(6), 120–125. DOI: 10.1109/MNET.011.2000064

Hossain, M. S., Muhammad, G., & Guizani, N. (2020). Explainable AI and mass surveillance system-based healthcare framework to combat COVID-I9 like pandemics. *IEEE Network*, *34*(4), 126–132. DOI: 10.1109/MNET.011.2000458

Hosseini, S. M., Sikaroudi, M., Babaie, M., & Tizhoosh, H. R. (2023). Proportionally fair hospital collaborations in federated learning of histopathology images. *IEEE Transactions on Medical Imaging*, *42*(7), 1982–1995. DOI: 10.1109/TMI.2023.3234450 PMID: 37018335

Hu, Y., Liyanage, M., Mansoor, A., Thilakarathna, K., Jourjon, G., & Seneviratne, A. (2018). Blockchain-based smart contracts-applications and challenges. *arXiv preprint arXiv:1810.04699.*

Huang, G., & Al Foysal, A. (2021). Blockchain in Healthcare. *Technology and Investment*, *12*(3), 168–181. DOI: 10.4236/ti.2021.123010

Huang, L., Shea, A. L., Qian, H., Masurkar, A., Deng, H., & Liu, D. (2019). Patient clustering improves efficiency of federated machine learning to predict mortality and hospital stay time using distributed electronic medical records. *Journal of Biomedical Informatics*, *99*, 103291. DOI: 10.1016/j.jbi.2019.103291 PMID: 31560949

Hu, H., Chen, K., He, J., & Du, L. (2019). Whole cycle disruption analysis of petroleum supply chain (PSC) based on UASNs monitoring. *EURASIP Journal on Wireless Communications and Networking*, *2019*(1), 119. DOI: 10.1186/s13638-019-1426-0

Hu, M., Ren, Y., & Chen, C. (2023). Privacy-Preserving Medical Data-Sharing System with Symmetric Encryption Based on Blockchain. *Symmetry*, *15*(5), 1010. DOI: 10.3390/sym15051010

Humayun, M., Jhanjhi, N., Hamid, B., & Ahmed, G. (2020). Emerging Smart Logistics and Transportation Using IoT and Blockchain. *IEEE Internet of Things Magazine*, *3*(2), 58–62. DOI: 10.1109/IOTM.0001.1900097

Hussain, A. A., & Al-Turjman, F. (2021). Artificial intelligence and blockchain: A review. *Transactions on Emerging Telecommunications Technologies*, *32*(9), e4268. DOI: 10.1002/ett.4268

Hu, Y., Niu, D., Yang, J., & Zhou, S. (2019). FDML: A collaborative machine learning framework for distributed features. In *Proceedings of the 25th ACM SIGKDD International Conference on Knowledge Discovery & Data Mining* (pp. 2232–2240). DOI: 10.1145/3292500.3330765

Hwang, M. S., Li, C. T., Shen, J. J., & Chu, Y. P. (2004). Challenges in e-government and security of information. *Information & Security*, *15*(1), 9–20. DOI: 10.11610/isij.1501

Ichikawa, D., Kashiyama, M., & Ueno, T. (2017). Tamper-resistant mobile health using blockchain technology. *JMIR mHealth and uHealth*, *5*(7), e7938. DOI: 10.2196/mhealth.7938 PMID: 28747296

IEEE. Computer Society, & Green University of Bangladesh. (n.d.). *2021 3rd International Conference on Sustainable Technologies for Industry 4.0 (STI) 18-19 December, Dhaka.*

Islam, I., Munim, K., Oishwee, S., Islam, A., & Islam, M. (2020). A Critical Review of Concepts, Benefits, and Pitfalls of Blockchain Technology Using Concept Map. *IEEE Access : Practical Innovations, Open Solutions*, *8*, 68333–68341. DOI: 10.1109/ACCESS.2020.2985647

Islam, M. R., & Nahiduzzaman, M. (2022). Complex features extraction with deep learning model for the detection of COVID-19 from CT scan images using ensemble-based machine learning approach. *Expert Systems with Applications*, *195*, 116554. DOI: 10.1016/j.eswa.2022.116554 PMID: 35136286

Jabarulla, M. Y., & Lee, H. N. (2021, August). A blockchain and artificial intelligence- based, patient-centric healthcare system for combating the COVID-19 pandemic: Opportunities and applications. []. Mdpi.]. *Health Care*, *9*(8), 1019. PMID: 34442156

Jabarulla, M. Y., & Lee, H. N. (2021, August). A blockchain and artificial intelligence-based, patient-centric healthcare system for combating the COVID-19 pandemic: Opportunities and applications. []. Mdpi.]. *Health Care*, *9*(8), 1019. PMID: 34442156

Jabeen, M., Hussain, M., & Rana Hassam Ahmed, H. A. (n.d.). *A BLOCKCHAIN-BASED IPFS AUGMENTED DISTRIBUTED INFORMATION SHARING PARADIGM FOR SECURE COMMUNICATION IN NETWORKED ENVIRONMENT.*

Jabeen, M., Hussain, M., & Rana Hassam Ahmed, H. A. A BLOCKCHAIN-BASED IPFS AUGMENTED DISTRIBUTED INFORMATION SHARING PARADIGM FOR SECURE COMMUNICATION IN NETWORKED ENVIRONMENT.

Jacob, C., Bourke, S., & Heuss, S. (2022). From Testers to Cocreators—the Value of and Approaches to Successful Patient Engagement in the Development of eHealth Solutions: Qualitative Expert Interview Study. *JMIR Human Factors*, *9*(4), e41481. DOI: 10.2196/41481 PMID: 36102548

Jagatheesaperumal, S. K., Pham, Q. V., Ruby, R., Yang, Z., Xu, C., & Zhang, Z. (2022). Explainable AI over the Internet of Things (IoT): Overview, state-of-the-art and future directions. *IEEE Open Journal of the Communications Society*, *3*, 2106–2136. DOI: 10.1109/OJCOMS.2022.3215676

Jaiman, V., & Urovi, V. (2020). A Consent Model for Blockchain-Based Health Data Sharing Platforms. *IEEE Access : Practical Innovations, Open Solutions*, *8*, 143734–143745. DOI: 10.1109/ACCESS.2020.3014565

Jaiswal, A., Gianchandani, N., Singh, D., Kumar, V., & Kaur, M. (2021). Classification of the COVID-19 infected patients using DenseNet201-based deep transfer learning. *Journal of Biomolecular Structure & Dynamics*, *39*(15), 5682–5689. DOI: 10.1080/07391102.2020.1788642 PMID: 32619398

Jalil, S., Rafi, S., LaToza, T. D., Moran, K., & Lam, W. (2023). Chatgpt and software testing education: Promises & perils. In *2023 IEEE International Conference on Software Testing, Verification and Validation Workshops (ICSTW)* (pp. 4130-4137). IEEE. DOI: 10.1109/ICSTW58534.2023.00078

Jamil, F., Ahmad, S., Whangbo, T. K., Muthanna, A., & Kim, D.-H. (2022). Improving blockchain performance in clinical trials using intelligent optimal transaction traffic control mechanism in smart healthcare applications. *Computers & Industrial Engineering*, *170*, 108327. DOI: 10.1016/j.cie.2022.108327

Jampani, R. (2024). *Blockchain Technology in Global Healthcare: A Paradigm Shift.*

Jaoude, J., & Saadé, R. (2019). Blockchain Applications – Usage in Different Domains. *IEEE Access : Practical Innovations, Open Solutions*, *7*, 45360–45381. DOI: 10.1109/ACCESS.2019.2902501

Javaid, M., Haleem, A., & Singh, R. P. (2023). ChatGPT for healthcare services: An emerging stage for an innovative perspective. BenchCouncil Transactions on Benchmarks. *Standards and Evaluations*, *3*(1), 100105.

Javed, A. R., Sarwar, M. U., Beg, M. O., Asim, M., Baker, T., & Tawfik, H. (2020). A collaborative healthcare framework for shared healthcare plan with ambient intelligence. *Human-centric Computing and Information Sciences*, *10*(1), 40. DOI: 10.1186/s13673-020-00245-7

Jayabalan, J., & Jeyanthi, N. (2022). Scalable blockchain model using off-chain IPFS storage for healthcare data security and privacy. *Journal of Parallel and Distributed Computing*, *164*, 152–167. DOI: 10.1016/j.jpdc.2022.03.009

Jiang, L. (2021). IoT Sensors for Smart Health Devices and Data security in Healthcare. *JJ Biomed. Sustain. Healthc. Appl*, 105-112.

Jiang, S., Cao, J., Wu, H., Yang, Y., Ma, M., & He, J. (2018, June). Blochie: a blockchain-based platform for healthcare information exchange. In *2018 ieee international conference on smart computing (smartcomp)* (pp. 49-56). IEEE. DOI: 10.1109/SMARTCOMP.2018.00073

Jodka, S. H. (2024). *HIPAA-free zone? Think again: the surprising state laws regulating collection of health and fitness data.* https://www.reuters.com/legal/litigation/hipaa-free-zone-think-again-surprising-state-laws-regulating-collection-health-2024-10-25/?utm_source=chatgpt.com

Johnson, A. E., Pollard, T. J., Shen, L., Lehman, L.-H., Feng, M., Ghassemi, M., Moody, B., Szolovits, P., Anthony Celi, L., & Mark, R. G. (2016). MIMIC-III, a freely accessible critical care database. *Scientific Data*, *3*(1), 1–9. DOI: 10.1038/sdata.2016.35 PMID: 27219127

Johnson, A. E., Pollard, T. J., Shen, L., Lehman, L.-H., Feng, M., Ghassemi, M., Moody, B., Szolovits, P., Celi, L. A., & Mark, R. G. (2016). Data descriptor: MIMIC-III, a freely accessible critical care database. *Scientific Data*, *3*(160035), 1–9.

Johnson, K. B., Wei, W. Q., Weeraratne, D., Frisse, M. E., Misulis, K., Rhee, K., Zhao, J., & Snowdon, J. L. (2021). Precision medicine, AI, and the future of personalized health care. *Clinical and Translational Science*, *14*(1), 86–93. DOI: 10.1111/cts.12884 PMID: 32961010

Jraisat, L., Jreissat, M., Upadhyay, A., & Kumar, A. (2023). *Blockchain technology: The role of integrated reverse supply chain networks in sustainability.* Paper presented at the Supply chain forum: An international journal. DOI: 10.1080/16258312.2022.2090853

Jum'a, L., Ikram, M., & Jabbour, C. J. C. (2024). Towards circular economy: A IoT enabled framework for circular supply chain integration. *Computers & Industrial Engineering*, *192*, 110194. DOI: 10.1016/j.cie.2024.110194

Junaid, M., Zhang, Q., Cao, M., & Luqman, A. (2023). Nexus between technology enabled supply chain dynamic capabilities, integration, resilience, and sustainable performance: An empirical examination of healthcare organizations. *Technological Forecasting and Social Change*, *196*, 122828. DOI: 10.1016/j.techfore.2023.122828

Junaid, S. B., Imam, A. A., Balogun, A. O., De Silva, L. C., Surakat, Y. A., Kumar, G., & Mahamad, S. (2022, October). Recent advancements in emerging technologies for healthcare management systems: A survey. [). MDPI.]. *Health Care*, *10*(10), 1940. PMID: 36292387

Kairouz, P., McMahan, H. B., Avent, B., Bellet, A., Bennis, M., Bhagoji, A. N., Bonawitz, K., Charles, Z., Cormode, G., & Cummings, R. (2021). Advances and open problems in federated learning. *Foundations and trends® in machine learning, 14*(1–2), 1-210.

Kalasin, S., & Surareungchai, W. (2023). Challenges of emerging wearable sensors for remote monitoring toward telemedicine healthcare. *Analytical Chemistry*, *95*(3), 1773–1784. DOI: 10.1021/acs.analchem.2c02642 PMID: 36629753

Kalsoom, A., Maqsood, M., Yasmin, S., Bukhari, M., Shin, Z., & Rho, S. (2022). A computer-aided diagnostic system for liver tumor detection using modified U-Net architecture. *The Journal of Supercomputing*, *78*(7), 1–23. DOI: 10.1007/s11227-021-04266-6

Kammerer, E., Fawcett-Arsenault, J., Iliscupidez, L., & Ali, S. (2024). Healthcare Professionals' Perspectives on Improving Family-Centred Pain Care in a Tertiary Pediatric Centre. *Canadian Journal of Nursing Research*, *56*(2), 171–177. Advance online publication. DOI: 10.1177/08445621241228063 PMID: 38258330

Kant, N., & Anjali, K. (2021). Blockchain Technology: A Strategic Resource. In Blockchain for Healthcare Systems (pp. 1-15). CRC Press. 13

Kaplan, R. M., & Hays, R. D. (2022). Health-related quality of life measurement in public health. *Annual Review of Public Health*, *43*(1), 355–373. DOI: 10.1146/annurev-publhealth-052120-012811 PMID: 34882431

Karunarathne, S. M., Saxena, N., & Khan, M. K. (2021). Security and privacy in IoT smart healthcare. *IEEE Internet Computing*, *25*(4), 37–48. DOI: 10.1109/MIC.2021.3051675

Kasat, K., Rani, D. L., Khan, B., Kirubakaran, M., & Malathi, P. (2022). A novel security framework for healthcare data through IOT sensors. *Measurement. Sensors*, *24*, 100535. DOI: 10.1016/j.measen.2022.100535

Kasneci, E., Seßler, K., Küchemann, S., Bannert, M., Dementieva, D., Fischer, F., Gasser, U., Groh, G., Günnemann, S., Hüllermeier, E., Krusche, S., Kutyniok, G., Michaeli, T., Nerdel, C., Pfeffer, J., Poquet, O., Sailer, M., Schmidt, A., Seidel, T., & Kasneci, G. (2023). ChatGPT for good? On opportunities and challenges of large language models for education. *Learning and Individual Differences*, *103*, 102274. DOI: 10.1016/j.lindif.2023.102274

Kassani, S. H., Kassani, P. H., Khazaeinezhad, R., Wesolowski, M. J., Schneider, K. A., & Deters, R. (2019). Diabetic retinopathy classification using a modified Xception architecture. In *2019 IEEE International Symposium on Signal Processing and Information Technology (ISSPIT)* (pp. 1–6). DOI: 10.1109/ISSPIT47144.2019.9001846

Kassani, S. H., Kassani, P. H., Wesolowski, M. J., Schneider, K. A., & Deters, R. (2021). Automatic detection of coronavirus disease (COVID-19) in X-ray and CT images: A machine learning-based approach. *Biocybernetics and Biomedical Engineering*, *41*(3), 867–879. DOI: 10.1016/j.bbe.2021.05.013 PMID: 34108787

Kasyapa, M. S., & Vanmathi, C. (2024). Blockchain integration in healthcare: A comprehensive investigation of use cases, performance issues, and mitigation strategies. *Frontiers in Digital Health*, *6*, 1359858. DOI: 10.3389/fdgth.2024.1359858 PMID: 38736708

Kayikci, S., & Khoshgoftaar, T. M. (2024). Blockchain meets machine learning: A survey. *Journal of Big Data*, *11*(1), 9. DOI: 10.1186/s40537-023-00852-y

Kelly, C. J., & Young, A. J. (2017). Promoting innovation in healthcare. *Future Healthcare Journal*, *4*(2), 121–125. DOI: 10.7861/futurehosp.4-2-121 PMID: 31098448

Kelsall-Knight, L., & Stevens, R. (2024). Exploring the implementation of person-centred care in nursing practice. *Nursing Standard (Royal College of Nursing (Great Britain) : 1987)*, *39*(1). DOI: 10.7748/ns.2023.e12190

Kendzerska, T., Zhu, D. T., Gershon, A. S., Edwards, J. D., Peixoto, C., Robillard, R., & Kendall, C. E. (2021). The effects of the health system response to the COVID-19 pandemic on chronic disease management: A narrative review. *Risk Management and Healthcare Policy*, *14*, 575–584. DOI: 10.2147/RMHP.S293471 PMID: 33623448

Kermany, D. (2018). Labeled optical coherence tomography (oct) and chest x-ray images for classification. *Mendeley data*.

Kfoury, E., & Khoury, D. (2018, July). Distributed public key infrastructure and PSK exchange based on blockchain technology. In *2018 IEEE International Conference on Internet of Things (iThings) and IEEE Green Computing and Communications (GreenCom) and IEEE Cyber, Physical and Social Computing (CPSCom) and IEEE Smart Data (SmartData)* (pp. 1116-1120). IEEE. DOI: 10.1109/Cybermatics_2018.2018.00203

Khadidos, A. O., Shitharth, S., Khadidos, A. O., Sangeetha, K., & Alyoubi, K. H. (2022). Healthcare data security using IoT sensors based on random hashing mechanism. *Journal of Sensors, 2022*(1), 8457116. DOI: 10.1155/2022/8457116

Khalid, S., Sajjad, S., Jabbar, S., & Chang, H. (2017). Accurate and efficient shape matching approach using vocabularies of multi-feature space representations. *Journal of Real-Time Image Processing, 13*(3), 449–465. DOI: 10.1007/s11554-015-0545-z

Khalilia, M., Chakraborty, S., & Popescu, M. (2011). Predicting disease risks from highly imbalanced data using random forest. *BMC Medical Informatics and Decision Making, 11*(1), 51. DOI: 10.1186/1472-6947-11-51 PMID: 21801360

Khalsa, U., Pooni, R., Sandborg, C., Balboni, I., Wayman, K., & Lee, T. (2021). Supporting patient-centered care in the pediatric rheumatology setting: Patient, family and provider experiences with ournotes. *Arthritis and Rheumatology, 73*(SUPPL 9).

Khan, A. U., Shahid, A., Tariq, F., Ghaffar, A., Jamal, A., Abbas, S., & Javaid, N. (2020). Enhanced Decentralized Management of Patient-Driven Interoperability Based on Blockchain. In *Lecture Notes in Networks and Systems* (Vol. 97). DOI: 10.1007/978-3-030-33506-9_74

Khan, A. A., Bourouis, S., Kamruzzaman, M., Hadjouni, M., Shaikh, Z. A., Laghari, A. A., Elmannai, H., & Dhahbi, S. (2023). Data security in healthcare industrial internet of things with blockchain. *IEEE Sensors Journal, 23*(20), 25144–25151. DOI: 10.1109/JSEN.2023.3273851

Khanh, H. H., & Khang, A. (2021). The role of artificial intelligence in blockchain applications. In *Reinventing Manufacturing and Business Processes through Artificial Intelligence* (pp. 19–38). CRC Press. DOI: 10.1201/9781003145011-2

Khan, M., & Salah, K. (2018, May). IoT security: Review, blockchain solutions, and open challenges. *Future Generation Computer Systems, 82*, 395–411. DOI: 10.1016/j.future.2017.11.022

Khan, S. N., Loukil, F., Ghedira-Guegan, C., Benkhelifa, E., & Bani-Hani, A. (2021). Blockchain smart contracts: Applications, challenges, and future trends. *Peer-to-Peer Networking and Applications, 14*(5), 2901–2925. DOI: 10.1007/s12083-021-01127-0 PMID: 33897937

Khatri, S., Alzahrani, F. A., Ansari, M. T. J., Agrawal, A., Kumar, R., & Khan, R. A. (2021). A systematic analysis on blockchain integration with healthcare domain: Scope and challenges. *IEEE Access : Practical Innovations, Open Solutions, 9*, 84666–84687. DOI: 10.1109/ACCESS.2021.3087608

Khatun, M. A., Memon, S. F., Eising, C., & Dhirani, L. L. (2023). Machine Learning for Healthcare-IoT Security: A Review and Risk Mitigation. *IEEE Access : Practical Innovations, Open Solutions, 11*, 145869–145896. DOI: 10.1109/ACCESS.2023.3346320

Khedr, A. M., & S, S. R. (2024). Enhancing supply chain management with deep learning and machine learning techniques: A review. *Journal of Open Innovation*, *10*(4), 100379. DOI: 10.1016/j.joitmc.2024.100379

Khezr, S., Moniruzzaman, M., Yassine, A., & Benlamri, R. (2019). Blockchain technology in healthcare: A comprehensive review and directions for future research. *Applied Sciences (Basel, Switzerland)*, *9*(9), 1736. DOI: 10.3390/app9091736

Khogali, H. O., & Mekid, S. (2023). The blended future of automation and AI: Examining some long-term societal and ethical impact features. *Technology in Society*, *73*, 102232. DOI: 10.1016/j.techsoc.2023.102232

Khorram-Manesh, A., Gray, L., Goniewicz, K., Cocco, A., Ranse, J., Phattharapornjaroen, P., Achour, N., Sørensen, J., Peyravi, M., Hertelendy, A. J., Kupietz, K., Bergholtz, J., & Carlström, E. (2024). Care in emergencies and disasters: Can it be person-centered? *Patient Education and Counseling*, *118*, 108046. Advance online publication. DOI: 10.1016/j.pec.2023.108046 PMID: 37924742

Khosravi, M., Zare, Z., Mojtabaeian, S. M., & Izadi, R. (2024). Artificial intelligence and decision-making in healthcare: A thematic analysis of a systematic review of reviews. *Health Services Research and Managerial Epidemiology*, *11*, 23333928241234863. DOI: 10.1177/23333928241234863 PMID: 38449840

Khyati Kapadiya, U. P. (2022). Blockchain and AI-Empowered Healthcare Insurance Fraud Detection: An Analysis, Architecture, and Future Prospects. *IEEE Access : Practical Innovations, Open Solutions*, *10*(7), 79606–79627. DOI: 10.1109/ACCESS.2022.3194569

Kifer, D., & Machanavajjhala, A. (2011). No free lunch in data privacy. *Proceedings of the 2011 ACM SIGMOD International Conference on Management of data*

Ko, H. Y. K., Tripathi, N. K., Mozumder, C., Muengtaweepongsa, S., & Pal, I. (2023). Real-Time Remote Patient Monitoring and Alarming System for Non Communicable Lifestyle Diseases. *International Journal of Telemedicine and Applications*, *2023*(1), 9965226. PMID: 38020047

Kopyto, M., Lechler, S., Heiko, A., & Hartmann, E. (2020). Potentials of blockchain technology in supply chain management: Long-term judgments of an international expert panel. *Technological Forecasting and Social Change*, *161*, 120330. DOI: 10.1016/j.techfore.2020.120330

Kotcher, J., Maibach, E., Miller, J., Campbell, E., Alqodmani, L., Maiero, M., & Wyns, A. (2021). Views of health professionals on climate change and health: A multinational survey study. *The Lancet. Planetary Health*, *5*(5), e316–e323. DOI: 10.1016/S2542-5196(21)00053-X PMID: 33838130

Kouba, P., Kohout, P., Haddadi, F., Bushuiev, A., Samusevich, R., Sedlar, J., Damborsky, J., Pluskal, T., Sivic, J., & Mazurenko, S. (2023). Machine Learning-Guided Protein Engineering. *ACS Catalysis*, *13*(21), 13863–13895. DOI: 10.1021/acscatal.3c02743 PMID: 37942269

Kovaleva, M. A., Nikolaeva, A. R., Uzdenova, B. R., Rafikova, N. F., Trostina, V. V., Marzieva, A. M., & Dorofeev, Y. N. (2024). Arterial blood pressure and its cerebral implications: A comprehensive examination of patient-centered approaches in clinical settings. *Revista Latinoamericana de Hipertensiòn*, *19*(1). Advance online publication. DOI: 10.5281/zenodo.10645465

Kraushaar, J., & Bohnet-Joschko, S. (2022). Smartphone use and security challenges in hospitals: A survey among resident physicians in Germany. *International Journal of Environmental Research and Public Health*, *19*(24), 16546.

Kruse, C. S., Smith, B., Vanderlinden, H., & Nealand, A. (2017). Security techniques for the electronic health records. *Journal of Medical Systems*, *41*(8), 1–9. DOI: 10.1007/s10916-017-0778-4 PMID: 28733949

Kshetri, N. (2023). Blockchain's role in enhancing quality and safety and promoting sustainability in the food and beverage industry. *Sustainability (Basel)*, *15*(23), 16223. DOI: 10.3390/su152316223

Kumar, A., Gupta, D. N., & Kumar, R. (2022). Integration Aspects of AI, IoT, Big Data, and Blockchain in Healthcare Industry. In *Transformation in Healthcare with Emerging Technologies* (pp. 81–104). Chapman and Hall/CRC. DOI: 10.1201/9781003201960-5

Kumar, K., Kumar, N., & Shah, R. (2020). Role of IoT to avoid spreading of COVID-19. *International Journal of Intelligent Networks*, *1*, 32–35. DOI: 10.1016/j.ijin.2020.05.002

Kumar, R., Javeed, D., Aljuhani, A., Jolfaei, A., Kumar, P., & Islam, A. N. (2023). Blockchain-based authentication and explainable AI for securing consumer IoT applications. *IEEE Transactions on Consumer Electronics*.

Kumar, R., Khan, A. A., Kumar, J., Golilarz, N. A., Zhang, S., Ting, Y., & Wang, W. (2021). Blockchain-federated-learning and deep learning models for covid-19 detection using ct imaging. *IEEE Sensors Journal*, *21*(14), 16301–16314. DOI: 10.1109/JSEN.2021.3076767 PMID: 35789224

Kumar, R., Wang, W., Kumar, J., Yang, T., Khan, A., Ali, W., & Ali, I. (2021). An integration of blockchain and AI for secure data sharing and detection of CT images for the hospitals. *Computerized Medical Imaging and Graphics*, *87*, 101812. DOI: 10.1016/j.compmedimag.2020.101812 PMID: 33279761

Kuo, T. T., Kim, H. E., & Ohno-Machado, L. (2017). Blockchain distributed ledger technologies for biomedical and health care applications. *Journal of the American Medical Informatics Association : JAMIA*, *24*(6), 1211–1220. DOI: 10.1093/jamia/ocx068 PMID: 29016974

Kvæl, L. A. H., Bergland, A., & Eldh, A. C. (2024). Preference-based patient participation in intermediate care: Translation, validation and piloting of the 4Ps in Norway. *Health Expectations*, *27*(1), e13899. Advance online publication. DOI: 10.1111/hex.13899 PMID: 37934200

Kwok, A. O., & Treiblmaier, H. (2023). Blockchain technology as a driver of economic development in small economies: A dynamic capabilities framework. *Journal of Decision Systems*, •••, 1–26.

Lan, Z.-C., Huang, G.-Y., Li, Y.-P., Rho, S., Vimal, S., & Chen, B.-W. (2022). Conquering insufficient/imbalanced data learning for the Internet of Medical Things. *Neural Computing & Applications*, •••, 1–10. DOI: 10.1007/s00521-022-06897-z

Laroiya, C., Saxena, D., & Komalavalli, C. (2020). Applications of blockchain technology. In *Handbook of research on blockchain technology* (pp. 213–243). Academic press. DOI: 10.1016/B978-0-12-819816-2.00009-5

Lashkari, B., & Musilek, P. (2021). A Comprehensive Review of Blockchain Consensus Mechanisms. *IEEE Access : Practical Innovations, Open Solutions*, *9*(3), 43620–43652. DOI: 10.1109/ACCESS.2021.3065880

Latif, R. M. A., Iqbal, S., Rizwan, O., Shah, S. U. A., Farhan, M., & Ijaz, F. (2019). *Blockchain transforms the retail level by using a supply chain rules and regulation.* Paper presented at the 2019 2nd International Conference on Communication, Computing and Digital systems (C-CODE).

Latif, R. M. A., Farhan, M., Rizwan, O., Hussain, M., Jabbar, S., & Khalid, S. (2020). Retail level Blockchain transformation for product supply chain using truffle development platform. *Cluster Computing*, •••, 1–16.

Latif, R. M. A., Hussain, K., Jhanjhi, N., Nayyar, A., & Rizwan, O. (2020). A remix IDE: Smart contract-based framework for the healthcare sector by using Blockchain technology. *Multimedia Tools and Applications*, •••, 1–24.

Lau, F., Bartle-Clar, J. A., Bliss, G., Boricky, E. M., Courtney, K. L., Kuo, A., Kushniruk, A., Monkman, H., & Roudsari, A. (2019). *Improving Usability, Safety and Patient Outcomes with Health Information Technology. From Research to Practice*. IOS Press.

Lee, J., Sun, J., Wang, F., Wang, S., Jun, C. H., & Jiang, X. (2018). Privacy-preserving patient similarity learning in a federated environment: Development and analysis. *JMIR Medical Informatics*, *6*(2), e7744. DOI: 10.2196/medinform.7744 PMID: 29653917

Leeming, G., Cunningham, J., & Ainsworth, J. (2019). A Ledger of Me: Personalizing Healthcare Using Blockchain Technology. *Frontiers in Medicine*, *6*, 171. Advance online publication. DOI: 10.3389/fmed.2019.00171 PMID: 31396516

Leffa, D. T., Grevet, E. H., Bau, C. H. D., Schneider, M., Ferrazza, C. P., da Silva, R. F., Miranda, M. S., Picon, F., Teche, S. P., Sanches, P., Pereira, D., Rubia, K., Brunoni, A. R., Camprodon, J. A., Caumo, W., & Rohde, L. A. (2022). Transcranial direct current stimulation vs sham for the treatment of inattention in adults with attention-deficit/hyperactivity disorder: The TUNED randomized clinical trial. *JAMA Psychiatry*, *79*(9), 847–856. DOI: 10.1001/jamapsychiatry.2022.2055 PMID: 35921102

Liang, X., Zhao, J., Shetty, S., Liu, J., & Li, D. (2017). Integrating blockchain for data sharing and collaboration in mobile healthcare applications. 2017 IEEE 28th annual international symposium on personal, indoor, and mobile radio communications (PIMRC), Lim, W. Y. B., Luong, N. C., Hoang, D. T., Jiao, Y., Liang, Y.-C., Yang, Q., Niyato, D., & Miao, C. (2020). Federated learning in mobile edge networks: A comprehensive survey. *IEEE Communications Surveys and Tutorials*, *22*(3), 2031–2063.

Li, C., Chen, Y., & Shang, Y. (2022). A review of industrial big data for decision making in intelligent manufacturing. *Engineering Science and Technology, an International Journal*, *29*, 101021. DOI: 10.1016/j.jestch.2021.06.001

Li, C., Wang, J., Wang, S., & Zhang, Y. (2024). A review of IoT applications in healthcare. *Neurocomputing*, *565*, 127017. DOI: 10.1016/j.neucom.2023.127017

Lichtfous, M., Yadav, V., & Fratino, V. (2018). Can blockchain accelerate financial inclusion globally. *Deloitte Inside Magazine*, *19*(02), 1–8.

Li, D., Gong, Y., Zhang, X., & Huang, M. (2022). An Exploratory Study on the Design and Management Model of Traditional Chinese Medicine Quality Safety Traceability System Based on Blockchain Technology. *Security and Communication Networks*, *2022*, 1–24. Advance online publication. DOI: 10.1155/2022/7011145

Li, J., Cai, J., Khan, F., Rehman, A. U., Balasubramaniam, V., Sun, J., & Venu, P. (2020). A secured framework for sdn-based edge computing in IOT-enabled healthcare system. *IEEE Access : Practical Innovations, Open Solutions*, *8*, 135479–135490. DOI: 10.1109/ACCESS.2020.3011503

Lin, H. (2024). Artificial intelligence with great potential in medical informatics: A brief review. *Medinformatics*, *1*(1), 2–9. DOI: 10.47852/bonviewMEDIN42022204

Liu, H., Crespo, R. G., & Martínez, O. S. (2020, July). Enhancing privacy and data security across healthcare applications using blockchain and distributed ledger concepts. []. MDPI.]. *Health Care*, *8*(3), 243. PMID: 32751325

Liu, J., Jiang, W., Sun, R., Bashir, A. K., Alshehri, M. D., Hua, Q., & Yu, K. (2022). Conditional anonymous remote healthcare data sharing over blockchain. *IEEE Journal of Biomedical and Health Informatics*, *27*(5), 2231–2242. DOI: 10.1109/JBHI.2022.3183397 PMID: 35704539

Liu, S., Zhang, R., Liu, C., & Shi, D. (2023). P-PBFT: An improved blockchain algorithm to support large-scale pharmaceutical traceability. *Computers in Biology and Medicine*, *154*, 106590. DOI: 10.1016/j.compbiomed.2023.106590 PMID: 36736098

Liu, X., Hong, Y., & Sun, J. (2022, August). Blockchain-based medical data storage and sharing system. In *2022 IEEE International Conference on Advances in Electrical Engineering and Computer Applications (AEECA)* (pp. 62-66). IEEE. DOI: 10.1109/AEECA55500.2022.9918841

Liu, Y., Liu, Z., Zhang, Q., Su, J., Cai, Z., & Li, X. (2024). Blockchain and trusted reputation assessment-based incentive mechanism for healthcare services. *Future Generation Computer Systems*, *154*, 59–71. DOI: 10.1016/j.future.2023.12.023

Liu, Y., Tian, J., Hu, R., Yang, B., Liu, S., Yin, L., & Zheng, W. (2022). Improved Feature Point Pair Purification Algorithm Based on SIFT During Endoscope Image Stitching. *Frontiers in Neurorobotics*, *16*, 840594. DOI: 10.3389/fnbot.2022.840594 PMID: 35242022

Liu, Z., & Zhang, X. (2023). Multimedia and multimodal sensing with edge computing for personalized healthcare supply chain system data optimization. *Personal and Ubiquitous Computing*, *27*(3), 955–972. DOI: 10.1007/s00779-022-01679-9

Lomotey, R. K., Pry, J., & Sriramoju, S. (2017). Wearable IoT data stream traceability in a distributed health information system. *Pervasive and Mobile Computing*, *40*, 692–707. DOI: 10.1016/j.pmcj.2017.06.020

Lou, M., Dong, X., Cao, Z., & Shen, J. (2021). SESCF: A Secure and Efficient Supply Chain Framework via Blockchain-Based Smart Contracts. *Security and Communication Networks*, *2021*, 1–18. Advance online publication. DOI: 10.1155/2021/8884478

Lu, W., Wang, J., Chen, Y., Qin, X., Xu, R., Dimitriadis, D., & Qin, T. (2022). Personalized federated learning with adaptive batchnorm for healthcare. *IEEE Transactions on Big Data*. https://doi.org//arXiv.2112.00734DOI: 10.48550

Lu, L. L. M., Henn, P., O'Tuathaigh, C., & Smith, S. (2024). Patient–healthcare provider communication and age-related hearing loss: A qualitative study of patients' perspectives. *Irish Journal of Medical Science*, *193*(1), 277–284. Advance online publication. DOI: 10.1007/s11845-023-03432-4 PMID: 37386348

Lu, Q., Link, E., Baumann, E., & Schulz, P. J. (2024). Linking patient-centered communication with cancer information avoidance: The mediating roles of patient trust and literacy. *Patient Education and Counseling*, *123*, 108230. Advance online publication. DOI: 10.1016/j.pec.2024.108230 PMID: 38484597

Lu, W.-J., Yamada, Y., & Sakuma, J. (2015). Privacy-preserving genome-wide association studies on cloud environment using fully homomorphic encryption. *BMC Medical Informatics and Decision Making*.

Lu, Y. (2019). The blockchain: State-of-the-art and research challenges. *Journal of Industrial Information Integration*, *15*, 80–90. DOI: 10.1016/j.jii.2019.04.002

Maariz, A., Wiputra, M. A., & Armanto, M. R. D. (2024). Blockchain technology: Revolutionizing data integrity and security in digital environments. [ITEE]. *International Transactions on Education Technology*, *2*(2), 92–98. DOI: 10.33050/itee.v2i2.435

Määttä, S., & Björkman, I. (2024). We are not even allowed to call them patients anymore: Conceptions about person-centred care. *Health Expectations*, *27*(1), e13887. Advance online publication. DOI: 10.1111/hex.13887 PMID: 37854003

Mackey, T. K., Liang, B. A., York, P., & Kubic, T. (2015). Counterfeit drug penetration into global legitimate medicine supply chains: A global assessment. *The American Journal of Tropical Medicine and Hygiene*, *92*(6_Suppl, Suppl 6), 59–67. DOI: 10.4269/ajtmh.14-0389 PMID: 25897059

Madanian, S., Chinbat, T., Subasinghage, M., Airehrour, D., Hassandoust, F., & Yongchareon, S. (2024). Health IoT Threats: Survey of Risks and Vulnerabilities. *Future Internet*, *16*(11), 389. DOI: 10.3390/fi16110389

Mahajan, P., Aujla, G. S., & Krishna, C. R. (2024, June). Explainable Edge Computing in a Distributed AI-Powered Autonomous Vehicular Networks. In *2024 IEEE International Conference on Communications Workshops (ICC Workshops)* (pp. 1195-1200). IEEE. DOI: 10.1109/ICCWorkshops59551.2024.10615824

Mahammad, A. B., & Kumar, R. (2023). *Scalable and security framework to secure and maintain healthcare data using blockchain technology.* Paper presented at the 2023 International Conference on Computational Intelligence and Sustainable Engineering Solutions (CISES). DOI: 10.1109/CISES58720.2023.10183494

Maleki Varnosfaderani, S., & Forouzanfar, M. (2024). The role of AI in hospitals and clinics: Transforming healthcare in the 21st century. *Bioengineering (Basel, Switzerland)*, *11*(4), 337. DOI: 10.3390/bioengineering11040337 PMID: 38671759

Mallick, S. R., & Sharma, S. "EMRI: A Scalable and Secure Blockchain-based IoMT Framework for Healthcare Data Transaction," 2021 *International Conference on Information and Communication Technology (OCIT)*, pp. 261-266, DOI: 10.1109/OCIT53463.2021.00060

Mangala, N., Naveen, D. R., Reddy, B. E., Buyya, R., Venugopal, K. R., Iyengar, S. S., & Patnaik, L. M. (2024). Secure pharmaceutical supply chain using blockchain in iot cloud systems. *Internet of Things : Engineering Cyber Physical Human Systems*, *26*, 101215. DOI: 10.1016/j.iot.2024.101215

Manogaran, G., Thota, C., Lopez, D., & Sundarasekar, R. (2017). Big data security intelligence for healthcare industry 4.0. *Cybersecurity for Industry 4.0: Analysis for Design and Manufacturing*, 103-126.

Manoharan, A. (n.d.). *BLOCKCHAIN TECHNOLOGY: REINVENTING TRUST AND SECURITY IN THE DIGITAL WORLD.*

Marito, D. R., & Widianto, S. (2024). Link of Infection Prevention Climate to Patient-Centered Care: Role of Workplace Safety and Risk Mitigation. *Risk Management and Healthcare Policy*, *17*, 329–340. Advance online publication. DOI: 10.2147/RMHP.S439907 PMID: 38352960

Marry, P., Yenumula, K., Katakam, A., Bollepally, A., & Athaluri, A. (2023, June). Blockchain based smart healthcare system. In *2023 International Conference on Sustainable Computing and Smart Systems (ICSCSS)* (pp. 1480-1484). IEEE. DOI: 10.1109/ICSCSS57650.2023.10169704

Masih, E. A. (2022). Feasibility of using QR code for registration & evaluation of training and its ability to increase response rate–The learners' perception. *Nurse Education Today*, *111*, 105305. DOI: 10.1016/j.nedt.2022.105305 PMID: 35220149

Maslove, D. M., Klein, J., Brohman, K., & Martin, P. (2018). Using blockchain technology to manage clinical trials data: A proof-of-concept study. *JMIR Medical Informatics*, *6*(4), e11949. DOI: 10.2196/11949 PMID: 30578196

Mathew, P. S., & Pillai, A. S. (2015, March). Big Data solutions in Healthcare: Problems and perspectives. In *2015 International conference on innovations in information, embedded and communication systems (ICIIECS)* (pp. 1-6). IEEE. DOI: 10.1109/ICIIECS.2015.7193211

Mayer, R., Tahir, S., & Smith, M. R. "Blockchain Technology in Healthcare: Enhancing Data Exchange and Interoperability," *Journal of Medical Systems*, vol. 43, no. 6, pp. 1-12, 2019. [Online]. Available: https://journals.sagepub.com/doi/pdf/10.1177/1460458219866350

Mayra Macas, C. W. (2024). Adversarial examples: A survey of attacks and defenses in deep learning-enabled cybersecurity systems. *Expert Systems with Applications*, *238*(3), 1–12. DOI: 10.1016/j.eswa.2023.122223

Mazlan, A., Abas, H., Abdul Rasid, S. Z., Mohd Sam, S., Yusof, M. F., & Mohd Daud, S. (2020, January). Scalability Challenges in Healthcare Blockchain System—A Systematic Review. *IEEE Access : Practical Innovations, Open Solutions*, *8*, 23663–23673. DOI: 10.1109/ACCESS.2020.2969230

McGhin, T., Choo, K. K. R., Liu, C. Z., & He, D. (2019). Blockchain in healthcare applications: Research challenges and opportunities. *Journal of Network and Computer Applications*, *135*, 62–75. DOI: 10.1016/j.jnca.2019.02.027

McGraw, D. (2013). Building public trust in uses of Health Insurance Portability and Accountability Act de-identified data. *Journal of the American Medical Informatics Association : JAMIA*, *20*(1), 29–34.

McMahan, B., Moore, E., Ramage, D., Hampson, S., & Arcas, B. A. (2017). Communication-efficient learning of deep networks from decentralized data. Artificial intelligence and statistics,

McMahan, B., Moore, E., Ramage, D., Hampson, S., & Arcas, B. A. (2017, April). Communication-efficient learning of deep networks from decentralized data. In *Artificial intelligence and statistics* (pp. 1273–1282). PMLR., DOI: 10.1109/ICDE51399.2021.00040

McSherry, R. O. B., & Douglas, M. (2011). Innovation in nursing practice: A means to tackling the global challenges facing nurses, midwives and nurse leaders and managers in the future. *Journal of Nursing Management*, *19*(2), 165–169. DOI: 10.1111/j.1365-2834.2011.01241.x PMID: 21375618

Megaro, A. (2023). Transparency in AI systems for value co-creation in healthcare. In *Big Data and Decision-Making*. Applications and Uses in the Public and Private Sector., DOI: 10.1108/978-1-80382-551-920231007

Mehrabi, N., Morstatter, F., Saxena, N., Lerman, K., & Galstyan, A. (2021). A survey on bias and fairness in machine learning. *ACM Computing Surveys*, *54*(6), 1–35.

Meidute-Kavaliauskiene, I., Yazdi, A. K., & Mehdiabadi, A. (2022). Integration of blockchain technology and prioritization of deployment barriers in the blood supply chain. *Logistics (Basel)*, *6*(1), 21. DOI: 10.3390/logistics6010021

Mele, G., Capaldo, G., Secundo, G., & Corvello, V. (2023). Revisiting the idea of knowledge-based dynamic capabilities for digital transformation. *Journal of Knowledge Management.*

Mertz, L. (2018). (Block) Chain Reaction: A Blockchain Revolution Sweeps into Health Care, Offering the Possibility for a Much-Needed Data Solution. *IEEE Pulse*, *9*(3), 4–7. DOI: 10.1109/MPUL.2018.2814879 PMID: 29757744

Mettler, M. (2016, September). Blockchain technology in healthcare: The revolution starts here. In 2016 IEEE 18th international conference on e-health networking, applications and services (Healthcom) (pp. 1-3). IEEE.

Mikula, T., & Jacobsen, R. H. (2018, August). Identity and access management with blockchain in electronic healthcare records. In *2018 21st Euromicro conference on digital system design (DSD)* (pp. 699-706). IEEE. DOI: 10.1109/DSD.2018.00008

Min, E., Guo, X., Liu, Q., Zhang, G., Cui, J., & Long, J. (2018). A Survey of Clustering With Deep Learning: From the Perspective of Network Architecture. *IEEE Access : Practical Innovations, Open Solutions*, *6*(7), 39501–39514. DOI: 10.1109/ACCESS.2018.2855437

Miotto, R., Wang, F., Wang, S., Jiang, X., & Dudley, J. T. (2018). Deep learning for healthcare: Review, opportunities and challenges. *Briefings in Bioinformatics*, *19*(6), 1236–1246. DOI: 10.1093/bib/bbx044 PMID: 28481991

Miriam, H., Doreen, D., Dahiya, D., & Rene Robin, C. (2023). Secured Cyber Security Algorithm for Healthcare System Using Blockchain Technology. *Intelligent Automation & Soft Computing*, *35*(2).

Mirin, K. (2021). Implementation of AI in Healthcare: Challenges and Potential.

Mistry, C., Thakker, U., Gupta, R., Obaidat, M. S., Tanwar, S., Kumar, N., & Rodrigues, J. J. 2021, June. MedBlock: An AI-enabled and blockchain-driven medical healthcare system for COVID-19. In *ICC 2021-IEEE International Conference on Communications* (pp. 1-6). IEEE.

Mittelstadt, B. D., Allo, P., Taddeo, M., Wachter, S., & Floridi, L. (2016). The ethics of algorithms: Mapping the debate. *Big Data & Society*, *3*(2), 2053951716679679. DOI: 10.1177/2053951716679679

Moglia, A., Georgiou, K., Georgiou, E., Satava, R. M., & Cuschieri, A. (2021). A systematic review on artificial intelligence in robot-assisted surgery. *International Journal of Surgery*, *95*, 106151. DOI: 10.1016/j.ijsu.2021.106151 PMID: 34695601

Mohamed Yaseen Jabarulla, H.-N. L. (2021). A Blockchain and Artificial Intelligence-Based, Patient-Centric Healthcare System for Combating the COVID-19 Pandemic: Opportunities and Applications. *Healthcare (Basel)*, *9*(8), 1–12. DOI: 10.3390/healthcare9081019 PMID: 34442156

Mohammed, M. A., Lakhan, A., Zebari, D. A., Abd Ghani, M. K., Marhoon, H. A., Abdulkareem, K. H., & Martinek, R. (2024). Securing healthcare data in industrial cyber-physical systems using combining deep learning and blockchain technology. *Engineering Applications of Artificial Intelligence*, *129*, 107612. DOI: 10.1016/j.engappai.2023.107612

Monrat, A., Schelén, O., & Andersson, K. (2019). A Survey of Blockchain From the Perspectives of Applications, Challenges, and Opportunities. *IEEE Access : Practical Innovations, Open Solutions*, *7*, 117134–117151. DOI: 10.1109/ACCESS.2019.2936094

Moosivand, A., Ghatari, A. R., & Rasekh, H. R. (2019). Supply Chain Challenges in Pharmaceutical Manufacturing Companies: Using Qualitative System Dynamics Methodology. *Iranian Journal of Pharmaceutical Research : IJPR*, *18*(2), 1103. PMID: 31531092

Moqurrab, S. A., Tariq, N., Anjum, A., Asheralieva, A., Malik, S. U., Malik, H., Pervaiz, H., & Gill, S. S. (2022). A deep learning-based privacy-preserving model for smart healthcare in Internet of medical things using fog computing. *Wireless Personal Communications*, *126*(3), 2379–2401. DOI: 10.1007/s11277-021-09323-0 PMID: 36059591

Mostafiz, M. I., Musteen, M., Saiyed, A., & Ahsan, M. (2022). COVID-19 and the global value chain: Immediate dynamics and long-term restructuring in the garment industry. *Journal of Business Research*, *139*, 1588–1603. DOI: 10.1016/j.jbusres.2021.10.078

Motamed, S., Rogalla, P., & Khalvati, F. (2021). RANDGAN: Randomized generative adversarial network for detection of COVID-19 in chest X-ray. *Scientific Reports*, *11*(1), 8602. DOI: 10.1038/s41598-021-87994-2 PMID: 33883609

Mukherjee, A., Singh, R., Mishra, R., & Bag, S. (2021). Application of blockchain technology for sustainability development in agricultural supply chain: Justification framework. *Operations Management Research : Advancing Practice Through Research*, *15*(1-2), 46–61. DOI: 10.1007/s12063-021-00180-5

Murthy, C. V. B., & Shri, M. L. (2024, February). Novel Architecture Integrating XAI with Blockchain and IoT Devices for Healthcare. In *2024 Second International Conference on Emerging Trends in Information Technology and Engineering (ICETITE)* (pp. 1-5). IEEE DOI: 10.1109/ic-ETITE58242.2024.10493418

Mwashuma, E. W. (2018). Towards universal healthcare coverage through adoption of blockchain technology: A literature review. *Journal of Health Informatics in Africa*, *5*(2).

Nabiyeva, A., & Wu, D. Z. (2017). Serialization of prescription drugs in the USA: a centralized view (Doctoral dissertation, Massachusetts Institute of Technology).

Naeem, H., & Bin-Salem, A. A. (2021). A CNN-LSTM network with multi-level feature extraction-based approach for automated detection of coronavirus from CT scan and X-ray images. *Applied Soft Computing*, *113*, 107918. DOI: 10.1016/j.asoc.2021.107918 PMID: 34608379

Naehrig, M. Improved Security for a Ring-Based Fully Homomorphic Encryption Scheme.

Nair, A. K., Sahoo, J., & Raj, E. D. (2023). Privacy preserving Federated Learning framework for IoMT based big data analysis using edge computing. *Computer Standards & Interfaces*, *86*, 103720. DOI: 10.1016/j.csi.2023.103720

Nakamoto, S. (2008). Bitcoin. *A peer-to-peer electronic cash system, 21260.*

Nakamoto, S. (2008). Bitcoin: A peer-to-peer electronic cash system.

Nakamoto, S. (2008). *Bitcoin: A peer-to-peer electronic cash system.*https://bitcoin.org/bitcoin.pdf

Nakamoto, S., & Bitcoin, A. (2008). A peer-to-peer electronic cash system. *Bitcoin.–URL: https://bitcoin. org/bitcoin. pdf, 4*(2), 15.

Nakamoto, S. (2008). *Bitcoin: A peer-to-peer electronic cash system*. Satoshi Nakamoto.

Narayanan, A., & Shmatikov, V. (2008). Robust de-anonymization of large sparse datasets. 2008 IEEE Symposium on Security and Privacy (sp 2008), Panayides, A. S., Amini, A., Filipovic, N. D., Sharma, A., Tsaftaris, S. A., Young, A., Foran, D., Do, N., Golemati, S., & Kurc, T. (2020). AI in medical imaging informatics: Current challenges and future directions. *IEEE Journal of Biomedical and Health Informatics*, *24*(7), 1837–1857.

Nasiri, S., Sadoughi, F., Tadayon, M. H., & Dehnad, A. (2019). Security requirements of internet of things-based healthcare system: A survey study. *Acta Informatica Medica*, *27*(4), 253. DOI: 10.5455/aim.2019.27.253-258 PMID: 32055092

Nassimbwa Kabanda, D. (n.d.). The Impact of AI on Reducing Medical Errors. *SSRN*.

National Academies of Sciences, Engineering, and Medicine. (2018). The Current State of Global Health Care Quality. In *Crossing the Global Quality Chasm: Improving Health Care Worldwide*. National Academies Press (US).

Nawaz, H., Maqsood, M., Afzal, S., Aadil, F., Mehmood, I., & Rho, S. (2021). A deep feature-based real-time system for Alzheimer's disease stage detection. *Multimedia Tools and Applications*, *80*(26), 35789–35807. DOI: 10.1007/s11042-020-09087-y

Nguyen, D. C., Ding, M., Pathirana, P. N., & Seneviratne, A. (2021). Blockchain and AI- based solutions to combat coronavirus (COVID-19)-like epidemics: A survey. *IEEE Access : Practical Innovations, Open Solutions*, *9*, 95730–95753. DOI: 10.1109/ACCESS.2021.3093633 PMID: 34812398

Nimmagadda, V. S. P. (2021). Artificial Intelligence and Blockchain Integration for Enhanced Security in Insurance: Techniques, Models, and Real-World Applications. *African Journal of Artificial Intelligence and Sustainable Development*, *1*(2), 187–224.

Nugent, T., Upton, D., & Cimpoesu, M. (2016). Improving data transparency in clinical trials using blockchain smart contracts. *F1000 Research*, *5*, 5. DOI: 10.12688/f1000research.9756.1 PMID: 28357041

O'Donnell, A., Gonyea, J., Wensley, T., & Nizza, M. (2024). High-quality patient-centered palliative care: Interprofessional team members' perceptions of social workers' roles and contribution. *Journal of Interprofessional Care*, *38*(1), 1–9. Advance online publication. DOI: 10.1080/13561820.2023.2238783 PMID: 37525994

O'Riordan, A., & Morin, A. (2023). Pandemic Patient Engagement Success: Maintaining Family Presence Through Partnership. *International Journal of Integrated Care*, *23*(S1), 703. Advance online publication. DOI: 10.5334/ijic.ICIC23270

Obaid, O. I., & Salman, S. A.-B. (2022). Security and privacy in IoT-based healthcare systems: A review. *Mesopotamian Journal of Computer Science*, *2022*, 29–39. DOI: 10.58496/MJCSC/2022/007

OECD. (2018). Innovation and Access to Medicines. *OECD*. https://www.oecd.org/content/dam/oecd/en/publications/reports/2018/11/pharmaceutical-innovation-and-access-to-medicines_g1g98d77/9789264307391-en.pdf

Office of the National Coordinator for Health Information Technology. (2018). *Blockchain and health IT: Algorithms, privacy, and data* (White paper). U.S. Department of Health and Human Services. https://www.healthit.gov/sites/default/files/1-78-blockchainandhealthitalgorithmsprivacydata_whitepaper.pdf

Okamura, M., Fujimori, M., Otsuki, A., Saito, J., Yaguchi-Saito, A., Kuchiba, A., Uchitomi, Y., & Shimazu, T. (2024). Patients' perceptions of patient-centered communication with healthcare providers and associated factors in Japan – The INFORM Study 2020. *Patient Education and Counseling*, *122*, 108170. Advance online publication. DOI: 10.1016/j.pec.2024.108170 PMID: 38308974

Omar, I. A., Jayaraman, R., Debe, M. S., Salah, K., Yaqoob, I., & Omar, M. (2021). Automating procurement contracts in the healthcare supply chain using blockchain smart contracts. *IEEE Access : Practical Innovations, Open Solutions*, *9*, 37397–37409. DOI: 10.1109/ACCESS.2021.3062471

Omar, M., Bhuiyan, M. Z. A., Basu, A., Kiyomoto, S., & Rahman, M. S. (2019). Bhuiyan, A. Basu, S. Kiyomoto, and M. Rahman, "Privacy-Friendly Platform for Healthcare Data in Cloud Based on Blockchain Environment,". *Future Generation Computer Systems*, *95*, 511–521. DOI: 10.1016/j.future.2018.12.044

Omidian, H. (2024). Synergizing blockchain and artificial intelligence to enhance healthcare. *Drug Discovery Today*, *29*(9), 104111. DOI: 10.1016/j.drudis.2024.104111 PMID: 39034026

Otoom, M., Otoum, N., Alzubaidi, M. A., Etoom, Y., & Banihani, R. (2020). An IoT-based framework for early identification and monitoring of COVID-19 cases. *Biomedical Signal Processing and Control*, *62*, 102149. DOI: 10.1016/j.bspc.2020.102149 PMID: 32834831

Pablo, R.-G. J., Roberto, D.-P., Victor, S.-U., Isabel, G.-R., Paul, C., & Elizabeth, O.-R. (2022). Big data in the healthcare system: A synergy with artificial intelligence and blockchain technology. *Journal of Integrative Bioinformatics*, *19*(1), 20200035. DOI: 10.1515/jib-2020-0035 PMID: 34412176

Panda, S. K., & Satapathy, S. C. (2021). Drug traceability and transparency in medical supply chain using blockchain for easing the process and creating trust between stakeholders and consumers. *Personal and Ubiquitous Computing*, •••, 1–17.

Pandey, P., & Litoriya, R. (2020). Securing and Authenticating Healthcare Records through Blockchain Technology. *Cryptologia*, *44*(4), 341–356. DOI: 10.1080/01611194.2019.1706060

Pant, H., Sharma, M., & Soman, S. (2019). Twin neural networks for the classification of large unbalanced datasets. *Neurocomputing*, *343*, 34–49. DOI: 10.1016/j.neucom.2018.07.089

Patil et al. (2022). "Utilization of Artificial Intelligence in Healthcare System, Pharmaceutical Industry & Education". International Journal of Advanced Research in Science, Communication and Technology.

Paul, M., Maglaras, L., Ferrag, M. A., & Almomani, I. (2023). Digitization of the healthcare sector: A study on privacy and security concerns. *ICT Express*, *9*(4), 571–588. DOI: 10.1016/j.icte.2023.02.007

Pawar, P., Edoh, T. O., Singh, M., & Parolia, N. (2021). Hitching medical iot devices to blockchain for personal health information management. *Blockchain Technology for IoT Applications*, 191-205.

Peng, S., Hu, X., Zhang, J., Xie, X., Long, C., Tian, Z., & Jiang, H. (2020). An Efficient Double-Layer Blockchain Method for Vaccine Production Supervision. *IEEE Transactions on Nanobioscience*, *19*(3), 579–587. DOI: 10.1109/TNB.2020.2999637 PMID: 32603300

Pereira, R., Bianchi, I. S., & Araújo, V. M. D. S. (2021). Multi-framework implementation of the problem management process. *Форсайт*, *15*(3, 3 (eng)), 94–104. DOI: 10.17323/2500-2597.2021.3.94.104

Pesqueira, A. M., Sousa, M., & Pereira, R. (2023). Individual dynamic capabilities influential factors in blockchain technology innovation from hospital settings.

Pesqueira, A., & Sousa, M. J. (2022). Life Sciences Industry Blockchain Value Management, Investments, and Finance Impact Assessment: Global Questionnaire Survey of 1524 Industry Professionals and Executives. In Incorporating AI Technology in the Service Sector (pp. 67-107). Apple Academic Press.

Pesqueira, A., & Sousa, M. J. (2022). *12 Social Analytics Influencing KOLs Profiling in the Dissemination of Innovations and Scientific Knowledge in the Life Sciences Industry*. Innovations and Social Media Analytics in a Digital Society.

Peterson, K., Deeduvanu, R., Kanjamala, P., & Boles, K. (2017). A Blockchain Approach to Health Information Exchange Networks. *Mayo Clinic. Disponível:*https://www. healthit. gov/sites/default/files/12-55-blockchain-based-approach-final. pdf

Pham, H. L., Tran, T. H., & Nakashima, Y. (2019, December 1). Practical Anti-Counterfeit Medicine Management System Based on Blockchain Technology. *TIMES-ICON 2019 - 2019 4th Technology Innovation Management and Engineering Science International Conference*. DOI: 10.1109/TIMES-iCON47539.2019.9024674

Pinto-Coelho, L. (2023). How artificial intelligence is shaping medical imaging technology: A survey of innovations and applications. *Bioengineering (Basel, Switzerland)*, *10*(12), 1435. DOI: 10.3390/bioengineering10121435 PMID: 38136026

Pisani, E., Hasnida, A., Rahmi, M., Kok, M. O., Harsono, S., & Anggriani, Y. (2021). Substandard and falsified medicines: Proposed methods for case finding and sentinel surveillance. In JMIR Public Health and Surveillance (Vol. 7, Issue 8). JMIR Publications Inc. DOI: 10.2196/29309

Ploug, T. (2020). In Defence of informed consent for health record research-why arguments from 'easy rescue','no harm'and 'consent bias' fail. *BMC Medical Ethics*, *21*(1), 75. DOI: 10.1186/s12910-020-00519-w PMID: 32819343

Prainsack, B., & Buyx, A. (2017). *Solidarity in biomedicine and beyond* (Vol. 33). Cambridge University Press. DOI: 10.1017/9781139696593

Pramesha Chandrasiri, G., Halgamuge, M. N., & Subhashi Jayasekara, C. (2019). A comparative study in the application of IoT in health care: data security in telemedicine. *Security, Privacy and Trust in the IoT Environment*, 181-202.

Pranav, R., Amanpreet, K., Sparsh, S., Mohammad, S., & Gaurav, D. (2021). Application of Blockchain and Internet of Things in Healthcare and Medical Sector: Applications, Challenges, and Future Perspectives. *Journal of Food Quality*, *21*(3), 1–20. Advance online publication. DOI: 10.1155/2021/7608296

Pranto Kumar Ghosh, A. C. (2024). Blockchain Application in Healthcare Systems: A Review. *Systems*, *11*(1), 1–44. DOI: 10.3390/systems11010038

PRNewswire. (2024, June). Medical Virtual Assistant Market. https://www.prnewswire.com/news-releases/medical-virtual-assistant-market-size-to-grow-usd-2668-4-million-by-2029-at-a-cagr-of-27-9--valuates-reports-302168403.html

Punia, A., Gulia, P., Gill, N. S., Ibeke, E., Iwendi, C., & Shukla, P. K. (2024). A systematic review on blockchain-based access control systems in cloud environments. *Journal of Cloud Computing (Heidelberg, Germany)*, *13*(1), 146. DOI: 10.1186/s13677-024-00697-7

Qayyum, A., Ahmad, K., Ahsan, M. A., Al-Fuqaha, A., & Qadir, J. (2022). Collaborative federated learning for healthcare: Multi-modal covid-19 diagnosis at the edge. *IEEE Open Journal of the Computer Society*, *3*, 172–184. DOI: 10.1109/OJCS.2022.3206407

Qin, X., Su, Q., Huang, S. H., Wiersma, U. J., & Liu, M. (2019). Service quality coordination contracts for online shopping service supply chain with competing service providers: Integrating fairness and individual rationality. *Operations Research*, *19*(1), 269–296. DOI: 10.1007/s12351-016-0288-z

Quayson, M., Avornu, E. K., & Bediako, A. K. (2024). Modeling the enablers of blockchain technology implementation for information management in healthcare supply chains. *Modern Supply Chain Research Applications*(ahead-of-print).

Rabah, K. (2017). Challenges & opportunities for blockchain powered healthcare systems: A review. *Mara res. j. med. health sci, 1*(1), 45-52.

Radanović, I., & Likić, R. (2018). Opportunities for use of blockchain technology in medicine. *Applied Health Economics and Health Policy, 16*(5), 583–590. DOI: 10.1007/s40258-018-0412-8 PMID: 30022440

Raghupathi, W., Raghupathi, V., & Saharia, A. (2023). *Analyzing Health Data Breaches: A Visual Analytics Approach.* AppliedMath., DOI: 10.3390/appliedmath3010011

Rahman, M. A., Hossain, M. S., Islam, M. S., Alrajeh, N. A., & Muhammad, G. (2020). Secure and provenance enhanced internet of health things framework: A blockchain managed federated learning approach. *IEEE Access : Practical Innovations, Open Solutions, 8*, 205071–205087. DOI: 10.1109/ACCESS.2020.3037474 PMID: 34192116

Rahman, M. A., Hossain, M. S., Showail, A. J., Alrajeh, N. A., & Alhamid, M. F. (2021). A secure, private, and explainable IoHT framework to support sustainable health monitoring in a smart city. *Sustainable Cities and Society, 72*, 103083. DOI: 10.1016/j.scs.2021.103083

Rajadevi, R., Devi, E. R., Latha, R. S., Harshini, S., Ajay, K., & Abinash, M. (2022, January). Secured storing and sharing of medical records based on blockchain. In *2022 International Conference on Computer Communication and Informatics (ICCCI)* (pp. 1-5). IEEE. DOI: 10.1109/ICCCI54379.2022.9741070

Rajkomar, A., Dean, J., & Kohane, I. (2019). Machine learning in medicine. *The New England Journal of Medicine, 380*(14), 1347–1358. DOI: 10.1056/NEJMra1814259 PMID: 30943338

Rajotte, J. F., Mukherjee, S., Robinson, C., Ortiz, A., West, C., Ferres, J. M. L., & Ng, R. T. (2021, September). Reducing bias and increasing utility by federated generative modeling of medical images using a centralized adversary. In *Proceedings of the conference on information Technology for Social Good* (pp. 79-84). DOI: 10.1145/3462203.3475875

Ramasamy, L. K., & Khan, F. (2024). *Blockchain for Global Education.* Springer. DOI: 10.1007/978-3-031-52123-2

Ram, H., Sahadevan, S., Gale, N., Caggiano, M. P., Yu, X., Ohno, C., & Heisler, M. G. (2020). An integrated analysis of cell-type specific gene expression reveals genes regulated by REVOLUTA and KANADI1 in the Arabidopsis shoot apical meristem. *PLOS Genetics, 16*(4), e1008661. DOI: 10.1371/journal.pgen.1008661 PMID: 32294082

Ramzan, S., Aqdus, A., Ravi, V., Koundal, D., Amin, R., & Ghamdi, M. A. (2023). Healthcare Applications Using Blockchain Technology: Motivations and Challenges. *IEEE Transactions on Engineering Management, 70*(8), 2874–2890. DOI: 10.1109/TEM.2022.3189734

Rane, N., Choudhary, S., & Rane, J. (2023). Explainable Artificial Intelligence (XAI) in healthcare: Interpretable Models for Clinical Decision Support. Available at *SSRN* 4637897. DOI: 10.2139/ssrn.4637897

Razzaq, A., Mohsan, S. A. H., Ghayyur, S. A. K., Al-Kahtani, N., Alkahtani, H. K., & Mostafa, S. M. (2022, December). Blockchain in healthcare: a decentralized platform for digital health passport of COVID-19 based on vaccination and immunity certificates. In Healthcare (Vol. 10, No. 12, p. 2453). MDPI.

Razzaq, A., Ahmad, A., Malik, A. W., Fahmideh, M., & Ramadan, R. A. (2023). Software engineering for internet of underwater things to analyze oceanic data. *Internet of Things : Engineering Cyber Physical Human Systems*, *24*, 100893. DOI: 10.1016/j.iot.2023.100893

Razzaq, A., Mohsan, S. A. H., Ghayyur, S. A. K., Alsharif, M. H., Alkahtani, H. K., Karim, F. K., & Mostafa, S. M. (2022). Blockchain-Enabled Decentralized Secure Big Data of Remote Sensing. *Electronics (Basel)*, *11*(19), 3164. DOI: 10.3390/electronics11193164

Razzaq, A., Zhang, T., Numair, M., Alreshidi, A., Jing, C., Aljaloud, A., & Qurat Ul Ain, M. (2024). Transforming academic assessment: The metaverse-backed Web 3 secure exam system. *Computer Applications in Engineering Education*, *32*(6), e22797.

Rehman, A., & Ilyas, M. (2024). Blockchain-Enhanced Privacy and Security in Medicare Data Sharing: Identifying Gaps and Solutions in Current Practices. *Internet of Things and Data Analytics*, *1145*(2), 432–442. DOI: 10.1007/978-3-031-53717-2_40

Rieke, N., Hancox, J., Li, W., Milletari, F., Roth, H. R., Albarqouni, S., Bakas, S., Galtier, M. N., Landman, B. A., Maier-Hein, K., Ourselin, S., Sheller, M., Summers, R. M., Trask, A., Xu, D., Baust, M., & Cardoso, M. J. (2020). The future of digital health with federated learning. *NPJ Digital Medicine*, *3*(1), 1–7. DOI: 10.1038/s41746-020-00323-1 PMID: 33015372

Rinehart-Thompson, L. A. (2013). *Health information management and compliance: Challenges in HIPAA implementat(2013)*.https://pmc.ncbi.nlm.nih.gov/articles/PMC3797550/

Roberta Bernardi, S. S. (2019). The Role of Affordances in the Deinstitutionalization of a Dysfunctional Health Management Information System in Kenya. *Management Information Systems Quarterly*, *43*(4), 1177–1200. Advance online publication. DOI: 10.25300/MISQ/2019/14187

Rodríguez-Barroso, N., Stipcich, G., Jiménez-López, D., Ruiz-Millán, J. A., Martínez-Cámara, E., González-Seco, G., Luzón, M. V., Veganzones, M. A., & Herrera, F. (2020). Federated Learning and Differential Privacy: Software tools analysis, the Sherpa. ai FL framework and methodological guidelines for preserving data privacy. *Information Fusion*, *64*, 270–292. DOI: 10.1016/j.inffus.2020.07.009

Rohila, V. S., Gupta, N., Kaul, A., & Sharma, D. K. (2021). Deep learning-assisted COVID-19 detection using full CT scans. *Internet of Things : Engineering Cyber Physical Human Systems*, *14*, 100377. DOI: 10.1016/j.iot.2021.100377 PMID: 38620521

Rumbold, J. M. M., & Pierscionek, B. (2017). The effect of the general data protection regulation on medical research. *Journal of Medical Internet Research*, *19*(2), e47. DOI: 10.2196/jmir.7108 PMID: 28235748

Rundle, J. (Dec. 27, 2024). *Healthcare Providers Face Stiffer Cyber Rules Even as They Cry for Help*. https://www.wsj.com/articles/healthcare-providers-face-stiffer-cyber-rules-even-as-they-cry-for-help-b466197a?utm_source=chatgpt.com

Sabri, Y., Harchi, S., & El Kamoun, N. (2022). Managing health supply chain using blockchain technology: State of art challenges and solution. *International Journal of Reconfigurable Embedded Systems*, *11*(3), 258. DOI: 10.11591/ijres.v11.i3.pp258-264

Sadhya, V., & Sadhya, H. (2018). Barriers to adoption of blockchain technology.

Sagi, O., & Rokach, L. (2018). Ensemble learning: A survey. *Wiley Interdisciplinary Reviews. Data Mining and Knowledge Discovery*, *8*(4), e1249. DOI: 10.1002/widm.1249

Saha, E., Rathore, P., & Gigi, A. (2021). Utilizing Blockchain Technology to Manage Functional Areas in Healthcare Systems. In *The Big Data-Driven Digital Economy: Artificial and Computational Intelligence* (pp. 125-139): Springer. DOI: 10.1007/978-3-030-73057-4_11

Saha, E., Rathore, P., Parida, R., & Rana, N. P. (2022). The interplay of emerging technologies in pharmaceutical supply chain performance: An empirical investigation for the rise of Pharma 4.0. *Technological Forecasting and Social Change*, *181*, 121768. DOI: 10.1016/j.techfore.2022.121768

Sai, S., Chamola, V., Choo, K. K. R., Sikdar, B., & Rodrigues, J. J. (2022). Confluence of blockchain and artificial intelligence technologies for secure and scalable healthcare solutions: A review. *IEEE Internet of Things Journal*, *10*(7), 5873–5897. DOI: 10.1109/JIOT.2022.3232793

Salah, K., Rehman, M. H. U., Nizamuddin, N., & Al-Fuqaha, A. (2019). Blockchain for AI: Review and Open Research Challenges. *IEEE Access : Practical Innovations, Open Solutions*, *7*, 10127–10149. DOI: 10.1109/ACCESS.2018.2890507

Salama, R., & Ragab, M. (2023). Blockchain with Explainable Artificial Intelligence Driven Intrusion Detection for Clustered IoT Driven Ubiquitous Computing System. *Computer Systems Science and Engineering*, *46*(3), 2917–2932. DOI: 10.32604/csse.2023.037016

Samala, A. D., & Rawas, S. (2024). Generative AI as Virtual Healthcare Assistant for Enhancing Patient Care Quality. *International Journal of Online & Biomedical Engineering*, *20*(5), 174–187. DOI: 10.3991/ijoe.v20i05.45937

Sarkar, S. (2022b). *International Journal of Advance Research in Computer Science and Management Studies Online Drug trade-a threat to pharmaceutical industry.* Retrieved from www.ijarcsms.com

Sarkar, S. (2022). Supply chain security act 2023: Interoperable data exchange for drug traceability. *Int. J. Sci. Res. Comput. Sci. Eng. Inf. Technol*, *8*(3), 471–477.

Sarkar, S. (2022a). Digital Traceability of pharmaceutical drugs in supply chain. *International Journal of Advance Research in Computer Science and Management Studies*, *10*(2). www.ijarcsms.com

Sarker, L., Islam, M. M., Hannan, T., & Ahmed, Z. (2020). COVID-DenseNet: A deep learning architecture to detect COVID-19 from chest radiology images. *arXiv preprint*, arXiv:2003.11055. https://doi.org/DOI: 10.20944/preprints202005.0151.v1

Sarker, M. (2024). Reinventing Wellness: How Machine Learning Transforms Healthcare. *Journal of Artificial Intelligence General Science (JAIGS) ISSN:3006-4023*, *3*(1). DOI: 10.60087/jaigs.v3i1.73

Sarode, R. P., Poudel, M., Shrestha, S., & Bhalla, S. (2021). Blockchain for committing peer-to-peer transactions using distributed ledger technologies. *International Journal on Computer Science and Engineering*, *24*(3), 215–227.

Sarthak Dhingra, R. R. (2023). Blockchain Technology Applications in Healthcare Supply Chains—A Review. *IEEE Access : Practical Innovations, Open Solutions*, *12*(1), 11230–11257. DOI: 10.1109/ACCESS.2023.3348813

Saxena, N., Thomas, I., Gope, P., Burnap, P., & Kumar, N. (2020). Pharmacrypt: Blockchain for critical pharmaceutical industry to counterfeit drugs. *Computer*, *53*(7), 29–44. DOI: 10.1109/MC.2020.2989238

Saygılı, A. (2021). A new approach for computer-aided detection of coronavirus (COVID-19) from CT and X-ray images using machine learning methods. *Applied Soft Computing*, *105*, 107323. DOI: 10.1016/j.asoc.2021.107323 PMID: 33746657

Schwartz, S. (2016). Does HIPAA hit its mark. *Medical Economics*.

Secinaro, , Calandra, D., Secinaro, A., Muthurangu, V., & Biancone, P. (2021). The role of artificial intelligence in healthcare: A structured literature review. *BMC Medical Informatics and Decision Making*, *21*(1), 125. DOI: 10.1186/s12911-021-01488-9 PMID: 33836752

Segal, G., Martsiano, Y., Markinzon, A., Mayer, A., Halperin, A., & Zimlichman, E. (2023). A blockchain-based computerized network infrastructure for the transparent, immutable calculation and dissemination of quantitative, measurable parameters of academic and medical research publications. *Digital Health*, *9*, 20552076231194851. Advance online publication. DOI: 10.1177/20552076231194851 PMID: 37654719

Seh, A. H., Zarour, M., Alenezi, M., Sarkar, A. K., Agrawal, A., & Khan, A. R. (2020). Healthcare Data Breaches: Insights and Implications. *Health Care*, *8*, 133. PMID: 32414183

Senna, P., Reis, A., Dias, A., Coelho, O., Guimarães, J., & Eliana, S. (2021). Healthcare supply chain resilience framework: Antecedents, mediators, consequents. *Production Planning and Control*, •••, 1–15.

Shafik, W. (2023). Wearable Medical Electronics in Artificial Intelligence of Medical Things. In *Handbook of Security and Privacy of AI-Enabled Healthcare Systems and Internet of Medical Things*. https://doi.org/DOI: 10.1201/9781003370321-2

Shafik, W. (2024a). Artificial Intelligence-Enabled Internet of Medical Things (AIoMT) in Modern Healthcare Practices. In *Clinical Practice and Unmet Challenges in AI-Enhanced Healthcare Systems* (pp. 42–69). IGI Global. DOI: 10.4018/979-8-3693-2703-6.ch003

Shafik, W. (2024f). Smart Health Revolution: Exploring Artificial Intelligence of Internet of Medical Things. In *Healthcare Industry Assessment: Analyzing Risks, Security, and Reliability* (pp. 201–229). Springer. DOI: 10.1007/978-3-031-65434-3_9

Shafik, W. (2025a). Artificial Intelligence Assisted Internet of Medical Things (AIoMTs) in Sustainable Healthcare Ecosystem. *Wellness Management Powered by AI Technologies*, 75–101.

Shafik, W. (2025b). Human-Artificial Intelligence Collaborations in Polycystic Ovary Syndrome (PCOS) Clinical Trials and Research. In *AI-Based Nutritional Intervention in Polycystic Ovary Syndrome (PCOS)* (pp. 307–330). Springer Nature Singapore. DOI: 10.1007/978-981-96-2120-0_13

Shafik, W. (2025d). Revolutionizing Skin Cancer Diagnosis With Artificial Intelligence: Insights Into Machine Learning Techniques. In *Impact of Digital Solutions for Improved Healthcare Delivery* (pp. 167–194). IGI Global.

Shafik, W., & Kalinaki, K. (2024). Societal and Ethical Implications of Technology-Enhanced Agriculture and Healthcare: An African Context. *2024 IST-Africa Conference (IST-Africa)*, 1–11. DOI: 10.23919/IST-Africa63983.2024.10569306

Shafik, W. (2024b). Artificial Intelligence-Enabled Internet of Medical Things for Enhanced Healthcare Systems. In *Smart Healthcare Systems* (pp. 119–134). CRC Press., DOI: 10.1201/9781032698519-9

Shafik, W. (2024c). Connected healthcare—the impact of Internet of Things on medical services. In *Artificial Intelligence and Internet of Things based Augmented Trends for Data Driven Systems* (pp. 181–217). CRC Press., DOI: 10.1201/9781003497318-10

Shafik, W. (2024d). Digital healthcare systems in a federated learning perspective. In *Federated Learning for Digital Healthcare Systems* (pp. 1–35). Elsevier., DOI: 10.1016/B978-0-443-13897-3.00001-1

Shafik, W. (2024e). IoT-Enabled Secure and Intelligent Smart Healthcare. In *Secure and Intelligent IoT-Enabled Smart Cities* (pp. 308–333). IGI Global., DOI: 10.4018/979-8-3693-2373-1.ch015

Shafik, W. (2024g). The Future of Healthcare: AIoMT—Redefining Healthcare with Advanced Artificial Intelligence and Machine Learning Techniques. In *Artificial Intelligence and Machine Learning in Drug Design and Development* (pp. 605–634). Wiley., DOI: 10.1002/9781394234196.ch19

Shafik, W. (2024h). The Future of Healthcare: Data-Driven Trends and Innovation. In *Advancing Healthcare through Data-driven Innovations* (pp. 166–185). CRC Press. DOI: 10.1201/9781003475392-11

Shafik, W. (2025c). Introduction to Machine Learning and Its Applications to Neuroscience. In *Machine Learning for Neurodegenerative Disorders* (pp. 1–32). CRC Press., DOI: 10.1201/9781032661025-1

Shafik, W. (2025e). Smart biomedical devices for smart healthcare. In *Machine Learning Models and Architectures for Biomedical Signal Processing* (pp. 421–448). Elsevier. DOI: 10.1016/B978-0-443-22158-3.00017-X

Shafik, W., Singh, R., & Kumar, V. (2025). Artificial Intelligence Transparency and Explainability in Sustainable Healthcare. In *Transforming Healthcare Sector Through Artificial Intelligence and Environmental Sustainability* (pp. 165–191). Springer.

Shah, Y., Verma, Y., Sharma, U., Sampat, A., & Kulkarni, V. (2023). *Supply chain for safe & timely distribution of medicines using blockchain & machine learning.* Paper presented at the 2023 5th International Conference on Smart Systems and Inventive Technology (ICSSIT). DOI: 10.1109/ICSSIT55814.2023.10061049

Shahid, J., Ahmad, R., Kiani, A. K., Ahmad, T., Saeed, S., & Almuhaideb, A. M. (2022). Data protection and privacy of the internet of healthcare things (IoHTs). *Applied Sciences (Basel, Switzerland)*, *12*(4), 1927. DOI: 10.3390/app12041927

Shah, P., Patel, C., Patel, J., Shah, A., Pandya, S., & Sojitra, B. (2024, October). Utilizing Blockchain Technology for Healthcare and Biomedical Research: A Review. *Cureus*, *16*(10). Advance online publication. DOI: 10.7759/cureus.72040 PMID: 39569280

Shah, V., Keniya, R., Shridharani, A., Punjabi, M., Shah, J., & Mehendale, N. (2021). Diagnosis of COVID-19 using CT scan images and deep learning techniques. *Emergency Radiology*, *28*(4), 497–505. DOI: 10.1007/s10140-020-01886-y PMID: 33523309

Shahzad, W., Chen, W., Shaheen, M., Zhang, Y., & Ahmad, F. (2024). Chen, M. Shaheen, Y. Zhang, and F. Ahmad, "A Robust Algorithm for Authenticated Health Data Access via Blockchain and Cloud Computing,". *PLoS One*, *19*(9), e0307039. Advance online publication. DOI: 10.1371/journal.pone.0307039 PMID: 39312513

Shan, F., Gao, Y., Wang, J., Shi, W., Shi, N., Han, M., ... (2020). Lung infection quantification of COVID-19 in CT images with deep learning. *arXiv preprint*, arXiv:2003.04655.

Shari, N. F. M., & Malip, A. (2024). Enhancing privacy and security in smart healthcare: A blockchain-powered decentralized data dissemination scheme. *Internet of Things : Engineering Cyber Physical Human Systems*, *27*, 101256. DOI: 10.1016/j.iot.2024.101256

Sheeraz, M. M., Mozumder, M. A. I., Khan, M. O., Abid, M. U., Joo, M. I., & Kim, H. C. (2023, February). Blockchain system for trustless healthcare data sharing with hyperledger fabric in action. In *2023 25th International Conference on Advanced Communication Technology (ICACT)* (pp. 437-440). IEEE. DOI: 10.23919/ICACT56868.2023.10079423

Sheetz, K. H., Claflin, J., & Dimick, J. B. (2020). Trends in the adoption of robotic surgery for common surgical procedures. *JAMA Network Open*, *3*(1), e1918911–e1918911. DOI: 10.1001/jamanetworkopen.2019.18911 PMID: 31922557

Sheller, M. J., Edwards, B., Reina, G. A., Martin, J., Pati, S., Kotrotsou, A., Milchenko, M., Xu, W., Marcus, D., Colen, R. R., & Bakas, S. (2020). Federated learning in medicine: Facilitating multi-institutional collaborations without sharing patient data. *Scientific Reports*, *10*(1), 12598. DOI: 10.1038/s41598-020-69250-1 PMID: 32724046

Shi, H., Han, X., Jiang, N., Cao, Y., Alwalid, O., Gu, J., Fan, Y., & Zheng, C. (2020). Radiological findings from 81 patients with COVID-19 pneumonia in Wuhan, China: A descriptive study. *The Lancet. Infectious Diseases*, *20*(4), 425–434. DOI: 10.1016/S1473-3099(20)30086-4 PMID: 32105637

Shinde, R., Patil, S., Kotecha, K., Potdar, V., Selvachandran, G., & Abraham, A. (2024). Securing AI-based healthcare systems using blockchain technology: A state-of-the-art systematic literature review and future research directions. *Transactions on Emerging Telecommunications Technologies*, *35*(1), e4884. DOI: 10.1002/ett.4884

Shini, S. G., Thomas, T., & Chithraranjan, K. (2012). Cloud Based Medical Image Exchange-Security Challenges. *Procedia Engineering*, *38*, 3454–3461. DOI: 10.1016/j.proeng.2012.06.399

Shivani, B., Vikram, B., Mohanty, R. P., & Dev, G. (2023). Analysis of critical success factors for blockchain technology implementation in healthcare sector. *Benchmarking*, *30*(4), 1367–1399. DOI: 10.1108/BIJ-07-2021-0433

Shiwlani, A., Khan, M., Sherani, A. M. K., & Qayyum, M. U. (2023). Synergies of AI and Smart Technology: Revolutionizing Cancer Medicine, Vaccine Development, and Patient Care. International Journal of Social. *Humanities and Life Sciences*, *1*(1), 10–18.

Shome, A., Amiri, S., & Belloum, A. S. Systematic Literature Review of Privacy-Preserving Deep Learning in Medical Image Analysis.

Shrobe, H., Shrier, D. L., & Pentland, A. (2018). Enigma: Decentralized computation platform with guaranteed privacy.

Shuker, C., Hamblin, R., Stolarek, I., & Simpson, A. (2018). Transparency in Healthcare 2017: Working with Consumers and Clinicians to Co-design a Transparent Future. *International Journal of Integrated Care*, *18*(s1), 34. Advance online publication. DOI: 10.5334/ijic.s1034

Silva, P., Luz, E., Silva, G., Moreira, G., Silva, R., Lucio, D., & Menotti, D. (2020). COVID-19 detection in CT images with deep learning: A voting-based scheme and cross-datasets analysis. *Informatics in Medicine Unlocked*, *20*, 100427. DOI: 10.1016/j.imu.2020.100427 PMID: 32953971

Singh, K., Krishna, C., & Kumar, D. (2024). Professional Ethics, Challenges and Opportunities for Blockchain Technology in Healthcare Sector: A Systematic Review. *Recent Advances in Computer Science and Communications (Formerly: Recent Patents on Computer Science)*, *17*(1), 72-86.

Singh, A. K., Anand, A., Lv, Z., Ko, H., & Mohan, A. (2021). A survey on healthcare data: A security perspective. *ACM Transactions on Multimedia Computing Communications and Applications*, *17*(2s), 1–26. DOI: 10.1145/3422816

Sinha, A., Patel, A., & Jagdish, M. (2022, March). Application of Blockchain in Healthcare. In *2022 First International Conference on Artificial Intelligence Trends and Pattern Recognition (ICAITPR)* (pp. 1-4). IEEE.

Sintunavarat, W., & Turab, A. (2022). Mathematical analysis of an extended SEIR model of COVID-19 using the ABC-fractional operator. *Mathematics and Computers in Simulation*, *198*, 65–84. DOI: 10.1016/j.matcom.2022.02.009 PMID: 35194306

Siyal, A. A., Aisha, Z. J., Muhammad, Z., Kainat, A., Aiman, K., & Georgia, S. (2019). Applications of blockchain technology in medicine and healthcare: Challenges and future perspectives. *Cryptography*, *3*(1), 3. DOI: 10.3390/cryptography3010003

Sneha, S., Panjwani, A., Lade, B., Randolph, J., & Vickery, M. (2021). Alleviating Challenges Related to FDA-Approved Medical Wearables Using Blockchain Technology. *IT Professional*, *23*(4), 21–27. DOI: 10.1109/MITP.2021.3072535

Soman, S., & Saxena, S. (2018). EigenSample: A non-iterative technique for adding samples to small datasets. *Applied Soft Computing*, *70*, 1064–1077. DOI: 10.1016/j.asoc.2017.08.017

Somasundaram, R., & Thirugnanam, M. (2017). IoT in Healthcare: Breaching Security Issues. In *Security Breaches and Threat Prevention in the Internet of Things* (pp. 174-188). IGI Global.

Soni, M., & Singh, D. K. (2021). Blockchain Implementation for Privacy preserving and securing the Healthcare data. *IEEE International Conference on Communication Systems and Network Technologies (CSNT)* (pp. 729-734). IEEE. DOI: 10.1109/CSNT51715.2021.9509722

Spiel, K., Hornecker, E., Williams, R. M., & Good, J. (2022). ADHD and technology research–investigated by neurodivergent readers. In *Proceedings of the 2022 CHI Conference on Human Factors in Computing Systems* (pp. 1-21). DOI: 10.1145/3491102.3517592

Stamatellis, C., Papadopoulos, P., Pitropakis, N., Katsikas, S., & Buchanan, W. (2020). A Privacy-Preserving Healthcare Framework Using Hyperledger Fabric. *Sensors (Basel)*, *20*(22), 6587. Advance online publication. DOI: 10.3390/s20226587 PMID: 33218022

statista. (2024). Bitcoin (BTC) price per day from April 6, 2022 to December 30, 2024 Retrieved from https://www.statista.com/statistics/326707/bitcoin-price-index/

Stausberg, J., & Harkener, S. (2023). High-Quality Data for Health Care and Health Research. Methods of Information in Medicine, 62, 001 - 004. DOI: 10.1055/a-2045-8287

Stripelis, D., Gupta, U., Saleem, H., Dhinagar, N., Ghai, T., Anastasiou, C., Sánchez, R., Ver Steeg, G., Ravi, S., & Naveed, M. (2024). A federated learning architecture for secure and private neuroimaging analysis. *Patterns (New York, N.Y.)*, *5*(8), 101031. DOI: 10.1016/j.patter.2024.101031 PMID: 39233693

Sumalatha, M., Raghuraman, D., Surya, S., & Monisha, V. (2024). *Secured Blockchain Technology for Medical Supply Chain (SB-MSC)*. Paper presented at the 2024 International Conference on Advances in Data Engineering and Intelligent Computing Systems (ADICS). DOI: 10.1109/ADICS58448.2024.10533582

Sumner, J., Bundele, A., Lim, H. W., Phan, P., Motani, M., & Mukhopadhyay, A. (2024). Developing an Artificial Intelligence-Driven Nudge Intervention to Improve Medication Adherence: A Human-Centred Design Approach. *Journal of Medical Systems*, *48*(1), 3. Advance online publication. DOI: 10.1007/s10916-023-02024-0 PMID: 38063940

Sun, W., Lei, S., Wang, L., Liu, Z., & Zhang, Y. (2020). Adaptive federated learning and digital twin for industrial internet of things. *IEEE Transactions on Industrial Informatics*, *17*(8), 5605–5614. DOI: 10.1109/TII.2020.3034674

Supriya, S., & Padaki, S. (2016). Data security and privacy challenges in adopting solutions for IOT. 2016 IEEE International Conference on Internet of Things (iThings) and IEEE Green Computing and Communications (GreenCom) and IEEE Cyber, Physical and Social Computing (CPSCom) and IEEE Smart Data (SmartData)

Sweeney, L. (2002). k-anonymity: A model for protecting privacy. *International Journal of Uncertainty, Fuzziness and Knowledge-based Systems*, *10*(05), 557–570. DOI: 10.1142/S0218488502001648

Syed, H. H., Khan, M. A., Tariq, U., Armghan, A., Alenezi, F., Khan, J. A., Rho, S., Kadry, S., & Rajinikanth, V. (2021). A rapid artificial intelligence-based computer-aided diagnosis system for COVID-19 classification from CT images. *Behavioural Neurology*, *2021*, 5588967. Advance online publication. DOI: 10.1155/2021/2560388 PMID: 34966463

Tagde, P., Tagde, S., Bhattacharya, T., Tagde, P., Chopra, H., Akter, R., Kaushik, D., & Rahman, M. H. (2021). Blockchain and artificial intelligence technology in e-Health. *Environmental Science and Pollution Research International*, *28*(38), 52810–52831. DOI: 10.1007/s11356-021-16223-0 PMID: 34476701

Tahamtan, A., & Ardebili, A. (2020). Real-time RT-PCR in COVID-19 detection: Issues affecting the results. *Expert Review of Molecular Diagnostics*, *20*(5), 453–454. DOI: 10.1080/14737159.2020.1757437 PMID: 32297805

Tahir, M., Sardaraz, M., Muhammad, S., & Saud Khan, M. (2020). A lightweight authentication and authorization framework for blockchain-enabled IoT network in health-informatics. *Sustainability*, *12*(17), 6960.

Tamemi, H. T., Rabayah, M., Raad, K. A., Kanaan, M., & Awad, A. (2022). A Low Cost Blockchain-Based Framework for Preserving Critical Data in Health-Care IoT Systems Using Classification. *2022 IEEE Conference on Dependable and Secure Computing (DSC)*

Tang, C., Liu, Z., Hu, Q., Jiang, Z., Zheng, M., Xiong, C., Wang, S., Yao, S., Zhao, Y., Wan, X., Liu, G., Sun, Q., Wang, Z. L., & Li, L. (2024). Unconstrained Piezoelectric Vascular Electronics for Wireless Monitoring of Hemodynamics and Cardiovascular Health. *Small*, *20*(3), 2304752. Advance online publication. DOI: 10.1002/smll.202304752 PMID: 37691019

Tang, H., Jiang, X., Wang, X., Wang, S., Sofia, H., Fox, D., Lauter, K., Malin, B., Telenti, A., Xiong, L., & Ohno-Machado, L. (2016). Protecting genomic data analytics in the cloud: State of the art and opportunities. *BMC Medical Genomics*, *9*(1), 1–9. DOI: 10.1186/s12920-016-0224-3 PMID: 27733153

Tan, S. Y., Sumner, J., Wang, Y., & Wenjun Yip, A. (2024). A systematic review of the impacts of remote patient monitoring (RPM) interventions on safety, adherence, quality-of-life and cost-related outcomes. [PubMed]. *NPJ Digital Medicine*, *7*(1), 192.

Tao, H., Bhuiyan, M. Z. A., Abdalla, A. N., Hassan, M. M., Zain, J. M., & Hayajneh, T. (2018). Secured data collection with hardware-based ciphers for IoT-based healthcare. *IEEE Internet of Things Journal*, *6*(1), 410–420. DOI: 10.1109/JIOT.2018.2854714

Tariq, M. H., Hussain, M., Zahid, S., & Ahmed, R. H. (n.d.). *DECENTRALIZED APPLICATION FOR AUTO-INSURANCE INDUSTRY: AN INTERPLANETARY FILE SYSTEM AND BLOCKCHAIN-BASED PARADIGM FOR OPTIMAL DATA AND CLAIM MANAGEMENT.*

Tariq, , Awan, M. J., Alshudukhi, J., Alam, T. M., Alhamazani, K. T., & Meraf, Z. (2022). Software Measurement by Using Artificial Intelligence. *Journal of Nanomaterials*, *2022*(1), 7283171. DOI: 10.1155/2022/7283171

Tatineni, S. (2022). INTEGRATING AI, BLOCKCHAIN AND CLOUD TECHNOLOGIES FOR DATA MANAGEMENT IN HEALTHCARE. [JCET]. *Journal of Computer Engineering and Technology*, *5*(01).

Taylor, P. J., Dargahi, T., Dehghantanha, A., Parizi, R. M., & Choo, K. K. R. (2020). A systematic literature review of blockchain cyber security. *Digital Communications and Networks*, *6*(2), 147–156. DOI: 10.1016/j.dcan.2019.01.005

Thantharate, P., & Thantharate, A. (2023, October). ZeroTrustBlock: Enhancing Security, Privacy, and Interoperability of Sensitive Data through ZeroTrust Permissioned Blockchain. *Big Data and Cognitive Computing*, *7*(4), 165. DOI: 10.3390/bdcc7040165

Thatikonda, R., Kempanna, M., Tatikonda, R., & Bhuvanesh, A. (2024, June). The Impact of Blockchain and AI in the Healthcare. In *2024 IEEE 3rd International Conference on Electrical Power and Energy Systems (ICEPES)* (pp. 1-6). IEEE. DOI: 10.1109/ICEPES60647.2024.10653522

Thiruthuvanathan, M. M., Kumar, K. P., Nasar, N., Swathikiran, K. K., & Joseph, P. M. (2024). Security and privacy aspects in intelligence systems through blockchain and explainable AI. In *XAI Based Intelligent Systems for Society 5.0* (pp. 365–400). Elsevier. DOI: 10.1016/B978-0-323-95315-3.00011-5

Tian, Y., Wang, S., Xiong, J., Bi, R., Zhou, Z., & Bhuiyan, M. Z. A. (2023). Robust and privacy-preserving decentralized deep federated learning training: Focusing on digital healthcare applications. *IEEE/ACM Transactions on Computational Biology and Bioinformatics*. Advance online publication. DOI: 10.1109/TCBB.2023.3243932 PMID: 37028039

Tith, J., Lee, J.-S., Suzuki, H., Wijesundara, W. M. A. B., Taira, N., Obi, T., & Ohyama, N. (2020). Lee, H. Suzuki, W. Wijesundara, N. Taira, T. Obi, and N. Ohyama, "Patient Consent Management by a Purpose-Based Consent Model for Electronic Health Record Based on Blockchain Technology,". *Healthcare Informatics Research*, *26*(4), 265–273. DOI: 10.4258/hir.2020.26.4.265 PMID: 33190460

Tiwari, S. (2017). An introduction to QR code technology. *Proceedings - 2016 15th International Conference on Information Technology, ICIT 2016*, 39–44. doi: DOI: 10.1109/ICIT.2016.38

Totzkay, D. (2024). The potential influence of patient-centered communication, online provider communication, and social determinants of health on cancer screening. *Patient Education and Counseling*, *123*, 108238. Advance online publication. DOI: 10.1016/j.pec.2024.108238 PMID: 38452686

Tseng, L., Yao, X., Otoum, S., Aloqaily, M., & Jararweh, Y. (2020). Blockchain-based database in an IoT environment: Challenges, opportunities, and analysis. *Cluster Computing*, *23*(3), 1–15. DOI: 10.1007/s10586-020-03138-7

Tseng, T. Y., Mitchell, M. M., Chander, G., Latkin, C., Kennedy, C., & Knowlton, A. R. (2024). Patient-centered Engagement as a Mediator in the Associations of Healthcare Discrimination, Pain Care Denial, and Later Substance Use Among a Sample of Predominately African Americans Living with HIV. *AIDS and Behavior*, *28*(2), 429–438. Advance online publication. DOI: 10.1007/s10461-023-04235-5 PMID: 38060111

Turab, A., Shafqat, R., Muhammad, S., Shuaib, M., Khan, M. F., & Kamal, M. (2024). Predictive modeling of hepatitis B viral dynamics: A Caputo derivative-based approach using artificial neural networks. *Scientific Reports*, *14*(1), 21853. DOI: 10.1038/s41598-024-70788-7 PMID: 39300092

Turab, A., Sintunavarat, W., Ullah, F., Zaidi, S. A., Montoyo, A., & Nescolarde-Selva, J. A. (2024). Computational modeling of animal behavior in T-mazes: Insights from machine learning. *Ecological Informatics*, *81*, 102639. DOI: 10.1016/j.ecoinf.2024.102639

Turk, F., Sweetman, J., Chew-Graham, C. A., Gabbay, M., Shepherd, J., & van der Feltz-Cornelis, C. (2024). Accessing care for Long Covid from the perspectives of patients and healthcare practitioners: A qualitative study. *Health Expectations*, *27*(2), e14008. Advance online publication. DOI: 10.1111/hex.14008 PMID: 38481384

Turki, M., Cheikhrouhou, S., Dammak, B., Baklouti, M., Mars, R., & Dhahbi, A. (2023). NFT-IoT Pharma Chain: IoT Drug traceability system based on Blockchain and Non Fungible Tokens (NFTs). *Journal of King Saud University. Computer and Information Sciences*, *35*(2), 527–543. Advance online publication. DOI: 10.1016/j.jksuci.2022.12.016

Turransky, A., & Amini, M. H. (2022). Artificial intelligence and cybersecurity: tale of healthcare applications. *Cyberphysical smart cities infrastructures: Optimal operation and intelligent decision making*, 1-11.

U.S. Department of Health and Human Services. (2020). *Breaches of Unsecured Protected Health Information* [Online]. Available. [link]

U.S. Department of Health and Human Services. (n.d.). *Health Information Privacy: Laws and regulations*. HHS.gov. https://www.hhs.gov/hipaa/for-professionals/privacy/laws-regulations/index.html

Ullah, F., Habib, M. A., Farhan, M., Khalid, S., Durrani, M. Y., & Jabbar, S. (2017). Semantic interoperability for big data in heterogeneous IoT infrastructure for healthcare. *Sustainable Cities and Society*, *34*, 90–96. DOI: 10.1016/j.scs.2017.06.010

Ullah, F., Moon, J., Naeem, H., & Jabbar, S. (2022). Explainable artificial intelligence approach in combating real-time surveillance of COVID19 pandemic from CT scan and X-ray images using ensemble model. *The Journal of Supercomputing*, *78*(17), 19246–19271. DOI: 10.1007/s11227-022-04631-z PMID: 35754515

Ullah, F., Turab, A., Ullah, S., Cacciagrano, D., & Zhao, Y. (2024). Enhanced network intrusion detection system for internet of things security using multimodal big data representation with transfer learning and game theory. *Sensors (Basel)*, *24*(13), 4152. DOI: 10.3390/s24134152 PMID: 39000931

Ullah, H., Manickam, S., Obaidat, M., Laghari, S. U. A., & Uddin, M. (2023). Exploring the Potential of Metaverse Technology in Healthcare: Applications, Challenges, and Future Directions. *IEEE Access : Practical Innovations, Open Solutions*, *11*, 69686–69707. DOI: 10.1109/ACCESS.2023.3286696

Umayal, K. (2024). Strategic Integration of Digital Health Technologies for Enhanced Patient-Centered Care in Modern Healthcare Management. *Shanlax International Journal of Management, 11*(iS1-Jan). DOI: 10.34293/management.v11iiS1-Jan.7142

Upadhyay, J., Singh, S. K., Kar, N. K., Pandey, M. K., Gupta, P., & Tiwari, P. (2024). Healthcare Data Security Using AI and Blockchain: Safeguarding Sensitive Information for a Safer Society. In *Next-Generation Cybersecurity: AI, ML, and Blockchain* (pp. 159–178). Springer Nature Singapore. DOI: 10.1007/978-981-97-1249-6_8

Uppal, S., Kansekar, B., Mini, S., & Tosh, D. (2023). HealthDote: A blockchain-based model for continuous health monitoring using an interplanetary file system. *Healthcare Analytics*, *3*, 100175. DOI: 10.1016/j.health.2023.100175

Valentin, J. B., Mainz, J., Johnsen, S. P., Kristensen, K., & Kristensen, S. (2024). Rasch analysis of a patient-reported outcome measure for self-perceived health among psychiatric patients in Denmark. *BMJ Open Quality*, *13*(1), e002519. Advance online publication. DOI: 10.1136/bmjoq-2023-002519 PMID: 38350672

Vallentin, A., Thórisson, K. R., & Latapie, H. (2023). Addressing the Unsustainability of Deep Neural Networks with Next-Gen AI. In International Conference on Artificial General Intelligence (pp. 296-306). Cham: Springer Nature Switzerland. DOI: 10.1007/978-3-031-33469-6_30

van Lummel, E. V. T. J., Ietswaard, L., Rigter, M., Tjan, D. H. T., van Delden, J. J. M., & Milota, M. (2024). Finding the balance between person-centred and treatment-centred discussions in advance care planning—A qualitative analysis of conversations within the MUTUAL (Multidisciplinary Timely Undertaken Advance Care Planning conversations) intervention using a narrative analysis. *Age and Ageing*, *53*(3), afae020. Advance online publication. DOI: 10.1093/ageing/afae020 PMID: 38452194

Vatambeti, R., Krishna, E. P., Karthik, M. G., & Damera, V. K. (2024). Securing the medical data using enhanced privacy preserving based blockchain technology in Internet of Things. *Cluster Computing*, *27*(2), 1625–1637. DOI: 10.1007/s10586-023-04056-0

Vazirani, A. A., O'Donoghue, O., Brindley, D., & Meinert, E. (2019). Implementing blockchains for efficient health care: Systematic review. *Journal of Medical Internet Research*, *21*(2), e12439. DOI: 10.2196/12439 PMID: 30747714

Venkatesh, V., & Davis, F. D. (2000). A theoretical extension of the technology acceptance model: Four longitudinal field studies. *Management Science*, *46*(2), 186–204. DOI: 10.1287/mnsc.46.2.186.11926

Vidhya, S., Siva Raja, P., & Sumithra, R. (2024). Blockchain-Enabled Decentralized Healthcare Data Exchange: Leveraging Novel Encryption Scheme, Smart Contracts, and Ring Signatures for Enhanced Data Security and Patient Privacy. *International Journal of Network Management*, *34*(5), e2289. Advance online publication. DOI: 10.1002/nem.2289

Viegas, C. V., Bond, A., Vaz, C. R., & Bertolo, R. J. (2019). Reverse flows within the pharmaceutical supply chain: A classificatory review from the perspective of end-of-use and end-of-life medicines. *Journal of Cleaner Production*, *238*, 117719. DOI: 10.1016/j.jclepro.2019.117719

Vinnarasi, P. R., and K. Vadivukkarasi, "Healthcare Data Security using Blockchain Technology," *2023 International Conference on Intelligent Systems for Communication, IoT and Security (ICISCoIS)*, pp. 298-303, 2023, DOI: 10.1109/ICISCoIS56541.2023.10100572

Vishwa, A. (2021). *MediBlock-A Privacy-aware Blockchain to store patients data and effective diagnosis methods*. University of Technology Sydney.

Vlasta, M. (2023). Methodological framework for European regulation of (artificial) intelligence and its limits.

Voigt, P., & Von dem Bussche, A. (2017). The eu general data protection regulation (gdpr). *A Practical Guide, 1st Ed., Cham: Springer International Publishing, 10*(3152676), 10-5555.

Vora, L. K., Gholap, A. D., Jetha, K., Thakur, R. R. S., Solanki, H. K., & Chavda, V. P. (2023). Artificial intelligence in pharmaceutical technology and drug delivery design. *Pharmaceutics*, *15*(7), 1916. DOI: 10.3390/pharmaceutics15071916 PMID: 37514102

Wada, M., Noda, Y., Iwata, Y., Tsugawa, S., Yoshida, K., Tani, H., Hirano, Y., Koike, S., Sasabayashi, D., Katayama, H., Plitman, E., Ohi, K., Ueno, F., Caravaggio, F., Koizumi, T., Gerretsen, P., Suzuki, T., Uchida, H., Müller, D. J., & Nakajima, S. (2022). Dopaminergic dysfunction and excitatory/inhibitory imbalance in treatment-resistant schizophrenia and novel neuromodulatory treatment. *Molecular Psychiatry*, *27*(7), 2950–2967. DOI: 10.1038/s41380-022-01572-0 PMID: 35444257

Wamba, S. F., Queiroz, M. M., Jabbour, C. J. C., & Shi, C. V. (2023). Are both generative AI and ChatGPT game changers for 21st-Century operations and supply chain excellence? *International Journal of Production Economics*, *265*, 109015. DOI: 10.1016/j.ijpe.2023.109015

Wang, B., Song, W., Lou, W., & Hou, Y. T. (2017). Privacy-preserving pattern matching over encrypted genetic data in cloud computing. IEEE INFOCOM 2017-IEEE Conference on Computer Communications

Wang, H., Pathak, M., Takami, T., Wiener, R. C., Shen, C., & Sambamoorthi, U. (2024). Ethnic Disparities in Patient-Centered Communication with Healthcare Providers: A Comparison of Non-Hispanic Asians and Non-Hispanic Whites. *Journal of Racial and Ethnic Health Disparities*. Advance online publication. DOI: 10.1007/s40615-023-01898-7 PMID: 38228862

Wang, S., Zha, Y., Li, W., Wu, Q., Li, X., Niu, M., Wang, M., Qiu, X., Li, H., Yu, H., Gong, W., Bai, Y., Li, L., Zhu, Y., Wang, L., & Tian, J. (2020). A fully automatic deep learning system for COVID-19 diagnostic and prognostic analysis. *The European Respiratory Journal*, *56*(2), 2000778. DOI: 10.1183/13993003.00775-2020 PMID: 32444412

Wang, W., Li, X., Qiu, X., Zhang, X., Brusic, V., & Zhao, J. (2023). A privacy preserving framework for federated learning in smart healthcare systems. *Information Processing & Management*, *60*(1), 103167. DOI: 10.1016/j.ipm.2022.103167

Wang, Y., Han, J. H., & Beynon-Davies, P. (2019). Understanding blockchain technology for future supply chains: A systematic literature review and research agenda. *Supply Chain Management*, *24*(1), 62–84. DOI: 10.1108/SCM-03-2018-0148

Wani, . (2022). Utilization of Artificial Intelligence in Disease Prevention: Diagnosis, Treatment, and Implications for the Healthcare Workforce. *Health Care*. PMID: 35455786

Wan, Y., & Huang, H. (2023). Adoption and optimization of blockchain technology in the regulation of Class II vaccines. *IEEE Access : Practical Innovations, Open Solutions*, *11*, 84607–84619. DOI: 10.1109/ACCESS.2023.3301772

Weber, D., & Nøhr, C. (2024). National Trial Overview: Towards Accessible and Patient-Centered Healthcare. *Studies in Health Technology and Informatics*, *310*. Advance online publication. DOI: 10.3233/SHTI231175 PMID: 38270025

Westphal, J., Singh, A. K., & Gupta, R. K. "Blockchain Integration in Healthcare: A Comprehensive Investigation," *Frontiers in Blockchain*, vol. 4, no. 1, pp. 1-15, 2021. [Online]. Available: https://www.frontiersin.org/journals/blockchain/articles/10.3389/fbloc.2021.732112/full

Williamson, S. M., & Prybutok, V. (2024). Balancing privacy and progress: A review of privacy challenges, systemic oversight, and patient perceptions in AI-driven healthcare. *Applied Sciences (Basel, Switzerland)*, *14*(2), 675. DOI: 10.3390/app14020675

Winnie, Y., Umamaheswari, E., & Ajay, D. (2018). Enhancing data security in IoT healthcare services using fog computing. *2018 International Conference on Recent Trends in Advance Computing (ICRTAC)*

Wong, H. H., Jessup, A., Sertkaya, A., Birkenbach, A., Berlind, A., & Eyraud, J. (2014). Examination of clinical trial costs and barriers for drug development final. *Office of the Assistant Secretary for Planning and Evaluation, US Department of Health & Human Services*, 1-92.

World Health Organization (WHO). (2016). Innovation. http://www.who.int/ topics/innovation/en/

Xia, Q. I., Sifah, E. B., Asamoah, K. O., Gao, J., Du, X., & Guizani, M. (2017). MeDShare: Trust-less medical data sharing among cloud service providers via blockchain. *IEEE Access : Practical Innovations, Open Solutions*, *5*, 14757–14767. DOI: 10.1109/ACCESS.2017.2730843

Xia, Q., Sifah, E. B., Asamoah, K. O., Gao, J., Du, X., & Guizani, M. (2017). MeDShare: Trust-Less Medical Data Sharing Among Cloud Service Providers via Blockchain. *Journal of Biomedical Informatics*, *76*, 39–52. DOI: 10.1016/j.jbi.2017.04.005

Xie, Y., Lu, L., Gao, F., He, S. J., Zhao, H. J., Fang, Y., Yang, J. M., An, Y., Ye, Z. W., & Dong, Z. (2021). Integration of artificial intelligence, blockchain, and wearable technology for chronic disease management: A new paradigm in smart healthcare. *Current Medical Science*, *41*(6), 1123–1133. DOI: 10.1007/s11596-021-2485-0 PMID: 34950987

Xu, S., Wu, H., & Bie, R. (2018). CXNet-m1: Anomaly detection on chest X-rays with image-based deep learning. *IEEE Access : Practical Innovations, Open Solutions*, *7*, 4466–4477. DOI: 10.1109/ACCESS.2018.2885997

Xu, X., Weber, I., & Staples, M. (2019). *Architecture for blockchain applications*. Springer. DOI: 10.1007/978-3-030-03035-3

Xu, Y., Liu, X., Cao, X., Huang, C., Liu, E., Qian, S., Liu, X., Wu, Y., Dong, F., Qiu, C.-W., Qiu, J., Hua, K., Su, W., Wu, J., Xu, H., Han, Y., Fu, C., Yin, Z., Liu, M., & Zhang, J. (2021). Artificial intelligence: A powerful paradigm for scientific research. *Innovation (Cambridge (Mass.))*, *2*(4), 100179. DOI: 10.1016/j.xinn.2021.100179 PMID: 34877560

Yang, H. M., Duan, T., Ding, D., Bagul, A., Langlotz, C., & Shpanskaya, K. (2017). CheXNet: radiologist-level pneumonia detection on chest x-rays with deep learning. *arXiv preprint arXiv:1711.05225*.

Yang, Q., Liu, Y., Chen, T., & Tong, Y. (2019). Federated machine learning: Concept and applications. [TIST]. *ACM Transactions on Intelligent Systems and Technology*, *10*(2), 1–19. DOI: 10.1145/3298981

Yaqoob, K. Salah, R. Jayaraman, and Y. Al-Hammadi, "Blockchain for healthcare data management: opportunities, challenges, and future recommendations," *Neural Computing and Applications*, vol. 34, pp. 11475-11490, 2021, doi: Azaria, A., Ekblaw, A., Vieira, T., & Lippman, A. (2016). MedRec: Using Blockchain for Medical Data Access and Permission Management. *Proceedings of the 2nd International Conference on Open and Big Data (OBD 2016)*. Available at: DOI: 10.1109/OBD.2016.11

Yaqoob, I., Salah, K., Jayaraman, R., & Al-Hammadi, Y. (2022). Blockchain for healthcare data management: Opportunities, challenges, and future recommendations. *Neural Computing & Applications*, *34*(14), 1–16. DOI: 10.1007/s00521-020-05519-w

Yele, S., & Litoriya, R. (2024). Blockchain-based secure dining: Enhancing safety, transparency, and traceability in food consumption environment. *Blockchain: Research and Applications*, 100187.

Ye, Z., Zhang, Y., Wang, Y., Huang, Z., & Song, B. (2020). Chest CT manifestations of new coronavirus disease 2019 (COVID-19): A pictorial review. *European Radiology*, *30*(8), 4381–4389. DOI: 10.1007/s00330-020-06801-0 PMID: 32193638

Yigzaw, K. Y., Olabarriaga, S. D., Michalas, A., Marco-Ruiz, L., Hillen, C., Verginadis, Y., De Oliveira, M. T., Krefting, D., Penzel, T., & Bowden, J. (2022). Health data security and privacy: Challenges and solutions for the future. *Roadmap to Successful Digital Health Ecosystems*, 335-362.

Yin, X. C., Liu, Z. G., Ndibanje, B., Nkenyereye, L., & Riazul Islam, S. (2019). An IoT-based anonymous function for security and privacy in healthcare sensor networks. *Sensors (Basel)*, *19*(14), 3146.

Yli-Huumo, J., Ko, D., Choi, S., Park, S., & Smolander, K. (2016). Where Is Current Research on Blockchain Technology?—A Systematic Review. *PLoS One*, *11*(10), e0163477. Advance online publication. DOI: 10.1371/journal.pone.0163477 PMID: 27695049

Yogesh, M. J., & Karthikeyan, J. (2022). Health informatics: engaging modern healthcare units: a brief overview. *Frontiers in Public Health*, *10*, 854688. DOI: 10.3389/fpubh.2022.854688 PMID: 35570921

Yue, X., Wang, H., Jin, D., Li, M., & Jiang, W. (2016). Healthcare data gateways: Found healthcare intelligence on blockchain with novel privacy risk control. *Journal of Medical Systems*, *40*(10), 1–8. DOI: 10.1007/s10916-016-0574-6 PMID: 27565509

Yulianti, T., & Sulistyawati, A. (2021). Enhancing public speaking ability through focus group discussion. [Pendidikan Dan Pengajaran]. *JURNAL PAJAR*, *5*(2), 287–295.

Zahid, S., Hussain, M., Ahmed, R. H., Shahid, M. R., & Abbas, H. (2023). Blockchain-based Health Insurance Model Using IPFS: A Solution for Improved Optimization, Trustability, and User Control. *2023 International Conference on IT and Industrial Technologies (ICIT)*, 1–7. DOI: 10.1109/ICIT59216.2023.10335701

Zhang, J., Xie, Y., Li, Y., Shen, C., & Xia, Y. (2020). COVID-19 screening on chest X-ray images using deep learning-based anomaly detection. arXiv preprint, arXiv:2003.12338.

Zhang, P., Walker, M. A., White, J., Schmidt, D. C., & Lenz, G. (2017, October). Metrics for assessing blockchain-based healthcare decentralized apps. In *2017 IEEE 19th international conference on e-health networking, applications and services (Healthcom)* (pp. 1-4). IEEE. DOI: 10.1109/HealthCom.2017.8210842

Zhang, P., Schmidt, D. C., White, J., & Lenz, G. (2018). Blockchain technology use cases in healthcare. [). Elsevier.]. *Advances in Computers*, *111*, 1–41. DOI: 10.1016/bs.adcom.2018.03.006

Zhang, P., Schmidt, D. C., White, J., & Lenz, G. (2018). Blockchain Technology Use Cases in Healthcare. *IEEE Access : Practical Innovations, Open Solutions*, *6*, 28126–28139. DOI: 10.1109/ACCESS.2018.2842265

Zhang, P., White, J., Schmidt, D. C., Lenz, G., & Rosenbloom, S. T. (2018). FHIRChain: Applying Blockchain to Securely and Scalably Share Clinical Data. *Computational and Structural Biotechnology Journal*, *16*, 267–278. DOI: 10.1016/j.csbj.2018.07.004 PMID: 30108685

Zhang, R., Xue, R., & Liu, L. (2021). Security and privacy for healthcare blockchains. *IEEE Transactions on Services Computing*, *15*(6), 3668–3686. DOI: 10.1109/TSC.2021.3085913

Zhao, J., Mortier, R., Crowcroft, J., & Wang, L. (2018). Privacy-preserving machine learning based data analytics on edge devices. Proceedings of the 2018 AAAI/ACM Conference on AI, Ethics, and Society DOI: 10.1145/3278721.3278778

Zhao, C. X., & Yam, M. (2024). Role of patient specific 3D printed models in patient confidence, understanding and satisfaction of care in Singapore. *Journal of Orthopaedics*, *52*, 28–32. Advance online publication. DOI: 10.1016/j.jor.2024.02.010 PMID: 38404701

Zheng, Z., Xie, S., Dai, H., Chen, X., & Wang, H. (2018). Blockchain challenges and opportunities: A survey. *International Journal of Web and Grid Services*, *14*(4), 352. DOI: 10.1504/IJWGS.2018.095647

Zhu, L., Wu, Y., Gai, K., & Choo, K. K. R. (2019). Controllable and trustworthy blockchain-based cloud data management. *Future Generation Computer Systems*, *91*, 527–535. DOI: 10.1016/j.future.2018.09.019

Ziavrou, K. S., Noguera, S., & Boumba, V. A. (2022). Trends in counterfeit drugs and pharmaceuticals before and during COVID-19 pandemic. *Forensic Science International*, *338*, 111382. DOI: 10.1016/j.forsciint.2022.111382 PMID: 35882074

Zubair, M., Ahmad, J., Alqahtani, F., Khan, F., Shah, S. A., Abbasi, Q. H., & Jan, S. U. (2022, May). Automated grading of diabetic macular edema using color retinal photographs. In *2022 2nd International Conference of Smart Systems and Emerging Technologies (SMARTTECH)* (pp. 1-6). IEEE. DOI: 10.1109/SMARTTECH54121.2022.00016

Zubair, M., Umair, M., & Owais, M. (2023, September). Automated brain tumor detection using soft computing-based segmentation technique. In *2023 3rd International Conference on Computing and Information Technology (ICCIT)* (pp. 211-215). IEEE. DOI: 10.1109/ICCIT58132.2023.10273963

Zubair, M., Ali, H., & Javed, M. Y. (2016). Automated Segmentation of Hard Exudates Using Dynamic Thresholding to Detect Diabetic Retinopathy in Retinal Photographs. *J. Multim. Process. Technol.*, *7*(3), 109–116.

Zubair, M., Ali, J., Alhussein, M., Hassan, S., Aurangzeb, K., & Umair, M. (2024). An improved machine learning-driven framework for cryptocurrencies price prediction with sentimental cautioning. *IEEE Access : Practical Innovations, Open Solutions*, *12*, 51395–51418. DOI: 10.1109/ACCESS.2024.3367129

Zubair, M., Khan, S. A., & Yasin, U. U. (2014). Classification of diabetic macular edema and its stages using color fundus image. *Journal of Electronic Science and Technology*, *12*(2), 187–190.

Zubair, M., Umair, M., Naqvi, R. A., Hussain, D., Owais, M., & Werghi, N. (2023). A comprehensive computer-aided system for an early-stage diagnosis and classification of diabetic macular edema. *Journal of King Saud University. Computer and Information Sciences*, *35*(8), 101719. DOI: 10.1016/j.jksuci.2023.101719

Zubair, M., Yamin, A., & Khan, S. A. (2013, October). Automated detection of optic disc for the analysis of retina using color fundus image. In *2013 IEEE International Conference on Imaging Systems and Techniques (IST)* (pp. 239-242). IEEE. DOI: 10.1109/IST.2013.6729698

Zyskind, G., & Nathan, O. (2015, May). Decentralizing privacy: Using blockchain to protect personal data. In 2015 IEEE security and privacy workshops (pp. 180-184). IEEE.

Zyskind, G., & Nathan, O. (2015, May). *Decentralizing privacy: Using blockchain to protect personal data. In 2015 IEEE security and privacy workshops*. IEEE.

About The Contributors

Abdul Ahad earned his PhD in Computer Science from Sunway University Malaysia (2018-2022), an M.S. in Computer Science from the Virtual University of Pakistan (2015-2017), and an M.Sc. in Computer Science from Swat University of Pakistan (2012-2014). Currently, Ahad enriches the scientific community as a Postdoctoral Researcher at Northwestern Polytechnical University in Xi'an, China, engaging in groundbreaking research in the Internet of Medical Things (IoMT) and federated deep learning. His journey before this role includes impactful tenures as an Assistant Professor at the University of Management and Technology in Pakistan, a Scientific Researcher at Istanbul Technical University, and a Data Processing Officer for the Government of Pakistan Revenue Department, among other notable positions. His research interests are vast and visionary, focusing on 5G and 6G technologies, smart healthcare, the Internet of Things (IoT), cyber security, machine learning, and deep learning. His work aims to bridge technological innovation with practical healthcare solutions, contributing to smarter, safer, and more efficient cities and communities. His academic and research excellence has been recognized through numerous awards and achievements, including being listed in the top 2\% of scientists worldwide by Stanford University in 2023. He has received merit awards for his Ph.D. and M.S. studies, grants for his contributions to journals and conferences, and several accolades for his teaching and research roles, illustrating a track record of excellence and dedication to his field. He has also contributed to the academic community through workshops, memberships in conferences such as IEEE, Elsevier, Springer, and EAI, and numerous publications in esteemed journals and conferences on subjects central to his research interests, including 5G, 6G, smart healthcare, cyber security, and the Internet of Things (IoT).

Farhan Ullah is an Associate Professor at the School of Software, Northwestern Polytechnical University (NPU), Xi'an Shaanxi, P.R. China. He received Ph.D. Computer Science degree in 2020 from College of Computer Science, Sichuan University Chengdu, P.R. China. He was awarded a full-time Chinese Government Scholarship (CGS) for his Ph.D. He works as editorial board member in several SCIE journals including KSII Transactions on Internet and Information Systems, Electronics, CMC Computers, Materials & Continua, CSSE Computer Systems Science and Engineering, etc. He received research landmark achievement award (2021) from School of Software, NPU, Xian, China. He also received Research Productivity Award (2016) from COMSATS Institute of Information Technology (CIIT), Sahiwal, Pakistan. He is an active researcher who works with well-known professors and scientists. His research work is published in various renowned journals of IEEE, Springer, Elsevier, Wiley, MDPI, and Hindawi.

***

Rana Hassam Ahmed received his Bachelor of Science degree in Computer Science (BSCS) from the University of Central Punjab, Lahore, Pakistan, in 2020. He went on to earn his Master of Science degree in Computer Science (MSCS) from The University of Faisalabad, Faisalabad, Pakistan, in 2023. During his MS studies, he de- veloped a keen interest in blockchain technology, specifically focusing on its applications in com- bating counterfeit medicine. His thesis work was dedicated to this field, and he has authored three papers presented at IEEE conferences. His certifications include membership in IEEE, participation in Innovative Lyallpur by TUF, XTC NTU 2017, and IEEE Expo 2017. He also holds a Diploma of Associate Engineering (DAE) in Electrical from Jinnah Poly Technical Institute Faisalabad, Pakistan completed between 2016 and 2019. In addition to his academic achievements, Rana Hassam Ahmed has two years of experience working as a Vice Principal at a private school. Currently, he is a Lecturer at The University of Faisalabad, where he teaches various computer science subjects. His research interests include blockchain and IoT technology, counterfeit medicine solutions, and other related areas in computer science.

Dora Almeida is an integrated researcher at Dynamic Capabilities Operational Progressive Institute, and a collaborator researcher at UE in Lisbon. She is graduated in Physiology and with a master's degree in management. She is a co-author of some papers and conference presentations. She is an academic reviewer of some scientific journals and guest editor in some special issues/research topics.

Noah Mike Barr is an accomplished professional with a dynamic career in technology and healthcare management. He holds advanced degrees that blend his expertise in computer science and health administration, which underpin his innovative approaches to solving industry challenges. Barr's career spans significant achievements across healthcare technology, financial systems, and administrative strategy. With a unique combination of technical expertise and management acumen, he has contributed to transformative projects, advancing innovation in critical sectors. Barr's dedication to improving systems through integrated methodologies has made him a respected voice in his fields of study and practice.

Hira Butt, I hold a Master's degree in Computer Science with a specialization in Machine Learning and currently serve as a professor at the University of Central Punjab. Additionally, I contributed as a researcher for the 2024 IEEE Globecom Workshops (GC Wkshps), further enhancing my academic and professional expertise in the field.

C. Bhuvaneswari has been Assistant Professor for 17 years, specializing in Artificial Intelligence, Machine Learning, and Blockchain. With numerous research publications and presentations at national and international conferences, she is deeply committed to advancing knowledge in these dynamic fields. Passionate about exploring emerging technologies, she continuously expands her expertise, making a significant impact on both her students and the academic community through her dedication to research and teaching.

M. Kazem Chamran received a B.Eng. degree (honor) in Electrical and Electronic Engineering from Sheffield Hallam University, in 2010, an M.Sc. degree in Network and Communication Engineering from University Putra Malaysia (UPM), in 2015, and PhD in Computing from Sunway University Malaysia in 2022. Currently, he is the head of research at City University Malaysia and a senior lecturer in the IT faculty. He is also a member of several national and international committees and scientific societies like IEEE and Malaysian Research Committees. His research interests are in Artificial Intelligence, 5G-6G, Energy harvesting, Machine Learning, and IoT.

Muhammad Arshad Shehzad Hassan received the Ph.D. degree in Electrical Engineering from Chongqing University, Chongqing, China, in 2019. He is currently an Associate Professor with The University of Faisalabad, Faisalabad, Pakistan. His research interests include intelligent modeling and control, optimization of microgrids, microgrid control, energy policy, high voltage technology, and transmission line fault location and protections.

Shoaib Hassan received the B.Sc. degree in computer system engineering from the University College of Engineering and Technology (UCET), The Islamia University of Bahawalpur (IUB), in 2012, and the M.S. degree in software engineering from the National University of Sciences and Technology (NUST), Pakistan, in 2015. He is currently pursuing the Ph.D. degree in computer science with the School of Computer Science and Engineering, NJUST, China. He has published various research papers in well-reputed conferences and journals. His research interests include software engineering, requirement engineering, machine learning, healthcare systems, software project management, and emotion modeling.

Majid Hussain has earned a Ph.D. in Computer Science with a specialization in Wireless Sensor Networks and has amassed approximately 20 years of academic, research, and administrative experience at reputed universities in Pakistan. Currently, he serves as the Dean of the Faculty of Information Technology at The University of Faisalabad. Throughout his career, he has played a pivotal role in research and academic leadership. He founded research groups in Blockchain, UAVs, Cybersecurity, and Machine Learning, leading to multiple significant research outputs. Under his leadership, his teams have secured one international research project and one NRPU project in Blockchain, an NRPU project in UAVs, and seven Ignite/HEC startup grants over the past two years. As an academic leader, he manages a team of approximately 60 faculty members (core and allied) and oversees a student body of 1,500 across programs in Computer Science, Software Engineering, Information Technology, Artificial Intelligence, and Data Science at the BS, MS, and Ph.D. levels. Beyond daily departmental operations, he has spearheaded major academic initiatives, including curriculum revisions, the launch of new MS and BS programs in Data Science and Artificial Intelligence, accreditation of BS (CS/SE) programs, and the organization of significant academic events such as the Advanced STEAM Education Conference, IEEE Summit on AI, and various national and international seminars. Additionally, he has actively facilitated collaborations with both private and public sector organizations, established final-year project (FYP) open houses, and strengthened industry linkages. Before joining The University of Faisalabad, he served at COMSATS University for approximately 12 years, where he led the Computer Science department as Head of Department (HoD) for several years. Under his leadership, the department grew to encompass around 70 faculty members, 1,400 students, and a dedicated support staff. He also held multiple administrative roles, including Warden Hostels, Convener of Event Management, Founder and Manager of the Cisco Networking Academy Program, and Library Manager. Additionally, he served as the Focal Person for the Pak-China Business Forum and received multiple awards and recognitions for his contributions. Prior to his tenure at COMSATS University, he worked at the University of Engineering and Technology (UET) Lahore as a team lead in the Visual Sensor Networks Lab alongside Prof. Dr. Ali Hamad Akbar. He played a key role in establishing the lab and led the development of the UET Surveillance System Project, culminating in research materialized as VISTA. Before UET, he served at Government College

University Faisalabad from 2007 to 2009 as HoD and Assistant Professor, where he led the establishment of multiple IT and Electrical Engineering laboratories. His early academic career includes teaching experience at the Institute of Engineering and Technology (IET) Lahore from 2005 to 2007 and Shiblee College of Commerce and Science, Faisalabad, from 2003 to 2005. With a profound commitment to research, education, and institutional development, Dr. Majid continues to make significant contributions to the fields of Information Technology, Computer Science, and interdisciplinary research.

Muhammad Ibrar is currently an Assistant Professor at The University of Faisalabad, Faisalabad, Pakistan. Before that, he was a Postdoctoral Fellow at the School of Software, Dalian University of Technology, China. He obtained his Ph.D. from the School of Software, Dalian University of Technology in 2021. He completed his MS in Telecommunication and Networking from Bahria University, Islamabad, Pakistan, in 2014. He earned his BS in Telecommunication and Networking from COMSATS University Islamabad, Abbottabad Campus, Pakistan, in 2010. His research interests include Software-Defined Networking (SDN), fog computing, wireless ad hoc networks, and sensor networks.

Ishal Imran, She is a recent graduate in Information Technology from the University of Management and Technology, Pakistan. She has a strong interest in exploring innovative technologies such as artificial intelligence and blockchain. She also has professional experience in digital marketing, including SEO and social media management. Her passion lies in leveraging technology to create impactful solutions for real-world challenges.

Muqadsa Jabeen is currently a Lecturer/ researcher at The University of Faisalabad, Faisalabad, Pakistan. She completed her MS in Computer Science from The University of Faisalabad in 2023. Before that, she obtained her MSc in Information Technology from Government College University Faisalabad in 2018. Her research interests focus on emerging technologies, including blockchain, Explainable AI (XAI), cybersecurity, and their applications in smart healthcare systems. She has actively participated in various international conferences and is working on several publications that explore the intersection of modern technology, education, and secure communication systems.

Abha Susan Jimmy, a Computer Science and Engineering student at Manav Rachna International Institute of Research and Studies (MRIIRS) in Faridabad, Haryana. I have written a manuscript titled "Case Studies of Blockchain and AI Integration in Medical Systems," which was submitted for inclusion in the book AI and Blockchain Applications for Privacy and Security in Smart Medical Systems. This manuscript was written in collaboration with two teammates, under the guidance of Mr. Bhanu Dwivedi.

Jipson Joseph has a PhD in Ethics from DVK Bangalore. Currently, he is a Research Scholar in the School of Law at Christ University, Bangalore. His research interests are in the fields of ethics, gender studies, constitutional law, human rights, human security, food security, environmental justice, developmental policies and global poverty.

Zunaira Rashid attends UMT Sialkot as an MS Computer Science student who focuses on Privacy-Preserving Machine Learning for Medical Data within smart healthcare systems. She obtained her BSCS degree from UMT while she specializes in Machine Learning and LLMs alongside distributed systems and Data Analytics.

Ashraf Khalil has a PhD in Computer Science from Indiana University, USA and has published notable research in Human Computer Interaction, Ubiquitous Computing, Social and Mobile Computing, Bioinformatics, and Privacy. Prof. Khalil actively applies diverse technological innovations in addressing pertinent problems. He has authored over 50 publications in top journals and conferences and achieved numerous accolades including many research grants from ADEK, Emi- rates Foundation, and Google. Prior to joining ZU, he worked at Abu Dhabi University as Director of Research and as Professor of Computer Science. During his tenure as Director of Research, he developed the university research strategy that led to a 6-fold increase in research productivity. He also established and directed the Center of Excellence for Smart, En- trepreneurial and Sustainable Cities. Prof. Khalil has played an instrumental role in promoting undergraduate research in the UAE as an integral part of university education through running the largest regional competition for undergraduate researchers for five consecutive years. Additionally, Prof. Khalil served as a usability consultant for major companies such as Nokia, HSBC, Microsoft, and Samsung.

Qianmu Li (Member, IEEE) received the B.Sc. and Ph.D. degrees from Nanjing University of Science and Technology, China, in 2001 and 2005, respectively. He is currently a full Professor with the School of Computer Science and Engineering, Nanjing University of Science and Technology. He is the author or co-author of more than 100 high-indexed (SCIE/E-SCI/EI) journal/conference articles and eight books. His research interests include information security, computing system management, and data mining. He was the recipient of China Network and Information Security Outstanding Talent Award in 2016; and the multiple Education Ministry Science and Technology Awards, in 2012.

Filipe Madeira is a Coordinator Professor at the Polytechnic Institute of Santarém, where he leads the Master's Program in Applied Informatics. He also holds key roles in the Technical-Scientific Council, Pedagogical Council, and the School Assembly of ESGTS. Additionally, he serves as the Editor-in-Chief of the *Scientific Journal of UI_IPSantarém* and as Vice-Coordinator and researcher at the Digital Literacy and Social Inclusion Hub (PLDIS) of CIAC, University of Algarve. Holding a Ph.D. in Computer Science from the University of Évora, his research interests span recommender systems, advanced educational technologies, and digital health literacy. His academic contributions include numerous peer-reviewed journal articles, book chapters on personalized learning systems and collaborative filtering, and a book exploring the impact of digital tools in education and health promotion. Filipe has also contributed to creating resources aimed at improving health empowerment and technology-enhanced learning. Beyond his academic and research endeavors, Filipe acts as a reviewer for doctoral fellowship programs in Computer Science at the Portuguese Foundation for Science and Technology (FCT). With over 30 years of experience in teaching and research, he has played a pivotal role in advancing technology in education and digital health, earning awards and widespread recognition for his scientific and academic contributions.

Amiti Mahajan, a Computer Science and Engineering student at Manav Rachna International Institute of Research and Studies (MRIIRS) in Faridabad, Haryana. I have written a manuscript titled "Case Studies of Blockchain and AI Integration in Medical Systems," which was submitted for inclusion in the book AI and Blockchain Applications for Privacy and Security in Smart Medical Systems. This manuscript was written in collaboration with two teammates, under the guidance of Mr. Bhanu Dwivedi.

Nandini Newar, a Computer Science and Engineering student at Manav Rachna International Institute of Research and Studies (MRIIRS) in Faridabad, Haryana. I have written a manuscript titled "Case Studies of Blockchain and AI Integration in Medical Systems," which was submitted for inclusion in the book AI and Blockchain Applications for Privacy and Security in Smart Medical Systems. This manuscript was written in collaboration with two teammates, under the guidance of Mr. Bhanu Dwivedi.

Muhammad Numair is a researcher at the Advanced Innovation Center for Future Education in China and holds a Ph.D. in Educational Technology from Beijing Normal University. His research focuses on the integration of blockchain technology, artificial intelligence, large language models, and the Internet of Things (IoT) in education. He also holds a master's degree in computer science, where his work centered on blockchain technology, AI, and large language models, particularly their applications in education and IoT. Muhammad has published research articles on blockchain applications in education and IoT and has completed projects emphasizing the practical implementation of blockchain in educational settings. His Ph.D. research delved into leveraging blockchain technology to enhance educational systems.

Ananya Pandey is a Research Scholar in School of Law at Christ University, Bangalore. She has her research interests in the field of Constitutional Law, Environment Law, Human Rights, Food Security, Intellectual Property Law and Jurisprudence.

Antonio Pesqueira is a healthcare and pharmaceutical commercial and supply chain management leader, with an emphasis on technological advancements and process improvement. Concurrently, he holds esteemed academic positions as a professor and research fellow at ISCTE/IUL. Within the Technology and Architecture Research Department, he contributes to the Ph.D. program, focusing his research on digital technologies, healthcare data management, blockchain, and the nexus of innovation and business management. He has notably chaired the Pharmaceutical Supply Chain & Security World Forum and is often invited as a keynote speaker at events such as the Pharma Track & Trace, and Serialization & Labeling Summit. Co-authored more than 20 scholarly articles and book chapters that have been featured in prestigious scientific journals. These include the Journal of Business Research, Future Generations Computer Systems, Journal of Medical Systems, Knowledge Management, WSEAS Transactions on Business and Economics, and Information Systems Frontiers, to name a few. Moreover, his outstanding contributions have been acknowledged at various peer-reviewed international conferences.

R. Gayathri, an Assistant Professor in Computer Science at various colleges in Coimbatore, has over 16 years of experience. Her areas of interest include machine learning, artificial intelligence, IoT, and blockchain. She has presented and published 28 research papers in national and international conferences and journals and has filed a design patent. She has received the Best Research Scholar Award and the Best Women Faculty Award for her contributions to academia. Dr. Gayathri also serves as a resource person, delivering expert talks and lectures to enhance knowledge sharing in her field.

Wasswa Shafik (Member, IEEE) received a Bachelor of Science degree in information technology from Ndejje University, Uganda, a Master of Engineering degree in Information Technology (Computer and Communication Networks) from Yazd University, Iran, and a PhD in Computer Science with the School of Digital Science, Universiti Brunei Darussalam, Brunei Darussalam. He is also the Founder and Research Director of the Dig Connectivity Research Laboratory (DCRLab) after serving as a Research

Associate at the Network Interconnectivity Research Laboratory at Yazd University. Prior to this, he worked as a Community Data Analyst at Population Services International (PSI-Uganda), a Community Data Officer at the Programme for Accessible Health Communication (PACE-Uganda), a Research Assistant at the Socio-Economic Data Centre (SEDC-Uganda), Uganda, an Assistant Data Officer at TechnoServe, Kampala, Uganda, and Asmaah Charity Organization as Cheif Executive Officer. He has hundreds of publications with renowned publishers. His research interests include Artificial Intelligence, Smart Agriculture, Digital Health, Green Computing, Security and Privacy.

Ali Turab, an Associate Professor at NPU, China, holds a PhD degree in Applied Mathematics from Thammasat University, Thailand. His postdoctoral research at TU and tenure as a Research Associate at UMP have honed his expertise in Mathematical Modelling, Animal Behaviors, and Psychological Learning Theory. With a focus on Chemical Graph Theory, Fractional Calculus, and Nonlinear Analysis, Dr. Turab has made significant contributions to scholarly discourse, boasting numerous publications and acclaimed presentations at international symposia. Committed to educational excellence, he actively participates in pedagogical enhancement workshops, underscoring his dedication to the forefront of teaching and research.

Farhan Ullah is an Associate Professor at the School of Software, Northwestern Polytechnical University, Xi'an Shaanxi, P.R. China. He received Ph.D. Computer Science degree in 2020 from College of Computer Science, Sichuan University Chengdu, P.R. China. He was awarded a full-time Chinese Government Scholarship (CGS) for his Ph.D. During his Ph.D. studies, he participated in different research projects which include, the National Key Research and Development Program, the National Natural Science Foundation of China, and the Technology Research and Development Program of Sichuan, China. He performed as a research member of the science and technology project of Taicang (2020), Jiangsu, China. He is the Special Issue Lead Guest Editor for Security and Communication Networks Journal in the CCF C category and CMC-Computers, Materials & Continua Journals. He also served as a Guest Editor (GE) for a special issue of Future Internet Journal, MDPI. He received Research Productivity Award (RPA) from COMSATS Institute of Information Technology (CIIT), Sahiwal, Pakistan in 2016. His research work is published in various renowned journals of IEEE, Springer, Elsevier, Wiley, MDPI, and Hindawi.

Muhammad Usman Akhtar, completed my Ph.D. in Software Engineering from Wuhan University, Hubei, China in the year 2024. I previously received my MS in Computer Science from the University of Engineering and Technology (UET), Peshawar, Pakistan, in the year 2018, and my BS in Software Engineering from Islamia College, Peshawar, Pakistan, in the year 2013. Then I started my professional career as a Research Assistant at the National Center for Big Data and Cloud Computing at UET, Peshawar. As far as my research publications are concerned, I have eight publications to my credit, with a cumulative impact factor of more than 37.7. In addition, I contributed to one chapter in the book EH-ARCUN: Energy Harvested Analytical Approach Towards Reliability with Cooperation for Underwater WSNs (Chapter 14, 147-157). I have contributed to NetworkX (an open-source Python library) used for creating, analyzing and visualizing complex graphs in various domains such as social networks, biological networks, and more. Besides my research contributions, I actively engage as an independent reviewer for top-ranked SCI and ESI journals and conferences, including Information Fusion, Engineering Applications of Artificial Intelligence, Knowledge-Based Systems, Arrays, The Journal of Supercomputing, Peer-to-Peer Networking and Applications, Social Network Analysis and Mining, and Cluster Computing. I have been honored as an excellent international scholar for three consecutive years during my doctoral studies at Wuhan University, China, and have received numerous national and international awards and honorary certificates for excellence in research and co-curricular activities. These include recognitions from the Chinese WUSHU Association, Wuhan International Students Union, United Nations Development Program, China University of Geosciences, Nanjing University, BRICS, and Wuhan University. My key research areas include Web 3.0-based Technologies, artificial intelligence, large language models, machine learning, deep learning, information fusion, embedding technologies, complex networks, recommendation systems, data analysis, semantics-search technologies, knowledge graphs-construction and their integration, extraction and completion.

Affan Yasin (Member, IEEE) received the Ph.D. degree in software engineering from Tsinghua University, Beijing, China. He is currently an Assistant Professor at the School of AI and Advanced Computing, Xi'an Jiaotong Liverpool University, Suzhou, China. Prior to this, he was a Postdoctoral researcher at Northwestern Polytechnical University, Xi'an, China, and a Postdoctoral Fellow at Tsinghua University. He is particularly interested in how these areas can be integrated to enhance learning outcomes and improve system security and usability. His work contributes to both academic advancements and practical applications in these fields. He has published over 35 research papers in reputable journals and conferences. His work has been well-received in the academic community. His research interests include the intersection of empirical software engineering and cutting-edge technologies, with a focus on game-based learning, serious games, social engineering, AI in education, and requirements engineering.

Index

E

F

H

I

L

M

P

R

S

T

V

www.ingramcontent.com/pod-product-compliance
Ingram Content Group UK Ltd.
Pitfield, Milton Keynes, MK11 3LW, UK
UKHW050845101026
15624UKWH00018B/585